Essentials of Geriatric Psychiatry

Essentials of Geriatric Psychiatry

Edited by

Dan G. Blazer, M.D., Ph.D.

David C. Steffens, M.D., M.H.S.

Ewald W. Busse, M.D.

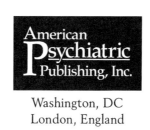

American Psychiatric Publishing, Inc.

Washington, DC
London, England

If you would like to buy between 25 and 99 copies of this or any other APPI title, you are eligible for a 20% discount; please contact APPI Customer Service at appi@psych.org or 800-368-5777. If you wish to buy 100 or more copies of the same title, please e-mail us at bulksales@psych.org for a price quote.

Manufactured in the United States of America on acid-free paper
11   10   09   08   07   5   4   3   2   1

Typeset in Adobe's Revival and Caecilia.

American Psychiatric Publishing, Inc.
1000 Wilson Boulevard
Arlington, VA 22209-3901
www.appi.org

Library of Congress Cataloging-in-Publication Data
Essentials of geriatric psychiatry / edited by Dan G. Blazer, David C. Steffens,
    Ewald W. Busse.
        p. ; cm.
    Includes bibliographical references and index.
    ISBN 1-58562-247-8 (pbk. : alk. paper)
    1. Geriatric psychiatry. I. Blazer, Dan G. (Dan German), 1944–   . II. Steffens,
David C., 1962–   . III. Busse, Ewald W., 1917–2004. [DNLM: 1. Mental Disorders.
2. Aged. 3. Aging—physiology. 4. Geriatric Psychiatry—methods. WT 150 E775
2007]
RC451.4.A5E87 2007
618.97′689—dc22

                                                                    2006020585

British Library Cataloguing in Publication Data
A CIP record is available from the British Library.

We dedicate this book to Ewald W. Busse, M.D., who died in March 2004. His influence on this book and on the field of geriatric psychiatry will continue for many years to come.

Contents

Part 1

Basic Issues in Geriatric Psychiatry

Part 2

The Diagnostic Interview in Late Life

Part 3

Psychiatric Disorders in Late Life

Part 4

Treatment of Psychiatric Disorders in Late Life

Contributors

Marc E. Agronin, M.D.
Director, Mental Health Services, Miami Jewish Home & Hospital for the Aged; Assistant Professor of Psychiatry, University of Miami Miller School of Medicine, Miami, Florida

Ann K. Aspnes, M.A.
Department of Psychology: Social and Health Sciences, Duke University, Durham, North Carolina

Deborah K. Attix, Ph.D.
Division of Neurology, Department of Medicine, and Division of Medical Psychology, Department of Psychiatry and Behavioral Sciences, Duke University Medical Center, Durham, North Carolina

John L. Beyer, M.D.
Assistant Professor of Psychiatry, Duke University Medical Center, Durham, North Carolina

Dan G. Blazer, M.D., Ph.D.
J.P. Gibbons Professor of Psychiatry, Department of Psychiatry and Behavioral Sciences, Duke University Medical Center, Durham, North Carolina

Lauren T. Bonner, M.D.
Private Practice, Glendale, Arizona

Harvey J. Cohen, M.D.
Professor of Medicine and Interim Chair, Department of Medicine; Director, Center for the Study of Aging and Human Development, Duke University School of Medicine, Durham, North Carolina

Marty Cusing, M.A.
Older Adult and Family Center, Department of Psychiatry and Behavioral Sciences, Stanford University School of Medicine, VA Palo Alto Health Care System, Menlo Park, California; Notre Dame de Namur University, Belmont, California

John Di Mario, B.S.
Older Adult and Family Center, Department of Psychiatry and Behavioral Sciences, Stanford University School of Medicine, VA Palo Alto Health Care System, Menlo Park, California

Christian R. Dolder, Pharm.D., B.C.P.S.
Assistant Professor, Wingate University School of Pharmacy, Wingate, North Carolina; Clinical Pharmacist, NorthEast Medical Center, Concord, North Carolina

P. Murali Doraiswamy, M.D.
Head, Division of Biological Psychiatry and Associate Professor, Department of Psychiatry and Behavioral Sciences, Duke University, Durham, North Carolina

Jack D. Edinger, Ph.D.
Professor of Psychiatry, Department of Psychiatry and Behavioral Sciences, Duke University Medical Center, Durham, North Carolina

Dolores Gallagher-Thompson, Ph.D., A.B.P.P.
Professor of Research, Department of Psychiatry and Behavioral Sciences, Stanford University School of Medicine, VA Palo Alto Health Care System, Menlo Park, California

Lisa P. Gwyther, M.S.W.
Associate Clinical Professor, Department of Psychiatry and Behavioral Sciences, Joseph and Kathleen Bryan Alzheimer's Disease Research Center, Duke Center for the Study of Aging, Duke University Medical Center, Durham, North Carolina

Judith C. Hays, R.N., Ph.D.
Associate Professor and Chair, Accelerated BSN Program, Duke University School of Nursing, Durham, North Carolina

Celia F. Hybels, Ph.D.
Assistant Research Professor, Department of Psychiatry and Behavioral Sciences, Duke University Medical Center, Durham, North Carolina

Dilip V. Jeste, M.D.
Estelle and Edgar Levi Chair in Aging; Director, Sam and Rose Stein Institute for Research on Aging; Distinguished Professor of Psychiatry and Neurosciences, University of California, San Diego, VA San Diego Healthcare System, San Diego, California

Robert M. Kaiser, M.D., M.H.Sc.
Associate Professor of Medicine, Geriatrics Institute, University of Miami Miller School of Medicine; GRECC Investigator, Miami VA Medical Center, Miami, Florida

Ira R. Katz, M.D., Ph.D.
Professor of Psychiatry, Section on Geriatric Psychiatry, University of Pennsylvania, Philadelphia, Pennsylvania

Harold G. Koenig, M.D., M.H.Sc.
Professor of Psychiatry and Behavioral Sciences, Department of Psychiatry and Behavioral Sciences, Duke University Medical Center, Durham, North Carolina

Andrew D. Krystal, M.D., M.S.
Associate Professor with Tenure, Department of Psychiatry and Behavioral Sciences, Duke University School of Medicine, Durham, North Carolina

Thomas R. Lynch, Ph.D.
Director, Cognitive Behavior Research and Treatment Program, Duke University Medical Center; Department of Psychology: Social and Health Sciences, Duke University, Durham, North Carolina

Benoit H. Mulsant, M.D., M.S., FRCPC
Professor, Department of Psychiatry, University of Toronto; Clinical Director, Centre for Addiction and Mental Health, Toronto, Ontario, Canada

Paul D. Nagy, M.S.
Program Director, Duke Addictions Program; Clinical Associate, Department of Psychiatry and Behavioral Sciences, Duke University Medical Center, Durham, North Carolina

Elaine R. Peskind, M.D.
Professor of Psychiatry and Behavioral Sciences, University of Washington School of Medicine, Seattle, Washington

Bruce G. Pollock, M.D., Ph.D., FRCPC
Sandra A. Rotman Chair in Neuropsychiatry and Head, Division of Geriatric Psychiatry, University of Toronto; Senior Scientist, Centre for Addiction and Mental Health, Toronto, Ontario, Canada

Murray A. Raskind, M.D.
Professor of Psychiatry and Behavioral Sciences, University of Washington School of Medicine, Seattle, Washington

Burton L. Scott, Ph.D., M.D.
Associate Professor of Medicine (Neurology), Duke University Movement Disorders Center, Durham, North Carolina

Joseph M. Sharpe, M.D.
Resident, Department of Psychiatry and Behavioral Sciences, Duke University School of Medicine, Durham, North Carolina

David C. Steffens, M.D., M.H.S.
Professor of Psychiatry, Department of Psychiatry and Behavioral Sciences, Duke University Medical Center, Durham, North Carolina

Joel E. Streim, M.D.
Professor of Psychiatry, Section on Geriatric Psychiatry, University of Pennsylvania, Philadelphia, Pennsylvania

Paulette C.Y. Tang, Ph.D.
Older Adult and Family Center, Department of Psychiatry and Behavioral Sciences, Stanford University School of Medicine, VA Palo Alto Health Care System, Menlo Park, California

Warren D. Taylor, M.D.
Assistant Professor, Department of Psychiatry and Behavioral Sciences, Duke University, Durham, North Carolina

Larry W. Thompson, Ph.D.
Pacific Graduate School of Psychology, Department of Psychiatry and Behavioral Sciences, Stanford University School of Medicine; VA Palo Alto Health Care System, Palo Alto, California

Kathleen A. Welsh-Bohmer, Ph.D.
Joseph and Kathleen Bryan Alzheimer's Disease Research Center, Department of Psychiatry and Behavioral Sciences, Division of Medical Psychology, Duke University Medical Center, Durham, North Carolina

William K. Wohlgemuth, Ph.D.
Assistant Professor, Department of Psychiatry and Behavioral Sciences, Duke University School of Medicine, Durham, North Carolina

Preface

Essentials of Geriatric Psychiatry is based on *The American Psychiatric Publishing Textbook of Geriatric Psychiatry*, 3rd Edition, published in 2004. (The first edition of the textbook, titled *Geriatric Psychiatry*, was published in 1989, and the second edition, retitled *The American Psychiatric Press Textbook of Geriatric Psychiatry*, appeared in 1996.) The decision to publish *Essentials of Geriatric Psychiatry* recognized the enormous expansion of scientific knowledge about aging and the diseases of late life, as well as the advances in biological psychiatry and neuropsychiatry that have greatly altered the practice of geriatric psychiatry. A version that captures "the essentials" is specifically designed to provide the clinician with the current state of scientific understanding as well as the practical skills and knowledge base required for dealing with mental disorders in late life.

As in the textbook, the chapters are presented in a sequential and integrated fashion, which we have found enhances the accessibility and usefulness of the information presented. The contributors have a clear ability to make complex material understandable to our readers. We maintained an eclectic orientation regarding theory and practice in geriatric psychiatry. Although most contributors are psychiatrists, we also called on colleagues from relevant biomedical and behavioral disciplines, because of their expertise and their ability to incorporate such knowledge into a comprehensive approach to patient care.

We have targeted this text to psychiatrists and other health professionals who have an interest in and a commitment to the diagnosis, treatment, and long-term management of older adults experiencing psychiatric problems. This book is of particular value to psychiatrists, neurologists, and geriatric psychiatrists sitting for their board examinations, as well as candidates seeking certification in geriatrics from the American Board of Internal Medicine and the American Board of Family Practice. Nonphysicians whose accreditation examinations recognize the critical role of working with the elderly, including psychologists and social workers, will also find this text useful. All of these examinations place considerable emphasis on geriatric psychiatry and the behavioral aspects of aging.

We wish to express our deepest appreciation for the assistance of our staff assistant, Jill Gabel, for her long hours typing, editing, and organizing the manuscripts.

Dan G. Blazer, M.D., Ph.D.
David C. Steffens, M.D., M.H.S.

PART

1

Basic Issues in Geriatric Psychiatry

Demography and Epidemiology of Psychiatric Disorders in Late Life

Dan G. Blazer, M.D., Ph.D.

Celia F. Hybels, Ph.D.

Judith C. Hays, R.N., Ph.D.

The epidemiology of psychiatric disorders in late life is the study of the distribution of psychiatric disorders among the elderly and those factors that influence this distribution (MacMahon and Pugh 1970). Roberts (1977) suggested that epidemiology is not only the basic science of preventive and community medicine but also may serve as the basic science of clinical practice. In this chapter, the findings of demographers and epidemiologists are reviewed as they relate to the care of the psychiatrically impaired older adult.

Demography

Of the more than 275 million persons enumerated during the United States census of 2000, nearly 35 million, or 13% of the population, are age 65 years or older (Fed-eral Interagency Forum on Aging Related Statistics 2000). The average age in the United States is now 36 years. Even more astounding, more than 4 million, or 1.6% of the United States population and 12.5% of the 65 and older age group, are age 85 years or older. These oldest old among us are projected to reach 20 million by the year 2050 and to make up 5% of the United States population at that time. The "old-old" are more likely to experience poverty, to have less education, and to receive far more federal transfer payments (Blazer 2000).

More than 50% of the nursing home residents in the United States are age 80 years or older, representing a cost of more than $30 million per year (Suzman 1995). At least half of these residents are placed in nursing homes because of psychiatric

disorders, especially the behavior problems that result from Alzheimer's disease.

The size of the elderly U.S. population
is expected to dramatically increase in the
next few decades, reaching 70 million by
the year 2030 (Federal Interagency Forum
on Aging Related Statistics 2000). Most of
these elders are women (58%) and white
(84%). Women are expected to continue to
survive longer than men, yet the racial/eth-
nic composition of the elderly will change
dramatically over the next few decades.
Currently, 8% of elders are non-Hispanic
black, 2% are non-Hispanic Asian and Pacific Islander, and fewer than 1% are non-
Hispanic American Indian/Alaska natives.
Hispanic elders make up 6% of the 65 and
older age group. By 2050, the percentage of
white non-Hispanic elders will decline to
64%, and Hispanic persons will account for
16% (a growth of 11 million persons), with
non-Hispanic blacks accounting for 12%
(Federal Interagency Forum on Aging Related Statistics 2000).

In 1900, the life expectancy at birth in
the United States was 49 years (Federal
Interagency Forum on Aging Related Statistics 2000). In 1997, the life expectancy at
birth was 79 years for women and 74 years
for men. Persons who survive to age 65 can
expect to live an average of nearly 18 more
years. Life expectancy of persons who survive to age 85 is 7 years for women and
6 years for men.

If an older person develops a psychiatric disorder, that disorder may become
chronic, and the years of life that are associated with a decreased quality of life
because of psychiatric morbidity are substantial. In addition, with increasing age,
the great majority of older persons with
psychiatric disorders experience a comorbid physical illness (Blazer 2000).

What can psychiatric epidemiological
studies contribute to mental health services
for older adults? Morris (1975) suggested
the following uses of epidemiology:

- Identify cases (e.g., can the symptom
  pattern of depression in elderly persons
  be readily identified in community-
  dwelling and clinical [e.g., hospitalized]
  populations of older adults?).
- Reveal the distribution of psychiatric
  disorders in the population (e.g., what
  is the prevalence and/or incidence of
  dementia?).
- Trace historical trends of mental illness
  among elderly persons (e.g., has the incidence of suicide increased among this
  population over the past 10 years?).
- Determine the etiology of psychiatric
  disorders in late life (e.g., do social factors contribute more to the etiology of
  late-life psychiatric disorders than to
  such disorders in midlife, given lower
  potential for genetic contributions?).
- Examine the use of psychiatric and
  other mental health services by elderly
  persons (e.g., do psychiatrically impaired older adults in the community
  underutilize psychiatric services?).

Each of these functions of epidemiology is reviewed in this chapter.

Case Identification

Clinicians constantly face the task of distinguishing abnormality from normality.
Although most epidemiologists and clinicians agree on the core symptoms of psychiatric disorders throughout the life cycle,
the absolute distinction between a case and
a noncase—that is, persons requiring psychiatric attention versus those who do not
require such care—is not easily established.

Many of the symptoms and signs of a
psychiatric disorder in late life may be ubiquitous with the aging process, thus blurring
the distinction between cases and noncases.
Epidemiologists can assist the clinician in
identifying meaningful clusters of symptoms and significant degrees of symptom

severity. Case identification is also the foundation of descriptive epidemiology: "cases" are the numerator of the equation from which prevalence and incidence estimates are derived in community and clinical samples (the denominator). For most clinicians the goal of case identification is to identify subjects experiencing uniform underlying psychopathology, as is implicit in DSM-IV and DSM-IV-TR (American Psychiatric Association 1994, 2000).

One method of case identification is the use of diagnostic instruments. These instruments (usually standardized interviews) have been developed and used in community- and clinic-based epidemiological studies to identify persons with symptoms that meet these criteria. The Structured Clinical Interview for DSM-IV (SCID; First et al. 1997) and Diagnostic Interview Schedule (DIS; Robins et al. 1981) are examples of the most frequently used interview schedules. For example, the DIS was used in the Epidemiologic Catchment Area (ECA) study, from which a 1-month national estimate of the prevalence of affective disorders in persons age 65 years and older was 2.5% (compared with 6.4% for persons age 25–44 years) (Regier et al. 1988).

A second approach to case identification is the use of self-administered symptom scales and personality inventories. Scales frequently used in epidemiological surveys include the Center for Epidemiologic Studies Depression Scale (CES-D; Radloff 1977) and the Geriatric Depression Scale (Yesavage et al. 1983), which screen for depressive symptoms, and the Short Portable Mental Status Questionnaire (Pfeiffer 1975) and the Mini-Mental State Exam (MMSE; Folstein et al. 1975), which screen for cognitive impairment. The advantage of these scales is that, unlike diagnostic interviews, they do not subjectively assign patients to a particular diagnostic category; a disadvantage is the lack of diagnostic specificity that can be achieved with their use.

Other authors define a case on the basis of severity of physical, psychological, and social impairment secondary to the symptoms. This approach to case identification is less popular among clinicians, who are more inclined to "treat a disease" than to "improve function." Improved function, in theory, should derive from remission of the disease. Nevertheless, function has special relevance in the care of older adults, especially the oldest old (Blazer 2000). When managing chronic psychiatric disorders, such as primary degenerative dementia of the Alzheimer's type, the improvement or maintenance of physical, psychological, and social functioning is a clinician's primary goal (Hazzard 1994). Family members are often more concerned with improved functioning than with alleviation of symptoms.

The epidemiological method depends, for the most part, on a clear distinction between cases and noncases (Kleinbaum et al. 1982), yet most older adults do not ideally fit the psychiatric diagnosis that they receive (Strauss et al. 1981). Regardless of the diagnostic system, unusual or borderline cases that cannot be clearly placed in a single category exist. This has led some investigators to consider the possibility of "fuzzy sets" as a means by which cases can be more realistically distinguished (Blazer et al. 1989). Not infrequently, older adults manifest more than one disease simultaneously—for example, major depression and primary degenerative dementia. In addition, the prescribed categories of DSM-IV-TR do not always match the symptoms that individuals in this population may be experiencing; generalized anxiety, for instance, is not easily disentangled from a major depressive episode in an agitated older adult.

Regardless of the approach taken to case identification, a diagnosis must be reliable and valid for it to be a useful means of communicating clinical information. To pass the test of reliability, a diagnosis must be consistent and repeatable. Standardized or operational methods for identifying psychiatric symptoms and the availability of specific criteria for psychiatric diagnoses have greatly improved the reliability of case identification by psychiatrists and by lay interviewers in psychiatric epidemiological surveys. Reliability, however, does not ensure validity—that is, the test of whether a case identified by a particular method reflects underlying reality (Blazer and Kaplan 2000).

Distribution of Psychiatric Disorders

The authors of descriptive studies of the epidemiology of psychiatric impairment in older adults have concentrated on either overall mental health functioning or the distribution of specific psychiatric disorders in the population. Reports from these studies usually begin as general observations of the relation of impairment or specific disorders to characteristics such as age, gender, race/ethnicity, and socioeconomic status. These trends provide the template for more in-depth studies of the hereditary, biological, and psychosocial contributors to the etiology of disorders and the effect of the distribution of the disorders on mental health care utilization.

Frequencies of disorders within the population are usually presented in terms of prevalence—the proportion or percentage of persons within the population with a defined impairment or specific disorder at a particular time or within a particular period. Almost all such studies provide estimates based on community samples of larger populations. Smaller studies of the prevalence of impairment or specific disorders in institutional or clinical settings provide important data about service use.

Longitudinal epidemiological studies of older adults also can provide data on the incidence of impairment or psychiatric disorders; that is, the proportion of persons who develop the disorder during a specified period of observation. In addition, longitudinal studies provide data on outcomes associated with impairment or specific psychiatric disorders.

The National Institute of Mental Health (NIMH) established the ECA program in the United States to determine the prevalence of specific psychiatric disorders in both community and institutional populations (Regier et al. 1984). Data were collected in five communities, and the DIS was used to identify persons who met criteria for specific disorders. Although conducted more than two decades ago, the ECA study remains the landmark study in the United States for addressing the prevalence of psychiatric impairment in older adults. More than 18,000 persons were interviewed in the ECA study, including 5,702 persons who were age 65 years or older. All disorders, with the exception of cognitive impairment, were more prevalent in younger or middle-aged adults, compared with older adults. A total of 12.3% (13.6% of the women and 10.5% of the men) of those age 65 or older met criteria for one or more psychiatric disorders in the month before the interview. The two most prevalent disorders in this age group were an anxiety disorder (5.5%) and severe cognitive impairment (4.9%) (Regier et al. 1988). Representative surveys also allow comparisons to be made across various age groups. For example, in the recently published data from the National Comorbidity Survey–Replication (NCS-R), the lifetime odds of major depressive disorder (MDD) were two times higher in younger adults compared with older adults. Among those adults reporting lifetime MDD, the odds of 12-month MDD were higher in younger adults compared with individuals 60 years or older (OR = 3.0 for those 18–29 and OR = 1.8

for those 30–44 years of age). Differences in 12-month MDD between those 45–59 and 60 or older were not significant. (Kessler et al. 2003).

Specific disorders will be addressed in detail in subsequent chapters, but the tables in this chapter provide a summary of the prevalence of psychiatric symptoms and specific disorders in both community and institutional samples based on studies conducted in the United States, Canada, Europe, and Australia over the last several decades.

The prevalence of cognitive impairment in selected community and institutional populations is presented in Table 1–1. While estimates in community studies can range from 1% to 6%, the prevalence of cognitive impairment among primary care patients and in institutional samples is higher, ranging from 15.7% in primary care patients to 59.4% in institutionalized Medicaid patients (Burns et al. 1988; Callahan et al. 1995; Teeter et al. 1976).

It is important to note that these studies reporting the prevalence of cognitive impairment are measuring cognitive function by standardized screening tests such as the Short Portable Mental Status Questionnaire and the MMSE. Therefore, these studies are not reporting the prevalence of dementia or Alzheimer's disease or actual cerebral impairment. The prevalence of cognitive impairment can be affected by educational level of the population being studied, as well as by other sociocultural factors that may affect performance on cognitive tasks.

The prevalence of dementia and Alzheimer's disease in both community and institutional samples is shown in Table 1–2. While the prevalence of dementia reported from community studies ranges from 5% to 10%, the prevalence of dementia is higher in institutional samples. In their sample of nursing home patients, Rovner et al. (1986) found that the prevalence of primary de-

generative dementia was 56%, whereas the prevalence of multi-infarct dementia was 18% and the prevalence of Parkinson's dementia was 4%. As expected, the prevalence of dementia in community-dwelling older adults is higher in older age groups.

Several studies have provided data on the prevalence of Alzheimer's disease, as shown in Table 1–2. Evans et al. (1989) reported that the prevalence of probable Alzheimer's disease was 10.3% in a sample of community-dwelling adults age 65 or older. The prevalence increased with age. Specifically, the prevalence was 3.0% in those age 65–74, 18.7% in those age 75–84, and 47.2% in those age 85 or older. That the prevalence of Alzheimer's disease is estimated to be higher than the prevalence of cognitive impairment may at first appear counterintuitive. Nevertheless, a careful diagnostic evaluation may establish Alzheimer's disease even when overall cognitive impairment is not severe.

The prevalence of psychiatric symptoms in community populations of older adults is presented in Table 1–3. The most frequently reported symptoms are problems with sleep and symptoms of anxiety. Numerous studies have reported a high prevalence of depressive symptoms among community-dwelling older adults. Copeland et al. (1999) found in the European Concerted Action on Depression of Older People (EURODEP) that 12.3% of the sample age 65 or older represented either cases or subcases of depression. Beekman et al. (1999) reviewed studies of major depression and depressive symptoms among persons age 55 or older and found that the average prevalence of depressive syndromes deemed clinically relevant was 13.5%.

Across the entire life cycle, many psychiatric symptoms, especially hypochondriasis and sleep disorders, have their highest frequencies among elderly adults. A relatively high frequency of certain symptoms in elderly populations, however, does not

TABLE 1–1. Prevalence of cognitive impairment in community and institutional populations of older adults

Study/Site	Reference	Sample	N	Age (years)	Measurement	Prevalence
ECA	Regier et al. 1988	Five U.S. communities	5,702	65+	MMSE	4.9%
				65–74	MMSE	2.9%
				75–84	MMSE	6.8%
				85+	MMSE	15.8%
New Haven EPESE	Cornoni-Huntley et al. 1986	Community	2,811	65+	SPMSQ	5.3%
Iowa EPESE	Cornoni-Huntley et al. 1986	Community	3,673	65+	SPMSQ	1.3%
East Boston EPESE	Cornoni-Huntley et al. 1986	Community	3,812	65+	SPMSQ	6.0%
Minnesota	Teeter et al. 1976	Institutionalized Medicaid patients	74	Mean age = 81	SPMSQ	59.4%
U.S. national sample	Burns et al. 1988	Institution	526	Mean age = 79	Chart review and nurse interview	39.0%
Canadian Study of Health and Aging	Graham et al. 1997	Community and institution	2,914	65+	Modified MMSE and clinical assessment	16.8% cognitive impairment, no dementia
Indiana	Callahan et al. 1995	Primary care patients	3,594	60+	SPMSQ	15.7%
Germany	Busse et al. 2003	Community	1,045	75+	SIDAM	3.1% mild cognitive impairment 8.8% age-associated cognitive decline

Note. ECA = Epidemiologic Catchment Area; EPESE = Established Populations for Epidemiologic Studies of the Elderly; MMSE = Mini-Mental State Exam (Folstein et al. 1975); SIDAM = Structured Interview for Diagnosis of Dementia of Alzheimer Type, Multi-Infarct Dementia and Dementias of Other Aetiology According to ICD-10 and DSM-III-R (Zaudig et al. 1991); SPMSQ = Short Portable Mental Status Questionnaire (Pfeiffer 1975).

TABLE 1–2. Prevalence of dementia and Alzheimer's disease in community and institutional populations of older adults

Study/Site	Reference	Sample	N	Age (years)	Measurement	Prevalence
England	Kay et al. 1970	Community	758	65+	Psychiatric interviews	6.2% chronic brain syndromes
Netherlands	Heeren et al. 1991	Community	1,259	85+	Standardized interviews	23% dementia (11% with moderate or severe dementia)
Maryland	Rovner et al. 1986	Institution	50	Mean age = 83	Standardized interviews	56% primary degenerative dementia; 18% multi-infarct dementia; 4% Parkinson's dementia
East Boston EPESE	Evans et al. 1989	Community	467	65+	Standardized interviews and clinical evaluation	10.3% probable Alzheimer's disease
Liverpool	Copeland et al. 1987	Community	1,070	65+	GMS-AGECAT	5.2% probable dementia
Liverpool	Copeland et al. 1992	Community	1,070	65+	GMS-AGECAT	3.3% Alzheimer's disease
Canada	Canadian Study of Health and Aging Working Group 1994	Community and institution	10,263	65+	3MS and clinical examination	8.0% dementia 5.1% Alzheimer's disease
Germany	Riedel-Heller et al. 2001	Community and institution	1,692	75+	SIDAM	17.4% DSM-III-R dementia 12.4% ICD-10 dementia
London	Stevens et al. 2002	Community	1,085	65+	Short-CARE	9.86% dementia

Note. EPESE = Established Populations for Epidemiologic Studies of the Elderly; GMS-AGECAT = Geriatric Mental State (Copeland et al. 1976); 3MS = Modified Mini-Mental State (Teng and Chui 1987); Short-CARE = Short Comprehensive Assessment and Referral Evaluation (Gurland et al. 1984); SIDAM = Structured Interview for Diagnosis of Dementia of Alzheimer Type, Multi-Infarct Dementia and Dementias of Other Aetiology According to ICD-10 and DSM-III-R (Zaudig et al. 1991).

TABLE 1–3. Prevalence of psychiatric symptoms in community populations of older adults

Study/Site	Reference	N	Age (years)	Measurement	Disorder/Syndrome	Prevalence
New Haven EPESE	Cornoni-Huntley et al. 1986	2,811	65+	CES-D	Depressive symptoms	15.1%
Durham County, NC	Blazer and Houpt 1979	997	65+	Selected questions	Hypochondriasis	14%
Durham County, NC	Christenson and Blazer 1984	997	65+	MMPI	Persecutory ideation	4%
Australia	Henderson et al. 1998	1,377	70+	Structured psychiatric interviews	Psychotic symptoms	5.7%
Iowa EPESE	Cornoni-Huntley et al. 1986	3,673	65+	Selected questions	Trouble falling asleep Awakens during night Sleepy during day	14.1% 33.7% 30.7%
EURODEP	Copeland et al. 1999	13,808	65+	GMS-AGECAT	Cases and subcases of depression	12.3% Males 8.6% Females 14.1%
Liverpool	P.A. Saunders et al. 1989	1,070	65+	GMS-AGECAT	Among drinkers, proportion exceeding sensible limits	Males 19.5% Females 19.6%
Stockholm	Forsell and Winblad 1998	966	78+	Selected questions	Feelings of anxiety	24.4%
LASA	Beekman et al. 1995	3,056	55–85	CES-D	Minor depression	12.9%

Note.   CES-D = Center for Epidemiologic Studies Depression Scale (Radloff 1977); EPESE = Established Populations for Epidemiologic Studies of the Elderly; EURODEP = European Concerted Action on Depression of Older People; GMS-AGECAT = Geriatric Mental State (Copeland et al. 1976); LASA = Longitudinal Aging Study Amsterdam; MMPI = Minnesota Multiphasic Personality Inventory (Hathaway and McKinley 1970).

necessarily signify an increased frequency of specific psychiatric disorders. The paradox of relatively high reports of depressive symptoms and relatively low reports of the prevalence of major depressive episodes illustrates this point (Blazer 1982). Diagnostic categories, such as those found in DSM-IV-TR, are clusters of symptoms and signs that derive their validity not from the overall weight of symptomatology but, rather, from regularities in the clustering of history, the persistence of symptoms over time, a predictable outcome, a common pathophysiology, and possibly common biochemical disturbances. As biological markers of psychiatric disorders are identified, laboratory diagnostic techniques will provide information that is complementary to the symptoms reported. As our knowledge progresses in the area of nomenclature, new categories of symptoms may be lumped together to define a particular syndrome.

Symptoms, the most objective clinical indicators of psychopathology, may reflect more than one diagnostic entity. On the other hand, symptoms may not be associated with any disorder of interest to the clinician. For example, decreased appetite can result from several sources. At a given time, grief reactions, more frequent in late life than at other stages of the life cycle, may be virtually indistinguishable from major depressive episodes if appetite alone is considered. Loss of appetite also accompanies major life adjustments such as a forced change of residence or a decline in economic resources. Most commonly, loss of appetite in late life is a result of poor physical health.

The prevalence of selected psychiatric disorders in community populations of older adults is shown in Table 1–4. The prevalence of psychiatric disorders is lower than the prevalence of related psychiatric symptoms. The most prevalent disorders, other than dementia disorders, are mood and anxiety disorders. Numerous studies of older adults have reported that the prevalence of major depression is approximately 1%–2%, with a higher prevalence in females (Beekman et al. 1995; Bland et al. 1988; Regier et al. 1988). Henderson et al. (1993) reported that the prevalence of ICD-10 (World Health Organization 1992) depressive episodes in persons age 70 or older was 3.3%. Kay et al. (1985) reported an increase in DSM depression with age, with a prevalence of 6.3% in those age 70–79 and 15.5% in those age 80 or older. The prevalence of any anxiety disorder in adults age 65 or older in the ECA study was 5.5%, with a higher prevalence in females (6.8%) compared with males (3.6%) (Regier et al. 1988). The prevalence of alcohol abuse or dependence was low in this population, with an overall 1-month prevalence of 0.9% reported from the ECA study (Regier et al. 1988). Similarly, the 1-month prevalence of schizophrenia reported from the ECA study in adults age 65 or older was 0.1% (Regier et al. 1988).

Overall, psychiatric disorders are found at a lower prevalence among the elderly than at other stages of the life cycle. The virtual absence of alcohol abuse or dependence and schizophrenia in those age 65 or older in the ECA data may reflect selective mortality or case-finding techniques used. The community data do not include individuals in institutions, and many persons in late life with chronic schizophrenia may be institutionalized.

Another question derives from these data: Do unique late-life symptom presentations render the Research Diagnostic Criteria (RDC; Spitzer et al. 1978) and DSM-IV-TR inadequate as systems of nomenclature? DSM-IV-TR provides age-specific categories for children but not for elderly persons. Clinicians who work with older adults, however, have often commented that depression may be masked

TABLE 1–4. Prevalence of selected psychiatric disorders in community populations of older adults

Study/Site	Reference	Sample	N	Age (years)	Measurement	Disorder	Prevalence
ECA	Regier et al. 1988	Five U.S. communities	5,702	65+	DIS	Major depression	Males 0.4% Females 0.9%
						Dysthymia	Males 1.0% Females 2.3%
						Alcohol abuse/dependence	Males 1.8% Females 0.3%
						Schizophrenia	Males 0.1% Females 0.1%
						Any anxiety disorder	Males 3.6% Females 6.8%
ECA	Blazer et al. 1991	Three U.S. communities	784	65+	DIS	Generalized anxiety	2.2%
LASA	Beekman et al. 1995	Netherlands	3,056	55–85	DIS	Major depression	2.0%
Edmonton	Bland et al. 1988	Canada	358	65+	DIS	Major depression	1.2%
						Phobic disorder	3.0%
						Panic disorder	0.3%
Liverpool	Copeland et al. 1987	England	1,070	65+	GMS-AGECAT	Depressive neurosis	8.3%
						Depressive psychosis	2.9%
Guy's/Age Concern Survey	Lindesay et al. 1989	London	890	65+	Structured interview	Phobic disorder	10.0%

Note. DIS = Diagnostic Interview Schedule (Robins et al. 1981); ECA = Epidemiologic Catchment Area; GMS-AGECAT = Geriatric Mental State (Copeland et al. 1976); LASA = Longitudinal Aging Study Amsterdam.

in late life by symptoms of poor physical health or pseudodementia. Yet there is no compelling evidence for developing a new diagnostic classification specific to older adults. Although DSM-IV-TR may not identify all persons with significant psychiatric symptoms, those who do qualify for a DSM-IV-TR diagnosis are not unlike persons at other stages of the life cycle (Blazer 1980b; Blazer et al. 1987a). The deficiency inherent in DSM-IV-TR is that it poorly differentiates psychiatric symptoms from those that signify the presence of physical illness and impaired cognition—a situation that also may occur in younger individuals, although it is far more common as a diagnostic problem in late life than in midlife.

The prevalence of psychiatric disorders, especially major depression, in treatment facilities is presented in Table 1–5. Burns et al. (1988) found among nursing home patients with mental disorders, excluding organic brain syndrome, an average of 1.3 mental disorder diagnoses per person. As is evident, the prevalence of both minor and major depression is much higher than that found in community populations. The prevalence of major depression is estimated to be 6.0%–14.4% (Koenig et al. 1988; Lyness et al. 1999; Parmelee et al. 1989; Rovner et al. 1986; Teresi et al. 2001) and the prevalence of minor depression to be as high as 30.5% (Parmelee et al. 1989). Many depressed older adults may be selectively admitted to medical inpatient units or long-term care facilities (because older adults are less likely to use specialty psychiatric care). The lower prevalence of these disorders in the community, therefore, should not lull clinicians into believing that psychiatric problems are of little consequence for older adults.

Fewer data regarding the incidence of psychiatric disorders in late life are available because most disorders begin earlier in adulthood. In a study of 875 nondepressed

older adults, the 3-year incidence of depression was 4.1% (Forsell and Winblad 1999). Henderson et al. (1997) reported that the 3- to 6-year incidence of depression in a sample of community-dwelling elders age 70 or older was 2.5%. The incidence of schizophrenia among older adults is estimated to be 3.0 per 100,000 persons per year for new cases (Copeland et al. 1998). Finally, the incidence of dementia increases with age. Bachman et al. (1993) reported from the Framingham data that the 5-year incidence of dementia was 7.0 per 1,000 in those age 65–69 and 118.0 per 1,000 at ages 85–89. A similar increase with age in the 1-year incidence of Alzheimer's disease was reported from the East Boston EPESE: 0.6% in those age 65–69 and 8.4% in those age 85 or older (Hebert et al. 1995).

Historical Studies

Psychiatrists typically follow up patients for relatively short periods during the course of their illnesses. In addition, they usually interact with each patient within a relatively brief window of historical time. Epidemiological studies add a historical perspective to current cross-sectional findings in population and clinical surveys. Historical studies in psychiatric epidemiology are rare, especially of the elderly. Unlike changes observed with infectious diseases, temporal changes that occur with most behaviors that are of psychiatric interest must be determined over years rather than months. Constructs of case identification have changed over the years, and so it is rare to find a study in which similar methods of case identification were applied at two points distant enough in time to establish historical trends. Longitudinal studies are also fraught with methodological problems, especially problems with follow-up.

TABLE 1–5. Prevalence of selected psychiatric disorders among older adults in selected treatment facilities

Study/Site	Reference	Sample	N	Age (years)	Measurement	Disorder	Prevalence
Intermediate-care facility	Rovner et al. 1986	Nursing home	50	Mean age = 83	Standardized interviews	Major depression	6.0%
Long-term care facility	Parmelee et al. 1989	Nursing home and congregate housing	708	Mean age = 84	DSM-III-R checklist GDS	Major depression Minor depression	12.4% 30.5%
Acute-care facility	Koenig et al. 1988	Hospital	171	65+	Screening and modified DIS	Major depression Minor depression	11.5% 23.0%
Primary care facility	Lyness et al. 1999	Primary care	224	60+	SCID Ham-D	Major depression Minor depression	6.5% 5.2%
Long-term care facility	Teresi et al. 2001	Nursing homes	319	Mean age = 85	Structured psychiatric interviews	Major depression	14.4%

Note.   DIS = Diagnostic Interview Schedule (Robins et al. 1981); GDS = Geriatric Depression Scale (Yesavage et al. 1983); Ham-D = Hamilton Rating Scale for Depression (Williams 1988); SCID = Structured Clinical Interview for DSM-III-R (Spitzer et al. 1992).

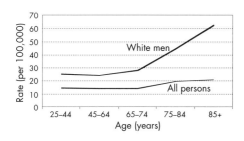

FIGURE 1–1. Suicide rates in the United States by age in 1998.

The study of changes in suicide frequency among older adults during the twentieth century illustrates the value of longitudinal studies, despite the methodological problems associated with these designs. Suicide rates have been positively correlated with age. The highest suicide rates are consistently evident among persons older than 65 (McIntosh et al. 1994; Moscicki 1997). As is shown in Figure 1–1, the correlation is largely explained by the elevated rates of suicide among white men older than 70 years. Rates among white men age 70 and older have fallen since 1940, from a high of 60–65 per 100,000 in 1940 (Bureau of the Census 1973) to a low of 39 per 100,000 in 2000 (data from WISQARS injury mortality report database, see Centers for Disease Control and Prevention 2003).

The century-long trend for suicide rates increasing with age has flattened. Why has this happened? The suicide rate at any point in time is determined by at least three factors: age, generational or cohort effects, and unique stressors for a particular age group at a particular point in time (i.e., period effects). Both age and generational effects were shown to be predictors of suicide in the United States since 1900 in a study by G.E. Murphy and Wetzel (1980). The generational effect was illustrated in a study by Haas and Hendin (1983). Age groups were studied at four points in time

from 1908 to 1970. Cohorts in the 15- to 24-year-old age group showed significantly different suicide rates. The 15- to 24-year-olds in 1908 showed a suicide rate of 13.5 per 100,000; in contrast, the rate of the same age group in 1923 showed a rate of 6.3 per 100,000. The 1908 cohort continued to show higher rates of suicide than the 1923 cohort at every age through life, although both cohorts showed increases in suicide rates with age.

In 2000, the suicide rate was 12.6 per 100,000 for those age 65–74, 17.7 per 100,000 for those age 75–84, and 19.4 per 100,000 for those age 85 or older (Centers for Disease Control and Prevention 2002). For all cohorts combined, annual national suicide rates have stabilized at about 10–13 per 100,000 since 1941 (McIntosh et al. 1994).

In a study of suicides in England and Wales, E. Murphy and colleagues (1986) were able to show a marked period effect. In a cohort analysis of recorded suicides from 1921 to 1980, a decline in suicide rates of successively older cohorts was identified. (This finding contrasts with figures in the United States.) Murphy postulated the effect of period events—specifically, World War II and the detoxification of domestic gas. As domestic gas was converted to a methane-based product in the 1960s, the rate of gas poisoning in the more elderly groups decreased dramatically. This decrease was not offset by increasing rates of suicide by other means, suggesting that withdrawal of a method of suicide could result in a net saving of life.

It is clear from these historical studies that many factors contribute to changing rates in at least one indicator of psychiatric disorder—that is, suicide. Concomitant changes in other factors are less well understood but may be especially relevant to the study of psychiatric disorders in elderly persons. Klerman et al. (1985) suggested that the relatively low prevalence of depression in the 1980s among late-life cohorts might have been the result of a cohort effect. Current cohorts of older adults appear remarkably protected against severe or clinically diagnosed depressive disorders. Younger cohorts, in contrast, have had higher rates of major depression over the life cycle. Because there is no reason to expect the rates for younger cohorts to decrease as they enter late life—that is, there is no evidence of a period effect—the prevalence of major depression in late life may increase in future years.

Age, period, and cohort effects on suicide rates also have been anticipated for future decades. Aging is assumed to be a risk factor for suicide, as in the past. Period effects could work for or against increased age effects. Proliferation of how-to manuals for suicide and dramatic erosion of economic conditions could elevate risk; enhanced pain management and palliative care services, improvement in economic conditions, and advances in treatment of depression and Alzheimer's disease could decrease risk (McIntosh et al. 1994). The sheer size of the baby-boom cohort may presage extremely high absolute frequency and rates of suicide in the decades ahead, although earlier elevated rates in this cohort may mean that surviving members are more suicide resistant (Manton et al. 1987; McIntosh et al. 1994). If the baby-boom cohort depletes economic resources, there is some concern for elevated suicide rates among subsequent cohorts (the baby busters, followed by the baby boomlet or echo cohort). A historical perspective enables public health workers to anticipate future needs and plan preventive services targeted to subgroups of the population at potentially high risk.

An additional historical consideration in the study of psychiatric disorders is the study of incidence and duration of these disorders, which together determine prevalence. Cumulative incidence, the probability of developing a disorder over a specified time (usually 1 year), is less important to the health care provider at a given point in time but is very relevant to planning for services in the future.

Etiological Studies

One of the more important tasks in epidemiology is to identify factors that can either predispose individuals to developing psychiatric disorders or precipitate such disorders (Blazer and Jordan 1985). Other factors can be identified that are associated with the prevalence of a disorder, but the antecedent/consequent relationship has not been established. For practical purposes in this discussion, we identify all of these as "risk factors." These factors generally fall into several categories, including genetic or biological factors, environmental or chemical factors, and social factors. Examples of each are provided below. In addition, the presence of a comorbid physical or mental condition or disorder often leads to the development of psychiatric symptoms or another disorder.

The contribution of epidemiology to uncovering hereditary trends in mental disorders is best illustrated by the work in senile dementia. Heston et al. (1981) studied the relatives of 125 probands who had dementia of the Alzheimer's type (as identified at autopsy). The risk of dementia in first-degree relatives varied with the age of the person at the onset of dementia. Those persons who were first-degree relatives of someone with Alzheimer's disease were more likely to develop the disease earlier in life, suggesting that the inherited form of Alzheimer's disease is associated with an accelerated onset. Barclay et al. (1986) reported that a family history for dementia was positive in 35.9% of the patients with Alzheimer's disease, compared with 5.6% of the individuals who were cognitively intact.

Folstein and Breitner (1981) suggested that a subtype of Alzheimer's disease may be transmitted as an autosomal dominant trait with complete penetrance (Chase et al. 1983). In their original investigation, Folstein and Breitner found that the presence of aphasia and apraxia distinguished patients with a primary degenerative dementia who had a family history of the disease from those who did not have such a history. In a study of 39 cases of Alzheimer's disease, patients with relatives who had the disease were less often able to complete a sentence on the MMSE than were those who did not have afflicted relatives (P<0.05). Among those individuals who were unable to write a sentence, the investigators found a fourfold increased risk of dementia compared with the general population. In a follow-up study, Folstein and colleagues (1985) found that among 54 nursing home patients diagnosed with Alzheimer's disease, 40 were considered aphasic and agraphic and 14 were not. The first-degree relatives of the aphasic and agraphic patients with primary degenerative disorder had a 44% risk of senile dementia by age 90, approaching the 50% rate for a genetic disorder that is autosomal dominant with complete penetrance.

Other biological risk factors have been identified. Research in Alzheimer's disease and dementia has focused on the ε4 allele of the APOE gene (Evans et al. 1997; A.M. Saunders et al. 1993). That is, the ε4 allele is a susceptibility gene in that some (but not all) persons with the allele develop dementia. Some studies have also found a relation between the APOE3 and APOE4 alleles and the onset of late-life depression (Krishnan et al. 1996), whereas

other studies did not find a link between genotype and change in the number of depressive symptoms (Mauricio et al. 2000).

Investigators have suggested an association between early-onset Alzheimer's disease and Down syndrome, suggesting a common biological or genetic mechanism. Heyman et al. (1983) studied 68 patients with Alzheimer's disease who had experienced clinical onset before age 70. Secondary cases of dementia were found in 17 (25%) of the families, affecting 22 of the probands' siblings and parents. An increased frequency of Down syndrome was observed among relatives of the probands, a rate of 3.6 per 1,000, compared with the expected rate of 1.3 per 1,000. Heston et al. (1981) not only found an excess of Down syndrome in the families of patients with Alzheimer's disease but also identified an increased frequency of lymphoma and immune system disorder diatheses among family members, suggesting that immune system disorders and an increased risk for Alzheimer's disease are associated.

Physical agents in the environment may lead to cognitive problems and other psychiatric symptoms. Two illustrative studies show the effect of such agents on the brain. Goodwin et al. (1983) studied 260 non-institutionalized men and women between ages 60 and 94. On clinical examination, these individuals were not found to have serious illness or to be clinically malnourished or vitamin deficient. Dietary intake for these subjects was calculated: the nutrients measured included protein, vitamin C, vitamin B_{12}, folic acid, riboflavin, thiamine, niacin, and pyridoxine. Blood samples were obtained to determine the blood levels of these specific nutrients. The investigators discovered a significant relation between scores on memory tests and blood levels of vitamin C and folic acid in these generally well-functioning older adults. Henderson et al. (1992) found a relation between Alzheimer's disease and starvation/malnutrition in a case-control study. These results suggest that variables, such as nutrient levels, may provide an opportunity for intervention in the relation between cognitive functioning and primary (innate) and secondary (environmentally induced) changes with aging. Gerontologists have long sought such intervening variables that may allow clinical intervention to prevent or mitigate deficits that were previously ascribed to primary aging.

Parker et al. (1983) investigated the relation between alcohol use and cognitive functioning. In the study, 1,937 employed men and women were asked about their alcohol consumption during the previous month. In addition, vocabulary skills and abstraction abilities were examined. Results from the study suggested a linear relation between the amount of alcohol consumption during the previous month and cognitive impairment. The relation held both for the men and for the women whose drinking patterns resembled the men's. This model suggests that cognitive performance may be decreased by alcohol consumption before the postintoxication period, and because this relationship is linear, even moderate alcohol intake may lead to impairment in cognitive functioning. The implications of these findings for the elderly are evident.

Environmental agents such as bodily injury also can be factors. Studies of the association between prior head trauma and the development of Alzheimer's disease have been inconclusive. Mortimer et al. (1991) pooled data from 11 retrospective studies and concluded that head trauma increased the risk of Alzheimer's disease (relative risk = 1.82). In a prospective study of 6,645 patients age 55 or older, however, mild head trauma was not a risk factor for dementia or Alzheimer's disease (Mehta et al. 1999). Other chemical agents such as medication have the potential to affect the brain.

Estrogen has been shown in some studies to have a protective effect against dementia (Kawas et al. 1997), yet other studies have found that estrogen was not protective against cognitive decline (Fillenbaum et al. 2001). Some research has found a protective effect for the use of nonsteroidal anti-inflammatory medication in Alzheimer's disease (Anthony et al. 2000).

By far the most frequently investigated environmental factors associated with psychiatric disorders are social factors. Many investigators believe that the changing roles and circumstances of older adults can cause stress and therefore contribute to the onset of psychiatric disorders and cognitive difficulties in older adults. In a study of 986 community-dwelling older adults, Blazer (1980a) found the crude estimate of relative risk for mental health impairment to be 2.14, given a life event score of 150 or greater on the Schedule of Recent Events (Holmes and Rahe 1967). A relative risk of 1.73 ($P < 0.01$) was estimated when a binary regression procedure was used, controlling for physical health, economic status, social support, and age. In a study of individuals age 55 or older, Murrell et al. (1983) found that social factors, including widowhood, divorce, separation, and decreased income, were related to depressive symptomatology in the community.

In the LASA study, major depression was associated with being unmarried; having functional limitation, perceived loneliness, internal locus of control, and poorer self-perceived health; and not receiving instrumental social support (Beekman et al. 1995). In the Duke ECA study, the recent experience of negative life events and poor social support were associated with major depression (Blazer et al. 1987b). Cognitive impairment has been shown to be associated with poorer self-rated health (Christensen et al. 1994). Impairment or dissatisfaction with the social network has been reported to be associated with anxiety symptoms in late life (Forsell and Winblad 1998). Patterson et al. (1997) found that older patients with schizophrenia had more impairments in social functioning compared with control subjects.

Finally, issues of comorbidity between psychiatric symptoms and disorders and physical health are important in late life. Psychiatric symptoms and physical and mental conditions may themselves lead to the development of other psychiatric symptoms and impairment. Depression has been shown to be a risk factor for declines in physical functioning (Penninx et al. 1998), and declines in physical functioning have been shown to be a risk factor for depression (Kennedy et al. 1990). Studies also have shown that disability in daily life is associated with hallucinations and delusions in late life (Ostling and Skoog 2002). In cross-sectional studies, cognitive impairment has been associated with depressive symptoms (Yaffe et al. 1999). In addition, some studies have shown depression to be a risk factor for decline in cognitive function (Devanand et al. 1996). Finally, a history of depression or anxiety has been shown to be a risk factor for depression or anxiety symptoms in late life (Forsell 2000).

From these examples, it is clear that both psychiatric disorders and symptoms in late life can have multiple causes and that these factors may interact with one another to produce adverse outcomes.

Health Service Utilization

Epidemiological studies provide a disturbing profile of the use of mental health services by elderly persons. Although older adults are less likely than those in any other age group to use community-based psychiatric services, they are more likely to use psychotropic medication. In a study of three of the ECA communities (New Ha-

ven, Connecticut; Baltimore, Maryland; and St. Louis, Missouri), Shapiro et al. (1984) found that 6%–7% of older adults had made a visit to a health care provider for mental health reasons during the previous 6 months. Those in the group age 65 or older infrequently received care from mental health specialists, even if they were identified in the community as having a DSM-III (American Psychiatric Association 1980) psychiatric disorder or severe cognitive impairment. German et al. (1985) analyzed the data from Baltimore in greater detail. Of those persons younger than 65, 8.7% had made a visit to a specialty or primary care provider for mental health care during the 6 months prior to the interview. For those age 64–74, the rate was 4.2%; of those age 75 or older, only 1.4% received such care. In the 75 or older age group, not one person among the 292 individuals interviewed saw a specialty mental health care provider. The investigators concluded that the likeliest source of care for older individuals with emotional or psychiatric problems is their primary care provider, within the context of a visit for physical medical problems.

In contrast, the use of psychotropic drugs is high among older adults. Hanlon et al. (1992) found that 12.5% of community-dwelling persons older than 65 years during 1986 were taking central nervous system drugs, and psychotropic medications were the second most frequently used therapeutic class of medication. Blazer et al. (2000a) recently reported that the use of antidepressants in community-dwelling older adults increased from 1986 to 1996. Blazer et al. (2000b) also noted a simultaneous increase in the use of antianxiety, sedative, and hypnotic medications in this population.

Even though a high proportion of older adults uses psychotropic medications, their disorders, such as depression, remain untreated. Unutzer et al. (2000) found in a study of health maintenance organization enrollees that 4%–7% of the older adults received treatment for depression, but most individuals with probable depression did not receive treatment. Similarly, Steffens et al. (2000) recently found in the Cache County Study that only 35.7% of the older adults with major depression were taking an antidepressant. A total of 27.4% of those with major depression were taking a sedative-hypnotic.

By sampling elderly community-dwelling populations, researchers can collect data on the proportion of older adults with impairment, need for services, and perceived needs or demands for services and the current use of services. This information can be used by government and private agencies to chart effective assessment, treatment, and prevention programs. This development is especially relevant to the care of older adults because they tend to be isolated, their psychiatric impairment may be masked, and they are less active advocates for their mental health needs than are younger persons. In summary, community studies of older adults have shown that the prevalence of psychiatric disorders and psychiatric symptoms in older adults is significant, which has implications for all types of health service utilization.

References

American Psychiatric Association: Diagnostic and Statistical Manual of Mental Disorders, 3rd Edition. Washington, DC, American Psychiatric Association, 1980

American Psychiatric Association: Diagnostic and Statistical Manual of Mental Disorders, 4th Edition. Washington, DC, American Psychiatric Association, 1994

American Psychiatric Association: Diagnostic and Statistical Manual of Mental Disorders, 4th Edition, Text Revision. Washington, DC, American Psychiatric Association, 2000

Anthony JC, Breitner JC, Zandi P, et al: Reduced prevalence of AD in users of NSAIDs and H2 receptor antagonists: the Cache County Study. Neurology 54:2066–2071, 2000

Bachman DL, Wolf PA, Linn RT, et al: Incidence of dementia and probable Alzheimer's disease in a general population: the Framingham Study. Neurology 43:515–519, 1993

Barclay LL, Kheyfets S, Zemcov A, et al: Risk factors in Alzheimer's disease, in Alzheimer's Disease and Parkinson's Disease: Strategies for Research and Development. Edited by Fisher A, Hanin I, Lachman C. New York, Plenum, 1986, pp 141–146

Beekman ATF, Deeg DJH, van Tilberg T, et al: Major and minor depression in later life: a study of prevalence and risk factors. J Affect Disord 36:65–75, 1995

Beekman ATF, Copeland JR, Prince MJ: Review of community prevalence of depression in late life. Br J Psychiatry 174:307–311, 1999

Bland RC, Newman SC, Orn H: Prevalence of psychiatric disorders in the elderly in Edmonton. Acta Psychiatr Scand Suppl 338:57–63, 1988

Blazer DG: Life events, mental health functioning and the use of health care services by the elderly. Am J Public Health 70:1174–1179, 1980a

Blazer DG: The diagnosis of depression in the elderly. J Am Geriatr Soc 28:52–58, 1980b

Blazer DG: The epidemiology of late life depression. J Am Geriatr Soc 30:587–592, 1982

Blazer DG: Psychiatry and the oldest old. Am J Psychiatry 157:1915–1924, 2000

Blazer DG, Houpt JL: Perception of poor health in the healthy older adult. J Am Geriatr Soc 27:330–334, 1979

Blazer DG, Jordan K: Epidemiology of psychiatric disorders and cognitive problems in the elderly, in Psychiatry, Vol 3. Edited by Michels R, Cavenar JO. Philadelphia, PA, JB Lippincott, 1985, pp 1–12

Blazer D, Kaplan B: Controversies in community-based psychiatric epidemiology. Arch Gen Psychiatry 57:227–228, 2000

Blazer D, Bachar JR, Hughes DC: Major depression with melancholia: a comparison of middle-aged and elderly adults. J Am Geriatr Soc 35:927–932, 1987a

Blazer D, Hughes DC, George LK: The epidemiology of depression in an elderly community population. Gerontologist 27:281–287, 1987b

Blazer D, Woodbury M, Hughes D, et al: A statistical analysis of the classification of depression in a mixed community and clinical sample. J Affect Disord 16:11–20, 1989

Blazer D, Hughes D, George L: Generalized anxiety disorder, in Psychiatric Disorders in America: The Epidemiologic Catchment Area Study. Edited by Robins L, Regier D. New York, Free Press, 1991, pp 180–203

Blazer DG, Hybels C, Simonsick E, et al: Marked differences in antidepressant use by race in elderly community sample: 1986–1996. Am J Psychiatry 157:1089–1094, 2000a

Blazer DG, Hybels CF, Simonsick E, et al: Sedative, hypnotic and anti-anxiety medication use in an aging cohort over ten years: a racial comparison. J Am Geriatr Soc 48:1073–1079, 2000b

Bureau of the Census: Vital Statistics Special Reports, Vol 15, No 21. Washington, DC, U.S. Census Bureau, 1973, pp 217–243

Burns BJ, Larson DB, Goldstrom ID, et al: Mental disorder among nursing home patients: preliminary findings from the National Nursing Home Survey Pretest. Int J Geriatr Psychiatry 3:27–35, 1988

Busse A, Bischkopf J, Riedel-Heller SG, et al: Mild cognitive impairment: prevalence and incidence according to different diagnostic criteria. Results of the Leipzig Longitudinal Study of the Aged (LEILA 75+). Br J Psychiatry 182:449–454, 2003

Callahan CM, Hendrie HC, Tierney WM: Documentation and evaluation of cognitive impairment in elderly primary care patients. Ann Intern Med 122:422–429, 1995

Canadian Study of Health and Aging Working Group: Canadian Study of Health and Aging: study methods and prevalence of dementia. CMAJ 150:899–912, 1994

Centers for Disease Control and Prevention, NCHS: Death rates for suicide, 1950–2000, in Health, United States, 2002. Centers for Disease Control and Prevention, National Center for Health Statistics. Available at: http://infoplease.com/ipaA0779940.html. Accessed August 18, 2003.

Centers for Disease Control and Prevention, National Center for Health Statistics: WISQARS injury mortality report, suicide injury deaths and rates per 100,000 white, non-Hispanic males, ages 70–85+, ICD-10 codes: X60–X84, Y87.0. Available at http://webapp.cdc.gov/sasweb/ncipc/mortrate10.html. Accessed September 23, 2003.

Chase GA, Folstein MF, Breitner JCS, et al: The use of life tables and survival analyses in testing genetic hypotheses with an application to Alzheimer's disease. Am J Epidemiol 7:590–597, 1983

Christensen H, Jorm AF, Henderson AS, et al: The relationship between health and cognitive functioning in a sample of elderly people in the community. Age Ageing 23:204–212, 1994

Christenson R, Blazer D: Epidemiology of persecutory ideation in an elderly population in the community. Am J Psychiatry 141:1088–1091, 1984

Copeland JRM, Kelleher MJ, Kellett JM, et al: A semi-structured clinical interview for the assessment of diagnosis and mental state in the elderly. Psychol Med 6:439–449, 1976

Copeland JRM, Dewey ME, Wood N, et al: Range of mental illness among the elderly in the community: prevalence in Liverpool using the GMS-AGECAT package. Br J Psychiatry 150:815–823, 1987

Copeland JRM, Davidson IA, Dewey ME, et al: Alzheimer's disease, other dementias, depression, and pseudodementia: prevalence, incidence, and three-year outcome in Liverpool. Br J Psychiatry 161:230–239, 1992

Copeland JRM, Dewey ME, Scott A, et al: Schizophrenia and delusional disorder in older age: community prevalence, incidence, comorbidity, and outcome. Schizophr Bull 24:153–161, 1998

Copeland JRM, Beekman ATF, Dewey ME, et al: Depression in Europe: geographic distribution among older people. Br J Psychiatry 174:312–321, 1999

Cornoni-Huntley J, Brock D, Ostfeld A, et al: Established Populations for Epidemiologic Studies of the Elderly. Bethesda, MD, National Institute on Aging, 1986

Devanand DP, Sano M, Tang M-X, et al: Depressed mood and incidence of Alzheimer's disease in elderly living in the community. Arch Gen Psychiatry 53:175–182, 1996

Evans DA, Funkenstein HH, Albert MS, et al: Prevalence of Alzheimer's disease in a community population of older persons: higher than previously reported. JAMA 262:2551–2556, 1989

Evans DA, Beckett LA, Field T: Apolipoprotein E e4 and incidence of Alzheimer's disease in a community population of older persons. JAMA 277:822–824, 1997

Federal Interagency Forum on Aging Related Statistics: Older Americans 2000: Key Indicators of Well-Being. Washington, DC, Federal Interagency Forum on Aging Related Statistics, 2000

Fillenbaum GG, Hanlon JT, Landerman LR, et al: Impact of estrogen use on decline in cognitive function in a representative sample of older community-resident women. Am J Epidemiol 153:137–144, 2001

First MB, Spitzer RL, Gibbon M, et al: Structured Clinical Interview for DSM-IV Axis I Disorders, Research Version. Washington, DC, American Psychiatric Association, 1997

Folstein MF, Breitner JCS: Language disorder predicts familial Alzheimer's disease. Johns Hopkins Medical Journal 149:145–147, 1981

Folstein MF, Folstein SE, McHugh P: Mini-Mental State: a practical method for grading the cognitive state of patients for clinicians. J Psychiatr Res 12:189–198, 1975

Folstein MF, Anthony JC, Parhad I, et al: The meaning of cognitive impairment in the elderly. J Am Geriatr Soc 33:228–235, 1985

Forsell Y: Predictors for depression, anxiety and psychotic symptoms in a very elderly population: data from a 3-year follow-up study. Soc Psychiatry Psychiatr Epidemiol 35:259–263, 2000

Forsell Y, Winblad B: Feelings of anxiety and associated variables in a very elderly population. Int J Geriatr Psychiatry 13:454–458, 1998

Forsell Y, Winblad B: Incidence of major depression in a very elderly population. Int J Geriatr Psychiatry 14:368–372, 1999

German PS, Shapiro S, Skinner EA: Mental health of the elderly: use of health and mental health services. J Am Geriatr Soc 33:246–252, 1985

Goodwin JS, Goodwin JM, Garry PJ: Association between nutritional status and cognitive functioning in a healthy elderly population. JAMA 249:2917–2921, 1983

Graham JE, Rockwood K, Beattie BL, et al: Prevalence and severity of cognitive impairment with and without dementia in an elderly population. Lancet 349:1793–1796, 1997

Gurland B, Golden RR, Teresi JA, et al: The SHORT-CARE: an efficient instrument for the assessment of depression, dementia and disability. J Gerontol 39:166–169, 1984

Haas AP, Hendin H: Suicide among older people: projections for the future. Suicide Life Threat Behav 13:147–154, 1983

Hanlon JT, Fillenbaum GG, Burchett B, et al: Drug-use patterns among Black and non-black community-dwelling elderly. Ann Pharmacother 26:679–685, 1992

Hathaway SR, McKinley JC: Minnesota Multiphasic Personality Inventory, Revised Edition. Minneapolis, University of Minnesota, 1970

Hazzard W: Introduction: the practice of geriatric medicine, in Principles of Geriatric Medicine and Gerontology. Edited by Hazzard W, Bierman E, Blass J, et al. New York, McGraw-Hill, 1994, pp xxiii–xxiv

Hebert LE, Scherr PA, Beckett LA, et al: Age-specific incidence of Alzheimer's disease in a community population. JAMA 273:1354–1359, 1995

Heeren TJ, Lagaay AM, Hijmans W, et al: Prevalence of dementia in the 'oldest old' of a Dutch community. J Am Geriatr Soc 39:755–759, 1991

Henderson AS, Jorm AF, Korten AE, et al: Environmental risk factors for Alzheimer's disease: the relationship to age of onset and to familial or sporadic types. Psychol Med 22:429–436, 1992

Henderson AS, Jorm AF, MacKinnon A, et al: Prevalence of depressive disorders and the distribution of depressive symptoms in later life: a survey using Draft ICD-10 and DSM-III-R. Psychol Med 23:719–729, 1993

Henderson AS, Korten AE, Jacomb PA, et al: The course of depression in the elderly: a longitudinal community-based study in Australia. Psychol Med 27:119–129, 1997

Henderson AS, Korten AE, Levings C, et al: Psychotic symptoms in the elderly: a prospective study in a population sample. Int J Geriatr Psychiatry 13:484–492, 1998

Heston LL, Mastri AR, Anderson E, et al: Dementia of the Alzheimer's type: clinical genetics, natural history, and associated conditions. Arch Gen Psychiatry 38:1085–1090, 1981

Heyman A, Wilkinson WE, Hurwitz BJ, et al: Alzheimer's disease: genetic aspects and associated disorders. Ann Neurol 14:507–515, 1983

Holmes TH, Rahe RH: The Social Readjustment Rating Scale. J Psychosom Res 11:213–218, 1967

Kawas C, Resnick S, Morrison A, et al: A prospective study of estrogen replacement therapy and risk of developing Alzheimer's disease: the Baltimore Longitudinal Study of Aging. Neurology 48:1517–1521, 1997

Kay DWK, Bergmann K, Foster EM, et al: Mental illness and hospital usage in the elderly: a random sample followed up. Compr Psychiatry 11:26–35, 1970

Kay DWK, Henderson AS, Scott R, et al: Dementia and depression among the elderly living in the Hobart community: the effect of the diagnostic criteria on the prevalence rates. Psychol Med 15:771–788, 1985

Kennedy GJ, Kelman HR, Thomas C: The emergence of depressive symptoms in late life: the importance of declining health and increasing disability. J Community Health 15:93–103, 1990

Kessler RC, Berglund P, Demler O, et al: The epidemiology of major depressive disorder. JAMA 289:3095–3105, 2003

Kleinbaum DG, Kupper LL, Morgenstern H: Epidemiologic Research. New York, Van Nostrand Reinhold, 1982, pp 320–376

Klerman GL, Lavori PW, Rice J, et al: Birth-cohort trends in rates of major depression among relatives of patients with affective disorder. Arch Gen Psychiatry 42:689–694, 1985

Koenig HG, Meador KG, Cohen HJ, et al: Depression in elderly hospitalized patients with medical illness. Arch Intern Med 148:1929–1936, 1988

Krishnan KRR, Tupler LA, Ritchie JC, et al: Apolipoprotein E-e4 frequency in geriatric depression. Biol Psychiatry 40:69–71, 1996

Lindesay J, Briggs K, Murphy E: The Guy's/Age Concern Survey: prevalence rates of cognitive impairment, depression and anxiety in an urban elderly community. Br J Psychiatry 155:317–329, 1989

Lyness JM, King DA, Cox C, et al: The importance of subsyndromal depression in older primary care patients: prevalence and associated functional disability. J Am Geriatr Soc 47:647–652, 1999

MacMahon B, Pugh TF: Epidemiology: Principles and Methods. Boston, MA, Little, Brown, 1970

Manton KG, Blazer DG, Woodbury MA: Suicide in middle age and later life: sex- and race-specific life table and cohort analyses. J Gerontol 42:219–227, 1987

Mauricio M, O'Hara R, Yesavage JA, et al: A longitudinal study of apolipoprotein-E genotype and depressive symptoms in community-dwelling older adults. Am J Geriatr Psychiatry 8:196–200, 2000

McIntosh JL, Santos JF, Hubbard RW, et al: Elder Suicide: Research, Theory, and Treatment. Washington, DC, American Psychological Association, 1994

Mehta KM, Ott A, Kalmijn S, et al: Head trauma and risk of dementia and Alzheimer's disease: the Rotterdam Study. Neurology 53:1959–1962, 1999

Morris JN: Uses of Epidemiology, 3rd Edition. London, Churchill Livingstone, 1975

Mortimer JA, van Duijn CM, Chandra V, et al: Head trauma as a risk factor for Alzheimer's disease: a collaborative re-analysis of case-control studies. EURODEM Risk Factors Research Group. Int J Epidemiol 20 (suppl 2):S28–S35, 1991

Moscicki EK: Identification of suicide risk factors using epidemiologic studies. Psychiatr Clin North Am 20:499–517, 1997

Murphy E, Lindesay J, Grundy E: Sixty years of suicide in England and Wales. Arch Gen Psychiatry 43:969–977, 1986

Murphy GE, Wetzel RD: Suicide risk by birth cohort in the United States, 1949–1974. Arch Gen Psychiatry 37:519–523, 1980

Murrell SA, Himmelfarb S, Wright K: Prevalence of depression and its correlates in older adults. Am J Epidemiol 117:173–185, 1983

Ostling S, Skoog I: Psychotic symptoms and paranoid ideation in a nondemented population-based sample of the very old. Arch Gen Psychiatry 59:53–59, 2002

Parker DA, Parker ES, Brody JA, et al: Alcohol use and cognitive loss among employed men and women. Am J Public Health 73:521–526, 1983

Parmelee PA, Katz IR, Lawton MP: Depression among institutionalized aged: assessment and prevalence estimation. J Gerontol A Biol Sci Med Sci 44:M22–M29, 1989

Patterson TL, Semple SJ, Shaw WS, et al: Self-reported social functioning among older patients with schizophrenia. Schizophr Res 27:199–210, 1997

Penninx BWJH, Guralnik JA, Ferrucci L, et al: Depressive symptoms and physical decline in community-dwelling older persons. JAMA 279:1720–1726, 1998

Pfeiffer E: A Short Portable Mental Status Questionnaire for the assessment of organic brain deficit in elderly patients. J Am Geriatr Soc 23:433–441, 1975

Radloff LS: The CES-D scale: a self-report depression scale for research in the general population. Applied Psychological Measurement 1:385–401, 1977

Regier DA, Myers JK, Kramer M, et al: The NIMH Epidemiologic Catchment Area Program: historical context, major objectives and study population characteristics. Arch Gen Psychiatry 41:934–994, 1984

Regier DA, Boyd JH, Burke JD, et al: One-month prevalence of mental disorders in the United States. Arch Gen Psychiatry 45:977–986, 1988

Riedel-Heller SG, Busse A, Aurich C, et al: Prevalence of dementia according to DSM-III-R and ICD-10: results of the Leipzig Longitudinal Study of the Aged (LEILA 75+) Part 1. Br J Psychiatry 179:250–254, 2001

Roberts CJ: Epidemiology for Clinicians. London, Pitman Medical, 1977

Robins LN, Helzer JE, Croughan J, et al: National Institute of Mental Health Diagnostic Interview Schedule: its history, characteristics, and validity. Arch Gen Psychiatry 38:381–389, 1981

Rovner BW, Kafonek S, Filipp L, et al: Prevalence of mental illness in a community nursing home. Am J Psychiatry 143:1446–1449, 1986

Saunders PA, Copeland JRM, Dewey ME, et al: Alcohol use and abuse in the elderly: findings from the Liverpool Longitudinal Study of Continuing Health in the Community. Int J Geriatr Psychiatry 4:103–108, 1989

Saunders AM, Schmader K, Breitner J: Apolipoprotein E epsilon 4 allele distributions in late-onset Alzheimer's disease and in other amyloid forming disease. Lancet 342:710–711, 1993

Shapiro S, Skinner EA, Kessler LG, et al: Utilization of health and mental health services. Arch Gen Psychiatry 41:971–982, 1984

Spitzer RL, Endicott J, Robins E: Research Diagnostic Criteria: rationale and reliability. Arch Gen Psychiatry 35:773–782, 1978

Spitzer R, Williams J, Gibbon M, et al: The Structured Clinical Interview for DSM-III-R (SCID), I: history, rationale, and description. Arch Gen Psychiatry 49:624–629, 1992

Steffens DC, Skoog I, Norton M, et al: Prevalence of depression and its treatment in an elderly population: Cache County Study. Arch Gen Psychiatry 57:601–607, 2000

Stevens T, Livingston G, Kitchen G, et al: Islington study of dementia subtypes in the community. Br J Psychiatry 180:270–276, 2002

Strauss J, Gabriel K, Kokes R: Do psychiatric patients fit their diagnoses? Patterns of symptomatology as described with a biplot. J Nerv Ment Dis 167:105–113, 1981

Suzman R: Oldest old, in Encyclopedia of Aging. Edited by Maddox G. New York, Springer, 1995, pp 712–715

Teeter RB, Garetz FK, Miller WR, et al: Psychiatric disturbances of aged patients in skilled nursing homes. Am J Psychiatry 133:1430–1434, 1976

Teng EL, Chui HC: The Modified Mini-Mental State (3MS) Examination. J Clin Psychiatry 48:314–318, 1987

Teresi J, Abrams R, Holmes D, et al: Prevalence of depression and depression recognition in nursing homes. Soc Psychiatry Psychiatr Epidemiol 36:613–620, 2001

Unutzer J, Simon G, Belin T, et al: Care for depression in HMO patients aged 65 or older. J Am Geriatr Soc 48:871–878, 2000

Williams JBW: A structured interview guide for the Hamilton Depression Rating Scale. Arch Gen Psychiatry 45:742–747, 1988

World Health Organization: International Statistical Classification of Diseases and Related Health Problems, 10th Revision. Geneva, World Health Organization, 1992

Yaffe K, Blackwell T, Gore R, et al: Depressive symptoms and cognitive decline in nondemented elderly women. Arch Gen Psychiatry 56:425–430, 1999

Yesavage JA, Brink TL, Rose TL, et al: Development and validation of a geriatric depression screening scale. J Psychiatr Res 17:37–49, 1983

Zaudig M, Mittelhammer J, Hiller W, et al: SIDAM—a structured interview for the diagnosis of dementia of the Alzheimer type, multi-infarct dementia and dementias of other aetiology according to ICD-10 and DSM-III-R. Psychol Med 21:225–236, 1991

Study Questions

Select the single best response for each question.

1. The "old-old" populace (older than age 85) is projected to reach what number of persons by the year 2050?

    A. 10 million.
    B. 12 million.
    C. 20 million.
    D. 25 million.
    E. 27 million.

2. The geriatric population is expected to increase to how many by the year 2030?

    A. 30 million.
    B. 40 million.
    C. 50 million.
    D. 60 million.
    E. 70 million.

3. Case identification in geriatrics is particularly germane because

    A. Distinction between a case and a noncase is easily established.
    B. Epidemiologists cannot assist the clinician in identifying meaningful clusters of symptoms.
    C. Many of the symptoms and signs of a psychiatric disorder in late life may be ubiquitous with the aging process.
    D. Clinicians particularly favor case identification based on severity of functional impediment.
    E. Most older adults ideally fit the psychiatric diagnosis they receive.

4. The NIMH ECA program (1984) established the two most prevalent disorders of the elderly as

    A. Depressive and anxiety disorders.
    B. Depressive and cognitive disorders.
    C. Depressive and psychotic disorders.
    D. Anxiety and cognitive disorders.
    E. Anxiety and psychotic disorders.

5. The most frequently reported psychiatric symptom(s) of the elderly is (are)

    A. Depression.
    B. Fatigue.
    C. Problems with sleep.
    D. Anxiety related.
    E. C and D.

6. Suicide in the elderly

    A. Is highest in the 65–74 sector.
    B. Is highest in the 78–84 sector.
    C. Is inversely correlated with age.
    D. Is most pronounced in white men older than 70.
    E. Has demonstrated a cohort effect of an increased rate with more modern manufacture of domestic gas.

7. Major depression has *not* been associated with

    A. Having functional limitation.
    B. External locus of control.
    C. Poorer self-perceived health.
    D. Perceived loneliness.
    E. Being unmarried.

Physiological and Clinical Considerations of Geriatric Patient Care

Robert M. Kaiser, M.D., M.H.Sc.

Harvey J. Cohen, M.D.

The burgeoning of the geriatric population is an unquestioned demographic fact in the early twenty-first century. People are living longer, and the numbers of elderly grow with each passing year (Hobbs 2001). The average life span has lengthened significantly (Fried 2000; W.J. Hall 1997; Vaillant and Mukamal 2001).

Careful and sophisticated longitudinal studies of elderly populations in the United States have addressed how and why people are living to the eighth decade and beyond (see Cornoni-Huntley et al. 1986; Shock 1984). Basic science has yielded fundamental anatomic, physiologic, and genetic information about the aging process, and a more complete picture of what aging entails has emerged.

How does aging occur? That perplexing question has been answered, to date incompletely, by two main theories: 1) a "programmed" theory of aging, in which genetics dictates how fast one ages and how long one lives; and 2) a "wear and tear" theory, in which continued injury overwhelms the organism's capacity to repair it (Armbrecht 2001). The hallmarks of physiological change in the elderly are two-fold: impaired homeostasis (also called *homeostenosis*) and increased vulnerability because of decreased reserve capacity (Armbrecht 2000; Taffet 1999). The ability of the organism to maintain a steady state—homeostasis—lessens with time. Consider two straightforward, representative examples:

1. In the elderly, the baroreceptor reflex, which triggers vasoconstriction in order to maintain normal blood pressure, is less robust, and the elderly are less able to respond quickly to intravascular volume depletion.
2. When faced with repelling an invading microorganism, an older patient's immune system is less able to mount a strong response, and thus it is more difficult for the immune system to fight infection effectively.

Age brings with it expected decrements in function. In this chapter, we detail the various physiological changes that occur with "normal aging"—namely, those progressive changes that take place over time but not as a result of disease. We discuss 1) physiological changes in the major organ systems, 2) geriatric syndromes, 3) special implications for prescribing medications in the elderly because of age-related physiological changes, 4) chronic disease in the elderly, and 5) fundamental principles of geriatric assessment that follow from those expected physiological changes.

Major Organ Systems

Central Nervous System

The central nervous system (CNS) undergoes a number of anatomic changes with age. In the brain, significant neuronal loss occurs in the locus coeruleus and the substantia nigra, and Purkinje cells decrease in the cerebellum. Other areas of the brain lose neurons, including the entorhinal cortex, hypothalamus, pons, medulla, and nucleus basalis of Meynert. Aging neurons nevertheless maintain the ability to make new synapses. Both increases and decreases in the production of neurotransmitters in the brain occur with age, but the effect on brain function is unclear. The deposition of the amyloid in neurons damages them and may hasten cell death (Mattson 2003; Taffet 1999; Whalley 2001).

Cognition and Aging

Various studies have documented a decline in cognitive function with age. Such decline may occur in a number of areas, including intelligence, language, memory, learning, visuospatial function, and psychomotor function. Crystallized intelligence remains stable, but fluid intelligence declines. Elderly adults are also less able to name items. Remote (long-term) memory,

sensory memory, and procedural memory are generally unchanged, but the elderly learn more slowly and retain less information. Visuospatial tasks are more difficult, while both motor speed and response times decline with aging. Psychomotor function is affected by age, including an increase in reaction time and a decrease in the speed of cognitive processing. Some evidence suggests that executive function, or the ability to conceive, organize, and carry out a plan or activity, may remain intact in the elderly (Craft et al. 2003; Oskvig 1999).

Vision and Hearing

The elderly develop significant changes in the eye, which have important effects on vision. The weakening of the ciliary muscle, combined with the loss of elasticity in the lens, results in presbyopia; it then becomes difficult for an individual to focus on near objects, and bifocals may be needed. It is also difficult for the elderly to adapt to light, because of rigidity of the pupil and increasing opacity of the lens. The elderly show a decline in their ability to view objects at rest (static acuity) and in motion (dynamic acuity). With age, the lens opacifies, and a cataract can form; the lens becomes less transparent as a result of protein aggregations. Elderly patients are also at risk for age-related macular degeneration, which causes loss of central vision when drusen (yellowish-white deposits) accumulate in the retina (Kalina 1999; Taffet 1999).

Along with changes in vision, the elderly can also expect alterations in the ear that may lead to hearing loss in both high and low frequencies. In the inner ear, cochlear neurons are lost, and there are changes in the organ of Corti, basilar membrane, stria vascularis, and spiral ligament that also affect hearing. The degeneration of the organ of Corti is associated with high frequency sensorineural hearing loss, while atrophy of the stria vascularis may cause hearing loss across all frequencies. The stiffening of the basilar membrane and atrophy of the spiral ligament can both result in loss of speech discrimination (Mills 2003; Taffet 1999).

Cardiovascular System

The heart and blood vessels in the aging patient undergo significant anatomic alterations. These structural changes lead to changes in function. In addition, age-associated changes occur in the autonomic nervous system, which have important physiological effects. Both cardiac output and cardiac reserve decrease (Lakatta 1999; Oskvig 1999; Taffet 1999). With age, human blood vessels stiffen; the vessels are thicker and less distensible. The physiological result is a greater pulse wave velocity, early reflected pulse waves, and higher systolic blood pressures in older individuals. Higher pressures can increase the load on the heart and lead to left ventricular enlargement (Lakatta 1999; Oskvig 1999).

The function of the heart during exercise, including the force and rate of contraction, is mediated by the sympathetic nervous system. Age-related changes in that system occur, and this in turn affects the adaptability of the heart and blood vessels to stress. The older heart dilates during exercise to increase end-diastolic volume and maintain stroke volume, but cardiac output nonetheless declines with age. Because the heart stiffens, it empties less completely. The decline in cardiac output also adversely affects oxygen utilization in the elderly adult. The decline in cardiac function with age may explain 50% of the reduction in maximum oxygen consumption that occurs (Lakatta 1999).

Respiratory System

Notable changes in the chest wall develop with age (Oskvig 1999; Taffet 1999). The thoracic cage becomes rounder; the cartilaginous conducting airways enlarge, resulting in an increase in dead space. A more rigid chest wall negatively affects the mechanical process of breathing. In the older individual, more work is required to expand the chest wall. Declining respiratory muscle strength, particularly in the intercostal muscles, and decreased endurance also affect the ability to breathe normally.

Changes in the lung itself and in the control of breathing negatively affect the respiratory system (Oskvig 1999; Taffet 1999). A loss of elastic tissue occurs in the lung, and the alveolar ducts and respiratory bronchioles enlarge. This enlargement leads to a loss of alveolar surface area; less tissue is available for gas exchange, and the partial pressure of oxygen (pO_2) decreases at a rate of 0.5% per year (Taffet 1999). The elderly lung is less able to guard itself against infection. The mucociliary tree lining the respiratory tract lacks the same speed in rapidly ridding the lung of invading particles and microorganisms. With age, the ability to generate a sufficiently strong cough declines.

Gastrointestinal System

As human beings age, numerous anatomic changes take place throughout the gastrointestinal tract, some of which are functionally significant (K. E. Hall and Wiley 2003; Majumdar et al. 1997; Taffet 1999). For the most part, the production of saliva is adequately maintained. There are fewer myenteric ganglion cells, which in turn affects the coordination of swallowing and may predispose some elderly patients to aspiration. The strength of esophageal contractions is diminished, but food nonetheless traverses the length of the esophagus uneventfully. The production of acid and pepsin by the stomach is mostly preserved. Both the stomach and the small intestine do not dilate as easily when a bolus of food enters, and transit through the large bowel may be slower. The small bowel less effectively absorbs vitamins and minerals (such as vitamin D, calcium, and iron) and sugars (such as xylose and lactose). The liver, gall bladder, and pancreas continue to function well in the elderly patient (K.E. Hall and Wiley 2003; Majumdar et al. 1997; Taffet 1999).

Endocrine System

Prolactin

Levels of prolactin in aging women have been reported to increase, decrease, or remain the same, whereas those in men are slightly increased. None of these changes are believed to have an effect on normal function (Gruenewald and Matsumoto 2003).

Antidiuretic Hormone

With aging, there are significant changes in antidiuretic hormone (ADH), and the body's response to it, which alter the older patient's ability to excrete free water (resulting in hyponatremia) or to prevent volume losses (resulting in dehydration). Basal ADH levels are normal to increased in the elderly; because renal free water clearance decreases with age, hyponatremia can more easily occur. However, when volume loss takes place, with subsequent hypotension, less ADH is released in older persons. In this particular clinical situation, other age-related changes are also at work to produce dehydration: 1) the kidney is less responsive to ADH, which impairs its effort to make more concentrated urine; and 2) aldosterone activity decreases, and natriuretic hormone activity increases, both of which inhibit renal conservation of sodium and restoration of normal volume. The impaired thirst mechanism in the elderly further exacerbates this scenario by preventing them from drinking adequate amounts of fluid to correct free water losses, thereby contributing further to de-

hydration (Gruenewald and Matsumoto 2003; Oskvig 1999; Perry 1999).

Corticotropin and Cortisol

Basal corticotropin levels are normal in the elderly. Neither the corticotropin pulse frequency nor its circadian rhythm of secretion is altered. Stimulation of the hypothalamic-pituitary-adrenal (HPA) axis by exogenous corticotropin produces the expected cortisol response, but the cortisol secretion rate actually declines. Cortisol levels remain the same because of a decrease in the cortisol metabolic clearance rate. When subjected to stress, the HPA axis produces higher peak cortisol levels that then dissipate more slowly; this occurs because the negative feedback of cortisol on the HPA axis is less effective (Gruenewald and Matsumoto 2003).

Adrenal Androgens

Both dehydoepiandosterone (DHEA) and dehydroepiandosterone sulfate (DHEA-S) levels decrease significantly in the elderly. DHEA production peaks at age 20 and then declines (Fried and Walston 1999; Gruenewald and Matsumoto 2003).

Adrenal Medulla and Sympathetic Nervous System

In the elderly, secretion of norepinephrine increases and clearance decreases; plasma levels therefore increase. Epinephrine secretion and clearance both increase with age, so the level of epinephrine does not change. The level of sympathetic nervous system activity is increased in older persons, but both α-adrenergic and β-adrenergic receptors are less sensitive to stimulation (Gruenewald and Matsumoto 2003; Oskvig 1999; Seals and Ensler 2000).

Renin, Angiotensin, and Aldosterone

An age-related decrease in plasma renin activity leads to reduced aldosterone secretion; aldosterone levels are thus reduced significantly. The rise in natriuretic hormone secretion in the elderly also serves to decrease aldosterone levels; higher levels of natriuretic hormone suppress renin secretion, plasma renin activity, and angiotensin II, further lowering aldosterone secretion. In addition, natriuretic hormone itself can inhibit aldosterone secretion. The ability of corticotropin to stimulate aldosterone secretion is unchanged in the aging adult. The overall decrease in aldosterone adversely affects sodium retention in the kidney and predisposes the elderly to dehydration. Another consequence of lower aldosterone levels is an increased likelihood of hyperkalemia (Gruenewald and Matsumoto 2003).

Growth Hormone

Growth hormone levels peak at puberty and then decrease by 14% per decade. Both a decrease in growth hormone–releasing hormone secretion and an increase in somatostatin levels are responsible for the decline in growth hormone. Insulin-like growth factor (IGF-1), which is produced by the liver and mediates the actions of growth hormone in the body, also diminishes gradually, at a rate of 7%–13% per decade. The falloff in growth hormone with age may result in a decrease in both lean body mass and bone mass (Gruenewald and Matsumoto 2003; Perry 1999).

Parathyroid Hormone, Vitamin D, and Calcium Regulation

The elderly generally consume insufficient calcium in the diet; in addition, calcium is less efficiently absorbed in the small intestine. Vitamin D is essential to that absorption, and levels of vitamin D, 25-hydroxy (25D) and vitamin D, 1,25-dihydroxy (1,25D) both decrease as a result of several factors, including 1) decreased sunlight exposure and less efficient photoconversion in the skin of 2-dehydrocholesterol to vitamin D3; 2) insufficient dietary intake of vitamin D; 3) intestinal malabsorption of, or resistance to, vitamin D; 4) decreased 1-α hydroxylase activity in the kidney; and 5) the use of medications that cause the liver to break down vitamin D. The decline in both serum calcium and 1,25D levels triggers a compensatory increase in parathyroid hormone (PTH). PTH then 1) stimulates osteoclasts to resorb bone, and 2) acts on the renal distal tubule to promote calcium reabsorption, thereby increasing serum calcium levels. PTH levels are higher in the elderly due to increased secretion and decreased renal clearance. This is thought to represent a form of secondary, rather than primary, hyperparathyroidism and can have a deleterious effect on bone mass in older patients (Baylink et al. 1999; Perry 1999).

Testosterone

As men age, the number of Leydig's cells in the testis declines, and testosterone secretion gradually decreases. Two other factors influence the age-related decline in testosterone: 1) a loss in the circadian variation in testosterone levels, and 2) an increase in sex-hormone binding globulin levels, which limits the amount of free testosterone available. The overall decline in testosterone causes a decrease in both the number of Sertoli's cells and daily sperm production. Both libido and fertility may decline. The effect of declining testosterone levels on sexual function is thought to be less important than chronic medical or psychiatric illness, vascular disease, neuropathy, or medications. Declining testosterone may adversely affect bone mass as well as muscle mass and strength in older men. The changes in testosterone secretion are common but not universal, and some men demonstrate normal serum testosterone levels as they age (Gruenewald and Matsumoto 2003; Perry 1999).

Estrogen

Estrogen declines precipitously with menopause. Both fibrosis and involution of the ovary, as well as atrophy of the uterus and vagina, take place. The number of ovarian follicles declines, and a corresponding decrease in the secretion of both estrogen and androgens occurs; after menopause the ratio of estrogens to androgens decreases. Menopause is also marked by an alteration in gonadotropin-releasing hormone secretion and high follicle-stimulating hormone levels, although luteinizing hormone levels remain the same. The lack of estrogen affects bone mass and places women at risk for osteoporosis. Women also lose the beneficial effects of estrogen on lipids, with rising low-density lipoprotein levels, and are at higher risk for cardiovascular disease. The lack of estrogen causes atrophy of the vaginal endothelium, the endothelium thins, less lubrication occurs with intercourse, and dyspareunia can result (Gruenewald and Matsumoto 2003; Perry 1999; Taffet 1999).

Thyroid

Although there are age-related changes in the thyroid gland, these have no corresponding effect on thyroid function. The aging thyroid is more fibrotic and nodular in composition. Although the thyroid continues to make sufficient amounts of thyroxine (T_4), it fails to metabolize T_4 as well. The synthesis of T_4 actually declines, but its level is unchanged. Peripheral deiodination of T_4 to triiodothyronine (T_3) also decreases and the level of T_3 declines by 10%–20% in the elderly. Reverse T_3 levels do not change. Thyroxine-binding globulin levels remain normal with age (Hassani and Hershman 2003; Perry 1999).

Insulin

Elderly patients have a tendency towards hyperglycemia. Circulating insulin levels may rise but are less efficiently utilized. Although insulin secretion by the pancreatic beta cells is preserved with age, insulin clearance declines, and insulin levels increase. Peripheral uptake of insulin is affected by insulin resistance in peripheral tissues; some of these tissues, particularly adipocytes, have fewer receptors, and thus their sensitivity to insulin is decreased. Elderly patients have decreased muscle mass and a higher percentage of fat and therefore an increased number of adipocytes. These notable changes in insulin secretion and tissue sensitivity in the periphery may lead to observed increases in fasting glucose in the elderly. In addition, there is another factor leading to higher glucose levels. IGF-1, which acts at insulin receptors to promote glucose uptake, is less abundant in the elderly (Halter 2003; Perry 1999; Taffet 1999).

Musculoskeletal System

In general, the elderly person is less muscular and weaker. A decline in skeletal muscle mass, or sarcopenia, occurs. In the fourth decade, both muscle mass and strength begin to decrease. There are smaller numbers of type II fast-twitch fibers and fewer motor units and synapses; slow muscle fibers predominate. Exercise may modify age-associated changes in muscle mass and strength. Sarcopenia places the elderly at risk for significant physical disability and a decline in their ability to perform activities of daily living, and may ultimately undermine their ability to live independently (Loeser and Delbono 2003; Taffet 1999).

The elderly also develop demonstrable changes in cartilage, tendons, and ligaments. Cartilage becomes less cellular with age. Alterations in the structure of proteoglycans affect the ability of these molecules to bind water and maintain the hydration of cartilage. Cartilage weakens as the number of proteoglycan monomers decreases and the protein links between the monomers are broken. The overall effect of age-related changes in cartilage is to decrease both its tensile strength and stiffness, adversely affecting its response to mechanical stress (see Loeser and Delbono 2003; Taffet 1999).

Age-related changes in the structure of both cortical and trabecular bone occur. Cortical bone becomes thinner and more porous; trabecular bone also thins, and whole trabeculae are lost. Bones are therefore weaker. The elderly are at increased risk for bone loss. Women can lose significant bone mass after menopause. Elderly men with testosterone deficiency may also develop osteoporosis. Other factors that contribute to bone loss in both men and women include low peak bone density, poor calcium intake and secondary hyperparathyroidism (as discussed earlier), and insufficient exercise (Baylink et al. 1999).

Hematologic and Immune Systems

The aging adult does not lose the ability to produce normal numbers of red cells, white cells, and platelets—despite a decrease in the bone marrow mass—but when challenged to produce more red blood cells by the occurrence of blood loss or by the presence of hypoxic conditions, the bone marrow is less able to respond quickly. Red cells and white cells retain normal function. The red cell's capacity to carry oxygen is essentially unchanged. The white blood cell continues to engulf and kill bacteria, but the respiratory burst activity of polymorphonuclear neutrophils decreases with age. Platelets, however, may be more sensitive to substances that trigger them to form blood clots (Chatta and Lipschitz 2003; Taffet 1999).

When confronted with a new infection, the elderly are less able to mount an adequate cell-mediated response. The humoral, or antibody, response in the elderly is also impaired. The elderly respond less vigorously to the first presentation of an antigen

as well as to the re-introduction of antigen. These decreased primary and secondary responses may explain why the elderly respond less well to vaccination (Miller 2003; Taffet 1999).

The body's primary defenses against infection are also affected by age. The thinner skin of the elderly is more vulnerable to injury. The mucous membranes of the genitourinary and respiratory tracts of the elderly may become more easily colonized with gram-negative organisms. The decreased concentration, acidity, and amount of urea in the urine itself deprive it of an intrinsic defense against possible bacterial infection. Elderly patients with swallowing dysfunction may aspirate bacteria from the oral cavity, or those unable to produce an adequate cough will leave infectious material in the airways (Taffet 1999).

Renal System

Aging brings with it a progressive decrease in the size of the kidney due to fatty infiltration, fibrosis, and the drop-out of cortical nephrons. The rate of decline of nephrons is 0.5%–1% per year; by age 60, 30%–50% of functioning glomeruli have been eliminated. Creatinine clearance, a widely accepted measure of kidney function, declines 7.5%–10% per decade (Oskvig 1999; Taffet 1999).

These anatomical changes have important physiological consequences, including the decreased ability of the kidney to acidify urine or to excrete an acid or a water load. The response of the renin-angiotensin-aldosterone system is less supple, renin activity declines, and less renin is produced in the face of decreased intravascular volume or a depletion of salt. The kidney is able to maintain its output of erythropoietin, but the hydroxylation of vitamin D declines. Levels of atrial natriuretic peptide rise. The kidney less reliably metabolizes hormones such as glucagon, calcitonin, and parathyroid hormone; drug metabolism is also significantly affected and will be discussed in the next section (Oskvig 1999; Taffet 1999).

Geriatric Syndromes

In addition, several common syndromes—known generally as *geriatric syndromes*—are found more frequently in older patients. Four of the most characteristic geriatric syndromes—dementia, falls, urinary incontinence, and polypharmacy—are discussed in the following subsections.

Dementia

Dementia is a prevalent condition in the elderly but not a result of normal aging (Morris 1999). It is defined as the development of significant deficits in two or more areas of cognition—an impairment of memory and at least one other area such as abstract thinking, judgment, language, or visuospatial ability—that are severe enough to affect day-to-day functioning of the individual (Nyenhuis and Gorelick 1998).

Two-thirds of all dementia is caused by Alzheimer's disease. Vascular dementia accounts for 15%–25% of disease, and Lewy body dementia constitutes 10%. The natural history and symptomatology of dementia vary according to its etiology (Marin et al. 2002).

- In Alzheimer's disease, symptoms begin gradually and steadily progress. Early on, a loss of short-term memory occurs; difficulty learning may also be evident. With progression, long-term memory is affected as well as orientation, judgment, word-finding, performance of motor tasks, and visuospatial function. In late stages of the disease, patients lose their ability to perform their activities of daily living; they may become increasingly depressed or agitated. They may develop motor or gait problems and urinary and fecal incontinence (Marin et al. 2002).
- Vascular dementia occurs in patients with underlying cerebrovascular disease. Its clinical course is more abrupt in onset and less linear than Alzheimer's disease; the progressive nature of vascular dementia has not been precisely defined. In some cases of vascular dementia, there may be some overlap with Alzheimer's disease (Nyenhuis and Gorelick 1998).
- Lewy body dementia is distinguished by its unique set of presenting symptoms. Patients not only present with cognitive deficits but also may report visual hallucinations. The neurological examination may identify rigidity, bradykinesia, and postural changes (Gomez-Tortosa et al. 1998).

The accurate diagnosis of dementia requires a comprehensive assessment by the clinician, including a detailed history, thorough physical, neurological, and mental status examinations, and a depression screen. Since the patient may have significant deficits, the history needs to be gathered from the patient along with someone who is familiar with the history of the patient's illness, their medications, and social history. The evaluating clinician should order laboratory studies to rule out B_{12} deficiency, syphilis, and hypothyroidism and check for evidence of anemia, electrolyte abnormalities, renal failure, and liver dysfunction. This laboratory evaluation enables the clinician to detect reversible causes of dementia and uncover evidence of metabolic abnormalities that might point to a diagnosis of delirium, rather than dementia (Marin et al. 2002).

Above all, the proper treatment of dementia involves the building of a proper support system for the patient. Pharmacologic treatment of Alzheimer's disease patients may be appropriate in some cases.

Acetylcholinesterase inhibitors, including donepezil, galantamine, and rivastigmine, have shown some effectiveness in clinical trials of patients with mild to moderate disease, with documented improvements in the Alzheimer's Disease Assessment Scale Cognitive Subscale score (Frisoni 2001; Lanctot et al. 2003; Sramek et al. 2001). Patients with moderate to severe dementia have shown benefit from treatment with memantine (McShane et al. 2006). Patients with Alzheimer's disease are at risk for the development of depressive symptoms as well as major depression, and clinicians can provide effective medical treatment for this. Because agitation is also a prevalent symptom, particularly in patients with late disease, this symptom may also require treatment; atypical antipsychotic agents such as risperidone may be helpful in this context (Defilippi and Crismon 2000; Tune 2001).

Falls

Falls are a common phenomenon in older patients; every year, half of all nursing home residents and one-third of all community-dwelling elderly have a fall. These falls produce notable morbidity: 2% cause hip fractures; 5% cause other fractures; and 10% cause head injuries or other significant injuries. In the aftermath of falls, disability may result. Those who fall frequently are at risk for a decline in their instrumental activities of daily living as well as their activities of daily living (assessment of such functions is discussed later in "Fundamentals of Geriatric Assessment"). A decline in these functions can ultimately undermine their independence; hospitalization might also result (Alexander 1999; Fried 2000; King and Tinetti 1995; Rubenstein et al. 1994).

Falls are generally multifactorial and are caused by 1) intrinsic factors, 2) situational factors, 3) extrinsic factors, and/or 4) medications (Alexander 1999; King and Tinetti 1995). *Intrinsic factors* are disease-specific deficits in an individual patient that might contribute to falling; these factors include neurological problems (central, neuromuscular, vestibular, visual, and proprioceptive) as well as systemic illness. *Situational factors* relate to the particular activity that is taking place. *Extrinsic factors* relate to the demands and hazards of a particular environment. *Medications* may adversely affect mental status, cognition, balance, circulation, and neuromuscular function and predispose patients to falls.

The proper evaluation of a fall requires 1) taking a detailed history and review of systems and 2) performing a thorough physical exam and neurological exam (Alexander 1999). The fall may indeed be a nonspecific presentation of a serious medical illness such as cardiac ischemia, infection, intravascular volume depletion, or hypothyroidism, and such illnesses should be initially considered. The clinician should ask about any symptoms, situational, or extrinsic factors that might have led to the fall, and determine exactly how the fall occurred. A medication list should be compiled. The physical exam should rule out any cardiac abnormalities; the neurological exams must carefully assess the patient for any deficits in vision, strength, sensation, joint mobility, balance, cerebellar function, gait, or proprioception.

The prevention of falls focuses on altering both intrinsic and extrinsic factors (Alexander 1999; Gillespie et al. 2003; King and Tinetti 1995). With regard to intrinsic factors, one can 1) prescribe medication appropriately, 2) optimally treat disease, 3) improve balance and gait through physical therapy, and 4) improve conditioning and strength through exercise. With regard to extrinsic factors, one can 1) improve the environment by reducing or eliminating hazards, 2) monitor patients more carefully by increasing staff supervision and using motion detection, 3) eliminate restraints and the risk of injury they pose, 4) encourage patients to wear hip protectors, and 5) install protective flooring. Preventing falls ultimately requires multiple steps to produce successful results. A recent systematic review suggests that population-based interventions can be effective in the prevention of falls (McClure et al. 2005).

Urinary Incontinence

Urinary incontinence is a prevalent condition in the elderly that causes significant morbidity and affects quality of life (DuBeau 1999; Tannenbaum et al. 2001). Half of all nursing home residents and up to one-third of persons older than 65 residing in the community carry the diagnosis. It is a condition with multiple causes, including age-related changes, genitourinary tract abnormalities, and coexisting illnesses.

Urinary incontinence can be classified into two main categories: 1) transient incontinence and 2) established incontinence. Transient incontinence is reversible and can be easily treated; for example, transient incontinence could be a consequence of an acute urinary tract infection, inadequately controlled diabetes mellitus, or recent prescription of a diuretic, and will resolve with the correction of those conditions.

Established incontinence is further subdivided into the following three subcategories:

1. *Urge incontinence.* This form of incontinence has the highest prevalence in older patients. Urge incontinence results from detrusor overactivity, sometimes with simultaneous impaired contractility. Detrusor overactivity is more common with aging, but can also occur for other reasons, including neurological dysfunction (such as stroke) or irritation of the bladder (secondary to cancer, urolithiasis, or infection); it can also occur in elderly patients without other illnesses. Patients usually complain of a sudden urge to urinate. They also classically have urinary frequency and nocturia. They experience varying amounts of leakage.

2. *Stress incontinence.* Stress incontinence occurs when increased abdominal pressure, triggered by cough or sneezing, results in urinary leakage. It happens commonly in women with weak pelvic muscles, though it may also occur as a consequence of failed anti-incontinence surgery or vaginal mucosal atrophy in women or prostatectomy in men. It is a frequent form of incontinence among elderly women, ranking second.

3. *Overflow incontinence.* Detrusor underactivity and bladder outlet obstruction can both produce overflow incontinence. Detrusor underactivity can be caused by fibrosis of the detrusor muscle, peripheral neuropathy, disc herniation, or spinal stenosis. Detrusor underactivity is an infrequent cause of urinary incontinence in the elderly. Urethral strictures, benign prostatic hypertrophy, and prostate cancer can cause bladder outlet obstruction in elderly men; this form of incontinence is the second most prevalent in this population. Bladder outlet obstruction in women occurs much less frequently; the etiology is either the presence of a large cystocele or a history of anti-incontinence surgery.

In general, the treatment of incontinence in the elderly begins with behavioral interventions and then is followed by medical treatment. Surgery is considered the last option and is only appropriate for stress incontinence or outlet obstruction. Because urinary incontinence in the elderly is invariably the result of more than one cause, clinicians must appreciate that a single intervention may not be effective. Medications must be reviewed to determine if they are contributing to incontinence. Patients must be cautioned against intake of fluids, like alcohol, coffee, tea, and soft drinks, which stimulate urination. Fluid restriction at bedtime may be appropriate to decrease nocturia.

There are a number of specific interventions that can be undertaken to treat the three forms of established incontinence:

1. Urge incontinence is best treated by frequent voluntary voiding and bladder retraining. Patients are placed on a voiding schedule that corresponds to their usual minimal interval of urination. They are taught how to voluntarily inhibit the urge to void. The goal of therapy is to increase gradually the interval between urination. For patients with cognitive impairment, bladder retraining is not appropriate; instead, timed voiding, scheduled voiding, or prompted voiding is instituted to decrease episodes of incontinence. For those who fail behavioral methods, medications such as oxybutinin, tolterodine, or imipramine, may be helpful, but patients should be monitored carefully for anticholinergic side effects.
2. Stress incontinence is also amenable to nonmedical therapy. The mainstay of this approach is to strengthen the pelvic muscles that support the urethra by performing repeated isometric exercises, thereby preventing urinary leakage. The patient should be referred to a physical therapist to initiate an exercise program. In some cases, medical treatment may also be helpful. In women, oral or topical estrogen has sometimes been beneficial. Propanolamine can also be a useful adjunct, although this is not an option in patients with hypertension. For women who fail physical therapy and medical treatment, surgery remains another option.

3. Overflow incontinence in men is most often due to outlet obstruction due to benign prostatic hypertrophy, which can be treated by both medical and surgical modalities. Alpha-blockers have been proven most effective for benign prostatic hypertrophy in clinical trials, although finasteride may be used as a second-line treatment. Transurethral resection and prostatectomy are available options for those who fail medical therapy. In women, previous vaginal or urethral surgery may be the cause of overflow incontinence; this is surgically correctable by lysis of adhesions or unilateral suture removal. For cases of overflow incontinence caused by detrusor underactivity, appropriate interventions include avoidance of constipation as well as careful management of medications to exclude those that adversely affect detrusor function. Intermittent catheterization is most often recommended for treatment for detrusor underactivity.

Incontinence can ultimately have harmful medical consequences, including pressure ulcers, cellulitis, falls, and fractures. It can interfere with sleep. It can also result in sexual dysfunction and depression. The proper treatment of incontinence is therefore important and can yield significant benefits.

Polypharmacy

Polypharmacy, defined as the simultaneous use of multiple medications or the prescribing of more medications than is clinically appropriate, is a common problem in the elderly (Hanlon et al. 2001; Stewart 2001). Their use of drugs is attributable to a number of factors. Chronic illness is more common in older patients, and they experience more symptoms. They are also more frequent consumers of medical care. Drug use is also influenced by individual physician prescribing practices and by drug advertising. According to studies conducted in outpatients, elderly patients use an average of approximately 3–8 prescription and nonprescription drugs simultaneously. Polypharmacy carries with it certain consequences, including adverse drug reactions, drug interactions, and patient noncompliance. It also increases the incidence of geriatric syndromes such as urinary incontinence, falls, cognitive impairment, and delirium.

Clinicians should take several steps to ensure that medicines are prescribed appropriately. They should take a careful, comprehensive medication history, including information on allergies and adverse drug reactions. Current use of alcohol, tobacco, and recreational drugs should be documented. Medicines should be prescribed only if there is a known benefit, and if so, they should be given at the lowest effective dose. Instructions regarding medication use should be communicated clearly to patients. Patients taking medication should be carefully monitored for therapeutic effectiveness and for side effects (Semla and Rochon 2002). Two randomized controlled trials have demonstrated a reduction of inappropriate prescribing and polypharmacy when clinical pharmacists were asked to review drug regimens, consult with physicians, and meet with patients (Hanlon et al. 2001).

Geriatric Prescribing: Effects of Aging on Pharmacokinetics and Pharmacodynamics

The effects of aging on pharmacokinetics (absorption, volume of distribution, clearance rate, and elimination half-life) and pharmacodynamics (the effect of a drug at a given dose) are crucial to understanding how drugs should be prescribed in the elderly patient (J.B. Schwartz 1999; Semla and Rochon 2002).

Age has no significant effect on absorption. The volume of distribution is significantly affected by the changes in body mass and total body water that occur with aging; older patients, with decreased lean body mass and total body water, have a smaller volume of distribution. This is particularly relevant when choosing proper doses for drugs, such as antibiotics or lithium, which are primarily distributed in water. Protein binding can also affect the volume of distribution; it is generally unaffected by age. With age, renal mass and renal blood flow are decreased, resulting in a decline in glomerular filtration rate and creatinine clearance. This decrease in clearance can alter the rate at which drugs are excreted, and dosages must be appropriately adjusted. Hepatic drug clearance is decreased by an age-related decline in hepatic blood flow; oxidative metabolism in the cytochrome P450 system is slower, thereby affecting elimination, but conjugation is not. Underlying hepatic disease and drug interactions may also significantly affect the metabolism of drugs by the liver.

The elimination half-life—the time period required for the drug concentration to decrease by half—of certain drugs increases in the elderly and may be affected by the relation between volume of distribution or clearance; this may require adjustment of the drug dosing interval. One must also consider the pharmacodynamic effects of drugs in the elderly. Frequently, elderly persons are more sensitive to medications, and drugs often must be given in lower doses. For example, the response to anticholinergic drugs in particular is increased.

Chronic Disease in the Elderly

Some chronic diseases are more prevalent in the elderly, and these predominantly occur as a result of "usual aging." The cumulative effect of environment and heredity on the individual over time makes these diseases more common, and they account for significant morbidity and mortality. Among the most formidable and omnipresent of these diseases are cardiovascular disease, cerebrovascular disease, and cancer.

Hypercholesterolemia and hypertension are frequently diagnosed. With age, weight and the incidence of obesity increase; patients are at higher risk for the development of type 2 diabetes mellitus. Age also brings an increased occurrence of joint problems, in particular osteoarthritis, which can result in chronic pain and the need for joint replacement. The elderly can develop cataracts and macular degeneration and therefore impaired vision; hearing loss in the elderly, either due to previous exposure to noise or age-related anatomic changes in the ear, is also prevalent. Postmenopausal women and some hypogonadal elderly men are prone to develop osteoporosis. Benign prostatic hypertrophy, often with resultant urinary frequency and nocturia, becomes more of a clinical problem as men age. Polymyalgia rheumatica and temporal arteritis are collagen vascular diseases that occur often in elderly patients.

The increasing prevalence of multisystem disease in the older patient can impose a substantial burden on the individual; in the face of already diminished physiological reserves, such an individual is considerably more vulnerable to declining health (Fried 2000).

Fundamentals of Geriatric Assessment

Effective evaluation and treatment of the geriatric patient—from the fully functioning community-dwelling older adult to the frail older adult in decline—require a global approach, which includes, but reaches beyond, a consideration of the patient's medical problems. This approach—geriatric assessment—will now be discussed in more detail.

Reuben (2003) has defined *geriatric assessment* as a comprehensive patient evaluation, conducted by an individual clinician or an interdisciplinary team, which considers the impact of key medical, social, psychological, and environmental factors on health and pays careful attention to function. During the medical assessment, the clinician performs a complete history and physical examination. He or she reviews the medication list for appropriateness and evidence of polypharmacy; checks for deficits in vision, hearing, ambulation, and balance; and screens for common geriatric problems such as falling, incontinence, and malnutrition. Vision is tested with Snellen's eye chart. Hearing is screened with the "whispering voice test" or a hand-held audiometer. The patient is weighed, the height is measured, and the body mass index is calculated. In addition to the standard neurologic exam, the patient's mobility and balance can be determined by a "get up and go" test; the patient is asked to stand, walk 10 feet, turn around, return, and be seated. The task is timed; a time greater than 20 seconds suggests more extensive evaluation is needed.

Cognitive assessment is performed with the Folstein Mini-Mental State Exam. The Geriatric Depression Scale is used to screen for depression. Fundamental day-to-day functioning is determined by documenting activities of daily living—bathing, dressing, toileting, feeding, transferring—and instrumental activities of daily living—driving, shopping, cooking, housekeeping, telephone use, and finances. The clinician also must gather other important information about function: 1) the extent, strength, and reliability of the patient's social support system (this is most often the patient's family); 2) the patient's economic resources; and 3) the safety of the patient's home and its proximity to medical care and other essential services. An assessment of the patient's spiritual preferences and needs are also obtained. After the assessment is completed, recommendations are developed and a care plan is implemented.

Although the results across clinical trials have not been consistent, the effectiveness of comprehensive geriatric assessment and management has been validated in a number of studies. Increased diagnostic accuracy has been noted. Patients have shown significant improvements in functional status. Affect and cognition have improved. The use of health care services, as measured by nursing home days, hospital services and medical costs, has been reduced. The use of medications has improved, with fewer drugs being prescribed (Hanlon et al. 2001; Reuben 2003; Stuck et al. 1993). A multi-institutional randomized controlled trial of geriatric evaluation and management units clearly showed a positive effect on functional status and quality of life for inpatients and on mental health and quality of life for outpatients, with overall costs equivalent to those of usual care (Cohen et al. 2002).

As suggested by the evidence, comprehensive geriatric assessment and management serves as a useful tool in both the diagnosis and care of older patients. The geriatrician therefore may serve as a valuable and essential resource in the evaluation and treatment of this population.

References

Alexander NB: Falls and gait disturbances, in Geriatrics Review Syllabus: A Core Curriculum in Geriatric Medicine. Edited by Cobbs E, Duthie EH, Murphy JB. Dubuque, IA, Kendall/Hunt, 1999, pp 145–149

Armbrecht HJ: The biology of aging. J Lab Clin Med 138:220–225, 2001

Baylink DJ, Jennings JC, Mohan S: Calcium and bone homeostasis and changes with aging, in Principles of Geriatric Medicine and Gerontology, 4th Edition. Edited by Hazzard WR, Blass JP, Ettinger WH, et al. New York, McGraw-Hill, 1999, pp 1041–1057

Chatta GS, Lipschitz D: Aging of the hematopoietic system, in Principles of Geriatric Medicine and Gerontology, 5th Edition. Edited by Hazzard W, Blass J, Halter J, et al. New York, McGraw-Hill, 2003, pp 763–770

Cohen HJ, Feussner JR, Weinberger M, et al: A controlled trial of inpatient and outpatient geriatric evaluation and management. N Engl J Med 346:905–912, 2002

Cornoni-Huntley J, Brock DB, Ostfield A, et al (eds): Established Populations for the Epidemiologic Study of the Elderly: Resource Data Book. Bethesda, MD, National Institutes of Health, 1986

Craft S, Cholerton B, Reger M: Aging and cognition: what is normal? in Principles of Geriatric Medicine and Gerontology, 5th Edition. Edited by Hazzard WR, Blass JP, Halter JB, et al. New York, McGraw-Hill, 2003, pp 1355–1372

Defilippi JL, Crismon ML: Antipsychotic agents in patients with dementia. Pharmacotherapy 20:23–33, 2000

DuBeau CW: Urinary incontinence, in Geriatrics Review Syllabus: A Core Curriculum in Geriatric Medicine. Edited by Cobbs E, Duthie EH, Murphy JB. Dubuque, IA, Kendall/Hunt, 1999, pp 115–123

Fried LP: Epidemiology of aging. Epidemiol Rev 22:95–106, 2000

Fried LP, Walston J: Frailty and failure to thrive, in Principles of Geriatric Medicine and Gerontology, 4th Edition. Edited by Hazzard WR, Blass JP, Ettinger WH, et al. New York, McGraw-Hill, 1999, pp 1387–1402

Frisoni GB: Treatment of Alzheimer's disease with acetylcholinesterase inhibitors: bridging the gap between evidence and practice. J Neurol 248:551–557, 2001

Gillespie LD, Gillespie WJ, Robertson MC, et al: Interventions for preventing falls in the elderly. Cochrane Database of Systematic Reviews, Issue 4. Art No CD000340, DOI 10.1002/14651858.CD000340, 2003

Gomez-Tortosa E, Ingraham AO, Irizarry MC, et al: Dementia with Lewy bodies. J Am Geriatr Soc 46:1449–1458, 1998

Gruenewald DA, Matsumoto A: Aging of the endocrine system, in Principles of Geriatric Medicine and Gerontology, 5th Edition. Edited by Hazzard WR, Blass JP, Halter JB , et al. New York, McGraw-Hill, 2003, pp 819–836

Hall KE, Wiley JW: Effect of aging on gastrointestinal function, in Principles of Geriatric Medicine and Gerontology, 5th Edition. Edited by Hazzard WR, Blass JP, Halter JB, et al. New York, McGraw-Hill, 2003, pp 593–600

Hall WJ: Update in geriatrics. Ann Intern Med 127:557–564, 1997

Halter JB: Diabetes mellitus, in Principles of Geriatric Medicine and Gerontology, 5th Edition. Edited by Hazzard WR, Blass JP, Halter JB, et al. New York, McGraw-Hill, 2003, pp 855–874

Hanlon JT, Schmader K, Ruby C, et al: Suboptimal prescribing in older inpatients and outpatients. J Am Geriatr Soc 49:200–209, 2001

Hassani S, Hershman JM: Thyroid diseases, in Principles of Geriatric Medicine and Gerontology, 5th Edition. Edited by Hazzard WR, Blass JP, Halter JB, et al. New York, McGraw-Hill, 2003, pp 837–854

Hobbs FB: The elderly population. U.S. Census Bureau, Population Division and Housing and Household Economic Statistics Division, 2001. Available at: http://www.census.gov/population/www/pop-profile/elderpop.html. Accessed May 4, 2006.

Kalina R: Aging and visual function, in Principles of Geriatric Medicine and Gerontology, 4th Edition. Edited by Hazzard WR, Blass JP, Ettinger WH, et al. New York, McGraw-Hill, 1999, pp 603–615

King MB, Tinetti ME: Falls in community-dwelling older persons. J Am Geriatr Soc 43:1146–1154, 1995

Lakatta EG: Cardiovascular aging research: the next horizons. J Am Geriatr Soc 47:613–625, 1999

Lanctot KL, Herrmann N, Yau KK, et al: Efficacy and safety of cholinesterase inhibitors in Alzheimer's disease: a meta-analysis. CMAJ 169(6):557–564, 2003

Loeser RF, Delbono O: Aging of the muscles and joints, in Principles of Geriatric Medicine and Gerontology, 5th Edition. Edited by Hazzard WR, Blass JP, Halter JB, et al. New York, McGraw-Hill, 2003, pp 905–918

Majumdar AP, Jaszewski R, Dubick MA: Effect of aging on gastrointestinal tract and the pancreas. Proc Soc Exp Biol Med 215:134–144, 1997

Marin DB, Sewell MC, Schlecter A: Alzheimer's disease: accurate and early diagnosis in the primary care setting. Geriatrics 57:36–40, 2002

Mattson MP: Cellular and neurochemical aspects of the aging human brain, in Principles of Geriatric Medicine and Gerontology, 5th Edition. Edited by Hazzard WR, Blass JP, Halter JB, et al. New York, McGraw-Hill, 2003, pp 1341–1354

McClure R, Turner C, Peel N, et al: Population-based interventions for the prevention of fall-related injuries in older people. Cochrane Database of Systematic Reviews, Issue 1, Art No CD004441, DOI 10.1002/14651858.CD004441, 2005

McShane R, Areosa Sastre A, Minakaran N: Memantine for dementia. Cochrane Database of Systematic Reviews, Issue 2, Art No CD003154, DOI: 10.1002/14651858.CD003154, 2006

Miller RA: The biology of aging and longevity, in Principles of Geriatric Medicine and Gerontology, 5th Edition. Edited by Hazzard WR, Blass JP, Halter JB, et al. New York, McGraw-Hill, 2003, pp 3–16

Mills JH: Age-related changes in the auditory system, in Principles of Geriatric Medicine and Gerontology, 5th Edition. Edited by Hazzard WR, Blass JP, Halter JB, et al. New York, McGraw-Hill, 2003, pp 1239–1251

Morris JC: Is Alzheimer's disease inevitable with age? Lessons from clinicopathologic studies of healthy aging and very mild Alzheimer's disease. J Clin Invest 104:1171–1173, 1999

Nyenhuis DL, Gorelick PB: Vascular dementia: a contemporary review of epidemiology, diagnosis, prevention and treatment. J Am Geriatr Soc 46:1437–1448, 1998

Oskvig RM: Special problems in the elderly: perioperative cardiopulmonary evaluation and management. Chest 155(suppl):158S–164S, 1999

Perry HM: The endocrinology of aging. Clin Chem 45:1369–1376, 1999

Reuben DB: Principles of geriatric assessment, in Principles of Geriatric Medicine and Gerontology, 5th Edition. Edited by Hazzard WR, Blass JP, Halter JB, et al. New York, McGraw-Hill, 2003, pp 99–110

Rubenstein LZ, Josephson KR, Robbins AS: Falls in the nursing home. Ann Intern Med 121:442–451, 1994

Schwartz JB: Clinical pharmacology, in Principles of Geriatric Medicine and Gerontology, 4th Edition. Edited by Hazzard WR, Blass JP, Ettinger WH, et al. New York, McGraw-Hill, 1999, pp 303–332

Seals DR, Esler MD: Human ageing and the sympathoadrenal system. J Physiol (Lond) 528:407–417, 2000

Semla TP, Rochon PA: Pharmacotherapy, in Geriatrics Review Syllabus: A Core Curriculum in Geriatric Medicine. Edited by Cobbs E, Duthie EH, Murphy JB. London, Blackwell Scientific, 2002, pp 37–44

Shock NW: Normal Human Aging: The Baltimore Longitudinal Study of Aging. Washington, DC, National Institute on Aging, U.S. Government Printing Office, 1984

Sramek JJ, Alexander BD, Cutler NR: Acetylcholinesterase inhibitors for the treatment of Alzheimer's disease. Annals of Long Term Care 9(10):15–22, 2001

Stewart RB: Drug use in the elderly, in Therapeutics in the Elderly, 3rd Edition. Edited by Delafuente JC, Stewart RB. Cincinnati, OH, Harvey Whitney, 2001, pp 235–256

Stuck AE, Siu AL, Wieland GD, et al: Comprehensive geriatric assessment: a meta-analysis of controlled trials. Lancet 342:1032–1036, 1993

Taffet GE: Age-related physiologic changes, in Geriatrics Review Syllabus: A Core Curriculum in Geriatric Medicine. Edited by Cobbs E, Duthie EH, Murphy JB. Dubuque, IA, Kendall/Hunt, 1999, pp 10–23

Tannenbaum C, Perrin L, DuBeau CE, et al: Diagnosis and management of urinary incontinence in the older patient. Arch Phys Med Rehabil 82:134–138, 2001

Tune LE: Risperidone for the treatment of behavioral and psychological symptoms of dementia. J Clin Psychiatry 62 (suppl 21):29–32, 2001

Vaillant GE, Mukamal K: Successful aging. Am J Psychiatry 158:839–847, 2001

Whalley LJ: The Aging Brain. New York, Columbia University Press, 2001

Study Questions

Select the single best response for each question.

1. Falls in the elderly
   A. Are frequently multifactorial.
   B. Involve one-third of all community-dwelling elderly every year.
   C. Predict considerable morbidity.
   D. Promote risk for decline in instrumental activities of daily living.
   E. All of the above.

2. Urinary incontinence in the elderly is
   A. Most frequently stress incontinence in men.
   B. Most frequently overflow incontinence.
   C. Most frequently urge incontinence.
   D. Seen in up to one-half of community-residing elderly.
   E. None of the above.

3. The musculoskeletal system is affected in which of the following ways?
   A. Decrease in skeletal muscle mass.
   B. Increase in number of type II fibers.
   C. Age-associated changes in muscle mass and strength may be modified by exercise.
   D. A and B.
   E. A and C.

4. Considerations in geriatric prescription should include all of the following *except*
   A. Volume of distribution.
   B. Absorption.
   C. Renal clearance.
   D. Oxidative metabolism in the cytochrome P450 system.
   E. Change in elimination half-life.

5. Which of the following is true of cognition in normal aging?
   A. Crystallized intelligence changes with age.
   B. Fluid intelligence begins to improve in the middle of the sixth decade and thereafter.
   C. Practical intelligence may be stable or even improve with age.
   D. Executive function deteriorates with age.
   E. Long-term memory is affected.

6. Ocular changes include which of the following?

    A. Weakening of the ciliary muscle.
    B. Rigidity of the pupil.
    C. Decline in ability to view objects at rest.
    D. A and B.
    E. A, B, and C.

7. Gastrointestinal system changes of the elderly include

    A. Fewer myenteric ganglion cells.
    B. Diminished acid and pepsin production by the stomach.
    C. Diminished function of liver, gallbladder, and pancreas.
    D. Increased transit of food through the large bowel.
    E. More effective absorption of vitamins and minerals by the small bowel.

8. Hormone levels are affected in all of the following ways *except*

    A. Decrease in growth hormone.
    B. Decrease in dehydroepiandrosterone.
    C. Decrease in cortisol.
    D. Increase in parathyroid hormone levels.
    E. Increase in sex-hormone binding globulin levels.

The Diagnostic Interview in Late Life

The Psychiatric Interview of Older Adults

Dan G. Blazer, M.D., Ph.D.

The foundation of the diagnostic workup of the older adult experiencing a psychiatric disorder is the diagnostic interview. Unfortunately, in this age of increasing technology in the laboratory and standardization of interview techniques, the art of the clinical interview has suffered. In this chapter the core of the psychiatric interview, including history taking, assessment of the family, and the mental status examination, is reviewed. To supplement the clinical interview, structured interview schedules and rating scales that are of value in the assessment of older adults are described. Finally, techniques for communicating effectively with older adults are outlined.

History

The elements of a diagnostic workup of the elderly patient are presented in Table 3–1. To obtain historical information, the clinician should first interview the patient, if it is feasible. Then permission can be asked of the patient to interview family members. Members from at least two generations, if available for interview, can expand the perspective on the older adult's impairment. If the patient has difficulty in providing an accurate or understandable history, the clinician should concentrate especially on eliciting the symptoms or problems that the patient perceives as being most disabling, then fill the historical gap with data from the family.

Present Illness

As many insightful clinicians, such as Eisenberg (1977), have recognized, physicians diagnose and treat diseases—that is, abnormalities in the structure and function of body organs and systems. Patients have illnesses—experiences of disvalued changes in states of being and in social function. Disease and illness do not maintain a one-to-one relationship. Factors that determine who becomes a patient and who does not can be understood only by expanding horizons beyond symptoms. In other words, patienthood is a social state (Eisenberg and Kleinman 1981). During the process of becoming a patient, the older adult, usually with the advice of others, forms a self-diagnosis of his or her problem and makes a judgment about the degree of ill-being perceived.

TABLE 3–1. Diagnostic workup of the elderly patient

History

Symptoms—present episode, including onset, duration, and change in symptoms over time

Past history of medical and psychiatric disorders

Family history of depression, alcohol abuse/dependence, psychoses, and suicide

Physical examination

Evaluation of neurologic deficits, possible endocrine disorders, occult malignancy, cardiac dysfunction, and occult infections

Mental status examination

Disturbance of consciousness

Disturbance of mood and affect

Disturbance of motor behavior

Disturbance of perception (hallucinations, illusions)

Disturbance of cognition (delusions)

Disturbance of self-esteem and guilt

Suicidal ideation

Disturbance of memory and intelligence (memory, abstraction, calculation, language, and knowledge)

For this reason, the clinician must take care to avoid accepting the patient's explanation for a given problem or set of problems. Statements such as "I guess I'm just getting old and there's nothing really to worry about" or "Most people slow down when they get to be my age" can lull the clinician into complacency about what may be a treatable psychiatric disorder. On the other hand, the advent of new and disturbing symptoms in an older adult between each office visit can exhaust the clinician's patience to the point at which adequate pursuit of the problem is derailed. For example, the older adult with hypochondria whose difficulty with awakenings during the night is increasing may insist that this symptom be treated with a sedative and plead with the clinician not to allow continual suffering. In the clinician's view, however, the symptom is a normal accompaniment of old age and therefore should be accepted.

To prevent attitudinal biases when eliciting reports by the older adult (which may result in missing the symptoms and signs of a treatable psychiatric disorder),

the clinician must include in the initial interview a review of the more important psychiatric symptoms in a relatively structured format. Common symptoms that should be reviewed include excessive weakness or lethargy; depressed mood or the blues; memory problems; difficulty concentrating; feelings of helplessness, hopelessness, and uselessness; isolation; suspicion of others; anxiety and agitation; sleep problems; and appetite problems. Critical symptoms that should be reviewed include the presence or absence of suicidal thoughts, profound anhedonia, impulsive behavior ("I can't control myself"), confusion, and delusions and hallucinations.

The review of symptoms is most valuable when it is considered in the context of symptom presentation. When did the symptoms begin? How long have they lasted? Has their severity changed over time? Are there physical or environmental events that precipitate the symptoms? What steps, if any, have been taken to try to correct the symptoms? Have any of these interventions proved successful? Do the symptoms vary during the day (diurnal variation)?

Do they vary during the week or with seasons of the year? Do the symptoms form clusters—that is, are they associated with one another? Which symptoms appear ego-syntonic and which symptoms appear ego-dystonic? As symptoms are reviewed, a specific time frame facilitates focus on the present illness. Having a 1-month or 6-month window enables the patient to review symptoms and events temporally, an approach not usually taken by distressed elders, who tend to concentrate on immediate sufferings.

Critical to the assessment of the present illness is an assessment of function and change in function. The two parameters that are most important (and not included in usual assessments of physical and psychiatric illness) are social functioning and activities of daily living (ADLs). Questions should be asked about the social interaction of the older adult, such as the frequency of his or her visits outside the home, telephone calls, and visits from family and friends. Many scales have been developed to assess ADLs; however, in the interview the clinician can simply ask about ability to get around (for example, walk inside and outside the house), to perform certain physical activities independently (such as bathe, dress, shave, brush one's teeth, and pick out one's clothes) and to do instrumental activities (such as cook, keep one's bank account, shop, and drive).

Past History

Next, the clinician must review the past history of symptoms and episodes. The patient should be asked if he or she has had a similar episode or episodes in the past. How long did the episodes last? When did they occur? How many times in the patient's lifetime have such episodes occurred? Other psychiatric and medical problems should be reviewed as well, especially med-ical illnesses that have led to hospitalization and the use of medication. Not infrequently, the older adult has experienced a major illness or trauma in childhood or as a younger adult, but he or she views this information as being of no relevance to the present episode and therefore dismisses it. Probes to elicit these data are essential. Older adults may ignore or even forget past psychiatric difficulties, especially if these difficulties were disguised. For example, mood swings in early or middle life may have occurred during periods of excessive and productive activity, episodes of excessive alcohol intake, or periods of vague, undiagnosed physical problems. Previous periods of overt disability in usual activities may flag those episodes.

Family History

The distribution of psychiatric symptoms and illnesses in the family should be determined next. The older person with symptoms consistent with senile dementia or primary degenerative dementia is highly likely to have a family history of dementia. The genogram remains one of the best means for evaluating the distribution of mental illness and other relevant behaviors throughout the family tree. This genogram should include both of the parents, blood-related aunts and uncles, brothers and sisters, spouse(s), children, grandchildren, and great-grandchildren. A history should be obtained about institutionalization, significant memory problems in family members, hospitalization for a nervous breakdown or depressive disorder, suicide, alcohol abuse and dependence, electroconvulsive therapy, long-term residence in a mental health facility (and possibly a diagnosis of schizophrenia), and use of mental health services by family members (Blazer 1984).

Mendlewicz and colleagues (1975) remind us that accurate genetic information can be better obtained when family members from more than one generation are interviewed. Many psychiatric disorders are characterized by a variety of symptoms, so asking the patient or one family member for a history of depression is insufficient. Research on the genetic expression of psychiatric disorders in families requires the psychiatric investigator to interview directly as many family members as possible to determine accurately the distribution of disorders throughout the family. Such detailed family assessment is not feasible for clinicians, yet a telephone call to a relative with permission from the patient may become a standard of clinical assessment as the genetics of psychiatric disorders are clarified.

Context

Psychiatric disorders occur in a biomedical and psychosocial context. The clinician, although he or she will of course determine what medical problems the patient has experienced, might overlook a variation in the relative contribution of these medical disorders to psychopathology. The psychosocial contribution to the onset and continuance of the problem is just as likely to be overlooked. Has the spouse of the older adult undergone a change? Are the middle-aged children managing high stress, such as caring for an emotionally disturbed child and the loss of employment simultaneously? Are the grandchildren placing emotional stress on the elderly patient, perhaps requesting money? Has the economic status of the older adult deteriorated? Has the availability of medical care changed?

Although many psychiatric disorders are biologically driven, they do not occur in a psychosocial vacuum. Environmental precipitants remain important in the web of causation leading to the onset of an episode of emotional distress and are critical to the assessment of the older adult.

Medication History

Next, it is essential to evaluate the medication history of the older adult. A careful review of medications by the clinician is essential, although this may be done by a nurse or a physician's assistant. The clinician should ask the older person to bring in all pill bottles as well as a list of medications taken and the dosage schedule. A double check between the written schedule and the pill containers will frequently expose some discrepancy. Both prescription and over-the-counter drugs, such as laxatives and vitamins, should be recorded. The clinician can then identify the medications that are potentially critical in terms of drug-drug interactions and ask about them during subsequent visits.

Older persons are less likely than younger persons to abuse alcohol, but a careful history of alcohol intake is essential to the diagnostic workup. Older persons do not usually volunteer information about their alcohol intake, but they are generally forthcoming when asked about their drinking habits.

Substance abuse beyond alcohol and prescription drugs is rare in older adults but not entirely absent.

Medical History

Given the high likelihood of comorbid medical problems associated with psychiatric disorders in late life, a comprehensive medical history is essential. Most older persons see a primary care physician fairly regularly (although decreasing payment by Medicare renders this assumption less accurate each year). The geriatric psychiatrist should obtain medical records, if possible. Major illnesses should be recorded. A brief phone call to the primary care physician can be extremely useful.

Family Assessment

Clinicians working with older adults must be equipped to evaluate the family—both its functionality and its potential as a resource for the older adult. Geriatric psychiatry, almost by definition, is family psychiatry. Just as an elevated white blood cell count is not pathognomonic for a particular infectious agent yet is critical to the diagnosis, the complaint that "my family no longer loves me" does not reveal the specific problems in the family yet does highlight the need to assess the potential of that family for providing care and support for the older adult (Blazer 1984). Determination of the nature of the family structure in interaction, the presence or absence of a crisis in the family, and the type and amount of support available to the older adult are the basic goals of a comprehensive diagnostic family workup.

The genogram detailing the distribution of illnesses across a family has already been described. A family tree review of individuals' roles in the family, as well as of members' availability to provide care to the older adult, is equally important. For clinical purposes, the family consists not only of individuals genetically related but also of those who have developed relationships and are living together as if they were related (Miller and Miller 1979). Many older adults, especially those who have been widowed, have close friendships that are virtually familial.

A primary goal of the clinician, as advocate for the psychiatrically disturbed older adult, is to facilitate family support for the elder during a time of disability. At least four parameters of support are important for the clinician to evaluate as the treatment plan evolves. These are 1) availability of family members to the older person over time; 2) the tangible services provided by the family to the disturbed older person;

3) the perception of family support by the older patient (and therefore the willingness of the patient to cooperate and accept support); and 4) tolerance by the family of specific behaviors that derive from the psychiatric disorder.

The clinician should ask the older person, "If you become ill, is there a family member who will take care of you for a short period of time?" Next, the availability of family members who can care for the older adult over an extended period can be determined. If a particular member is designated as the primary caregiver, plans for respite care should be discussed. Given the increased focus on short hospital stays and the documented higher levels of impairment on discharge, the availability of family members becomes essential to the effective care of the older adult after hospitalization for a psychiatric, or combined medical and psychiatric, disorder.

What specific, tangible services can be provided to the older adult by family members? Even the most devoted spouse can be limited in the delivery of certain services because he or she may not drive a car, and therefore cannot provide transportation, or is not physically strong enough to provide certain types of nursing care. Generic services of special importance in the support of the psychiatrically impaired older adult at home include transportation; nursing services (such as administering medications at home); physical therapy; checking on or continuous supervision of the patient; homemaker and household services; meal preparation; administrative, legal, and protective services; financial assistance; living quarters; and coordination of the delivery of services. These services have been termed generic because they can be defined in terms of their activities, regardless of who provides the service. Assessing the range and extent of service delivery by the family to the functionally impaired older person provides a convenient barometer of the economic, social, and emotional burdens placed on the family.

Regardless of the level of service provided by the family to the older person, if these services are to be effective, it is beneficial for the older person to perceive that he or she lives in a supportive environment. These intangible supports include the perception of a dependable network, participation or interaction in the network, a sense of belonging to the network, intimacy with network members, and a sense of usefulness to the family (Blazer and Kaplan 1983).

Family tolerance of specific behaviors may not correlate with overall support. Every person has a level of tolerance for specific behaviors that are especially difficult. Sanford (1975) found that the following behaviors were tolerated by families of impaired older persons (in decreasing percentages): incontinence of urine (81%), personality conflicts (54%), falls (52%), physically aggressive behavior (44%), inability to walk unaided (33%), daytime wandering (33%), and sleep disturbance (16%). This frequency may appear counterintuitive, for incontinence is generally considered particularly aversive to family members. Yet the outcome of incontinence can be corrected easily enough. A few nights of no sleep, however, can easily extend family members beyond their capabilities for serving a parent, sibling, or spouse.

Mental Status Examination

Physicians and other clinicians are at times hesitant to perform a structured mental status examination, fearing the effort will insult or irritate the patient or that the patients will view it as an unnecessary waste of time. Nevertheless, the mental status examination of the psychiatric patient in later life is central to the diagnostic workup.

Appearance may be determined by the psychiatric symptoms of the older person (e.g., the depressed patient may neglect grooming), cognitive status (e.g., the patient with dementia may not be able to match clothes or even put on clothes appropriately) and the environment of the patient (e.g., a nursing home patient may not be groomed as well as a patient living at home with a spouse).

Affect and mood can usually be assessed by observing the patient during the interview. Affect is the feeling tone that accompanies the patient's cognitive output (Linn 1980). Affect may fluctuate during the interview; however, the older person is more likely to demonstrate a constriction of affect. Mood, the state that underlies overt affect and is sustained over time, is usually apparent by the end of the interview. For example, the affect of a depressed older adult may not reach the degree of dysphoria seen in younger persons (as evidenced by crying spells or protestations of uncontrollable despair), yet the depressed mood is usually sustained and discernible from beginning to end.

Psychomotor activity may be agitated or retarded. Psychomotor retardation or underactivity is characteristic of major depression and severe schizophreniform symptoms, as well as of some variants of primary degenerative dementia. Psychiatrically impaired older persons, except some who have advanced dementia, are more likely to exhibit hyperactivity or agitation. Those who are depressed will appear uneasy, move their hands frequently, and have difficulty remaining seated through the interview. Patients with mild to moderate dementia, especially those with vascular dementia, will be easily distracted, rise from a seated position, and/or walk around the room or even out of the room. Pacing is often observed when the older adult is admitted to a hospital ward. Agitation can usually be distinguished from anxiety, for the agitated individual does not complain of a sense of impending doom or dread. In patients with psychomotor dysfunction, movement generally relieves the immediate discomfort, although it does not correct the underlying disturbance. Occasionally the older adult with motor retardation may actually be experiencing a disturbance in consciousness and may even reach an almost stuporous state. The patient may not be easily aroused, but when aroused, he or she will respond by grimacing or withdrawal.

Perception is the awareness of objects in relation to each other and follows stimulation of peripheral sense organs (Linn 1980). Disturbances of perception include hallucinations—that is, false sensory perceptions not associated with real or external stimuli. For example, a paranoid older person may perceive invasion of his or her house at night by individuals who disarrange belongings and abuse him or her sexually. Hallucinations often take the form of false auditory perceptions, false perceptions of movement or body sensation (such as palpitations), and false perceptions of smell, taste, and touch. The severely depressed older patient may have frank auditory hallucinations that condemn or encourage self-destructive behavior.

Disturbances in thought content are the most common disturbances of cognition noted in the psychotic older patient. The depressed patient often develops beliefs that are inconsistent with the objective information obtained from family members about the patient's abilities and social resources. Even after elderly persons recover from depression, they may still experience periodic recurrences of delusional thoughts, which can be most disturbing to an otherwise rational older adult. Older patients appear less likely to experience delusional remorse, guilt, or persecution.

Even if delusions are not obvious, preoccupation with a particular thought or idea is common among depressed elderly persons. Such preoccupation is closely associated with obsessional thinking or irresistible intrusion of thoughts into the conscious mind. Although the older adult rarely acts on these thoughts compulsively, the guilt-provoking or self-accusing thoughts may occasionally become so difficult to bear that the person considers, attempts, or succeeds in committing suicide.

Disturbances of thought progression accompany disturbances of content. Evaluation of the content and process of cognition may uncover disturbances such as problems with the structure of associations, the speed of associations, and the content of thought. Thinking is a goal-directed flow of ideas, symbols, and associations initiated in response to environmental stimuli, a perceived problem, or a task that requires progression to a logical or reality-based conclusion (Linn 1980). The compulsive or schizophrenic older adult may pathologically repeat the same word or idea in response to a variety of probes, as may the patient who has primary degenerative dementia. Some older adults with dementia exhibit circumstantiality—that is, the introduction of many apparently irrelevant details to cover a lack of clarity and memory problems. Interviews with patients who have this problem can be most frustrating because they proceed at such a slow pace. On other occasions, elderly patients may appear incoherent, with no logical connection to their thoughts, or they may produce irrelevant answers. The intrusion of thoughts from previous conversations into current conversation is a prime example of the disturbance in association found in patients with primary degenerative dementia (for example, Alzheimer's disease). This symptom is not typical of other dementias, such as the dementia of Huntington's disease. However, in the absence of dementia, even paranoid older adults do not generally demonstrate a significant disturbance in the structure of associations.

Suicidal thoughts are critical to the assessment of the psychiatrically impaired elderly patient. Although thoughts of death are common in late life, spontaneous revelations of suicidal thoughts are rare. A stepwise probe is the best means of assessing the presence of suicidal ideation (Blazer 1982). First, the clinician should ask the patient if he or she has ever thought that life was not worth living. If so, has the patient considered acting on that thought? If so, how would the patient attempt to inflict such harm? If definite plans are revealed, the clinician should probe to determine whether the implements for a suicide attempt are available. For example, if a patient has considered shooting himself, the clinician should ask, "Do you have a gun available and loaded at home?" Suicidal ideation in an older adult is always of concern, but intervention is necessary when suicide has been considered seriously and the implements are available.

Assessment of memory and cognitive status is most accurately performed through psychological testing. However, the psychiatric interview of the older adult must include a reasonable assessment. Although older adults may not complain of memory dysfunction, they are more likely than younger patients to have problems with memory, concentration, and intellect. There are brief, informal means of testing cognitive functioning that should be included in the diagnostic workup. The clinician proceeding through an evaluation of memory and intellect must also remember that poor performance may reflect psychic distress or a lack of education, as opposed to mental retardation or dementia. In addition, to rule out the potential confounding of agitation and anxiety, testing can be performed on more than one occasion.

Testing of memory is based on three essential processes: 1) registration (the ability to record an experience in the central nervous system); 2) retention (the persistence and permanence of a registered experience); and 3) recall (the ability to summon consciously the registered experience and report it) (Linn 1980). *Registration*, apart from recall, is difficult to evaluate directly. Occasionally, events or information that the older adult denies remembering will appear spontaneously during other parts of the interview. Registration usually is not impaired except in patients with one of the more severely dementing illnesses.

Retention, on the other hand, can be blocked by both psychic distress and brain dysfunction. Lack of retention is especially relevant to the unimportant data often asked for on a mental status examination. For example, requesting the older adult to remember three objects for 5 minutes will frequently reveal a deficit if the older adult has little motivation to attempt the task. Disturbances of recall can be tested directly in a number of ways. The most common are *tests of orientation* to time, place, person, and situation. Most persons continually orient themselves through radio, television, and reading material, as well as through conversations with others. Some elderly persons may be isolated through sensory impairment or lack of social contact; poor orientation in these patients may represent deficits in the physical and social environment rather than brain dysfunction. *Immediate recall* can be tested by asking the older person to repeat a word, phrase, or series of numbers, but it can also be tested in conjunction with cognitive skills by requesting that a word be spelled backward or that elements of a story be recalled.

During the mental status examination, intelligence can be assessed only superficially. Tests of simple arithmetic calculation and fund of knowledge, supplemented by portions of well-known psychiatric tests, are helpful. The classic test for calculation is to ask a patient to subtract 7 from 100 and to repeat this operation on the succession of remainders. Usually five calculations are sufficient to determine the ability of the older adult to complete this task. If the older adult fails the task, a less exacting test is to request the patient to subtract 3 from 20 and to repeat this operation on the succession of remainders until 0 is reached. These examinations must not be rushed, for older persons may not perform as well when they perceive time pressure. A capacity for *abstract thinking* is often tested by asking the patient to interpret a well-known proverb, such as "A rolling stone gathers no moss." A more accurate test of abstraction, however, is classifying objects in a common category. For example, the elder is asked to state the similarity between an apple and a pear. Whereas naming objects from a category (such as fruits) is retained despite moderate and sometimes marked declines in cognition, the opposite process of classifying two different objects in a common category is not retained as well.

Rating Scales and Standardized Interviews

Rating scales and standardized or structured interviews have progressively been incorporated into the diagnostic assessment of the elderly psychiatric patient. Such rating procedures have increased in popularity as the need has increased for systematic, reproducible diagnoses for third-party carriers (part of the impetus for the dramatic change in nomenclature evidenced in DSM-IV) and for a standard means of assessing change in clinical status. A thorough review in this chapter of all instruments that are used is not possible. Therefore, selected instruments are presented and evaluated in this section, chosen either because they have special relevance to the geriatric patient or because they are widely used.

Cognitive Dysfunction and Dementia Schedules

Two interviewer-administered cognitive screens for dementia have been popular in both clinical and community studies. The first is the Short Portable Mental Status Questionnaire (SPMSQ; Pfeiffer 1975), a derivative of the Mental Status Questionnaire developed by Kahn and colleagues (1960). The SPMSQ consists of 10 questions designed to assess orientation, memory, fund of knowledge, and calculation. For most community-dwelling older adults, two or fewer errors indicate intact functioning; three or four errors, mild impairment; five to seven errors, moderate impairment; and eight or more errors, severe impairment. The ease of administration of this instrument and its reliability as supported by accumulated epidemiological data make it useful for both clinical and community screens.

The Mini-Mental State Examination (Folstein et al. 1975) is a 30-item instrument that assesses orientation, registration, attention/calculation, recall, and language. It requires 5–10 minutes to administer and includes more items of clinical significance than does the SPMSQ. Seven to 12 errors suggest mild to moderate cognitive impairment and 13 or more errors severe impairment. This instrument is perhaps the most frequently used standardized screening instrument in clinical practice.

A more recent and comprehensive scale is the Alzheimer's Disease Assessment Scale (Rosen et al. 1984). This clinical rating scale includes ratings of spoken language, language comprehension, recall, ability to follow commands, word-finding difficulty in spontaneous speech, ability to name objects, constructional praxis, ideational praxis, orientation, word recall, word recognition, and a series of noncognitive behaviors, such as tearfulness, distractibility, depression, and motor activity.

A dementia scale for assessing the probability that dementia is secondary to multiple infarcts was suggested by Hachinski et al. (1975). In the study, cerebral blood flow in patients with primary degenerative dementia was compared with those who had multi-infarct dementia. Certain clinical features were determined to be more associated with multi-infarct dementia, and each of these features was assigned a score. Those clinical features, along with their scores, are as follows: abrupt onset = 2, stepwise deterioration = 1, fluctuating course = 2, nocturnal confusion = 1, relative preservation of personality = 1, depression = 1, somatic complaints = 1, emotional incontinence = 1, history of hypertension = 1, history of strokes = 2, evidence of associated atherosclerosis = 1, focal neurological symptoms = 2, and focal neurological signs = 2. A score of 7 or greater was highly suggestive of multi-infarct dementia. However, given the frequent overlap of multiple small infarcts and primary degenerative dementia, as well as the difficulty of assessing these items effectively, most investigators have ceased to rely on the Hachinski scale for clinical use.

Depression Rating Scales

A number of self-rating depression scales have been used to screen for depression in patients at all stages of the life cycle; most of these scales have been studied in older populations. The most widely used of the current instruments in community studies is the Center for Epidemiologic Studies Depression Scale (CES-D; Radloff 1977). This instrument, because of the normative population data available for it, has replaced the Zung scale in recent years as a common instrument for screening for depression. The CES-D scale is similar in format to the Zung scale. In a factor-analytic study of the CES-D in a community population, three factors were identified: enervation, positive affect, and interpersonal relationships (Ross and Mirowsky 1984). The disaggregation of these factors and the exploration of their interaction are significant steps forward in understanding the results derived from symptom scales such as the CES-D in older populations. For example, the enervation items (e.g., loss of interest, poor appetite) are more likely to be associated with a course of depressive episodes similar to that described for major depression with melancholia, and the positive-affect items more likely to be associated with life satisfaction scores.

A scale that has been widely used in clinical studies, although less studied in community populations, is the Beck Depression Inventory (BDI; Beck et al. 1961). The reliability of the BDI has been shown to be good in both depressed and nondepressed samples of older people (Gallagher et al. 1982). The instrument consists of 21 symptoms and attitudes, rated on a scale of 0 to 3 in terms of intensity. In another study by Gallagher et al. (1983), the BDI misclassified only 16.7% of subjects who had been diagnosed on the basis of Research Diagnostic Criteria (RDC; Spitzer et al. 1978) as having major depression.

The Geriatric Depression Scale (GDS) was developed because the scales discussed above present problems for older persons who have difficulty in selecting one of four forced-response items (Yesavage et al. 1983). The GDS is a 30-item scale that permits patients to rate items as either present or absent; it includes questions about symptoms such as cognitive complaints, self-image, and losses. Items selected were thought to have relevance to late-life depression. The GDS has not been used extensively in community populations and is not as well standardized as the CES-D, but its yes/no format is preferred to the CES-D by many clinicians.

Of the interviewer-rated scales, the Hamilton Rating Scale for Depression (Ham-D; Hamilton 1960) is by far the most commonly used. The advantage of having ratings based on clinical judgment has made the Ham-D a popular instrument for rating outcome in clinical trials. For example, a reduction in the score to one-half the initial score or to a score below a certain value would indicate partial or complete recovery from an episode of depression.

A scale that has received considerable attention clinically, standardized in clinical but not community populations, is the Montgomery-Åsberg Rating Scale for Depression (Montgomery and Åsberg 1979). This scale follows the pattern of the Hamilton scale and concentrates on 10 symptoms of depression; the clinician rates each symptom on a scale of 0 to 6 (for a range of scores between 0 and 60). The symptoms include apparent sadness, reported sadness, inattention, reduced sleep, reduced appetite, concentration difficulties, lassitude, inability to feel, pessimistic thoughts, and suicidal thoughts. This scale, theoretically, is an improvement over the Hamilton scale in that it appears to better differentiate between responders and nonresponders to intervention for depression. The instrument does not include many somatic symptoms that tend to be more common in older adults, and therefore it may be of greater value in tracking the symptoms of depressive illness that would be expected to change with therapy.

General Assessment Scales

A number of general assessment scales of psychiatric status (occasionally combined with functioning in other areas) have been found to be useful in both community and clinical populations.

One of the more frequently used scales is the Global Assessment of Functioning Scale (GAF; American Psychiatric Associa-tion 2000). Using this scale, the rater makes a single rating, ranging from 0 to 100, that best describes—on the basis of his or her clinical judgment—the lowest level of the subject's functioning in the week before the rating. The scale has not been standardized for older adults, but its common use in psychiatric studies suggests the need for standardization. The scale was incorporated as Axis V in DSM-IV to measure overall functioning.

The Geriatric Mental State Schedule (Copeland et al. 1976), an adaptation of the Present State Exam (PSE; Wing et al. 1974) and the Psychiatric Status Schedule (Spitzer et al. 1968), is a semistructured interviewing guide that allows the rater to inventory symptoms associated with psychiatric disorders. More than 500 ratings are made on the basis of information obtained by a highly trained interviewer, who elicits reports of symptoms from the month preceding the evaluation. Data are computerized to derive psychiatric diagnoses (Copeland et al. 1986). The instrument measures depression, impaired memory, selected neurological symptoms such as aphasia, and disorientation.

Any discussion of clinical rating scales is not complete without a discussion of the Abnormal Involuntary Movement Scale (AIMS; National Institute of Mental Health 1975). There has been an increased incidence of tardive dyskinesia among older adults, coupled with the need for better documentation of this dreaded outcome of prolonged use of antipsychotic agents. Regular rating of patients on the AIMS by clinicians has therefore become essential to the practice of inpatient and outpatient geriatric psychiatry. The scale consists of seven movement disorders; the presence and severity of each is rated from "none" to "severe." Three items require a global judgment: severity of abnormal movements, incapacitation due to abnormal movements, and the patient's awareness of abnormal movements. Current problems with teeth or dentures are also assessed. Procedures are described to increase the reliability of this rating scale.

Structured Diagnostic Interviews

A number of structured interview schedules are now available for both clinical and community diagnosis. These interview schedules have allowed increased reliability of the identification of particular symptoms and psychiatric diagnoses. Unfortunately, if one adheres closely to the structured interview, the richness inherent in the unstructured interview tends to be lost. Comments made by the patient during the evaluation that could be used to trace relevant associations must be ignored to push through the interview schedule. Most of these interviews require more time than the traditional unstructured first session with the patient.

The most frequently used instrument in the United States is the Structured Clinical Interview for DSM-IV (SCID; First et al. 1997). This instrument is easily adaptable to the RDC, DSM-IV, and DSM-IV-TR (American Psychiatric Association 1994, 2000). Although specific questions are suggested for probing most areas of interest, the interviewer using the SCID has the flexibility to ask additional questions and can use any available data to assign a diagnosis. The interviewer must have clinical training but does not have to be a psychiatrist. Many of the symptoms may not be relevant to older adults (especially the extensive probes for psychotic symptoms), and the interview frequently takes 2½–3 hours to administer. Nevertheless, the experience gained by the clinician in using this instrument can contribute to a more effective clinical practice.

A relatively recent addition to the schedules available is the Diagnostic Interview Schedule (DIS; Robins et al. 1981).

This highly structured, computer-scored interview, which can be administered by a lay interviewer, allows psychiatric diagnoses to be made according to DSM-IV criteria, Feighner criteria (Feighner et al. 1972), and RDC. The DIS questions probe for the presence or absence of symptoms or behaviors relevant to a series of psychiatric disorders, the severity of the symptoms, and the putative cause of the symptoms. Diagnoses of cognitive impairment, schizophrenia or schizophreniform disorder, major depression, generalized anxiety disorder, panic disorder, agoraphobia, obsessive-compulsive disorder, dysthymic disorder, somatization disorder, alcohol abuse and/or dependence, and other substance abuse and/or dependence can be made from Axis I of DSM-IV. A diagnosis of antisocial personality disorder (Axis II) can also be made. The instrument has proved reasonably reliable in clinic populations for both current and lifetime diagnoses.

The range of disorders probed by the DIS questions, coupled with the instrument's relative ease of administration (it generally takes 45–90 minutes to administer to an older adult), has made it popular for use in clinical studies. In addition, community-based comparative data are available on a large sample from the Epidemiologic Catchment Area study (Myers et al. 1984; Regier et al. 1984). The DIS can be supplemented with additional questions to probe for specific symptoms, such as melancholic symptoms and additional data on sleep disorders for depressed older adults. No problems have arisen when the instrument is used among older adults in the community. The memory decay that occurs in elderly persons in general is no more of a problem with this instrument than with others. Nevertheless, the DIS is of less value in the study of institutional populations and in reconstruction of lifetime history regardless of setting, because memory problems cannot be circumvented by clinical judgment. Supplementary data can be added to the instrument for developing a standardized diagnosis. A shortened version of the DIS, which has been used in recent epidemiological surveys, is the Composite International Diagnostic Interview (CIDI; World Health Organization 1989).

Effective Communication With the Older Adult

The clinician who works with the older adult should be cognizant of factors relating to both the patient and the clinician that may produce barriers to effective communication (Blazer 1978). Many older persons experience a relatively high level of anxiety yet do not complain of this symptom. Stress deriving from a new situation, such as visiting a clinician's office or being interviewed in a hospital, may intensify such anxiety and subsequently impair effective communication. Perceptual problems, such as hearing and visual impairment, may exacerbate disorientation and complicate the communication of problems to the clinician. Elderly persons are more likely to withhold information than to hazard answers that may be incorrect—in other words, older persons tend to be more cautious. Elderly persons frequently take longer to respond to inquiries and resist the clinician who attempts to rush through the history-taking interview.

The elderly patient may perceive the physician unrealistically, on the basis of previous life experiences (that is, transference may occur). Although the older patient will sometimes accept the role of child, viewing the physician as parent, the patient is initially more likely to view the clinician as the idealized child who can provide reciprocal care to the previously capable but now impaired parent. Splitting

between the physician and the children of the patient may subsequently occur. The clinician may perceive the older adult patient incorrectly because of fears of aging and death or because of previous negative experiences with his or her own parents. For a clinician to work effectively with older adults, these personal feelings should be discussed during training—and afterward.

Once physician and patient attitudes have been recognized and acknowledged, certain techniques have generally proved to be valuable in communicating with the elderly patient. These techniques should not be implemented indiscriminately, however, for the variation among the population of older adults is significant. First, the older person should be approached with respect. The clinician should knock before entering a patient's room and should greet the patient by surname (Mr. Jones, Mrs. Smith) rather than by a given name, unless the clinician also wishes to be addressed by a given name.

After taking a position near the older person—near enough to reach out and touch the patient—the clinician should speak clearly and slowly and use simple sentences in case the person's hearing is impaired. Because of hearing problems, older patients may understand conversation better over the telephone than in person. By placing the receiver against the mastoid bone, the patient with otosclerosis can take advantage of preserved bone conduction.

The interview should be paced so that the older person has enough time to respond to questions. Most elders are not uncomfortable with silence, because it gives them an opportunity to formulate their answers to questions and elaborate certain points they wish to emphasize. Nonverbal communication is frequently a key to effective communication with elderly persons, because they may be reticent about revealing affect verbally. The patient's changes in facial expression, gestures, postures, and long silences may provide clues to the clinician about issues that are unspoken.

One key to successful communication with an older adult is a willingness to continue working as a professional with that person. Older adults—possibly unlike some of their children and grandchildren—place a great deal of stress on loyalty and continuity. Most elderly patients do not require large amounts of time from clinicians, and those who are more demanding can usually be controlled through structure in the interview.

References

American Psychiatric Association: Diagnostic and Statistical Manual of Mental Disorders, 4th Edition. Washington, DC, American Psychiatric Association, 1994

American Psychiatric Association: Diagnostic and Statistical Manual of Mental Disorders, 4th Edition, Text Revision. Washington, DC, American Psychiatric Association, 2000

Beck AT, Ward CH, Mendelson M, et al: An inventory for measuring depression. Arch Gen Psychiatry 4:561–571, 1961

Blazer DG: Techniques for communicating with your elderly patient. Geriatrics 33:79–80, 83–84, 1978

Blazer DG: Depression in Late Life. St Louis, MO, CV Mosby, 1982

Blazer DG: Evaluating the family of the elderly patient, in A Family Approach to Health Care in the Elderly. Edited by Blazer D, Siegler IC. Menlo Park, CA, Addison-Wesley, 1984, pp 13–32

Blazer DG, Kaplan BH: The assessment of social support in an elderly community population. Am J Soc Psychiatry 3:29–36, 1983

Copeland JRM, Kelleher MJ, Kellet JM, et al: A semi-structured clinical interview for the assessment and diagnosis of mental state in the elderly: the Geriatric Mental State Schedule. Psychol Med 6:439–449, 1976

Copeland JRM, Dewey ME, Griffiths-Jones HM, et al: A computerized psychiatric diagnostic system and case nomenclature for elderly subjects: GMS and AGECAT. Psychol Med 16:89–99, 1986

Eisenberg L: Disease and illness: distinctions between professional and popular ideas of sickness. Cult Med Psychiatry 1:9–23, 1977

Eisenberg L, Kleinman A: Clinical social science, in The Relevance of Social Science for Medicine. Edited by Eisenberg L, Kleinman A. Boston, MA, D Reidel, 1981, pp 1–26

Feighner JP, Robins E, Guze SB, et al: Diagnostic criteria for use in psychiatric research. Arch Gen Psychiatry 26:57–63, 1972

First MB, Spitzer RL, Gibbon M: Structured Clinical Interview for DSM-IV. Washington, DC, American Psychiatric Press, 1997

Folstein MF, Folstein SE, McHugh PR: Mini-Mental State: a practical method for grading the cognitive state of patients for the clinician. J Psychiatr Res 12:189–198, 1975

Gallagher D, Nies G, Thompson LW: Reliability of the Beck Depression Inventory with older adults. J Consult Clin Psychol 50:152–153, 1982

Gallagher D, Breckenridge J, Steinmetz J, et al: The Beck Depression Inventory and Research Diagnostic Criteria: congruence in an older population. J Consult Clin Psychol 51:945–946, 1983

Hachinski VC, Iliff LD, Zilhka E, et al: Cerebral blood flow in dementia. Arch Neurol 32:632–637, 1975

Hamilton M: A rating scale for depression. J Neurol Neurosurg Psychiatry 23:56, 1960

Kahn RL, Goldfarb AI, Pollack M, et al: Brief objective measures for the determination of mental status in the aged. Am J Psychiatry 117:326–328, 1960

Linn L: Clinical manifestations of psychiatric disorders, in Comprehensive Textbook of Psychiatry, 3rd Edition, Vol 1. Edited by Kaplan HI, Freedman AM, Sadock BJ. Baltimore, MD, Williams & Wilkins, 1980, pp 990–1034

Mendlewicz J, Fleiss JL, Cataldo M, et al: Accuracy of the family history method in affective illness: comparison with direct interviews in family studies. Arch Gen Psychiatry 32:309–314, 1975

Miller KT, Miller JL: The family as a system. Paper presented at the annual meeting of the American College of Psychiatrists, New York, February 1979

Montgomery SA, Åsberg M: A new depression scale designed to be sensitive to change. Br J Psychiatry 134:382–389, 1979

Myers JK, Weissman MM, Tischler GL, et al: Six-month prevalence of psychiatric disorders in three communities: 1980 to 1982. Arch Gen Psychiatry 41:959–967, 1984

National Institute of Mental Health: Development of a Dyskinetic Movement Scale (Publ No 4). Rockville, MD, National Institute of Mental Health, Psychopharmacology Research Branch, 1975

Pfeiffer E: A Short Portable Mental Status Questionnaire for the assessment of organic brain deficit in elderly patients. J Am Geriatr Soc 23:433–441, 1975

Radloff LS: The CES-D Scale: a self-report depression scale for research in the general population. Applied Psychological Measurement 1:385–401, 1977

Regier DA, Myers JK, Kramer M, et al: The NIMH Epidemiologic Catchment Area program: historical context, major objectives, and study population characteristics. Arch Gen Psychiatry 41:934–941, 1984

Robins LN, Helzer JE, Croughan J, et al: National Institute of Mental Health Diagnostic Interview Schedule: its history, characteristics, and validity. Arch Gen Psychiatry 38:381–389, 1981

Rosen WG, Mohs RC, Davis KL: A new rating scale for Alzheimer's disease. Am J Psychiatry 141:1356–1362, 1984

Ross CE, Mirowsky J: Components of depressed mood in married men and women: the CES-D. Am J Epidemiol 119:997–1004, 1984

Sanford JRA: Tolerance of debility in elderly dependents by supporters at home: its significance for hospital practice. BMJ 3:471–473, 1975

Spitzer RL, Endicott J, Cohen GM: Psychiatric Status Schedule, 2nd Edition. New York, New York State Department of Mental Hygiene, Evaluation Unit, Biometrics Research, 1968

Spitzer RL, Endicott J, Robins E: Research Diagnostic Criteria: rationale and reliability. Arch Gen Psychiatry 35:773–782, 1978

Wing JK, Cooper JE, Sartorius N: The Measurement and Classification of Psychiatric Symptoms. London, Cambridge University Press, 1974

World Health Organization: Composite International Diagnostic Interview. Geneva, Switzerland, World Health Organization, 1989

Yesavage JA, Brink TL, Rose TL, et al: Development and validation of a geriatric depression screening scale: a preliminary report. J Psychiatr Res 17:37–49, 1983

Study Questions

Select the single best response for each question.

1. Medication history of the older adult
   A. Should involve having the older person bring in all pill bottles.
   B. Should involve a double check between the written schedule and pill containers.
   C. Should assess alcohol intake.
   D. Should assess substance abuse.
   E. All of the above.

2. Evaluation of the family of the psychiatrically ill older adult would include all of the following parameters of support *except*
   A. Availability of the family member.
   B. Tangible services provided by the family.
   C. Patient's perception of family support.
   D. Tolerance by the family of specific behaviors derived from the psychiatric disorder.
   E. Consideration of only those individuals genetically related to the patient.

3. A dementia scale for assessing the probability that dementia is secondary to multiple infarcts was suggested by Hachinski et al. (1975). Among the clinical features noted to be more associated with multi-infarct dementia were all of the following *except*
   A. Stepwise deterioration.
   B. Gradual onset.
   C. Fluctuating course.
   D. Focal neurological symptoms.
   E. Focal neurological signs.

4. Barriers to effective communication between the older patient and clinician can include
   A. Physician perceiving the older adult patient incorrectly because of personal fears of aging and death.
   B. The patient's perceptual problems.
   C. Patient taking longer to respond to inquiries, resisting the physician who attempts to hurry through the interview.
   D. Patient perceiving the physician unrealistically.
   E. All of the above.

CHAPTER 4

Use of the Laboratory in the Diagnostic Workup of Older Adults

Warren D. Taylor, M.D.

P. Murali Doraiswamy, M.D.

Laboratory testing is an essential component of the psychiatric evaluation in elderly individuals, who often present with comorbid medical illnesses. Laboratory testing—although it cannot replace the clinical history and physical examination—does aid in the evaluation of comorbidities that complicate or contribute to a psychiatric diagnosis. It may even assist in identifying medical problems that mimic psychiatric illnesses, such as hypothyroidism masquerading as depression. To best use the laboratory, the clinician must be aware of the indications for and limitations of such tests.

Serologic Tests

Basic clinical chemistry and hematologic screens are routine for all hospital admissions and many outpatient evaluations. Although the yield from these screens is low for identifying causes of psychiatric disorders such as anxiety or depression, the screens are critical to identifying previously undiagnosed or poorly controlled medical illnesses that may contribute to mental status changes. These screens are vital for the initial evaluation of dementia or delirium and should be considered in individuals with complicated medical histories. These tests should also be monitored when patients are taking medications that may result in dangerous abnormalities.

Hematologic Tests

A complete blood count (CBC) is a standard part of any evaluation. It screens for multiple problems, including infections and anemia. It also provides a platelet count, a value important to monitor in psychiatric medications associated with thrombocytopenia, such as divalproex sodium or carbamazepine. This concern is particularly important in elderly patients, because there is some evidence that the risk of drug-induced thrombocytopenia may increase with age (Trannel et al. 2001). Lithium, in contrast, may result in mild leukocytosis. Weekly or biweekly CBC testing is required for patients taking clozapine, because of the risk of agranulocytosis, and may be needed more frequently if the patient develops signs of infection.

Chemistry Tests

Most general chemistry panels have a variety of values that may be helpful in medical evaluations. Blood glucose values may reveal hyperinsulinemia and hypoglycemia, which may produce anxiety and weakness; more commonly it shows hyperglycemia, which may be associated with diabetes and result in lethargy, or in severe cases, delirium, diabetic coma, or ketoacidosis. It is critical for the diagnosis of diabetes, which can be diagnosed with 1) an overnight fasting glucose greater than 126 mg/dL, 2) a random plasma glucose greater than 200 mg/dL with symptoms of diabetes, or 3) an oral glucose tolerance test resulting in a plasma glucose greater than 200 mg/dL 2 hours after a 75-g glucose load (Dagogo-Jack 2001).

Kidney function tests are equally important. Blood urea nitrogen (BUN) and creatinine will be elevated in kidney failure and hypovolemic states such as dehydration. These tests also must be performed before initiating lithium therapy because of lithium's potential for nephrotoxicity. General chemistry panels also measure serum sodium and potassium. Hyponatremia is reported with selective serotonin reuptake inhibitors (SSRIs). Potassium disorders may rarely cause psychiatric symptoms and result in severe cardiac arrhythmias. Although calcium and magnesium levels are not always included in routine chemistry screens, it is also worthwhile to check these levels, because abnormal levels may result in paranoid ideation or frank psychosis.

Serologic Tests for Syphilis

Syphilis should be considered in any case of new-onset psychosis; the patient's being elderly does not exclude this disease from the differential. The Venereal Disease Research Laboratory (VDRL) and the rapid plasmin reagin (RPR) tests are screening tools for infection with *Treponema pallidum*, the cause of syphilis. These tests are unfortunately nonspecific; false-positive results may occur in acute infections and chronic illnesses such as systemic lupus erythematosus. More specific tests, the fluorescent treponemal antibody (FTA) and the microhemagglutination–*Treponema pallidum* (MHA-TP) may distinguish false-positive from true-positive results and may aid in diagnosing late syphilis when blood and even cerebrospinal fluid (CSF) reagin tests are negative.

HIV Testing

It is also important to consider testing for human immunodeficiency virus (HIV) infection. In 1996, the Centers for Disease Control and Prevention reported that 11% of all acquired immunodeficiency syndrome (AIDS) cases occurred in patients older than age 50 (Centers for Disease Control and Prevention 1998). The diagnosis of AIDS in elderly persons is complicated; the disease has been described as the great imitator because its clinical presentation, as with syphilis, may mimic that of other diseases (Sabin 1987). AIDS may mimic not only medical illnesses but also neuropsychiatric disorders, and AIDS may result in dementia. Investigators have identified several differences between AIDS-related dementia and Alzheimer's disease (see Table 4–1), but often the clinical distinction may be less clear.

TABLE 4–1. Differences between AIDS-related dementia and Alzheimer's disease

	AIDS-related dementia	Alzheimer's disease
Clinical presentation	Subcortical dementia preceded by subacute encephalitis	Cortical dementia; no preceding encephalitis
	Attention and concentration deficits common; aphasia and other cortical deficits uncommon	Attention and concentration deficits common; aphasia and other cortical deficits common
	Associated with physical complaints, including neuropathies, myelopathies, weight loss, and fatigue	Less commonly, directly associated with physical complaints
Progression	Rapid progression over months	Slower progression over years
Cerebrospinal fluid (CSF) analysis	Mild protein elevation	Not typically associated with CSF abnormalities
	May have mononuclear CSF pleocytosis	
Treatment	No evidence for cholinesterase inhibitors	Cholinesterase inhibitors may result in improvement
	Antiretroviral therapy may improve cognitive deficits	No role for antiretroviral therapy

Note. AIDS = acquired immunodeficiency syndrome; CSF = cerebrospinal fluid.
Source. Data summarized from multiple sources (Chiao et al. 1999; Sabin 1987; Wallace et al. 1993; Weiler et al. 1988).

The role of the geriatric psychiatrist is to assist the internist by screening for risk factors—such as a history of sexually transmitted diseases, intravenous drug use, risky sexual behavior, or a history of blood transfusions. We recommend HIV testing in individuals with these risk factors or those who present with atypical neuropsychiatric symptoms. For patients for whom testing is warranted, the geriatric psychiatrist will also play an important role in counseling the patient about the testing and its results.

Thyroid Function Tests

A serum TSH (thyroid-stimulating hormone) test is most commonly used as a screen for thyroid disease; it is an excellent screening test because of its high negative predictive value (Klee and Hay 1997). However, an abnormal TSH does not definitively diagnose thyroid disease; a physical examination and measurement of T_4, T_3, and thyroxine-binding globulin are required for a diagnosis. Many medications may result in increased TSH levels (amiodarone, estrogens) or decreased TSH levels (glucocorticoids, phenytoin) (Kaplan 1999). Abnormal levels of T_4 or T_3 may result in psychological symptoms mimicking depression (low energy, fatigue) in hypothyroidism, and mimicking anxiety disorders or even psychosis in hyperthyroidism.

Vitamin B_{12}, Folate, and Homocysteine

The prevalence of B_{12} deficiency increases with age and may have various clinical signs, including macrocytic anemia and neuropathy. Unfortunately, these clinical presentations are unreliable, because only a minority of individuals exhibit these manifestations.

B_{12} and folate deficiencies may result in neuropsychiatric disturbances, including depression, psychosis, and cognitive deficits. In dementia, B_{12} deficiencies often result in delirium or disorientation (Carmel et al. 1995). Deficits may also result in specific neuropsychological problems, including visuospatial and word fluency deficits (Wahlin et al. 2001) and even greater behavioral disturbances than are standard in patients with Alzheimer's disease (Meins et al. 2000). Supplementation may result in mild improvements in memory function and processing speed, particularly in individuals with mild to moderate levels of cognitive impairment, but individuals with severe dementia are unlikely to demonstrate significant cognitive improvement.

Serum homocysteine levels may serve as a functional indicator of B_{12} and folate status (Selhub et al. 2000), because vitamin B_{12} is needed to convert homocysteine to methionine in one-carbon metabolism in brain tissue. Hyperhomocystinemia is prevalent in elderly persons, and high serum levels of homocysteine can be attributed to an inadequate supply of B_{12} and folate, even in the presence of low normal serum levels (Selhub et al. 2000). Hyperhomocystinemia is also associated with cognitive dysfunction (Leblhuber et al. 2000; Selhub et al. 2000). Vitamin replacement can reduce plasma homocysteine levels and may also produce improvement in individuals with mild cognitive dysfunction, although individuals with severe dementia may show little improvement (Nilsson et al. 2000). Because hyperhomocystinemia may occur even in individuals with low normal serum B_{12} levels, it is worthwhile to check for this complication and if present to treat with vitamin B_{12}.

Toxicology

When there is an acute change in an individual's mental status, an investigation of the cause of the change must include ingestion

TABLE 4–2. Common electrocardiographic changes associated with psychotropic medications

Medication	Electrocardiographic change
Antipsychotics (typical or atypical agents)	Increased QTc interval Potential for torsades de pointes
Beta-blockers	Bradycardia
Lithium	Sick sinus syndrome Sinoatrial block
Tricyclic antidepressants	Increased PR, QRS, or QT interval AV block

of a substance. In circumstances when an individual is taking medications such as lithium, phenytoin, tricyclic antidepressants, or any medication that requires monitoring of blood levels, those levels should be checked. Toxic levels of many pharmacologic agents may cause a variety of psychiatric or life-threatening medical conditions. Likewise, levels for common over-the-counter medications such as acetaminophen and salicylates are available. Concomitantly, a serum alcohol level should also be drawn. Depending on the individual's history, even a negative result may be critical if there is the possibility of withdrawal. Finally, urine tests can show prescription medications, such as benzodiazepines, barbiturates, and opioids, and can also test for illicit substances such as cocaine and marijuana. Advanced age does not preclude addiction.

Urinalysis

Urinalysis is an inexpensive, noninvasive test that provides a large amount of information. It determines the urine's specific gravity, which may indicate dehydration, and also tests for glucose and ketones, important in the evaluation of diabetic patients.

Identification of a urinary tract infection (UTI) is critical in the elderly population, particularly in those with dementia.

Approximately 20% of the persons admitted from the community to a geropsychiatry unit may have a UTI, and in many cases it may result in a delirium; however, the condition improves with appropriate antibiotic treatment (Manepalli et al. 1990). Timely identification and treatment can improve outcomes and shorten or avoid hospitalizations.

Electrocardiography

In psychiatry, the most important roles of the electrocardiogram (ECG) include screening for cardiovascular disease that may preclude the use of specific medications and monitoring for drug-induced electrocardiographic changes, either from standard doses or from overdose. Electrocardiographic changes associated with specific psychotropic medications are summarized in Table 4–2.

The tricyclic antidepressants (TCAs) are well known to be cardiotoxic in overdose; even at therapeutic doses, their use is considered unsafe in patients with cardiovascular disease, particularly ischemic disease (Roose 2000). Although the most common cardiovascular complication of TCAs is orthostatic hypotension (Glassman and Bigger 1981), TCAs have the same pharmacologic properties as type IA antiarrhythmics (such as quinidine and procainamide). TCAs slow conduction at the bundle of His; individuals with preexisting bundle branch block who take TCAs are at increased risk for AV block. Even therapeutic levels are associated with prolonged PR intervals and QRS complexes; these results may be more pronounced in elderly individuals as the incidence and severity of adverse drug reactions increase with age (Pollock 1999). These results may be more pronounced in elderly individuals as the incidence and severity of adverse drug reactions increase with age (Pollock 1999). If TCAs are used, baseline and frequent follow-up ECGs should be obtained.

Lithium may also result in electrocardiographic changes, and along with evaluations of thyroid and renal function, an ECG is recommended before the patient begins taking lithium and regularly while taking it. Lithium appears to most affect the sinus node, and even at therapeutic levels it may result in sick sinus syndrome or sinoatrial block, either of which may occur early or later in treatment. At higher levels, there have been reports of sinus arrest and asystole.

Antipsychotics also result in electrocardiographic changes; about 25% of individuals receiving antipsychotics exhibit ECG abnormalities (Thomas 1994). Although many of these changes have historically been considered benign, there is increased concern that prolongation of the QT interval (when corrected for heart rate, the QTc interval) may contribute to potentially fatal ventricular arrhythmias, particularly torsades de pointes. It is important to note that other medications also affect the QTc interval and produce an additive effect when combined with an antipsychotic. Routine ECGs for all patients receiving antipsychotics are not currently recommended, but it is wise to be prudent. A careful history of cardiac illness, family history, and syncope should be obtained for all patients. ECGs should be considered more carefully in older individuals, particularly those with a history of cardiac illness and those receiving other medications that may affect the QTc interval.

The last consideration is medication overdose. With few exceptions, an ECG should always be obtained, even in cases where the medication used is not associated with arrhythmias. Obtaining an ECG is a reasonable choice because ECGs are easy to perform, noninvasive, and relatively inexpensive. ECGs are also important because some medications may affect heart rhythm in overdose when they would not do so at usual doses. Finally, it is not uncommon that suicidal patients do not report all the medications that they have used to overdose: suicide attempts may be impulsive, and patients who have an altered mental status may be unable to provide a complete report.

Imaging Studies

Plain film radiographs remain an integral piece of the diagnostic imaging performed today in geriatric psychiatry. Such techniques are most commonly used to detect 1) lung pathology that may contribute to mental status changes and 2) bone fractures. Plain film radiographs are critical for individuals who have both severe dementia and either a recent history of falls or newly developed limb immobility.

This section does not discuss functional imaging techniques—those such as positron emission tomography (PET) and single photon emission computed tomography (SPECT) that play a role in examining brain metabolic rates or regional blood flow. At present, these imaging procedures have a limited clinical use and are primarily for research. PET imaging may prove to have a role in the clinical evaluation of dementia (Silverman et al. 2001), but it is still premature to recommend this modality for routine clinical practice.

Computed Tomography

CT, originally called computerized axial tomography (CAT), was introduced into clinical practice as "the ultimate X ray" in the 1970s. *CT* is a general term for several radiographic techniques resulting in the computer-assisted generation of a series of images showing slices of an organ or body region, such as the brain or the abdomen.

When used to examine brain structure, CT can allow for the ready identification of many structures, although it does have limitations. By measuring differences in density, it can distinguish among CSF, blood, bone, gray matter, and white matter. The test is particularly useful for demonstrating bone abnormalities (such as skull fractures), areas of hemorrhage (such as a subdural hematoma), and the mass effect of various lesions. It can also display atrophy or ventricular enlargement. However, because of surrounding bone, the test does not well visualize posterior fossa or brain stem structures.

Magnetic Resonance Imaging

Whereas CT scanners rely on radiation, the MRI scanner creates a magnetic field that is 3,000–25,000 times the strength of the earth's natural magnetic field. The underlying principle behind MRI is that the nuclei of endogenous identifiable isotopes (such as hydrogen or phosphorus) behave like tiny spinning magnets. Strong magnetic fields alter this behavior, and an MRI scanner can identify the resultant change.

MRI has advantages and disadvantages compared with CT imaging. It produces higher-resolution images and can obtain good detail in regions that are poorly visualized on CT, such as the posterior fossa. Additionally, no radiation is involved. Un-

fortunately, the procedure is more grueling than CT: the patient must remain motionless for a longer period of time in a smaller, enclosed space. This requirement may be difficult for claustrophobic individuals. Moreover, MRI tends to be more costly than CT imaging in most institutions.

In the psychiatric workup of a geriatric patient, MRI should be considered for patients in whom the clinician suspects small lesions in regions difficult to visualize or for patients with demyelinating diseases such as multiple sclerosis. MRI can easily identify pathology in vascular dementia, although the findings in other types of dementia are less specific. Currently, the routine use of brain MRI in these patients is questionable, because findings are unlikely to affect treatment.

Electroencephalography

Electroencephalography is a technique in which scalp electrodes allow the measurement of cortical electrical activity. A skilled reader can interpret the waveforms on an electroencephalogram (EEG) to identify the presence of epileptic activity, the slowing of electrical activity, or a patient's sleep stage. It is most useful in a psychiatric evaluation of individuals with known or suspected seizure disorders. A history of brain injury or trauma with mental status changes or psychosis may be a particularly important indication for an electroencephalographic evaluation. Certain types of epilepsy, specifically temporal lobe epilepsy, are also associated with psychotic or manic symptoms.

For indications other than these, the use of EEGs in the psychiatric evaluation of elderly patients is limited. Electroencephalographic changes occur in both delirium and dementia, but these changes are not specific to a given diagnosis. In delirium, except that caused by alcohol or sedative-hypnotic withdrawal, electroencephalographic testing typically displays slowing of the posterior dominant rhythm and increased generalized slow-wave activity (Jacobson and Jerrier 2000). Electroencephalography has limited clinical use in this area because the diagnosis of delirium is typically made clinically, increased slow-wave activity is seen in other disorders, and the EEG provides minimal information about the causes of delirium.

Likewise, there are electroencephalographic changes in dementia; Alzheimer's disease results in multiple changes in electroencephalographic parameters, and the degree of change is correlated with cognitive impairment (Kowalski et al. 2001). Various treatments, including cholinesterase inhibitors, may mitigate electroencephalographic changes in individuals with mild dementia (Kogan et al. 2001). This finding is not universal; there are also reports that worsening of the EEG does not always parallel clinical deterioration. Despite this, electroencephalography has limited clinical utility in most dementing syndromes.

The exception may occur when Creutzfeldt-Jakob disease is a consideration in the differential diagnosis. Creutzfeldt-Jakob disease is a rare, rapidly progressive prion disease characterized by dementia and neurologic signs that may include gait disturbances and myoclonus. Electroencephalography may play an important role in diagnosing this disease: periodic sharp-wave complexes are strongly associated with Creutzfeldt-Jakob disease, with a sensitivity of 67% and a specificity of 86% (Steinhoff et al. 1996). However, although electroencephalography is an important diagnostic tool when considering Creutzfeldt-Jakob disease, it is important to remember that periodic sharp-wave complexes may also occur in Alzheimer's disease and dementia with Lewy bodies (Tschampa et al. 2001).

Polysomnography

Sleep disorders are a common problem in elderly persons. Although sleep disturbances are most often associated with psychiatric disorders such as dementia, delirium, and depression, the disturbances can exist without any other obvious psychiatric diagnoses. The polysomnogram is an all-night procedure, and the full evaluation may require more than one night. It monitors cerebral and somatic functioning and has proved reliable and sensitive for recording the stages of sleep and concomitant physiological functioning. It incorporates three basic variables: the sleep EEG, the electro-oculogram (which measures eye motion), and the electromyogram (which measures air exchange and respiratory effort). Additional monitoring used in specific investigations includes hemoglobin oxygen saturation using pulse oximetry, an ECG, and electrodes placed over the anterior tibialis muscles to measure leg movement. Video recording of sleep behaviors and monitoring of penile tumescence may also be available.

The polysomnogram, although essential for the evaluation of sleep disorders, is less useful in depression and dementia. These disorders do result in polysomnographic changes, but the polysomnogram contributes little toward an appropriate diagnosis or treatment decision. The polysomnogram should be reserved for patients in whom a specific sleep disorder is suspected or patients who have unexplained sleep disturbances in the absence of a primary psychiatric illness.

Genetic Testing

Genetic testing is at the forefront of a new wave of available laboratory tests. Research is currently investigating the genetic basis behind such diverse neuropsychiatric illnesses as dementia, narcolepsy, schizophrenia, and substance addiction. Similar research has already had success in Huntington's disease, an autosomal dominant disorder caused by a trinucleotide repeat; testing for the length of this repeat can predict whether an individual is susceptible to the illness.

APOE Testing

Extensive research has attempted to identify genetic markers for Alzheimer's disease. Mutations on chromosomes 1, 14, and 21 have been linked to rare forms of early-onset familial Alzheimer's disease; such findings may help counsel families in making decisions about pregnancies (Verlinsky et al. 2002). One of the most studied genes for Alzheimer's disease is *APOE*. This gene encodes for an astrocyte-secreted plasma protein that is involved in cholesterol transport. Apolipoprotein E may also play a role in the regeneration of injured nerve tissue. There are three possible alleles (ε2, ε3, ε4) of the *APOE* gene that may be combined heterozygously (ε2/ε3, ε2/ε4, ε3/ε4) or homozygously (ε2/ε2, ε3/ε3, ε4/ε4).

Multiple epidemiological studies have documented that the presence of the ε4 allele is a risk factor for Alzheimer's disease (Roses 1997). Additionally, the presence of ε4 alleles increases the specificity of the diagnosis of Alzheimer's disease. Despite these associations, the presence of an ε4 allele, even a homozygous ε4/ε4 genotype, is not diagnostic for Alzheimer's disease. Other causes of dementia would have to be explored as clinically indicated. *APOE* testing is not currently recommended to predict dementia risk in asymptomatic individuals.

Arguments against routine testing are lack of an effective treatment that modifies the disease course and lack of evidence

that *APOE* status may influence current supportive treatments. Current treatments for cognitive dysfunction are limited to cholinesterase inhibitors, but response to these drugs is not dependent on *APOE* status. Although some evidence suggested that tacrine may be better for individuals who lack the ε4 allele than for those who have the ε4 allele (Farlow et al. 1998; Poirier et al. 1995; Sjogren et al. 2001), other studies using both tacrine and galantamine did not find such an association (Aerssens et al. 2001; McGowan et al. 1998; Raskind et al. 2000; Rigaud et al. 2000).

Ethical and Psychological Concerns

Genetic testing is more than a simple blood draw; its implications are farther ranging than the results of simple serum chemistry. Genetic testing is similar to HIV testing in that results may have significant psychological, social, and personal repercussions. For this reason, genetic testing should be considered only in the context of supportive counseling.

There has been considerable debate on the psychological repercussions of testing for Huntington's disease, because testing for this disorder has been available longer than for any other adult-onset genetic disease. Huntington's disease is therefore a useful model to consider. Testing can result in transient heightened anxiety and depression; in the long term, a positive test may result in hopelessness (Tibben et al. 1994). The test also has a significant impact on decisions to marry or bear children; although only the individual can decide how a test result may affect these decisions, he or she needs to be counseled about these considerations before taking the test.

There are also financial concerns, as the inappropriate release of genetic information could result in job loss or lack of insurability. Medical and life insurance in particular could be exceedingly difficult to obtain if insurance agencies had access to the information.

Genetic testing is another tool at our disposal, with much untapped potential. It also carries risks that are different from the risks associated with the other laboratory tests described in this chapter. As with the other procedures, clinicians must make sure that their patients or patients' families understand clearly not only the benefits but also the risks before they proceed.

References

Aerssens J, Raeymaekers P, Lilienfeld S, et al: apoE genotype: no influence on galantamine treatment efficacy nor on rate of cognitive decline in Alzheimer's disease. Dement Geriatr Cogn Disord 12:69–77, 2001

Carmel R, Gott PS, Waters CH, et al: The frequently low cobalamin levels in dementia usually signify treatable metabolic, neurologic and electrophysiologic abnormalities. Eur J Haematol 54:245–253, 1995

Centers for Disease Control and Prevention: AIDS among persons aged >50 years—United States, 1991–1996. MMWR Morb Mortal Wkly Rep 47:21–27, 1998

Chiao EY, Ries KM, Sande MA: AIDS and the elderly. Clin Infect Dis 28:740–745, 1999

Dagogo-Jack S: Diabetes mellitus and related disorders, in The Washington Manual of Medical Therapeutics. Edited by Ahya SN, Flood K, Paranjothi S. Philadelphia, Lippincott Williams & Wilkins, 2001, p 455

Farlow MR, Lahiri DK, Poirier J, et al: Treatment outcome of tacrine therapy depends on apoliprotein genotype and gender of the subjects with Alzheimer's disease. Neurology 50:669–677, 1998

Glassman AH, Bigger JT: Cardiovascular effects of therapeutic doses of tricyclic antidepressants: a review. Arch Gen Psychiatry 38:815–820, 1981

Jacobson S, Jerrier H: EEG in delirium. Semin Clin Neuropsychiatry 5:86–92, 2000

Kaplan MM: Clinical perspectives in the diagnosis of thyroid disease. Clin Chem 45:1377–1383, 1999

Klee GG, Hay ID: Biochemical testing of thyroid function. Endocrinol Metab Clin North Am 26:763–775, 1997

Kogan EA, Korczyn A, Virchovsky R, et al: EEG changes during long-term treatment with donepezil in Alzheimer's disease patients. J Neural Transm 108:1167–1173, 2001

Kowalski JW, Gawel M, Pfeffer A, et al: The diagnostic value of EEG in Alzheimer disease: correlation with the severity of mental impairment. J Clin Neurophysiol 18:570–575, 2001

Leblhuber F, Walli J, Artner-Dworzak E, et al: Hyperhomocysteinemia in dementia. J Neural Transm 107:1469–1474, 2000

Manepalli J, Grossberg GT, Mueller C: Prevalence of delirium and urinary tract infection in a psychogeriatric unit. J Geriatr Psychiatry Neurol 3:198–202, 1990

McGowan SH, Wilcock GK, Scott M: Effect of gender and apolipoprotein E genotype on response to anticholinesterase therapy in Alzheimer's disease. Int J Geriatr Psychiatry 13:625–630, 1998

Meins W, Muller-Thomsen T, Meier-Baumgartner H-P: Subnormal serum vitamin B12 and behavioural and psychological symptoms in Alzheimer's disease. Int J Geriatr Psychiatry 15:415–418, 2000

Nilsson K, Gustafson L, Hultberg B: Improvement of cognitive functions after cobalamin/folate supplementation in elderly patients with dementia and elevated plasma homocysteine. Int J Geriatr Psychiatry 16:609–614, 2000

Poirier J, Delisle M-C, Quirion R, et al: Apolipoprotein E4 allele as a predictor of cholinergic deficits and treatment outcome in Alzheimer disease. Proc Natl Acad Sci USA 92:12260–12264, 1995

Pollock BG: Adverse reactions of antidepressants in elderly patients. J Clin Psychiatry 60:4–8, 1999

Raskind MA, Peskind ER, Wessel T, et al: Galantamine in AD: a 6-month randomized, placebo-controlled trial with a 6-month extension. Neurology 54:2261–2268, 2000

Rigaud AS, Traykov L, Caputo L, et al: The apolipoprotein E epsilon4 allele and response to tacrine therapy in Alzheimer's disease. Eur J Neurol 7:255–258, 2000

Roose SP: Considerations for use of antidepressants in patients with cardiovascular disease. Am Heart J 140 (suppl 4):S84–S88, 2000

Roses AD: A model for susceptibility polymorphisms for complex diseases: apolipoprotein E and Alzheimer disease. Neurogenetics 1:3–11, 1997

Sabin TD: AIDS: the new "great imitator." J Am Geriatr Soc 35:460–464, 1987

Selhub J, Bagley LC, Miller J, et al: B vitamins, homocysteine, and neurocognitive function in the elderly. Am J Clin Nutr 71 (suppl): 614S–620S, 2000

Silverman DH, Small GW, Chang CY, et al: Positron emission tomography in evaluation of dementia: regional brain metabolism and long-term outcome. JAMA 286: 2120–2127, 2001

Sjogren M, Hesse C, Basun H, et al: Tacrine and rate of progression in Alzheimer's disease—relation of ApoE allele genotype. J Neural Transm 108:451–458, 2001

Steinhoff BJ, Racker S, Herrendorf G, et al: Accuracy and reliability of periodic sharp wave complexes in Creutzfeldt-Jakob disease. Arch Neurol 53:162–166, 1996

Thomas SHL: Drugs, QT interval abnormalities, and ventricular arrhythmias. Adverse Drug React Toxicol Rev 13:77–102, 1994

Tibben A, Duivenvoorden HJ, Niermeijer MF, et al: Psychological effects of presymptomatic DNA testing for Huntington's disease in the Dutch program. Psychosom Med 56:526–532, 1994

Trannel TJ, Ahmed I, Goebert D: Occurrence of thrombocytopenia in psychiatric patients taking valproate. Am J Psychiatry 158:128–130, 2001

Tschampa HJ, Neumann M, Zerr I, et al: Patients with Alzheimer's disease and dementia with Lewy bodies mistaken for Creutzfeldt-Jakob disease. J Neurol Neurosurg Psychiatry 71:33–39, 2001

Verlinsky Y, Rechitsky S, Verlinsky O, et al: Preimplantation diagnosis for early onset Alzheimer disease caused by V717L mutation. JAMA 287:1018–1021, 2002

Wahlin T-BR, Wahlin A, Winblad B, et al: The influence of serum vitamin B12 and folate status on cognitive functioning in very old age. Biol Psychol 56:247–265, 2001

Wallace J, Paauw D, Spach D: HIV infection in older patients: when to expect the unexpected. Geriatrics 48:61–70, 1993

Weiler P, Mungas D, Pomerantz S: AIDS as a cause of dementia in the elderly. J Am Geriatr Soc 36:139–141, 1988

Study Questions

Select the single best response for each question.

1. Serum vitamin B_{12} and folate levels

   A. Are rarely important in the evaluation of the elderly patient.
   B. May point to etiologies of a range of neuropsychiatric disturbances.
   C. May produce microcytic anemia when levels are deficient.
   D. Are not related to hyperhomocysteinemia.
   E. Are not related to one-carbon metabolism in brain tissue.

2. Approximately what percentage of persons admitted from the community to a geropsychiatry unit may have a urinary tract infection that may result in a delirium?

   A. 10%.
   B. 20%.
   C. 35%.
   D. 45%.
   E. 55%.

3. Lithium is most likely to demonstrate which of the following ECG changes?

   A. AV block.
   B. Prolonged PR interval.
   C. Sick sinus syndrome.
   D. Bradycardia.
   E. QTc prolongation.

4. *APOE* testing has shown that

   A. A homozygous epsilon 4/epsilon 4 genotype is diagnostic for Alzheimer's disease.
   B. It is valuable in modifying the disease course and influencing current supportive treatments for Alzheimer's disease.
   C. It predicts response to cholinesterase inhibitors.
   D. It lacks hierarchy of the alleles for prediction or risk for development of Alzheimer's disease.
   E. None of the above.

5. Which of the following statements about genetic testing is *not* true? Genetic testing

   A. Results in transient heightened anxiety and depression.
   B. Can possibly result in hopelessness.
   C. Results in job loss or lack of insurability.
   D. Proves to be a valuable tool with untapped potential.
   E. Is recommended to predict dementia risk in asymptomatic individuals.

Neuropsychological Assessment of Dementia

Kathleen A. Welsh-Bohmer, Ph.D.

Deborah K. Attix, Ph.D.

Alzheimer's disease is by far the most common disorder of aging causing dementia. The disorder affects nearly 10% of the population over age 65 and is found to affect at least 25%–40% of individuals over age 85 (Breitner et al. 1999; Evans et al. 1991). Because of its slow and insidious onset, the early stages of the illness can be confused with relatively benign memory impairments that are associated with normal aging.

Neuropsychological assessment plays a central role in the diagnosis of early dementing disorders, such as mild cognitive impairment (Petersen et al. 2001) and in the differentiation among the many cognitive disorders that can interfere with functional ability and quality of life (Knopman et al. 2001). The neuropsychological assessment offers a sensitive, reliable, and noninvasive approach to early symptom verification as well as a potentially cost-effective means for managing patients with memory disorders (Welsh-Bohmer et al. 2003).

The goals of this chapter are 1) to describe the instances in which neuropsychological assessment can be most useful in geriatric settings, 2) to detail the neuro-

psychological examination process, and 3) to summarize the neurobehavioral presentations of common disorders in geriatric practice, specifically the profiles of various common dementias, normal aging, and depression.

Neuropsychological Assessment in Geriatric Settings

In geriatric practices, the neuropsychological evaluation is useful in four common situations, none of which are mutually exclusive. The first and by far the most frequent use of the evaluation is to assist in diagnosing a cognitive disorder. Specifically, the evaluation is used to verify the presence or absence of a cognitive syndrome (e.g., dementia) and to determine the likely differential diagnostic possibilities based on the behavioral profile (e.g., Alzheimer's disease vs. vascular dementia). Second, neuropsychological testing results are also commonly used as an objective baseline for tracking changes in mentation over time. These baselines are useful in clarifying diagnostic classifications of dementia due to Alzheimer's disease and similar disorders, in which the establishment of progression is essential. The neuropsychological examination in this context can also be used to monitor treatment response. A third common use is for guiding clinical care decisions, including the determination of functional capacities and competency (see Koltai and Welsh-Bohmer 2000 for review). Issues typically confronted by a geriatric evaluation are ability to live independently, financial capacity, medication management, and driving safety. Finally, the neuropsychological evaluation can be used to guide appropriate therapeutic interventions. On the basis of test results, identified cognitive strengths and weaknesses can be used for designing appropriate rehabilitation approaches, such as those involving compensatory strategies or psychotherapy (for a full discussion of this topic, see Attix and Welsh-Bohmer 2006).

The neuropsychological evaluation process itself can vary in form across clinical practices, depending in part on the populations typically served (e.g., Spanish speakers or native English speakers) and in part on the training emphasis of the neuropsychologist administering the examination. The approach can use a fixed battery or more flexible methods tailored to the referral issue. Regardless of the testing choices, there are standard features uniformly applied across neuropsychological settings to ensure that all testable areas of cognition are assessed (Lezak 1995). The evaluation typically begins with a diagnostic interview to identify the major referral issues and obvious symptoms. In this interview, a patient's orientation to situation, language, behavioral organization, memory, mood, and affect are observed in a naturalistic context. Family members are generally also interviewed separately, with the patient's consent, to determine changes in functional

ability and to clarify historical and medical information. In the formal testing session, 10 central domains of cognition and behavior are generally assessed: orientation, intelligence, memory, attention and concentration, higher executive functions, language, visuoperception and spatial abilities, sensory-motor integration, mood, and personality. The tests commonly used to assess these functional domains are listed in Table 5–1. From the battery of tests, a profile of performance can be constructed, examined in reference to normative standards, and interpreted relative to the established behavioral profiles of known neurobehavioral syndromes.

Simplifying the geriatric assessment is the availability of a number of neuropsychological batteries designed for use with elderly persons for which appropriate normative information has been obtained. Among these are the Mattis Dementia Rating Scale (Mattis et al. 2002) and the neuropsychological battery from the Consortium to Establish a Registry for Alzheimer's Disease (CERAD; Morris et al. 1989). Both are relatively brief and are sensitive to early stages of Alzheimer's disease dementia. Additionally, the tests offer presentation formats, such as the use of large print and an oral format, to minimize the influences of sensory confounding (Welsh-Bohmer and Mohs 1997).

It must be emphasized that the neuropsychological examination is not simply a process of actuarial comparisons to normative tables. The neuropsychological evaluation, like other forms of clinical diagnosis, rests on an inferential process. The diagnosis is an iterative process that incorporates multiple sources of information to arrive at diagnostic impressions (see Potter and Attix 2006). In assessing the geriatric patient, the psychologist must first determine the patient's likely premorbid ability in order to evaluate whether observed behaviors are newly acquired or re-

TABLE 5–1.   Common neuropsychological tests used in geriatric assessment

Domain	Tests commonly used	References
Orientation/global mental status	Temporal Orientation Test	Benton et al. 1964
	Mini-Mental State Exam	Folstein et al. 1975
	Alzheimer's Disease Assessment Scale—Cognitive (ADAS-COG)	Mohs and Cohen 1988
Intellect	Wechsler Adult Intelligence Scale, 3rd Edition (WAIS-III)	Wechsler 1997a
Language	Multilingual Aphasia Examination	Benton and Hamsher 1983
	Category Fluency	Spreen and Strauss 1996
	Boston Naming Test	Kaplan et al. 1978
Memory	Wechsler Memory Scale, 3rd Edition (WMS-III)	Wechsler 1997b
	California Verbal Learning Test–II	Delis et al. 1987
	Selective Reminding Test	Buschke and Fuld 1974
	Consortium to Establish a Registry for Alzheimer's Disease (CERAD) Word List Memory Test	Welsh-Bohmer and Mohs 1997
	Rey Auditory Verbal Learning Test	Ivnik et al. 1992
Attention/concentration	Subtests from the WMS-III and WAIS-III	Lezak 1995
Executive function	Trail Making Test	Reitan 1958
	Symbol Digit Modalities Test	Smith 1968
	Short Category Test	Wetzel and Boll 1987
	Wisconsin Card Sorting Test	Berg 1948
Visuoperception	Benton Facial Recognition Test	Benton et al. 1983
	Judgment of Line Orientation Test	Benton et al. 1981
	Tests of constructional praxis	Lezak 1995
Sensory-motor	Grooved Pegboard Test	Spreen and Strauss 1996
	Finger Oscillation	Heaton et al. 1991
Personality and mood	Minnesota Multiphasic Personality Inventory–2 (MMPI-2)	Butcher et al. 1989
	Geriatric Depression Scale	Yesavage et al. 1983
	Beck Depression Inventory–II	Beck et al. 1996

flect long-standing weaknesses. Once that determination has been made, the presence of cognitive impairment is determined in reference to appropriate normative values from similarly aged individuals with comparable education level or intellectual function (Steinberg and Bieliauskas 2005).

Consideration is given to any potential confounding influences on test performance, including patient motivation factors, extratest factors (such as interruptions), and other test behaviors that might interfere with optimal functioning (e.g., anxiety).

The interpretation of the likely medical and psychological contributions to the cognitive profile requires a good appreciation of brain-behavior organization. The neuropsychologist must consider whether the results make sense from a functional anatomical perspective and then analyze the profile to determine its conformity to known neurobehavioral syndromes, such as normal aging, mild cognitive impairment, Alzheimer's disease, and depression. Before final diagnostic determination, consideration is given to other attendant data such as medical history, ancillary studies (including imaging data), and informants' report of functional change. On the basis of the combined information, the designation of normal aging or early dementia can be more comfortably supported, leading to improved diagnostic accuracy (Tschanz et al. 2000). In the next sections of this chapter, we summarize the neuropsychology of normal aging and the differentiation of various forms of late-life dementia. We also consider in some detail the neuropsychology of geriatric depression and the contribution of mood disorders to the presentation of dementing disorders.

Neuropsychology of Normal Aging

By far the most common cause for cognitive change after age 50 is normal aging of the nervous system (Ebly et al. 1994). Compared with young adults, older individuals show selective losses in functions related to the speed and efficiency of information processing. Particularly vulnerable are memory retrieval abilities, attentional capacity, executive skills, and divergent thinking, such as working memory and multitasking (Cullum et al. 1990; Salthouse et al. 1996). On formal neuropsychological testing, memory measures involving delayed free recall are typically affected (Craik 1984), although not to the pronounced extent seen in Alz-

heimer's disease (Welsh et al. 1991). Unlike the patient with Alzheimer's disease, the older adult without the disease typically shows normal performance on other memory procedures, such as cued recall and delayed recognition. This profile of performance suggests that different mechanisms underlie the memory loss of aging and that of Alzheimer's disease. In Alzheimer's disease, the problem resides in the consolidation or storage of new information in long-term memory stores. In normal aging, the principal problem appears to be primarily in the efficient accessing of recently stored information. As such, procedures providing structural support for recall (e.g., recognition) facilitate the retrieval process. Besides memory problems, older adults without dementing disorders also show some decrements compared with younger cohorts on tests of visuoperceptual, visuospatial, and constructional functions (Eslinger et al. 1985; Howieson et al. 1993; Koss et al. 1991). These modest declines are evident on tests involving visual analysis and integration, such as the Block Design subtest of the Wechsler Adult Intelligence Scale, 3rd Edition (WAIS-III; Wechsler 1997a) and similar tests involving visual integration. Performance on measures of executive control (e.g., the Trail Making Test; Reitan 1958), language retrieval (verbal fluency), and divided attention (e.g., the Digit Span test from WAIS-III; Wechsler 1997a) also tend to be lower in older groups than in their younger counterparts (Salthouse et al. 1996).

A number of explanations for age-related cognitive change have been suggested, and none of these are mutually exclusive. All basically support the premise of a broad explanatory mechanism for age-related cognitive change rather than unique and specific changes in restricted cognitive domains. Speed of central processing has been one popular unifying notion, given that the majority of tasks affected in aging involve motor responses or reaction times (Salthouse 1985). Another explanation posits that the profile of cognitive change in normal aging is the result of a loss in "fluid" abilities, that is, skills that require novel problem solving and flexible thought (Botwinick 1977; Horn 1982). Well-rehearsed verbal abilities (so-called crystallized skills), by contrast, are less susceptible to age-associated change. More recent refinements of this hypothesis conceptualize normal aging as a selective vulnerability in frontal dysexecutive processes (Daigneault and Braun 1993; Mittenberg et al. 1989; Van Gorp et al. 1990). This notion is consistent with observed behavioral difficulties that suggest subtle impairments in integrative and retrieval functions and is also supported by neuroimaging (Coffey et al. 1992; Gur et al. 1987; Langley and Madden 2000) and histopathological findings (Haug et al. 1983) within the frontal-subcortical brain connections. However, although the frontal hypothesis is conceptually appealing and capable of explaining much of the changes observed with aging, other work suggests that the deficits may not be localizable in their entirety to a single brain system (Salthouse et al. 1996). To this end, a significant problem in the interpretation of any of the earlier studies is that many did not routinely screen for nervous system disorders or operationalize their criteria for normal aging. Work continues to identify the nature of the mechanisms that underlie age-related cognitive change and the association of these mechanisms with brain diseases common to aging, specifically Alzheimer's disease.

Differentiation of Alzheimer's Dementia From Normal Aging

Alzheimer's disease is the leading cause of dementia in elderly persons, accounting for nearly 50%–75% of all cases in Western countries (Ebly et al. 1995; Fratiglioni et al. 1999). The second most common cause of dementia, accounting for 15%–30% of cases, is vascular dementia, which includes disorders arising from either large- or small-vessel strokes (Lobo et al. 2000). Far less common are the frontal lobe disorders (Geldmacher and Whitehouse 1997), Lewy body dementia and related movement disorders of the basal ganglia, and rare illnesses such as hydrocephalus, metabolic disorders, and infectious dementias (Hanson et al. 1990; Holman et al. 1995; Savolainen et al. 1999).

The cognitive profiles of these various dementing disorders overlap to some extent, but there are unique features to many of them that can be of diagnostic utility (see Table 5-2 for a summary of these features).

The presentation of Alzheimer's disease dementia is dominated by a pronounced impairment in recent-memory processing, which remains the most affected area of mentation in the majority of cases. This difficulty is now understood to arise from the selective involvement of the medial temporal lobe early in the illness (Braak and Braak 1991; Hyman et al. 1984), giving rise to impaired consolidation of newly learned information into the more permanent memory stores located across interconnected neocortical structures. On formal neuropsychological testing, the memory problem of Alzheimer's disease is manifest as a rapid forgetting of new information after very brief delays of 5–10 minutes (Welsh et al. 1991).

Patients in the mild prodrome of the illness, mild cognitive impairment, generally show only this isolated memory problem (see Hayden et al. 2005; Petersen et al. 2001 for review). However, as the disease progresses, other areas of cognition are involved, reflecting the specific spread of neuropathological involvement to the lateral temporal areas, parietal cortex, and

TABLE 5–2. Clinical cognitive syndromes and associated neuropsychological profiles

Cognitive syndrome and characteristics	Neuropsychological profile
Normal aging	
Subjective memory complaints	Impaired fluid abilities (novel problem solving)
Annoying but not disabling problems	Deficiencies in memory retrieval
Frequent problems with name retrieval	Decreased general speed of processing
Minor difficulties in recalling detailed events	Lowered performance on executive tasks and visuospatial skills/ visuomotor speed
Mild cognitive impairment/amnesic type prodromal AD	
Subjective memory complaints	Memory performance 1.5 standard deviations below age-matched peers
Noticeable change in memory as noted by informants	Otherwise intact neurocognitive function
Clinical Dementia Rating score of 0.5 (mild, questionable dementia) (Hughes et al. 1982)	Functional disorder limited to mild interference from the memory difficulty
Problem is not disabling	
Alzheimer's disease	
Insidious onset	Impaired memory consolidation with rapid forgetting
Progressive impairment	Diminished executive skills
Prominent memory impairment	Impaired semantic fluency and naming
Possible disorders: aphasia, apraxia, agnosia	Impaired visuospatial analysis and praxis
Frontotemporal dementia	
Prominent personality/behavioral change	Pronounced executive impairments
Disinhibition or apathy	Cognitive inflexibility
Impaired judgment, insight	Impaired sequencing
Normal mental status initially	Perseverative, imitative, utilization behaviors
	Poor use of feedback
	Prone to interference
	Less obvious memory impairments
Lewy body dementia	
Fluctuations in alertness/ acute confusional state	Memory impairment of Alzheimer's disease but with some partial saving
Visual hallucinations	Pronounced apraxia, visuospatial difficulties
Memory impairment	Rapidly increasing quantifiable deficits in many cases
Parkinsonian signs	
Neuroleptic sensitivity	
Falls resulting from orthostatic hypotension	
Vascular dementia	
Variation of symptoms with subtype	Language/memory retrieval difficulties common
Focality on examination	Benefit from structural support/cueing
Abrupt onset	Asymmetric motor speed/dexterity
In multi-infarct dementia, stepwise progression	Executive inefficiencies

TABLE 5–2. Clinical cognitive syndromes and associated neuropsychological profiles *(continued)*

Cognitive syndrome and characteristics	Neuropsychological profile
Parkinson's disease dementia	
Extrapyramidal motor disturbance	Slowed performance
Gait dysfunction and frequent falls	Retrieval memory deficit
Bradykinesia	Executive deficiencies
Bradyphrenia	(slowed sequencing, impaired lexical fluency)
	Impaired fine motor speed (asymmetry common)
	Constructional deficits
Huntington's disease	
Early age at onset (midlife)	Slowed performance
Choreiform movements	Memory difficulty in retrieval
Dementia	Benefit from retrieval supports (recognition OK)
Bradyphrenia	Executive compromises
	Poor verbal fluency/preserved naming
Progressive supranuclear palsy	
Extrapyramidal syndrome but no tremor	Mild dysexecutive symptoms: impaired sequencing, fluency, flexibility
Ophthalmic abnormalities (limited downgaze)	
Axial rigidity	Motor slowing
Pseudobulbar palsy	Memory weakness characterized as inefficiencies in storage and retrieval
Frequent falls	
Hydrocephalus	
Memory impairment	Slowed information processing
Gait disturbance	Memory retrieval problems
Incontinence	Benefit from retrieval supports
Creutzfeldt-Jakob disease	
Rare	Rapidly evolving dementia
Typically, rapid onset and course	Subtypes include a profile akin to Alzheimer's disease, or pronounced complex visuospatial disorder (Balint's syndrome)
Dementia with pyramidal and extrapyramidal signs	
Transient spikes on electroencephalogram	
Dementia of geriatric depression	
Affective disorder	Impaired performance on tasks involving effortful processing
Psychomotor slowing	
Memory complaints	Impaired attention, concentration, sequencing, cognitive flexibility, and executive control
Cognitive complaints linked temporally to the depressive disorder	
	Retrieval memory difficulty
	Memory improvement with cueing/recognition
	Behavioral tendencies to abandon tasks, poor motivation

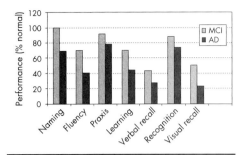

FIGURE 5–1. Profiles of neuropsychological test performance by patients with mild cognitive impairment and by patients with moderate Alzheimer's disease.

Bars indicate the performance of patients with mild cognitive impairment (*n* = 153; MCI in figure) and moderately impaired Alzheimer's disease patients (*n* = 277; AD in figure) on the subtests of the Consortium to Establish a Registry for Alzheimer's Disease (CERAD; Tariot 1996) neuropsychological battery, compared to the performance of normal elderly control subjects (*n* = 158) of similar age, sex, and education. The overall neuropsychological test performance of the Alzheimer's disease patients is well below that of both subjects with mild cognitive impairment and subjects experiencing normal aging. Patients with mild cognitive impairment perform at normal levels on naming and praxis. Learning and verbal fluency are mildly affected in this group, falling at 71% of normal. Memory is particularly affected in both Alzheimer's disease and mild cognitive impairment. Verbal recall on the CERAD Word List Memory test was 45% of normal in the sample with mild cognitive impairment and only 28% for the Alzheimer's disease patients. Visual memory was 51% of normal in mild cognitive impairment and 23% in Alzheimer's disease.

MCI = moderate cognitive impairment; AD = Alzheimer's disease.

Source. Data are derived from the Cache County Study of Memory sample (K.A. Welsh-Bohmer, unpublished).

frontal neocortical areas (Welsh et al. 1992). Prototypical changes occur in expressive language, visuospatial function, higher executive controls, and semantic knowledge. At these latter stages of the illness, anomia with impaired semantic fluency (e.g., generation of names of animals) is generally seen on examination. Word search and cir-

cumlocution tendencies are common in conversational speech, whereas speech comprehension itself is better preserved, as are all other fundamental elements of communication (Bayles et al. 1989). Visuospatial problems become more prominent in later stages of the illness, resulting in dressing apraxia, difficulty in recognizing objects or people, and problems in performing familiar motor acts (Benke 1993). Subtle problems in spatial processing can occur early and may be detectable only on formal examination. The problem can be illuminated by tests of spatial judgment and visual organization (Rizzo et al. 2000). In everyday settings, the problem may manifest as intermittent topographical disorientation, leading to difficulties in finding familiar routes while driving (Rizzo et al. 1997). An example of the profound memory loss differentiating Alzheimer's disease and mild cognitive impairment from normal aging appears in Figure 5–1.

Vascular Dementia

The neuropsychological profile of vascular dementia differs in many respects from that of Alzheimer's disease, with the largest difference being the absence of the profound memory impairment classic in Alzheimer's disease (Tierney et al. 2001). The presentation will vary according to the type and extent of the vascular disorder—multiple infarctions, a single strategic stroke, microvascular disease, cerebral hypoperfusion, hemorrhage, or combinations of these etiologies (Cohen et al. 2002).

Multi-infarct dementia, arising from multiple large- and small-vessel strokes, demonstrates a pattern of multifocal impairments on testing that relates to the cerebral territories involved in the infarctions (Chui et al. 1992; Roman et al. 1993). In dementias attributable to diffuse small-vessel disease (e.g., Binswanger's disease), test results follow a pattern reflecting the disruption in the dorsolateral prefrontal and subcortical circuitry (Kramer et al. 2002). Memory is involved, but deficits are often patchy in nature. Patients may show impaired recollection of some recent event but show a surprising memory of some other event occurring during the same time frame. On formal neuropsychological testing, the pattern in results of memory testing is one of inefficient acquisition of new information, leading to a flattened learning curve over repeating trials (Looi and Sachdev 1999; Padovani et al. 1995). Recall performance can be quite low—similar to that seen with Alzheimer's disease and mild cognitive impairment—but typically there is no rapid forgetting as there is in Alzheimer's disease (Matsuda et al. 1998). The information acquired, though little, is generally retained; as a result, savings scores between a final learning trial and a later delayed recall trial are generally high. Finally, memory recollection improves dramatically with a recognition format, suggesting a primary difficulty in retrieval rather than in storage or consolidation of new information (Hayden et al. 2005). Besides memory, dysexecutive functions are typically involved, leading to slowed sequencing, cognitive inflexibility, and decreased verbal fluency (Kertesz and Clydesdale 1994). Asymmetries in sensory motor function and deficits in coordination are also frequently demonstrated.

Frontotemporal Dementia

Frontotemporal dementia refers to a heterogeneous group of neurodegenerative conditions that are now recognized as a major non–Alzheimer's disease dementia, although the exact prevalence of these conditions remains inconclusive (Hodges and Miller 2001). The neuropathological features of these groups of illnesses are disparate, but the histological changes and atrophy are uniformly confined to the frontal and anterior temporal cortices.

Clinically, from the outset, the disorders are distinct from Alzheimer's disease and other forms of dementia. Typically, there are prominent early changes in behavior, personality, and/or language rather than impairments in memory and other aspects of cognition. As a consequence of impaired judgment and social inappropriateness, patients may have tremendous difficulties in their everyday lives, but on formal psychometric screening they may score entirely within normal limits.

A number of investigations that have delineated the cognitive profile characteristic of these disorders (Pachana et al. 1996) indicate double dissociations between frontotemporal dementia and Alzheimer's disease. In Alzheimer's disease there is classic rapid forgetting; in frontotemporal dementia there is impairment in executive function. This dysexecutive syndrome is characterized by slowed information processing, cognitive rigidity, diminished abstract reasoning, poor response inhibition, and impaired planning. At the neurobehavioral level there are major changes in personality and general social decorum. Disinhibition or its converse, behavioral apathy and inertia, frequently occurs. Patients' insight into their condition is also impaired, usually early in the course of the disorder. This pattern is in contrast to that seen in Alzheimer's disease, in which insight is generally lost later in the dementia process. In fact, appreciation of memory and other symptoms may be quite acute early in Alzheimer's disease and may be a harbinger of the progressive disorder (Geerlings et al. 1999).

Clinically, the presentation of frontotemporal dementia varies considerably (see McKhann et al. 2001; Snowden et al.

2002), and at least three subtypes are now recognized based on common clinical and neuropsychological features (see Hodges 2001). These subtypes are described behaviorally as 1) a so-called frontal variant, with the prominent behavioral disorder; 2) a semantic variant, which includes primary progressive aphasia (Weintraub et al. 1990); and 3) a rare form involving behavioral inertia and mutism (Hodges 2001). The disorder can also be segregated into two subtypes based on regional brain involvement of predominantly the frontal or temporal neocortices (e.g., Seeley et al. 2005). Regardless of subtype, the neuropathology appears heterogeneous (Brun et al. 1994; Jackson and Lowe 1996), with Alzheimer's disease–like pathology (tangles) in approximately half of the cases, Pick-like pathology (e.g. cortical thinning and gliosis)—but almost invariably without the Pick bodies—in the other half of the cases.

It should be underscored that the subtypes do not always present distinctly and that a combination of symptoms can occur. Other types of frontal lobe dementia also exist; they include presenile dementia associated with motor neuron disease, such as amyotrophic lateral sclerosis (ALS) with dementia. There are also a variety of degenerative conditions with secondary frontal lobe effects. Vascular conditions, such as subcortical ischemic vascular dementia or Binswanger's disease (mentioned previously), often manifest with frontal lobe impairments, which are probably secondary to the disruption of subcortical white matter pathways.

Parkinson's Disease and Related Disorders

Patients with Parkinson's disease and other neurological disorders involving the extrapyramidal motor system (basal ganglia)

commonly have cognitive complaints and in some instances a fulminate dementia syndrome (e.g. diffuse Lewy body dementia [DLB]). The cognitive profile common to the family of extrapyramidal disorders is a pattern of retrieval problems and mild dysexecutive disturbances, which in the early stages of disorder may be less dramatic or globally impairing than the cognitive deficits of early-stage AD (Butters et al. 1988).

In Parkinson's disease, unlike Alzheimer's disease, in which cognitive impairment is central to the diagnosis, neurocognitive deficits are not universally observed over the course of illness. When cognition is affected, it can be quite variable in both the nature and extent of symptoms. In some cases the cognitive problems bear some resemblance to normal aging, whereas in others dementia is manifest. The presence of cognitive loss does not necessarily herald dementia. Typically, only 20%–40% of Parkinson's disease patients are reported to have dementia (Cummings 1988; Pillon et al. 1991), and there is some evidence that age at illness onset is a risk factor for Parkinson's disease dementia (Friedman and Barcikowska 1994; Reid 1992).

In patients with idiopathic Parkinson's disease, cognitive changes are commonly noted as similar to those of Huntington's disease, probably reflecting similar regional localization of the major neuropathology. However, carefully controlled investigations have shown that reduction of the cognitive profile of Parkinson's disease to a single subtype may be an oversimplification (Filoteo et al. 1997). Part of the heterogeneity in presentation probably reflects an admixture of several similar syndromes with overlapping but not identical pathological and neurochemical etiologies (Cummings 1988). Diffuse Lewy body dementia and the Lewy body variant of Alzheimer's disease are now recognized forms of dementia (Zaccai et al. 2005) that share cognitive features common to Alzheimer's disease and Parkinson's disease (Geser et al. 2005). These disorders all show elements of rapid forgetting, albeit with some partial savings, and visuospatial disturbances (Ballard et al. 1996; Hanson et al. 1990; Salmon et al. 1996). Other conditions closely related to Parkinson's disease and diffuse Lewy body dementia include progressive supranuclear palsy, corticobasal degeneration, and multisystem atrophy. All these conditions are considered synucleinopathies, involving the pathological accumulation of the protein alpha-synuclein in midbrain structures of the nigrostriatal system. The prevailing features in these related conditions are parkinsonism, akinetic rigidity, and generalized slowing in motor movement/motor initiation and thought processes (bradykinesia and bradyphrenia, respectively). The core features distinguishing diffuse Lewy body dementia include fluctuations in cognition and attention, recurrent and persistent visual hallucinations, and extrapyramidal motor symptoms.

When the overall level of dementia is controlled, some clinical differentiation between the similar conditions can be made; but the process of differential diagnosis should include, at a minimum, careful attention to the history of symptoms, the cognitive deficits manifest, and the presence or absence of defined behavioral impairments (Pillon et al. 1991; Geser et al. 2005). Making a solid differential diagnosis based solely on cognitive profile is difficult (Monza et al. 1998; Soliveri et al. 2000; Testa et al. 2001). Some differentiation, however, is possible. For example, cognitively impaired patients with Parkinson's disease can be differentiated from patients with Alzheimer's disease by the relatively increased apathy observed in the former group and the memory impairment in the latter (Cahn-Weiner et al. 2002). Likewise, the neurop-

sychiatric profiles of the dementias of Alzheimer's disease and of Parkinson's disease differ (Aarsland et al. 2001). However, it is necessary to integrate the clinical examination findings—which include history and review of symptoms, cognitive findings, behavioral ratings, psychiatric interview, and supportive laboratory findings such as neuroimaging— to differentiate these disorders from each other.

Geriatric Depression and Mood Disorders

Among the most common uses of neuropsychological assessment in elderly persons are in evaluating memory disorders and determining the role of depression. By itself, serious mood depression in elderly persons can result in disabling cognitive impairment, or what has been called the dementia of depression or "pseudodementia" (Breitner and Welsh 1995). The problem of geriatric depression is fairly common, with some more recent epidemiology-based studies suggesting that 28% of elderly populations over age 65 exhibit prominent affective syndromes (Lyketsos et al. 2001). Depression also frequently co-occurs in the context of a range of medical disorders, including Alzheimer's disease, stroke, and Parkinson's disease, and this complicates the diagnosis of these disorders and exacerbates the functional loss associated with each (Ballard et al. 1996; Krishnan 2000; Migliorelli et al. 1995; Reichman and Coyne 1995). Distinguishing between depression and other conditions in elderly patients can be challenging, but it can be assisted by a thorough screening of both depressive symptoms and cognitive status.

When such screening fails to give a clear picture of the contribution of depression to the cognitive picture, neuropsychological examination can help. To this end, it must be noted that depression in late life is clinically heterogeneous, with variable concordance between severity of depressive symptoms and level of cognitive impairment (Alexopoulos et al. 2002; Krishnan 1993).

Despite this heterogeneity, some distinctive neurocognitive and behavioral changes appear to be ascribable to the condition of late-life depression and are characteristic of a rather large subgroup of patients (Beats et al. 1996; Lockwood et al. 2002). The neurocognitive profile appears to be one of a dysexecutive syndrome with impairments in planning, organization, initiation, sequencing, working memory, and behavioral shifting in response to feedback. Short-term memory and visuospatial skills are also disturbed, in part as a result of the attentional and organizational compromises. Behaviorally, the depression-dysexecutive syndrome of geriatric depressed patients is characterized by apathy and psychomotor retardation, as opposed to the prominent mood dysphoria of younger counterparts.

On formal neuropsychological testing, geriatric depressed patients show impairments on tests sensitive to frontal lobe function. Difficulties can be readily seen on tests of selective and sustained attention, verbal fluency, inhibitory control, and set shifting (Boone et al. 1995; Lockwood et al. 2002). Memory is impaired in both acquisition and recall, leading to a profile characterized by a flattened learning curve and impaired free recall, after brief delays, of previously learned information (Hart et al. 1987). Recognition memory is better preserved but can be characterized by false negative tendencies (i.e., not recognizing previous target material). The memory disturbance of depression is distinguished from that of Alzheimer's disease by the impaired acquisition and recognition elements in depression. In Alzheimer's disease, acquisition is relatively better preserved, whereas recog-

nition is characterized by false-positive tendencies (i.e., recognizing foils incorrectly as previously presented targets). The profile of impairment in depression gives the impression of generalized cognitive inefficiency and suppression of performance. Other qualitative differences between the performance of these two groups may also be seen; depressed patients often have a heightened tendency to abandon effortful tests.

It is important to note that, even with treatment, not all the cognitive impairments associated with geriatric depression remit. In older patients, these continuing impairments may be due to the co-occurrence of another disease process, such as Alzheimer's disease or vascular dementia. Although far from conclusive, a number of studies have reported that depression in elderly persons exerts a discernible additional effect on cognition and functional independence and that depression may be a risk factor for later cognitive decline (Steffens et al. 2006). Therefore, neuropsychological evaluation of elderly patients can provide critical information about the nature of their cognitive failures, differential diagnostic information, and a baseline for future comparisons. This information has obvious implications for diagnosis and management of these patients, regardless of whether all the cognitive change detected is reversible.

Conclusion

The neuropsychological evaluation provides a useful and cost-effective approach to diagnosis and management in the growing geriatric population with memory complaints. Although a neuropsychological evaluation is not needed in the majority of dementia cases, in which the patient's symptoms are obvious and the diagnosis is secure, the evaluation can be enormously useful in more complex, less straightforward diagnostic situations, such as early Alzheimer's disease detection or geriatric depression. Because of its objective nature, the neuropsychological examination has strong applications in medical management, providing information about patients' capacities and deficits that is important to intervention approaches and to guiding future decision making about competency and safety.

References

Aarsland D, Cummings JL, Larsen JP: Neuropsychiatric differences between Parkinson's disease with dementia and Alzheimer's disease. Int J Geriatr Psychiatry 16:184–191, 2001

Alexopoulos GS, Kiosses DN, Klimstra S, et al: Clinical presentation of the "depression-executive dysfunction syndrome" of late life. Am J Geriatr Psychiatry 10:98–106, 2002

Attix DK, Welsh-Bohmer KA: Geriatric Neuropsychology: Assessment and Intervention. Edited by Attix DK, Welsh-Bohmer KA. New York, Guilford, 2006

Ballard C, Bannister C, Solis M, et al: The prevalence, associations and symptoms of depression amongst dementia sufferers. J Affect Disord 36:135–144, 1996

Bayles KA, Boone DR, Tomoeda CK, et al: Differentiating Alzheimer's patients from the normal elderly and stroke patients with aphasia. J Speech Hear Disord 54:74–87, 1989

Beats BC, Sahakian BJ, Levy R: Cognitive performance in tests sensitive to frontal lobe dysfunction in the elderly depressed. Psychol Med 26:591–603, 1996

Beck AT, Steer RA, Brown GK: Beck Depression Inventory, II. San Antonio, TX, The Psychological Corporation, 1996

Benke T: Two forms of apraxia in Alzheimer's disease. Cortex 29:715–725, 1993

Benton AL, Hamsher K de S: Multilingual Aphasia Examination. Iowa City, IA, AJA Associates, 1983

Benton AL, Van Allen MW, Fogel ML: Temporal orientation in cerebral disease. J Nerv Ment Dis 139:110–119, 1964

Benton AL, Eslinger PJ, Damasio AR: Normative observations on neuropsychological test performance in old age. J Clin Neuropsychol 3:33–42, 1981

Benton AL, Hamsher K de S, Varney NR, et al: Contributions to Neuropsychological Assessment. New York, Oxford University Press, 1983

Berg EA: A simple objective treatment for measuring flexibility in thinking. J Gen Psychol 39:15–22, 1948

Boone KB, Lesser I, Miller B, et al: Cognitive functioning in older depressed outpatients: relationship of presence and severity of depression on neuropsychological test scores. Neuropsychology 9:390–398, 1995

Botwinick J: Intellectual abilities, in The Handbook of the Psychology of Aging. Edited by Birren JE, Schaie KW. New York, Van Nostrand Reinhold, 1977, pp 508–605

Braak H, Braak E: Neuropathological staging of Alzheimer-related changes. Acta Neuropathol (Berl) 82:239–259, 1991

Breitner JCS, Welsh KA: An approach to diagnosis and management of memory loss and other cognitive syndromes of aging. Psychiatr Serv 46:29–35, 1995

Breitner JC, Wyse BW, Anthony JC, et al: APOE-epsilon4 count predicts age when prevalence of AD increases, then declines: the Cache County Study. Neurology 53:321–331, 1999

Brun A, Englund B, Gustafson L, et al: Consensus statement: clinical and neuropathological criteria for frontotemporal dementia: the Lund and Manchester groups. J Neurol Neurosurg Psychiatry 57:416–418, 1994

Buschke H, Fuld P: Evaluation of storage, retention and retrieval in disordered memory and learning. Neurology 24:1019–1025, 1974

Butcher JN, Dahlstrom WG, Graham JR, et al: Minnesota Multiphasic Personality-2 (MMPI-2): Manual for Administration and Scoring. Minneapolis, University of Minnesota Press, 1989

Butters N, Salmon DP, Cullum M, et al: Differentiation of amnesic and demented patients with Wechsler Memory Scale—Revised. Clin Neuropsychol 2:133–148, 1988

Cahn-Weiner DA, Grace J, Ott BR, et al: Cognitive and behavioral features discriminate between Alzheimer's and Parkinson's disease. Neuropsychiatry Neuropsychol Behav Neurol 15:79–87, 2002

Chui HC, Victoroff JI, Margolin D, et al: Criteria for the diagnosis of ischemic vascular dementia proposed by the State of California Alzheimer's Disease Diagnostic and Treatment Centers. Neurology 42 (3, pt 1): 473–480, 1992

Coffey CE, Wilkinson WE, Parashos IA, et al: Quantitative cerebral anatomy of the aging human brain: a cross-sectional study using magnetic resonance imaging. Neurology 43:527–536, 1992

Cohen RA, Paul RH, Ott BR, et al: The relationship of subcortical MRI hyperintensities and brain volume to cognitive function in vascular dementia. J Int Neuropsychol Soc 8:743–752, 2002

Craik FIM: Age differences in remembering, in Neuropsychology of Memory. Edited by Squire L, Butters N. New York, Guilford, 1984, pp 3–12

Cullum CM, Butters N, Troster AL, et al: Normal aging and forgetting rates on the Wechsler Memory Scale—Revised. Arch Clin Neuropsychol 5:23–30, 1990

Cummings JL: Intellectual impairment in Parkinson's disease: clinical, pathologic, and biochemical correlates. J Geriatr Psychiatry Neurol 1:24–36, 1988

Daigneault S, Braun CM: Working memory and the Self-Ordered Pointing Task: further evidence of early prefrontal decline in normal aging. J Clin Exp Neuropsychol 15:881–895, 1993

Delis DC, Kramer JH, Kaplan E, et al: California Verbal Learning Tests: Adult Version. San Antonio, TX, Psychological Corporation, 1987

Ebly EM, Parhad IM, Hogan DB, et al: Prevalence and types of dementia in the very old: results from the Canadian Study of Health and Aging. Neurology 44:1593–1600, 1994

Ebly EM, Hogan DB, Parhad IM: Cognitive impairment in the nondemented elderly: results from the Canadian Study of Health and Aging. Arch Neurol 52:612–619, 1995

Eslinger PJ, Damasio AR, Benton AL, et al: Neuropsychologic detection of abnormal mental decline in older persons. JAMA 253:670–674, 1985

Evans DA, Smith LA, Scherr PA, et al: Risk of death from Alzheimer's disease in a community population of older persons. Am J Epidemiol 134:403–412, 1991

Filoteo JV, Rilling LM, Cole B, et al: Variable memory profiles in Parkinson's disease. J Clin Exp Neuropsychol 19:878–888, 1997

Folstein MF, Folstein S, McHugh P: "Mini-mental state." J Psychiatr Res 12:189–198, 1975

Fratiglioni L, De Ronchi D, Aguero-Torres H: Worldwide prevalence and incidence of dementia. Drugs Aging 15:365–375, 1999

Friedman A, Barcikowska M: Dementia in Parkinson's disease. Dementia 5:12–16, 1994

Geerlings MI, Jonker C, Bouter LM, et al: Association between memory complaints and incident Alzheimer's disease in elderly people with normal baseline cognition. Am J Psychiatry 156:531–537, 1999

Geldmacher DS, Whitehouse PJ Jr: Differential diagnosis of Alzheimer's disease. Neurology 48 (5, suppl 6):S2–S9, 1997

Geser F, Wenning GK, Poewe W, et al: How to diagnose dementia with Lewy Bodies: state of the art. Movement Disord 20(suppl): S11–S20, 2005

Gur RC, Gur RE, Obrist WD, et al: Age and regional cerebral blood flow at rest and during cognitive activity. Arch Gen Psychiatry 44:617–621, 1987

Hanson L, Salmon D, Galasko D, et al: The Lewy body variant of Alzheimer's disease: a clinical and pathological entity. Neurology 40:1–8, 1990

Hart RP, Kwentus JA, Taylor JR, et al: Rate of forgetting in dementia and depression. J Consult Clin Psychol 55:101–105, 1987

Haug H, Barmwater U, Eggers R, et al: Anatomical changes in aging brain: morphometric analysis of the human prosencephalon, in Neuropharmacology, Vol 21: Aging. Edited by Cervos-Navarro J, Sarkander HI. New York, Raven Press. pp 1–12, 1983

Hayden KM, Warren LH, Pieper CF, et al: Identification VaD and AD prodromes: The Cache County Study. Alzheimer's & Dementia: The Journal of the Alzheimer's Association 1:19–29, 2005

Heaton RK, Grant I, Matthews CG: Comprehensive Norms for an Expanded Halstead-Reitan Battery: Demographic Corrections, Research Findings and Clinical Applications. Odessa, FL: Psychological Assessment Resources, 1991

Hodges JR: Frontotemporal dementia (Picks disease). Clinical features and assessment. Neurology 56 (suppl):S6–S10, 2001

Hodges JR, Miller B: The classification, genetics and neuropathology of frontotemporal dementia. Introduction to the special topic papers: Part I. Neurocase 7(1):31–35, 2001

Holman RC, Khan AS, Kent J, et al: Epidemiology of Creutzfeldt-Jakob disease in the United States 1979–1990: analysis of national mortality data. Neuroepidemiology 14:174–181, 1995

Horn J: The theory of fluid and crystallized intelligence in relation to concepts of cognitive psychology and aging in adulthood, in Aging and Cognitive Processes. Edited by Craik F, Trehub S. New York: Plenum, 1982, pp 237–278

Howieson D, Holm L, Kaye J, et al: Neurologic function in the optimally healthy oldest old: neuropsychological evaluation. Neurology 43:1882–1886, 1993

Hughes CP, Berg L, Danziger WL, et al: A new clinical scale for the staging of dementia. Br J Psychiatry 140:566–572, 1982

Hyman BT, Van Horsen GW, Damasio AR, et al: Alzheimer's disease: cell-specific pathology isolates the hippocampal formation. Science 225:1168–1170, 1984

Ivnik RJ, Malec JF, Smith GE, et al: Mayo's older Americans normative studies: updated AVLT norms for ages 56–97. Clin Neuropsychol 6:83–104, 1992

Jackson M, Lowe J: The new neuropathology of degenerative frontotemporal dementias. Acta Neuropathologica 91:127–134, 1996

Kaplan EF, Goodglass H, Weintraub S: The Boston Naming Test, 2nd Edition. Philadelphia, PA, Lea & Febiger, 1978

Kertesz A, Clydesdale S Neuropsychological deficits in vascular dementia vs Alzheimer's disease. Frontal lobe deficits prominent in vascular dementia. Arch Neurol 51:1226–1231, 1994

Knopman DS, DeKosky ST, Cummings JL, et al: Practice parameter: diagnosis of dementia (an evidence based review). Report of the Quality Standards Subcommittee of the American Academy of Neurology. Neurology 56:1143–1153, 2001

Koltai DC, Welsh-Bohmer KA: Geriatric neuropsychological assessment, in Clinician's Guide to Neuropsychological Assessment, 2nd Edition. Edited by Vanderploeg RD. Mahwah, NJ, Lawrence Erlbaum, 2000, pp 383–415

Koss E, Haxby JV, DeCarli C, et al: Patterns of performance preservation and loss in healthy aging. Dev Neuropsychol 7:99–113, 1991

Kramer JH, Reed BR, Mungas D, et al: Executive dysfunction in subcortical ischaemic vascular disease. J Neurol Neurosurg Psychiatry 72:217–220, 2002

Krishnan KR: Neuroanatomic substrates of depression in the elderly. J Geriatr Psychiatry Neurol 6:39–58, 1993

Krishnan KR: Depression as a contributing factor in cerebrovascular disease. Am Heart J 140:70–76, 2000

Langley LK, Madden DJ: Functional neuroimaging of memory: implications for cognitive aging. Microsc Res Tech 51:75–84, 2000

Lezak MD: Neuropsychological Assessment, 3rd Edition. New York, Oxford University Press, 1995

Lobo A, Launer LJ, Fratiglioni L, et al: Prevalence of dementia and major subtypes in Europe: a collaborative study of population-based cohorts. Neurologic Diseases in the Elderly Research Group. Neurology 54 (11, suppl 5):S4–S9, 2000

Lockwood KA, Alexopoulos GS, Van Gorp WG: Executive dysfunction in geriatric depression. Am J Psychiatry 159:1119–1126, 2002

Looi J, Sachdev PS: Differentiation of vascular dementia from AD on neuropsychological tests. Neurology 53:670–678, 1999

Lyketsos CG, Sheppard JM, Steinberg M, et al: Neuropsychiatric disturbance in Alzheimer's disease clusters into three groups: the Cache County study. Int J Geriatr Psychiatry 16:1043–1053, 2001

Matsuda O, Saito M, Sugishita M: Cognitive deficits of mild dementia: a comparison between dementia of the Alzheimer's type and vascular dementia. Psychiatry Clin Neurosci 52:87–91, 1998

Mattis S, Jurica PJ, Leitten CL: Dementia Rating Scale-2™ (DRS-2™): Professional Manual. Odessa, FL, Psychological Assessment Resources, 2002

McKhann GM, Albert MS, Grossman M, et al: Clinical and pathological diagnosis of frontotemporal dementia: report of Work Group on Frontotemporal Dementia and Pick's Disease. Arch Neurol 58:1803–1809, 2001

Migliorelli R, Teson A, Sabe L, et al: Prevalence and correlates of dysthymia and major depression among patients with Alzheimer's disease. Am J Psychiatry 152:37–44, 1995

Mittenberg W, Seidenberg M, O'Leary DS, et al: Changes in cerebral functioning associated with normal aging. J Clin Exp Neuropsychol 11:918–932, 1989

Mohs RC, Cohen L: Alzheimer's Disease Assessment Scale (ADAS). Psychopharmacol Bull 24:627–628, 1988

Monza D, Soliveri P, Radice D, et al: Cognitive dysfunction and impaired organization of complex motility in degenerative parkinsonism syndromes. Arch Neurol 55:372–378, 1998

Morris JC, Heyman A, Mohs RC, et al: The Consortium to Establish a Registry for Alzheimer's Disease (CERAD). Part I. Clinical and neuropsychological assessment of Alzheimer's disease. Neurology 39:1159–1165, 1989

Pachana NA, Boone KB, Miller BL, et al: Comparison of neuropsychological functioning in Alzheimer's disease and frontotemporal dementia. J Int Neuropsychol Soc 2:505–510, 1996

Padovani A, Di Piero V, Bragoni M, et al: Patterns of neuropsychological impairment in mild dementia: comparison between Alzheimer's disease and multi-infarct dementia. Acta Neurol Scand 92:433–442, 1995

Petersen RC, Stevens JC, Ganguli M, et al: Practice parameter: early detection of dementia: mild cognitive impairment (an evidence based review). Report of the Quality Standards Subcommittee of the American Academy of Neurology. Neurology 56:1133–1142, 2001

Pillon B, Dubois B, Agid Y: Severity and specificity of cognitive impairment in Alzheimer's, Huntington's, and Parkinson's diseases and progressive supranuclear palsy. Ann N Y Acad Sci 640:224–227, 1991

Potter GG, Attix DK: Integrated model for geriatric neuropsychological assessment, in Geriatric Neuropsychology: Assessment and Intervention. Edited by Attix DK, Welsh-Bohmer KA. New York, Guilford, 2006

Reichman WE, Coyne AC: Depressive symptoms in Alzheimer's disease and multi-infarct dementia. J Geriatr Psychiatry Neurol 8:96–99, 1995

Reid WG: The evolution of dementia in idiopathic Parkinson's disease: neuropsychological and clinical evidence in support of subtypes. Int Psychogeriatr 4:147–160, 1992

Reitan RM: Validity of the Trail Making Test as an indicator of organic brain damage. Percept Mot Skills 8:271–276, 1958

Rizzo M, Reinach S, McGehee D, et al: Simulated car crashes and crash predictors in drivers with Alzheimer disease. Arch Neurol 54:545–551, 1997

Rizzo M, Anderson SW, Dawson J, et al: Vision and cognition in Alzheimer's disease. Neuropsychologia 38:1157–1169, 2000

Roman GC, Tatemichi TK, Erkinjuntti T, et al: Vascular dementia: diagnostic criteria for research studies. Report of the NINDS-AIREN International Workshop. Neurology 43:250–260, 1993

Salmon DP, Galasko D, Hansen LA, et al: Neuropsychological deficits associated with diffuse Lewy body disease. Brain Cogn 31:148–165, 1996

Salthouse T: Speed of behavior and its implications for cognition, in Handbook for the Psychology of Aging, 2nd Edition. Edited by Birren JE, Shaie KW. New York, Van Nostrand Reinhold, 1985, pp 400–426

Salthouse TA, Fristoe N, Rhee SH: How localized are age-related effects on neuropsychological measures? Neuropsychology 10:272–285, 1996

Savolainen S, Palijarvi L, Vapalahti M: Prevalence of Alzheimer's disease in patients investigated for presumed normal pressure hydrocephalus: a clinical and neuropathological study. Acta Neurochir (Wien) 141:849–853, 1999

Seeley WW, Bauer AM, Miller BL, et al: The natural history of temporal variant frontotemporal dementia. Neurology 64:1384–1390, 2005

Smith A: The Symbol Digit Modalities Test: a neuropsychologic test for economic screening of learning and other cerebral disorders. Learning Disorders 3:83–91, 1968

Snowden JS, Neary D, Mann DM: Frontotemporal dementia. Br J Psychiatry 180:140–143, 2002

Soliveri P, Monza D, Paridi D, et al: Neuropsychological follow up in patients with Parkinson's disease, striatonigral degeneration type multisystem atrophy and progressive supranuclear palsy. J Neurol Neurosurg Psychiatry 69:313–318, 2000

Spreen O, Strauss E. A Compendium of Neuropsychological Tests: Administration, Norms, and Commentary, 2nd Edition. New York, Oxford University Press, 1996

Steffens DC, Otey E, Alexopoulos GS, et al: Perspectives on depression, mild cognitive impairment, and cognitive decline. Arch Gen Psychiatry 63:130–138, 2006

Steinberg B, Bielauskas L: IQ based MOANS norms for multiple neuropsychological instruments. Clin Neuropsychol 19:277–279, 2005

Tariot PN: CERAD behavior rating scale for dementia. Int Psychogeriatr 8 (suppl 3):317–320, 1996

Testa D, Monza D, Ferrarini M, et al: Comparison of natural histories of progressive supranuclear palsy and multiple system atrophy. Neurol Sci 21:247–251, 2001

Tierney MC, Black SE, Szalai JP, et al: Recognition memory and verbal fluency differentiate probable Alzheimer disease from subcortical ischemic vascular dementia. Arch Neurol 58:1654–1659, 2001

Tschanz JT, Welsh-Bohmer KA, West N, et al: Identification of dementia cases derived from a neuropsychological algorithm: comparisons with clinically derived diagnoses. Neurology 54:1290–1296, 2000

Van Gorp WG, Mahler ME: Subcortical features of normal aging, in Subcortical Dementia. Edited by Cummings JL. New York, Oxford University Press, 1990, pp 231–250

Wechsler D: Wechsler Intelligence Scale, 3rd Edition, Manual. San Antonio, TX, Psychological Corporation, 1997a

Wechsler D: Wechsler Memory Scale, 3rd Edition, Manual. San Antonio, TX, Psychological Corporation, 1997b

Weintraub S, Rubin NP, Mesulam MM: Primary progressive aphasia: longitudinal course, profile and language features. Arch Neurol 47:1329–1335, 1990

Welsh K, Butters N, Hughes JP, et al: Detection of abnormal memory decline in mild Alzheimer's disease using CERAD neuropsychological measures. Arch Neurol 48:278–281, 1991

Welsh KA, Butters N, Hughes JP, et al: Detection and staging of dementia in Alzheimer's disease: use of the neuropsychological measures developed for the Consortium to Establish a Registry for Alzheimer's Disease (CERAD). Arch Neurol 49:448–452, 1992

Welsh-Bohmer KA, Mohs RC: Neuropsychological assessment of Alzheimer's disease. Neurology 49 (3 suppl 3): S11–S13, 1997

Welsh-Bohmer KA, Koltai DC, Mason DJ: The clinical utility of neuropsychological evaluation of patients with known or suspected dementia, in Demonstrating Utility and Cost Effectiveness in Clinical Neuropsychology.. Edited by Prigatano G, Pliskin N. Philadelphia, PA, Psychology Press—Taylor & Francis Group, 2003, pp 177–200

Wetzel L, Boll TJ: Short Category Test, Booklet Format. Los Angeles, CA, Western Psychological Services, 1987

Yesavage J, Brink TL, Rose TL, et al: Development and validation of a geriatric depression scale: a preliminary report. J Psychiatr Res 17:37–49, 1983

Zaccai J, McCracken C, Brayne C: A systematic review of prevalence and incidence studies of dementia with Lewy bodies. Age Ageing 34:561–566, 2005

Study Questions

Select the single best response for each question.

1. The most common cause for cognitive change after age 50 is

   A. Alzheimer's disease.
   B. Frontotemporal dementia.
   C. Normal aging of the nervous system.
   D. Vascular dementia.
   E. None of the above.

2. The differences underlying memory loss of normal aging and that of Alzheimer's disease include

   A. Consolidation or storage of new information in long-term memory stores.
   B. Efficient accessing of recently stored information.
   C. Difficulty with visuospatial tasks.
   D. A and B.
   E. A, B, and C.

3. The leading cause of dementia in elderly persons is

   A. Vascular disease.
   B. Alzheimer's disease.
   C. Lewy body disease.
   D. Frontotemporal disease.
   E. Corticobasal degeneration.

4. The earliest manifestation of Alzheimer's disease is

   A. Rapid forgetting of new information after very brief delays.
   B. Expressive language difficulty.
   C. Visuospatial difficulty.
   D. Apraxia.
   E. Circumlocution.

5. Patients with vascular dementia could be expected to show all of the following *except*

   A. Memory deficits often patchy in nature.
   B. Impaired recollection of some recent event but surprisingly good memory of some other event occurring during the same time frame.
   C. Flattened learning curve over repeated trials.
   D. Low recall performance as well as rapid forgetting.
   E. Recognition improving dramatically with a recognition format.

6. What percentage of patients with Parkinson's disease are reported to have dementia?

    A. 5%–10%.
    B. 10%–20%.
    C. 20%–40%.
    D. 50%–60%.
    E. 70%–80%.

7. Geriatric depression shows which of the following deficits?

    A. Impairments on tests sensitive to frontal lobe function.
    B. Difficulties on sustained and selective attention.
    C. Set shifting.
    D. Verbal fluency.
    E. All of the above.

PART

3

Psychiatric Disorders
in Late Life

CHAPTER 6

Cognitive Disorders

Murray A. Raskind, M.D.

Lauren T. Bonner, M.D.

Elaine R. Peskind, M.D.

The cognitive disorders are the most prevalent psychiatric disorders of later life. The predominant problem in these disorders is a clinically meaningful deficit in cognition that represents a decline from a previous level of functioning. The cognitive disorder focused on in this chapter is dementia; also discussed are delirium, amnestic disorder, alcoholic dementia, and Wernicke-Korsakoff syndrome. In this chapter, we attempt to use nomenclature that is consistent with DSM-IV-TR (American Psychiatric Association 2000).

Dementia is a syndrome of acquired impairment of memory and other cognitive functions caused by structural neuronal damage. Dementia is induced by a variety of specific diseases that damage and destroy neurons (e.g., Alzheimer's disease [AD], cerebrovascular disease). Delirium may either complicate dementia or impair cognition on its own. It is a syndrome of impaired attention and consciousness caused by disrupted brain physiology. Delirium results from a variety of specific disturbances that disrupt brain function (e.g., adverse effects of medications on the central nervous system [CNS], electrolyte imbalance). The presence of dementia lowers the threshold for delirium. Thus, delirium commonly occurs in the setting of dementia (Levkoff et al. 1992; Marcantonio et al. 2000; Rahkonen et al. 2000).

Dementia is particularly costly to society, both in terms of financial resources dedicated to patient care and in terms of morbidity, mortality, and the stress that patients place on caregivers and the broader community. One-half of the beds in community long-term-care facilities are devoted to patients with dementia, most of whom have AD (Katzman 1986). The prevalence and burden of the cognitive disorders of later life will further increase as the proportion of elderly persons in the United States population increases over the next 50 years.

Supported in part by the Department of Veterans Affairs, National Institute on Aging Alzheimer's Disease Research Center grant AG05316, and a minority faculty supplement to grant AG18644.

Dementia

Dementia is a syndrome—that is, a group of signs and symptoms that cluster together and are caused by a number of underlying diseases. These diseases produce neuronal loss or other structural brain damage. The central feature of dementia is acquired impairment of memory. In addition, at least one of the following cognitive deficits must be present: aphasia (language impairment secondary to disruption of brain function), apraxia (inability to perform complex motor activities despite intact motor abilities), agnosia (failure to recognize or identify objects despite intact sensory function), and disturbance in executive functions such as planning, organizing, sequencing, and abstracting. To meet formal criteria, the dementia must be severe enough to interfere with social or occupational functioning. Dementia resulting from any brain disorder has the aforementioned features in common.

Clinical Features

Although all disorders causing dementia must produce acquired impairment of memory and impairment of other cognitive functions—impairments that are severe enough to interfere with daily activities—and must represent a substantial decline from a previous level of functioning, the specific dementia disorders have distinguishing features that reflect the nature of the underlying disease. Recognizing the likely disorder underlying dementia can have important treatment implications.

Because AD is the most common dementia disorder of later life (Katzman 1976), the course of AD is often assumed to be the course of dementia in general. In fact, the course of AD is a relatively specific diagnostic feature of the disease (Khachaturian 1985; McKhann et al. 1984). The typical course of AD is one of insidious onset, with gradual but inexorable progression of cognitive deficits over a period ranging from 5 to 15 years or even longer.

Other diseases causing dementia may have quite different clinical courses. For example, dementia due to head trauma has a sudden onset, and the course is stable or the patient may improve over time. Dementia due to anoxia (such as in older persons resuscitated not soon enough after cardiac arrest to prevent hypoxic brain damage) has a similar course. Vascular dementia can progress in a stepwise manner, reflecting new episodes of cerebral infarction, or can progress gradually in a manner indistinguishable from AD (Chui et al. 1992). In the case of persons with dementia due to alcohol use who subsequently abstain from alcohol, a substantial number show meaningful improvements in cognitive function (Victor and Adams 1971).

Differential Diagnosis

Dementia and Delirium

A common problem in the differential diagnosis of dementia is mistaking a delirium for dementia. An even more common problem is failing to recognize a delirium superimposed on an underlying dementia. Both delirium and dementia manifest as impairment in cognitive functions, but the two conditions differ in the pattern of deficits and the cognitive domains primarily involved. In at least the early and middle stages of dementia, the patient is alert and attentive, whereas in delirium the patient shows decreased attention to the environment and has an altered level of arousal. The delirious patient's cognitive deficits fluctuate, whereas those of the patient with dementia are usually stable. Unfortunately, in the more advanced stages of progressive dementia disorders of late life such as AD, attention is impaired. However, even in the late stages of AD, a fluctuating level of consciousness is cause for concern—concern that a superimposed delirium may exist.

Dementia and Depression

A differential diagnostic problem that has received much attention involves the differentiation of a major depressive episode from dementia in a cognitively impaired older person. Although the term *depressive pseudodementia* (Kiloh 1961) was justly criticized by Reifler (1982), the concept has some heuristic value. It is unusual for a major depressive episode to produce such severe cognitive impairment that distinction of the impairment from a specific dementia disorder such as AD is persistently difficult. However, depressive pseudodementia secondary to a primary major depressive episode does occur. It usually begins with dysphoric mood, loss of interest and pleasure, and other typical signs and symptoms of primary depression, with subsequent cognitive impairment. Furthermore, patients with depressive pseudodementia often have a history of primary affective disorder earlier in life. The clinical examination is helpful in this differential diagnostic problem. The patient with a primary depression is inattentive, excessively aroused (in agitated depression) or lethargic (in retarded depression), poorly motivated during a mental status examination, and frequently answers "I don't know" to questions probing cognitive function. Aphasia, apraxia, and anomia are not present in the patient with cognitive symptoms secondary to a primary depression. Depressive pseudodementia might be more accurately classified as depressive delirium, given that depression is a manifestation of disrupted brain physiology at the biochemical level and that impaired attention and level of arousal are prominent symptoms.

More common than depressive pseudodementia are depressive signs and symptoms complicating a preexisting dementia (Zubenko and Moossy 1988). Such depressive signs and symptoms, as well as a diagnosable major depressive episode, frequently complicate the clinical courses of vascular dementia and AD. Recent studies suggest that treatment of such major depressive episodes with selective serotonin reuptake inhibitors (SSRIs) and behavioral approaches is effective (see "Abnormalities of Brain Neurotransmitters").

Differentiating Specific Disorders Causing Dementia

Differential diagnosis of dementia does not end with the exclusion of delirium and depression. It is also important to make the diagnosis of a specific dementia disorder with as great a degree of certainty as possible, because prognosis varies among dementia disorders and there are specific treatments for several diseases causing dementia. The essential elements of the clinical evaluation of the older patient with acquired cognitive impairment are listed in Table 6–1. By far the most important part of the evaluation is a careful history, obtained not only from the patient (whose insight into and recollection of signs, symptoms, and clinical course are usually unreliable) but also from friends, relatives, or other persons familiar with the patient. A mental status examination focusing on the patient's level of awareness and attention, memory, calculation, language, praxis, visual-spatial skills, and executive functioning must be performed. Observation of the patient's affect during the examination usually is more helpful, in evaluating for depression, than the memory-impaired patient's subjective response to questions about his or her mood status in the recent past.

A physical examination—including a screening neurological evaluation, with special attention given to localizing neurolog-

TABLE 6–1. Evaluation of cognitive impairment in later life

History from patient and from relative or friend
Mental status examination
Physical examination, including neurological examination
Medication inventory and urinalysis
Head CT or MRI
Complete blood count
Serum VDRL test
Measurement of serum sodium, potassium, chloride, bicarbonate, and calcium levels
Measurement of serum blood urea nitrogen, creatinine, bilirubin, and albumin/globulin levels
Measurement of serum B_{12} level
Measurement of serum triiodothyronine, thyroxine, and thyroid-stimulating hormone levels
Brief cognitive test (e.g., Mini-Mental State Exam)

Note. CT = computed tomography; MRI = magnetic resonance imaging; VDRL = Venereal Disease Research Laboratory.

ical signs—is also essential. An inventory of current medications, both prescribed and over-the-counter, should routinely be taken in the evaluation, and a urine specimen should be obtained and analyzed for the presence of drugs if there is a question about the reliability of the drug history. This part of the evaluation is particularly important if the clinical picture suggests delirium. Behavioral toxicity associated with pharmacotherapy is the most common etiology of reversible delirium and behavioral impairments in the elderly patient (Larson et al. 1984). Serum electrolyte levels, blood urea nitrogen levels, and serum B_{12} levels should be measured and thyroid function tests (including a thyroid-stimulating hormone test) should be performed to rule out correctable causes of delirium and/or dementia. Early in their courses, both thyroid deficiency (Whybrow et al. 1969) and B_{12} deficiency (Lindenbaum et al. 1988; Strachan and Henderson 1965) can manifest as a reversible delirium. However, if thyroid deficiency or B_{12} deficiency persists, neuronal loss and dementia ensue, and full recovery of cognitive function rarely occurs (Clarnette and Patterson 1994; Martin et al. 1992; Nilsson et al. 2000; Wang et al. 2001).

Although the routine inclusion of a computed tomography (CT) scan or magnetic resonance image of the brain in the evaluation of late-life cognitive impairment has been debated since Larson and colleagues' (1986) evaluation of the cost-effectiveness of these neuroimaging diagnostic procedures, they continue to be part of the standard diagnostic evaluation in most centers, particularly the evaluation of patients with early onset of cognitive impairment or with an atypical presentation.

Cognition Evaluation

Use of a formal cognitive rating scale should be part of the standard evaluation of an older patient with acquired cognitive impairment. The Mini-Mental State Exam (MMSE; Folstein et al. 1975) is a brief and easily performed test that has proved to be widely useful. The MMSE permits the clinician to obtain data about orientation, registration and recall of information, attention, calculation, language, praxis, basic executive functioning, and visual-spatial skills. Although the MMSE is not designed for the differential diagnosis of the various specific dementia disorders, it provides a useful snapshot of overall cognitive function. Despite psychometric shortcomings, the MMSE has gained extremely wide acceptance as a means both of estimating cognitive function and of following changes in cognitive function over time. Longer cognitive evaluation instruments such as the Mattis Dementia Rating Scale (Mattis 1976) allow a more comprehensive evaluation of cognitive function and are useful if neuropsychological testing resources are available. The Mattis Dementia Rating Scale is a reliable instrument that correlates well with the functional capacity of patients with AD (Vitaliano et al. 1984). The Alzheimer's Disease Assessment Scale—Cognitive subscale (ADAS-Cog; Rosen et al. 1984) has been widely used in clinical trials of cognition-affecting drugs and allows reference of an individual patient's cognitive status to large published data sets from these studies.

Reversible Causes of Dementia

The search for reversible causes of cognitive impairment in the older patient must be actively continued. Unfortunately, such reversible disorders are the exception rather than the rule. Although early reports suggested that potentially correctable disorders causing cognitive impairment would be detected by a careful evaluation in up to 30% of patients with acquired cognitive loss (Fox et al. 1975; Freeman 1976; Victoratos et al. 1977), Larson and co-workers (1984) reported a more realistic yield of truly correctable disorders impairing cognitive function. These investigators conducted comprehensive outpatient diagnostic evaluations of patients with late-onset cognitive disorders. Of 107 unselected elderly outpatients referred for evaluation of global cognitive impairment of at least 3 months' duration, only 15 had potentially reversible disorders possibly related to their cognitive loss. Six patients with apparent cognitive loss secondary to adverse effects of medications formed the largest single group. Other potentially reversible causes of cognitive loss that were identified included hypothyroidism, subdural hematoma, and rheumatoid or lupus cerebrovasculitis. In only 3 of the 107 patients evaluated was there a proven reversible cause of cognitive loss, as demonstrated by return to normal cognitive function after treatment. One of these patients had a subdural hematoma, another had mixed-drug toxicity, and the third had rheumatoid cerebrovasculitis. Two of these 3 patients presented with only subtle and mild cognitive deficits. Furthermore, of the 13 patients in the series who were judged to have reversible cognitive deficits at intake evaluation and who were available for follow-up over a 2-year period, 3 of the 4 patients with hypothyroidism, 1 patient with subdural hematoma, and 4 of the 6 patients with behavioral toxicity associated with pharmacotherapy subsequently developed progressive cognitive deterioration consistent with AD.

The results of this study suggest that the most important parts of the diagnostic evaluation of a cognitively impaired older person are the attempt a) to delineate the specific disease causing dementia and b) to uncover the treatable or general medical and psychiatric disorders that may be exacerbating the cognitive deficits caused by a primary dementia disorder. However, clinicians should always keep in mind that unusual medically or surgically reversible disorders resembling dementia caused by a neurodegenerative disorder will occasionally present in a busy geriatric practice. Examples of such reversible disorders include frontal meningioma (Avery 1971), NPH (Adams et al. 1965), hypothyroidism (Larson et al. 1984), cerebrovasculitis (Larson et al. 1984), and subdural hematoma (Ishikawa et al. 2002). These disorders will be overlooked unless clinicians continue to carefully evaluate atypical presentations of cognitive impairment.

TABLE 6–2. DSM-IV-TR diagnostic criteria for dementia of the Alzheimer's type

A. The development of multiple cognitive deficits manifested by both

(1) memory impairment (impaired ability to learn new information or to recall previously learned information)

(2) one (or more) of the following cognitive disturbances:

(a) aphasia (language disturbance)

(b) apraxia (impaired ability to carry out motor activities despite intact motor function)

(c) agnosia (failure to recognize or identify objects despite intact sensory function)

(d) disturbance in executive functioning (i.e., planning, organizing, sequencing, abstracting)

B. The cognitive deficits in Criteria A1 and A2 each cause significant impairment in social or occupational functioning and represent a significant decline from a previous level of functioning.

C. The course is characterized by gradual onset and continuing cognitive decline.

D. The cognitive deficits in Criteria A1 and A2 are not due to any of the following:

(1) other central nervous system conditions that cause progressive deficits in memory and cognition (e.g., cerebrovascular disease, Parkinson's disease, Huntington's disease, subdural hematoma, normal-pressure hydrocephalus, brain tumor)

(2) systemic conditions that are known to cause dementia (e.g., hypothyroidism, vitamin B_{12} or folic acid deficiency, niacin deficiency, hypercalcemia, neurosyphilis, HIV infection)

(3) substance-induced conditions

E. The deficits do not occur exclusively during the course of a delirium.

F. The disturbance is not better accounted for by another Axis I disorder (e.g., Major Depressive Disorder, Schizophrenia).

Code based on presence or absence of a clinically significant behavioral disturbance:

294.10 Without Behavioral Disturbance: if the cognitive disturbance is not accompanied by any clinically significant behavioral disturbance.

294.11 With Behavioral Disturbance: if the cognitive disturbance is accompanied by a clinically significant behavioral disturbance (e.g., wandering, agitation).

Specify subtype:

With Early Onset: if onset is at age 65 years or below

With Late Onset: if onset is after age 65 years

Coding note: Also code 331.0 Alzheimer's disease on Axis III. Indicate other prominent clinical features related to the Alzheimer's disease on Axis I (e.g., 293.83 Mood Disorder Due to Alzheimer's Disease, With Depressive Features, and 310.1 Personality Change Due to Alzheimer's Disease, Aggressive Type).

Specific Diseases Causing Dementia

Alzheimer's Disease

The majority of patients with late-life dementia of insidious onset and a progressive deteriorating course have AD (Katzman 1976). In DSM-IV-TR, the term *dementia of the Alzheimer's type* is used, but *Alzheimer's disease* is the much more generally accepted term for this devastating disease. Diagnostic criteria for AD are presented in Table 6–2. Technically, AD is a combined clinical and neuropathological diagnosis that can be made definitively only when a patient meeting antemortem clinical criteria for AD is found at postmortem examination to have the histopathological changes of AD (numerous neuritic plaques and neurofibrillary tangles in the hippocampus and neocortex). A work group convened by the National Institute of Neurological Disorders and Stroke and by the Alzheimer's Disease and Related Disorders Association (now known as the Alzheimer's Association) developed the term *probable AD* to denote the condition of persons meeting antemortem clinical criteria for AD (McKhann et al. 1984).

A clinician of the 1960s would be mystified today at the emphasis placed on what was considered then to be a relatively uncommon "presenile" dementia disorder. That AD is now regarded as the most important neuropsychiatric disorder of later life would be difficult for the 1960s clinician to comprehend. This "epidemic" of AD can be attributed largely to increased knowledge of the etiology of dementia in later life. Before the landmark studies by Blessed et al. (1968), the large number of persons who developed dementia after age 65—"senile dementia"—were believed to have cerebrovascular insufficiency. Blessed et al. (1968) performed a careful neuropathological and neurohistological study of senile dementia in elderly patients. In 70% of these patients, the only neuropathological lesions found were the neuritic plaques and neurofibrillary tangles described by Alzheimer in 1907 (Alzheimer 1907/1987) in his patient with early-onset dementia. Only in approximately 15% of patients with late-onset dementia could cognitive impairment be attributed to sequelae of cerebrovascular disease—specifically, infarcted brain tissue, which caused vascular dementia. Another 15% had neuropathology of both AD and vascular dementia. Multiple studies have confirmed that a dementia of insidious onset and with a gradually progressive course—whether beginning before or after age 65—is usually AD (Katzman 1986).

The likelihood that an antemortem diagnosis of AD by current DSM-IV-TR criteria or by National Institute of Neurological Disorders and Stroke–Alzheimer's Disease and Related Disorders Association criteria will be confirmed at postmortem examination is at least 85% (Joachim et al. 1988; Morris et al. 1988; Tierney et al. 1988). This is an excellent rate of antemortem diagnostic accuracy, and it compares favorably with that for many common general medical disorders in which the high probability of an accurate antemortem clinical diagnosis is widely accepted. The clinician should not think that AD is a difficult diagnosis that can be made only after exclusion of a long list of both common and uncommon disorders with the potential to produce dementia. In an older person in whom dementia begins insidiously and progresses gradually but inexorably, the diagnostic plaques and tangles of AD are highly likely to be found at neuropathological examination. Diagnostic certainty is further enhanced if the patient has no history of stroke, alcoholism, preexistent Parkinson's disease, or poorly controlled hypertension.

Relatively recent studies have added new complexity to the specific diagnosis of late-life dementia. First, careful neuroimaging and neuropathological studies of predominantly old-old (mean age > 80 years) persons with dementia suggest that vascular lesions together with AD lesions commonly contribute to the clinical expression of dementia (i.e., mixed dementia) (Skoog et al. 1994; Snowdon et al. 1997). Second, more sensitive immunostains for Lewy bodies (the classic substantia nigra lesions of Parkinson's disease) have frequently revealed Lewy bodies in limbic brain and neocortex together with the plaques and tangles of AD—a condition called *dementia with Lewy bodies* (DLB) (Kotzbauer et al. 2001; McKeith et al. 1996; R.H. Perry et al. 1990). Mixed dementia and DLB are discussed more fully later in the chapter (see "Vascular Dementia" and "Dementia With Lewy Bodies").

Course

AD begins insidiously. Subtle difficulties in recent memory are almost always the first sign. Personality changes also occur early and manifest most often as apathy and loss of interest in persons and activities. Memory impairment gradually becomes more severe, and deficits in other cognitive domains—particularly executive functioning and visual-spatial skills—appear. Usually after several years of cognitive impairment, a fluent type of aphasia begins, characterized by difficulty in naming objects or choosing the right word to express an idea. Apraxia often occurs concurrently, and this loss of the ability to perform often routine motor activities, such as eating with utensils or dressing, places care burdens on the patient's family and other care providers. In the later stages of AD, many patients develop disrupted sleep-wake cycles; wander; have episodes of irritability, agitation, and psychosis; and lose their ability to attend to personal care needs such as dressing, feeding, and personal hygiene. Motor signs, such as rigidity and myoclonic jerks and seizures, occur in subgroups of patients, particularly those with early-onset AD (i.e., beginning before age 70) (Risse et al. 1990a). The duration of the illness is rarely less than 5 years and may extend to more than 15 years.

Epidemiology

Prevalence studies suggest that approximately 5% of persons older than 65 years and 20% of persons older than 80 years have dementia severe enough to impair their ability to live independently (Mortimer 1983). It can be assumed that the majority of these persons have AD. The results of a classic study performed in East Boston, Massachusetts, suggest that the prevalence of AD in later life may be even higher (Evans et al. 1989). Evaluation of all non-institutionalized persons age 65 or older in this geographically defined community of 32,000 individuals revealed an estimated AD prevalence rate of 10% among those older than 65 years and 47% among those older than 85 years. Even when data from persons with mild cognitive impairment were excluded, fully 8% of the individuals older than 65 years and 36% of those older than 85 years had moderate to severe cognitive impairment sufficient to limit their ability to live independently.

Pathogenesis and Pathophysiology

Attempts to understand basic mechanisms underlying AD have focused on several areas. One of these areas is the neurobiology of the formation and potential neurotoxic effects of the histopathological hallmarks of AD: neuritic plaques and neurofibrillary tangles (and their component proteins). In addition, studies have identified rare genetic mutations on chromosomes 1, 14, and 21 that cause AD in families with early-onset autosomal dominant heritable AD (Levy-Lahad et al. 1995; Mullan et al. 1992; Schellenberg et al. 1992; Sherrington et al. 1995). Also, a polymorphism has been identified in the *APOE* gene in which the ε4 allele increases the risk of AD in families with the more common late-onset sporadic AD (Corder et al. 1993). Epidemiologic studies continue to be conducted for the purpose of determining which environmental exposures or biologic variables have increased prevalence among persons with AD. An extensive discussion of these neurobiologic, genetic, and epidemiologic studies is beyond the scope of this chapter, but we will review some aspects of this research that are pertinent to a general understanding of AD.

Abnormalities of brain proteins beta-amyloid and tau. Efforts in multiple laboratories have been directed toward understanding the possible role of β-amyloid (the major protein constituent of neuritic plaques) and the cytoskeleton protein tau (the major component of neurofibrillary tangles) in the pathogenesis of AD. β-Amyloid was first sequenced by Glenner and Wong (1984) from congophilic angiopathic deposits in postmortem brain tissue from patients with AD. β-Amyloid is a cleavage product of a normally expressed brain protein that is possibly involved in neuronal repair, amyloid precursor protein (APP) (Rosenberg 1993). The hypothesis that β-amyloid is involved in the pathogenesis of AD (Selkoe 2000) is supported by data from the rare families in whom point mutations in the APP gene on chromosome 21 (Mullan et al. 1992), the presenilin 1 gene on chromosome 14 (Schellenberg et al. 1992), and the presenilin 2 gene on chromosome 1 (Levy-Lahad et al. 1995) segregate with AD. Each of these mutations is associated with increased concentrations of β-amyloid (particularly the more neurotoxic β-amyloid 42).

The major constituent of neurofibrillary tangles is a hyperphosphorylated form of the microtubule-associated phosphoprotein tau. Several factors have increased interest in the protein chemistry of tau and tau's role in neuronal degeneration in AD. The correlation between the density of postmortem neurofibrillary tangles and antemortem cognitive deficits is more robust than that between neuritic plaques and cognitive deficits (Snowdon et al. 1997). Normal tau function enhances the formation and stability of intraneuronal microtubules. Dysfunctional tau, therefore, would disrupt critically important aspects of neuronal function. The tau in neurofibrillary tangles

(and in the dystrophic neurites associated with senile plaques) is hyperphosphorylated (Mitchell et al. 2002). It appears that this hyperphosphorylation results from the failure of phosphatases to normally remove phosphate moieties from the tau molecule (Trojanowski and Lee 1995). Therefore, enhancing appropriate phosphatase activity is one potential AD therapeutic goal (Iqbal et al. 1999). That abnormal tau function can produce dementia in the absence of β-amyloid plaque deposition has been demonstrated convincingly in patients with familial frontotemporal dementia (FTD) (Sumi et al. 1992). In such patients, mutations in the tau gene on chromosome 17 are sufficient to produce dementia (Hutton et al. 1998; Poorkaj et al. 1998; Wilhelmsen et al. 1999), and deposits of β-amyloid are absent histologically.

Hypothalamic-pituitary-adrenal axis. It has been suggested that identification of the hypothalamic-pituitary-adrenal (HPA) axis changes that occur in patients with primary major depression would be helpful in the differential diagnosis of dementia and depression. Specifically, it was hypothesized that administration of the dexamethasone suppression test (DST) would be useful (McAllister et al. 1982; Rudorfer and Clayton 1981). Because resistance to suppression of the HPA axis by the potent synthetic glucocorticoid dexamethasone had been demonstrated in patients with a severe major depressive episode (Carroll et al. 1981), it was suggested that positive DST results—failure of a late-evening dose of dexamethasone to suppress plasma cortisol to below a predetermined level the following day—in a patient with acquired cognitive impairment and depressive signs and symptoms would favor the diagnosis of either primary major depressive episode or secondary major depressive episode complicating dementia. Unfortunately, it soon became apparent that such positive DST findings occurred as frequently in patients with AD uncomplicated by depression as in those with a primary major depressive episode (Raskind et al. 1982; Spar and Gerner 1982).

Although the demonstrations of increased HPA axis activity in AD (and in vascular dementia) negated the diagnostic utility of the DST, it remains possible that this neuroendocrine abnormality plays a role in the pathophysiology of AD. A growing body of evidence suggests that increased HPA axis activity in aging (Raskind et al. 1994)—a phenomenon that is exaggerated in patients with AD or vascular dementia (Balldin et al. 1983; Davis et al. 1986)—may lower the threshold for the neuronal loss of AD (Peskind et al. 2001; Sapolsky et al. 1987) (see "Abnormalities of Brain Neurotransmitters" following discussion of genetic risk factors below).

APOE epsilon-4 genetic risk factor.
Apolipoprotein E (apoE) has long been of interest to cardiologists for its involvement in cholesterol and lipid transport and for the effect of the genetic polymorphisms of *APOE* (*APOE* ε2, *APOE* ε3, and *APOE* ε4) on the risk of heart disease (Mahley and Huang 1999). Observations initially made at the Duke University Alzheimer's Disease Research Center (Corder et al. 1993) and repeatedly confirmed by many other investigators (Mahley and Huang 1999) demonstrated that *APOE* genotype has a major effect on the expression of AD. Specifically, the ε4 allele (the second most common *APOE* allele) clearly increases the risk of AD, and the ε2 allele (the least common allele) appears to decrease the risk of AD. It is important to recognize that presence of one or two ε4 alleles increases AD risk but is not causative of AD. Some persons carrying one or even two copies of the ε4 allele never develop AD, and many persons not carrying

the ε4 allele do develop AD. In contrast, persons who carry the rare causative mutations for familial AD on chromosome 21 (in the APP gene), chromosome 14 (in the presenilin 1 gene), or chromosome 1 (in the presenilin 2 gene) will certainly develop AD if they live to the age of risk.

Despite intensive investigation, the mechanism by which the ε4 allele increases the risk of AD remains unclear. Differential effects of *APOE* alleles on β-amyloid deposition and on cytoskeletal stabilization are among the proposed mechanisms. Peskind et al. (2001) recently reported a potential mechanism for *APOE* genotype effects on AD risk that builds on the reported neurotoxic effect of high levels of cortisol (corticosterone in rodents) on hippocampal neurons (Sapolsky et al. 1987) and the aging-dependent effect of the ε4 allele to increase corticosterone concentrations in rodents (Raber et al. 2000). Peskind and colleagues (2001) measured cortisol concentrations in cerebrospinal fluid (CSF) of healthy older persons who had unimpaired cognition and of persons with AD. CSF cortisol levels varied by *APOE* genotype: subjects with the ε4 allele had higher CSF cortisol levels than did those homozygous for the ε3 allele, who in turn had higher CSF cortisol concentrations than did subjects with an ε2 allele. This pattern is consistent with the risk of AD that these alleles confer (Corder et al. 1993).

Abnormalities of brain neurotransmitters

Serotonin deficiency and SSRI treatment of depression. In patients with AD, there is a clear deficiency in brain serotonergic systems, manifested by loss of serotonergic neurons in the brain stem raphe nuclei (Mann and Yates 1983; Yamamoto and Hirano 1985), decreased concentrations of serotonin and its metabolite in brain tissue (Arai et al. 1984; D'Amato et al. 1987) and CSF (Blennow et al. 1991; Volicer et al. 1985), and decreased serotonin receptor concentrations (Cross et al. 1984). This serotonin deficiency may be relevant to the pathophysiology and treatment of depressive signs and symptoms seen in some patients with AD. Scandinavian studies demonstrated that in persons with AD or vascular dementia, the selective serotonin reuptake inhibitor (SSRI) citalopram is more effective than placebo for signs and symptoms of depression as well as for anxiety and other nonpsychotic behavioral disturbances (Nyth et al. 1992). A preliminary study of sertraline therapy in AD patients with depression found that this SSRI reduced depression ratings more effectively than did placebo (Lyketsos et al. 2000). In these studies, SSRI adverse effects were uncommon. Although outcome data from well-designed treatment trials remain scant, SSRIs have become the first choice for management of depressive signs and symptoms complicating AD. That nonpharmacological approaches can reduce depressive signs and symptoms in AD patients was confirmed by a trial in which behaviorally oriented psychotherapy effectively reduced depression in both AD patients and their caregivers (Teri 1994).

The noradrenergic system: possible contribution of compensatory upregulation to disruptive agitation.   Another major neurotransmitter system affected in AD is the brain noradrenergic system. Studies of postmortem brain tissue have consistently demonstrated neuronal loss in the locus coeruleus (the major source of noradrenergic neurons innervating the CNS) in patients with AD (Bondareff et al. 1982; Mann et al. 1980; Tomlinson et al. 1981). Locus coeruleus neuronal loss at first suggests a brain noradrenergic deficiency in AD. On the other hand, studies

measuring levels of both norepinephrine and its major metabolite, methoxyhydroxyphenylglycol (MHPG), in postmortem brain tissue have demonstrated an increased ratio of MHPG to norepinephrine in AD, suggesting increased norepinephrine turnover in locus coeruleus projection areas (Francis et al. 1985; Palmer et al. 1987; Winblad et al. 1982). Furthermore, norepinephrine and MHPG concentrations in CSF are normal or even increased in patients with AD, particularly in those who are in the later stages of the disease (Gibson et al. 1985; Raskind et al. 1984). An increased ratio of MHPG to locus coeruleus noradrenergic neuronal number in AD postmortem tissue suggests that compensatory upregulation of surviving locus coeruleus neurons might explain the above findings (Hoogendijk et al. 1999).

A recent study by Szot et al. (2000) using postmortem brain tissue supported that compensatory upregulation of locus coeruleus noradrenergic neurons occurs in AD and is associated with antemortem disruptive agitation. These investigators found increased messenger RNA expression for tyrosine hydroxylase (the rate-limiting synthetic enzyme for norepinephrine) in surviving locus coeruleus neurons in AD subjects with a history of disruptive agitation. Taken together with the finding of increased density of adrenergic postsynaptic receptors in AD subjects with antemortem aggressive behavior (Russo-Neustadt and Cotman 1997), these data suggest that enhanced responsiveness to brain noradrenergic outflow may contribute to the pathophysiology of disruptive agitation in AD. Support for this hypothesis in living AD patients was provided by Peskind et al. (1995), who demonstrated robust increases in CSF norepinephrine levels after yohimbine administration in both AD subjects and older subjects without dementia, but only AD subjects had meaningful increases in agitation ratings after CNS noradrenergic stimulation. These findings suggest that antagonism of locus coeruleus noradrenergic outflow with an α_2-adrenergic agonist (e.g., guanfacine, clonidine), blockade of postsynaptic β-adrenoceptors (e.g., with propranolol), or blockade of postsynaptic α_1-adrenoceptors (e.g., with prazosin) might relieve disruptive agitation in AD. Studies of these approaches are currently under way.

The presynaptic cholinergic deficit. The search for abnormalities in brain neurotransmitter systems in AD that might be correctable by pharmacological treatment (that would result in subsequent symptomatic improvement) received impetus from the successful use of L-dopa to correct the brain dopamine deficiency in Parkinson's disease. That such a strategy might succeed in AD became plausible in the late 1970s with the discovery of a deficit in the brain presynaptic cholinergic system in postmortem brain tissue from patients with AD (Davies and Maloney 1976; E.K. Perry et al. 1978). This hypothesis regarding cholinergic deficiency received further support when Whitehouse and colleagues (1982) demonstrated extensive neuronal loss in the cholinergic nucleus basalis of Meynert in patients with AD. This basal forebrain magnicellular nucleus is the primary source of cholinergic projections to the neocortex and hippocampus. A brain presynaptic cholinergic deficit has also been demonstrated in vascular dementia (Erkinjuntti et al. 2002) and dementia with Lewy bodies (DLB) (E.K. Perry et al. 1994); see also "Dementia With Lewy Bodies" later in the chapter.

Advances in Therapeutics: Cholinesterase Inhibitors and NMDA Receptor Antagonists

A major step forward in AD therapeutics has been the demonstration that acetylcholinesterase inhibitors, which increase intrasynaptic acetylcholine levels, produce modest symptomatic improvement in AD and appear to slow symptomatic deterioration. Cholinesterase inhibitors have been demonstrated to be effective and are indicated for the mild to moderate stages of AD (usually defined arbitrarily as stages when the patient has an MMSE score of 10–24) (Farlow et al. 1992; Raskind et al. 2000; Rogers et al. 1998). These drugs improve cognitive function only modestly. They are best conceptualized as drugs that "stabilize" cognition, activities of daily living, and behavioral function and that slow clinical deterioration in AD. Stabilization of cognition and functioning for approximately 1 year has been demonstrated with both galantamine and donepezil (Raskind et al. 2000; Winblad et al. 2001).

The fact that cholinesterase inhibitors are formally indicated for only the mild to moderate stages of AD does not preclude their having positive effects in patients with more advanced disease; more severely impaired patients also seem to benefit from these agents (Feldman et al. 2001; Tariot et al. 2000).

It also appears that cholinesterase inhibitors are effective in DLB (McKeith et al. 2000), vascular dementia, and mixed dementia (combined vascular dementia and AD) (Erkinjuntti et al. 2002). A consensus is emerging that cholinesterase inhibitor therapy should be started as soon as AD, DLB, vascular dementia, or mixed dementia becomes apparent and that treatment should be continued at least into moderately advanced stages of disease, provided the drug is well tolerated. The broadening spectrum of dementia disorders for which cholinesterase inhibitors are effective simplifies the differential diagnosis.

Tacrine was the first cholinesterase inhibitor demonstrated to be effective in AD (Knapp et al. 1994). However, hepatic toxicity has rendered this drug obsolete in AD treatment. Second-generation cholinesterase inhibitors have been shown to be as effective as tacrine and are free of hepatic toxicity. They are discussed here in the order of their introduction into clinical practice.

Donepezil was demonstrated to have positive effects on cognitive and overall function in several placebo-controlled trials involving AD patients with mild to moderate disease (Rogers and Friedhoff 1996; Rogers et al. 1998). Mean differences between active treatment and placebo approached 3 points on the Alzheimer's Disease Assessment Scale–Cognitive subscale (ADAS-Cog) in these multicenter studies. A northern European multicenter study compared donepezil and placebo, given for 12 months (Winblad et al. 2001). The condition of donepezil-treated patients remained significantly superior to the condition of patients who received placebo, and on average, scores on the MMSE did not significantly deteriorate from baseline. The 10-mg dose of donepezil administered once daily offers some advantage in terms of efficacy, but the 5-mg dose is also effective and is better tolerated. As is the case with all cholinesterase inhibitors, gastrointestinal symptoms—particularly nausea and vomiting (CNS cholinergic effects) and diarrhea (likely a peripheral cholinergic effect)—are the most frequent adverse effects (occurring in 10%–20% of patients given the 10-mg dose). Several recent studies demonstrated that donepezil is effective for maintaining levels of cognition and behavior in AD patients (including persons in long-term care) with dementia that is more severe than that of subjects who participated in the original Phase III trials (Feldman et al. 2001; Tariot et al. 2000). Donepezil may also be effective in vascular dementia (Pratt and Perdomo 2002). It remains the most frequently prescribed cholinesterase inhibitor.

Rivastigmine has been demonstrated to be more effective than placebo for main-taining cognitive function, global function, and activities of daily living in patients with AD. In multicenter placebo-controlled studies, there was approximately a 4-point difference on the ADAS-Cog between high-dose rivastigmine (6–12 mg/day) and placebo (Corey-Bloom 1998; Rösler et al. 1999). At these doses, gastrointestinal adverse effects such as nausea, vomiting, and diarrhea were relatively common (occurring in 40% of patients). In addition to inhibiting acetylcholinesterase, rivastigmine inhibits butyrylcholinesterase. The clinical meaningfulness of this latter effect remains to be determined, but butyrylcholinesterase appears to regulate brain acetylcholine levels in animal studies (Mesulam et al. 2002). Rivastigmine is the only cholinesterase inhibitor to have been compared with placebo in DLB. McKeith et al. (2000) found that rivastigmine was superior to placebo with regard to effects on cognitive deficits and on behavioral problems that are particularly prominent in DLB.

Galantamine is a reversible cholinesterase inhibitor that has the additional pharmacological effect of positively modulating nicotinic acetylcholine receptor responsiveness at an allosteric binding site (Maelicke et al. 2001). Because there is a prominent nicotinic cholinergic deficiency in AD (E.K. Perry et al. 1985), this additional action is potentially meaningful clinically. In large multicenter placebo-controlled trials (Raskind et al. 2000; Wilcock et al. 2000), galantamine was significantly superior to placebo in terms of effects on cognitive function, with an almost 4-point difference from placebo on the ADAS-Cog (Raskind et al. 2000). On average, ADAS-Cog scores of subjects who continued taking galantamine (24 mg/day) for an additional 6 months in an open extension of the United States study (Raskind et al. 2000) remained at the pretreatment baseline for the 1-year treatment trial, a finding that supports the concept of long-term symptomatic stabilization by galantamine. Activities of daily living, such as dressing and participating in activities, also remained stable for 12 months in patients receiving galantamine 24 mg/day for 1 year. AD subjects originally randomized to placebo for 6 months and then administered open-label galantamine failed to catch up with those who received galantamine for the entire 12 months. This finding is consistent with slowing of disease progression by galantamine therapy.

Similar long-term follow-up data suggesting slowed disease progression have emerged from studies of donepezil (Doody et al. 2001; Mohs et al. 2001) and rivastigmine (Farlow et al. 2000). In another multicenter placebo-controlled trial, patients randomized to either 16 or 24 mg of galantamine per day demonstrated better cognitive function and activities of daily living status than did AD patients randomized to placebo (Tariot et al. 2000). This study used a slow-dose titration schedule (increasing 8 mg every 4 weeks to a maximum of 24 mg/day), which minimized gastrointestinal adverse effects to a level comparable to that associated with administration of 10 mg of donepezil (10%–20%). In addition, galantamine decreased the emergence of behavioral problems as quantified by the Neuropsychiatric Inventory. Erkinjuntti et al. (2002) conducted a 6-month, multicenter, placebo-controlled study of galantamine in vascular dementia and mixed dementia. Galantamine was significantly superior to placebo with regard to effects on cognition, functioning, and behavior.

Memantine

Memantine is an uncompetitive low-to-moderate-affinity N-methyl-D-aspartate (NMDA) receptor antagonist. Its mechanism of action may be related to regulation of activity of glutamate, a neurotransmitter involved in information processing, storage, and retrieval. Glutamate stimulation of NMDA receptors increases neuronal calcium influx, presumably leading to information storage. Excessive glutamate stimulation of NMDA receptors dramatically increases calcium flow into neurons, leading to pathway disruption and cell death. Memantine may protect against the effects of excess glutamate by partially blocking NMDA receptors.

Memantine has been shown to be efficacious in moderate-to-severe Alzheimer's disease. In one study, 252 patients were randomly assigned to receive placebo or 20 mg of memantine daily for 28 weeks (Reisberg et al. 2003). Of these, 181 (72%) completed the study and were evaluated at week 28. Seventy-one patients discontinued treatment prematurely (42 taking placebo and 29 taking memantine). Patients receiving memantine had a better outcome than those receiving placebo, as measured by the Clinician's Interview-Based Impression of Change Plus Caregiver Input, Severe Impairment Battery, and Alzheimer's Disease Cooperative Study Activities of Daily Living Inventory, which was modified for more severe dementia. In this study memantine was not associated with a significant frequency of adverse events.

Memantine has also been studied as an adjunctive therapy in AD. In one 24-week study of 404 patients with moderate to severe AD receiving stable doses of donepezil, memantine resulted in significantly better outcomes than placebo on measures of cognition, activities of daily living, global outcome, and behavior (Tariot et al. 2004). The combination was well tolerated.

Other Approaches to Cognitive Enhancement

Vitamin E and selegiline.   Oxidative damage may contribute to neuronal degeneration and death in AD (reviewed in Sano et al. 1997). On the basis of this putative pathogenic mechanism, drugs with antioxidant activity have been evaluated for their effects on both cognitive and functional decline. In a large multicenter trial, the National Institute on Aging–supported Alzheimer's Disease Cooperative Study evaluated two such drugs—vitamin E and selegiline—singly and in combination, in AD outpatients with moderately advanced disease (Sano et al. 1997). Both vitamin E and selegiline were more effective than placebo in delaying deterioration to functional end points that included nursing home placement, progression to severe dementia, and substantial loss of basic activities of daily living or death. The combination of vitamin E and selegiline was no more effective than either agent alone. Neither agent had beneficial effects on cognitive function per se. Given its low toxicity and low cost, vitamin E should be considered as a part of the regimen of persons with AD. The dose of vitamin E used in this study, 1,000 U given twice daily, was well tolerated.

Ginkgo biloba. Extracts of the leaf of the ginkgo biloba tree have been used in traditional Chinese medications and may have antioxidant as well as stimulant and anti-inflammatory properties. In a multicenter, randomized, double-blind, placebo-controlled trial involving outpatients with AD or vascular dementia, a standardized extract of ginkgo biloba had small (less than half the effect of cholinesterase inhibitors) but statistically significant effects on cognitive function as measured by the ADAS-Cog (Le Bars et al. 1997). However, there was no effect on clinicians' ratings of global function. Interpreting the study results is difficult because the drop-out rate was very high (>50% in both groups) and because possible positive effects on mood that could have contributed to the slightly positive cognitive results were not reported. In a second multicenter, placebo-controlled study of ginkgo, involving persons with either AD, vascular dementia, or age-associated memory impairment, all of whom lived in Dutch homes for the elderly, results were negative. No significant differences were found in outcome measures between persons randomized to ginkgo and those randomized to placebo. Currently under way is a large, multicenter, National Institute on Aging–supported, AD prevention trial of ginkgo in healthy elderly subjects.

Estrogen replacement therapy. Estrogens have neuroprotective effects in preclinical studies, and most (but not all) epidemiologic studies suggest that estrogen replacement therapy decreases the risk of AD in postmenopausal women (reviewed in Mulnard et al. 2000). A small placebo-controlled trial of estradiol in AD demonstrated positive effects on cognitive function (Asthana et al. 1999). However, a recently reported 1-year, multicenter, randomized placebo-controlled trial performed by the Alzheimer's Disease Cooperative Study demonstrated no benefit from treatment with Premarin (a preparation of mixed conjugated equine estrogens that is widely used clinically) in persons with AD (Mulnard et al. 2000). A similar negative result was achieved in a 16-week trial of Premarin in AD subjects (Henderson et al. 2000). Large placebo-controlled prevention studies are under way to determine whether administration of Premarin to cognitively intact postmenopausal women reduces the incidence of AD and age-associated memory impairment. The results of the trial conducted by Asthana et al. (1999) raise the possibility that transdermal estradiol may be more effective than Premarin in counteracting the pathophysiology of AD.

Nonsteroidal anti-inflammatory drugs (NSAIDs). Neuropathological data demonstrate an intense immune response associated with β-amyloid–containing neuritic plaques (McGeer and McGeer 1999; Wyss-Coray and Mucke 2000). This response raises the possibility that an autoimmunity-like phenomenon contributes to neuronal damage in AD. This hypothesis is supported by epidemiologic studies suggesting that NSAIDs decrease the risk of AD in cognitively intact older persons (Breitner and Zandi 2001; in t' Veld et al. 2001; McGeer et al. 1996). Unfortunately, a multicenter placebo-controlled trial of the anti-inflammatory steroid prednisone failed to demonstrate positive effects on cognition or disease progression in AD (Aisen et al. 2000). Similarly, a recently completed placebo-controlled trial of the standard NSAID naproxen and the cyclo-oxygenase-2–specific NSAID rofecoxib yielded negative results (Thal 2002). However, the following hypothesis remains viable: NSAIDs reduce the risk of expression of AD in unaffected elders but the drugs are no longer effective after AD is clinically expressed (Breitner and Zandi 2001). Furthermore, the protective mechanism may not be the suppression of inflammation. A recent study demonstrated that the NSAIDs ibuprofen, indomethacin, and sulindac decreased β-amyloid production, whereas the NSAIDs naproxen, celecoxib, and rofecoxib did not (Weggen et al. 2001). A large-scale, prevention trial of naproxen and celecoxib in older healthy individuals is currently under way (Breitner and Zandi 2001). However, the recent preclinical demonstration that naproxen and celecoxib do not decrease β-amyloid production raises concern that the wrong NSAIDs may have been selected for evaluation.

Reducing beta-amyloid generation.
Given the multiple levels of evidence supporting a pathogenic role of β-amyloid aggregation and deposition in the expression of AD (Selkoe 2000), substantial resources have been directed toward basic studies

designed to develop approaches to reduce generation of β-amyloid from APP, its precursor protein molecule. APP has alternate cleavage pathways. Cleavage by the enzyme α-secretase occurs within the β-amyloid fragment, preventing β-amyloid production. In contrast, cleavage by the enzymes β-secretase (or BACE; β site APP cleavage enzyme) and then γ-secretase generates β-amyloid. With the recent identification of β-secretase and γ-secretase, which are necessary for the generation of β-amyloid (Selkoe 2000), opportunities now exist for inhibiting these enzymes in order to redirect APP metabolism toward nonamyloidogenic and presumably nonneurotoxic APP fragments. Protease inhibitors of β-secretase and γ-secretase are in the preclinical stages of development.

Beta-amyloid immunization.
β-Amyloid immunization is a particularly novel approach to both preventing brain β-amyloid deposition and removing β-amyloid already deposited in the brain. Substantial enthusiasm has been generated for this approach as a potentially powerful AD therapeutic. In a transgenic mouse model in which an inserted human mutated amyloid precursor protein gene led to overexpression of APP and dense amyloid plaque deposition by age 18 months, immunization with β-amyloid 1–42 early in life prevented formation of amyloid plaques (Peskind et al. 2001). In addition, immunization of these mice in middle life resulted in dramatic reductions in the amyloid plaque deposition already present. Whether this approach will be applicable in humans remains to be seen. Unfortunately, an initial clinical trial of immunization with β-amyloid in AD patients was suspended after a substantial number of β-amyloid–vaccinated AD subjects developed meningitis. Passive immunization strategies currently being developed may prove less neurotoxic than the active vaccine.

Vascular Dementia

Even in the classic studies by Blessed et al. (1968) that established AD neuritic plaques and neurofibrillary tangles as the predominant neuropathology of late-onset dementia, a subgroup of patients (approximately 25%) were found to have cerebrovascular lesions (infarcts) as the apparent primary or contributing etiology of their dementia (Tomlinson et al. 1970). Recent studies have confirmed the importance of infarcts in the etiology of dementia in the demographic group most at risk for dementia: the old-old (persons older than 80 years) (Skoog et al. 1994; Snowdon et al. 1997). Pure vascular dementia (the multi-infarct dementia of DSM-III-R [American Psychiatric Association 1987]) is relatively uncommon, characterized by stepwise progression of patchy cognitive deterioration, focal neurological signs and symptoms (other than fluent aphasia and apraxia), and a history of inadequately controlled hypertension (Zubenko 1990).

More frequently, dementia with a cerebrovascular contribution is mixed dementia—that is, progressive dementia with neuropathological findings of both cerebral infarcts and the plaques and neurofibrillary tangles of AD. Clinical-neuropathological correlation studies in community-based samples (in contrast to less representative samples derived from Alzheimer's disease center cohorts selected for antemortem characteristics) suggest that mixed dementia is more common than previously believed and may make up 10% to 30% of late-life dementia (Lim et al. 1999). It is often difficult to differentiate mixed dementia from pure AD clinically. Neuroradiologic evidence of infarcts is helpful.

Snowdon et al. (1997) described a provocative relationship between cognitive function and both AD and cerebrovascular neuropathological lesions (studied postmortem) in a carefully followed cohort of Catholic nun educators (mean age at death, 83 years) with similar life experiences and environments. Of 61 subjects meeting neuropathological criteria for AD, the 24 with infarcts had poorer cognitive function and a higher prevalence of dementia than did the 37 without infarcts. Infarcts in the basal ganglia, thalamus, or deep white matter were associated with an especially high prevalence and severity of dementia. Subjects with subcortical infarcts also had fewer postmortem AD lesions for a given amount of antemortem cognitive impairment than did subjects without subcortical infarcts. These findings suggest that infarcts lower the threshold for and increase the magnitude of dementia caused by AD.

Clinical differentiation of mixed dementia may be difficult, and this distinction appears to be increasingly irrelevant to the decision to prescribe a cholinesterase inhibitor. Galantamine was clearly demonstrated to be more effective than placebo in a large study involving persons with vascular dementia or mixed dementia (Erkinjuntti et al. 2002). A preliminary report suggests that donepezil has similar efficacy (Pratt and Perdomo 2002).

Dementia With Lewy Bodies

Lewy bodies are synaptophysin-containing cytoplasmic inclusions that are the defining histologic lesions in the substantia nigra in Parkinson's disease. During the past 15 years, it has become clear that Lewy bodies outside the substantia nigra are present in a subgroup of patients with late-onset dementia who do not have clinically typical Parkinson's disease (Kosaka et al. 1988; Leverenz and Sumi 1986). Fluctuating cognitive function, visual hallucinations, and mild parkinsonism-like bradykinesia and rigidity (but rarely tremor) often present early in the disease course in these patients, who are now regarded as having dementia with Lewy bodies (DLB) (McKeith et al. 2005). Neuropathologically, these persons have Lewy bodies in limbic and neocortical areas, in addition to having modest amounts of the neuritic plaques and neurofibrillary tangles of AD. In unusual cases, diffuse forebrain Lewy bodies are the only demonstrable neuropathological lesions. To make matters more complex, a subgroup of persons with classic Parkinson's disease develop dementia in the later stages of the disease (Mayeux et al. 1988).

Several important features of DLB are relevant to pharmacological management. Treatment of the disturbing visual hallucinations, delusions, and agitation commonly expressed in the early stages of DLB is complicated by marked sensitivity to induction or exacerbation of extrapyramidal symptoms by typical antipsychotics such as haloperidol and even by atypical antipsychotics with some dopamine D_2 receptor affinity (e.g., risperidone and even olanzapine) (Graham et al. 1998). Use of an atypical antipsychotic with a very low incidence of extrapyramidal symptom induction, such as quetiapine or low-dose clozapine (Parkinson Study Group 1999), is a reasonable approach to treating psychotic symptoms in DLB. Another important feature of DLB is a substantial presynaptic cholinergic deficit, apparently even more profound than that in AD (E.K. Perry et al. 1994). A multicenter placebo-controlled trial of the cholinesterase inhibitor rivastigmine in patients with DLB demonstrated superiority of rivastigmine over placebo with regard to effects on both cognitive and behavioral symptoms (McKeith et al. 2000).

Dementia in Parkinson's Disease

The dementia that occurs in the later stages of Parkinson's disease is manifested by impaired memory and slowness of thinking. In general, language function and praxis are preserved, although aphasia and apraxia may occur (E.K. Perry et al. 1985). In an extensive review of the prevalence of dementia among patients with Parkinson's disease, Brown and Marsden (1984) conservatively estimated that some degree of dementia occurs in 20% of such patients. Mayeux and colleagues (1988), using standardized criteria for dementia and idiopathic Parkinson's disease, found a dementia prevalence of 11% among 339 patients with idiopathic Parkinson's disease. In this study, dementia was associated with older age, later onset of motor manifestations, more rapid progression of physical disability, and relatively poor response to L-dopa therapy. Regardless of the estimate of the prevalence of dementia in Parkinson's disease, dementia is clearly more common among such patients than among neurologically intact adults of the same age (Rajput et al. 1987). The difficult task of distinguishing between parkinsonian dementia and DLB in persons who develop dementia within a few years of developing parkinsonian motor signs is an area of ongoing investigation (Kotzbauer et al. 2001).

Frontotemporal Dementia

Frontotemporal dementia (FTD) is an evolving diagnostic category that includes a group of dementia disorders with several clinical and neurobiologic features in common but also with substantial clinical and neuropathological variability. The diagnostic category includes Pick's disease, frontal lobe degeneration of non-Alzheimer type, amyotrophic sclerosis with frontal lobe degeneration linked to chromosome 17 (FTDP-17), and corticobasal degeneration. FTD typically presents with symptoms of frontal lobe dysfunction such as impaired judgment, perseveration, impulsivity, socially inappropriate behavior, and executive dysfunction. This frontal lobe syndrome (Neary and Snowden 1996) occurs early in the disease course (when memory is only mildly impaired) and can be mistaken for substance abuse, hypomania, or personality disorder. As the disease progresses, memory and speech become severely impaired, and full dementia develops. Although this clinical course commonly occurs in Pick's disease (the classically described form of FTD [Sjogren et al. 1952]), early symptoms often vary and can resemble those of AD, depression, or even schizophrenia. Brain neuroimaging may reveal frontal and anterior temporal atrophy, but neuroradiologic findings also can be variable.

Classically described Pick's disease is a progressive disorder of middle and late life that is often difficult to distinguish from AD (Heston et al. 1987). Although rare in most neuropathological series, it may have accounted for up to 5% of the cases of late-life progressive dementia that occurred in studies in Scandinavia (Sjogren et al. 1952) and Minnesota (Heston et al. 1987). The marked cholinergic deficit of AD does not appear to occur in Pick's disease (Wood et al. 1983). Frontotemporal atrophy and microscopic changes are present in Pick's disease; the latter include neuronal cell loss, gliosis, and the presence of massed cytoskeletal elements called Pick bodies. Although affective lability and excessive eating and other oral behaviors have been described in Pick's disease (Cummings and Duchen 1981), Heston et al. (1987) often could not easily clinically distinguish patients with Pick's disease from those with AD.

It is increasingly clear that abnormal function of the cytoskeletal protein tau ("taupathy") is a central feature of most forms of FTD (Wilhelmsen et al. 1999). In an FTDP-17 family in which tau inclusion bodies were morphologically and immunochemically indistinguishable from the neurofibrillary tangles of AD (Sumi et al. 1992), Poorkaj et al. (1998) found a causative mutation in the chromosome 17q21-22 region by sequencing the tau gene. Additional tau mutations were soon described by others (Hutton et al. 1998). Because these tau mutations demonstrated that tau dysfunction is sufficient to cause neurodegenerative dementia even in the absence of brain amyloid deposits such as neuritic plaques, there is increased interest in the role of tau abnormalities in the pathogenesis of the much more common dementia disorder, AD.

Dementia Due to Normal-Pressure Hydrocephalus

Normal-pressure hydrocephalus (NPH) was described by Adams et al. (1965) as an acquired disorder characterized by a triad of signs and symptoms—dementia, gait disturbance, and urinary incontinence associated with dilation of the cerebral ventricles—but with no evidence of persistently increased intracranial pressure. Although NPH is an unusual disorder, it is an important one to identify because of the potential for neurosurgical treatment and reversibility of the dementia and other symptoms. In most cases, the etiology of NPH is unclear, but previous subarachnoid hemorrhage or meningitis probably accounts for a sizable proportion of cases. A cerebroventricular shunting procedure can markedly improve cognitive function in some cases (Friedland 1989).

Clinical factors associated with a better postoperative outcome are the complete triad of signs and symptoms, with early gait disturbance; absence of gyral atrophy; and a known etiology (Hebb and Cusimano 2001; Thomasen et al. 1986). A factor associated with poor outcome is concomitant cerebrovascular disease (Boon et al. 1999). Despite these prognostic factors, it is difficult to predict which patients with NPH will respond well to a neurosurgical shunting approach and which will not. Interestingly, the presence of brain biopsy–determined AD histopathological changes and associated cognitive deficits did not substantially affect the outcome of a shunt procedure (Golomb et al. 2000). Drainage of 20–40 mL of CSF by lumbar puncture followed by transient clinical improvement may be an indication that the patient is likely to respond to neurosurgical intervention (Wikkelso et al. 1982). The cerebroventricular shunting procedure for NPH needs to be evaluated in controlled clinical trials. That such trials have not been done is understandable, given the invasive nature of this surgical procedure, but lack of such studies limits the ability to evaluate the therapeutic benefits of neurosurgical shunting for NPH (Clarfield 1989).

Dementia Due to Hypothyroidism or Vitamin B$_{12}$ Deficiency

Although early in their course, hypothyroidism and vitamin B$_{12}$ deficiency produce a syndrome more appropriately described as a delirium, persistent deficiencies result in neuronal loss and can produce a dementia that is irreversible. Hypothyroidism classically produces a cognitive syndrome of dementia accompanied by irritability, paranoid ideation, and depression. Unfortunately, it appears that once dementia is established, even aggressive thyroid replacement therapy does not result in a return to the patient's previous level of functioning (Larson et al. 1984). Vitamin B$_{12}$ deficiency can produce dementia even in the absence of anemia or megaloblastic bone marrow changes (Strachan and Henderson 1965). Anecdotal reports suggest that B$_{12}$ replacement in dementia that is apparently secondary to B$_{12}$ deficiency may produce some cognitive improvement (Gross et al. 1986; Rajan et al. 2002;

Wieland 1986) but dementia persists. Lindenbaum et al. (1988) suggested that B$_{12}$ deficiency complicated by cognitive and other neuropsychiatric problems may be responsive to treatment with exogenous vitamin B$_{12}$. It is likely that observed improvement after B$_{12}$ treatment in older patients with dementia represents resolution of concomitant B$_{12}$-induced delirium (Nilsson et al. 2000). Increased plasma homocysteine levels may be involved in the pathophysiology of B$_{12}$-induced cognitive impairment (Wang et al. 2001), and increased plasma homocysteine concentrations may be a marker of response to treatment of B$_{12}$ deficiency in persons with dementia (Nilsson et al. 2001).

Dementia Due to Creutzfeldt-Jakob Disease

Creutzfeldt-Jakob disease is caused by a transmissible nonnucleic acid protein called a prion body. This rare disease, which affects multiple neurological systems, is characterized by a prolonged latency from exposure to expression of the disease (Prusiner and DeArmond 1990). It is rapidly fatal: death usually occurs within 2 years of the time symptoms first appear. It is rare in the elderly population, mainly occurring in persons in midlife. Dementia—an almost universal feature of this infection—is rapidly progressive and is accompanied by myoclonus, seizures, ataxia, rigidity, and other signs of widespread CNS involvement. Because AD patients (particularly those with early onset) may also demonstrate myoclonic jerks and seizures, the rapid clinical course and multiple motor system involvement that is characteristic of Creutzfeldt-Jakob disease help to differentiate between this transmissible disease (transmitted by direct contact with infected nervous system tissue) and nontransmissible AD (Mayeux et al. 1985; Risse et al. 1990b). Creutzfeldt-Jakob neurohistological changes include spongiform encephalopathy, neuronal loss, and gliosis.

Dementia Due to Neurosyphilis

Although neurosyphilis was once a common cause of dementia in later life, it has become almost unknown since the advent of widespread use of antibiotics. Given the recent increase in sexually transmitted diseases, however, neurosyphilis should be considered in the differential diagnosis of dementia. The latency from infection to development of paralytic dementia can be as long as 20 years. Considering that Venereal Disease Research Laboratory (VDRL) test results are negative in nearly one-third of patients with late syphilitic infection, the more sensitive fluorescent treponemal antibody absorption test is more likely to be diagnostic. Unfortunately, neurosyphilis may progress despite what appears to be adequate antibiotic therapy with ultrahigh-dose penicillin (Wilner and Brody 1968).

Delirium

The criteria for delirium in DSM-IV-TR emphasize disturbance of consciousness, impairment of attention, and fluctuation over the course of the day. Delirium is due to disturbance of brain physiology, usually caused by a medical disorder or an ingested substance. In contrast, diseases that produce dementia cause neuronal damage and loss. One aspect of the new DSM-IV-TR criteria for delirium should be applied cautiously: the requirement that the disturbance must have developed over a short period, usually hours to days. In the elderly patient, a delirium secondary to drugs such as long-acting benzodiazepines or to illnesses such as renal failure may have a much longer prodromal period and an insidious onset. On the other hand, it is commendable that

in DSM-IV-TR, brief duration is not specified as a criterion for delirium. In a careful study, Levkoff et al. (1992) demonstrated that incident delirium in elderly persons hospitalized for medical or surgical reasons usually persists for months. Full resolution of symptoms of delirium in a short time was the exception rather than the rule in this study.

The disturbance in level of consciousness can range from reduced wakefulness or even stupor to severe insomnia and hyperarousal. Etiological factors for delirium are numerous and include systemic medical illnesses, toxic effects of both prescribed and nonprescribed medications, metabolic disorders, and a host of other illnesses and environmental stressors (e.g., intensive care unit syndrome) (see Table 6–3). Delirium due to withdrawal from alcohol (delirium tremens) and/or sedative-hypnotic drugs can occur in older persons, and denial of drug abuse is not restricted to the young.

Treatment of delirium should be directed toward correcting the underlying disorder when that disorder can be detected. Frequently, however, symptomatic treatment becomes necessary if disruptive behaviors such as agitation, delusions, hallucinations, or angry outbursts interfere with patient management or threaten the safety of the patient or others in the environment. Reassurance from a family member or a health care professional can sometimes be helpful in managing the manifestations of delirium; however, pharmacological intervention to resolve an acute crisis may be needed. Low doses of antipsychotic medication can be helpful. Delirium secondary to withdrawal from a CNS-depressive drug such as ethanol or a benzodiazepine should be treated with a cross-tolerant sedative-hypnotic drug. An episode of delirium often is the initial presentation of an underlying dementia. In a prospective 2-year study involving previously healthy, community-dwelling

---

TABLE 6–3. Etiologies of delirium

Systemic illness
  Acquired immunodeficiency syndrome
  Burns and multiple trauma
  Congestive heart failure
  Hepatic insufficiency
  Infection
  Lupus erythematosus
  Pulmonary insufficiency
  Renal insufficiency

Metabolic disorders
  Hyperadrenocorticism
  Hypercalcemia
  Hypoadrenocorticism
  Hypoglycemia
  Hypothyroidism

Miscellaneous
  Intensive care unit syndrome
  Postoperative state (particularly cardiac
    surgery and cataract surgery)
  Withdrawal from alcohol, sedatives,
    hypnotics

Neurological disorders
  Cerebrovascular accident
  Head trauma
  Intracranial mass lesion
  Meningitis (acute and chronic)
  Neurosyphilis
  Seizure
  Subarachnoid hemorrhage

Pharmacological adverse effects
  Anticholinergic drugs
  Antiparkinsonian agents
  Antipsychotics (e.g., phenothiazines)
  Antispasmodics (e.g., belladonna)
  Bromide
  Cimetidine
  Corticosteroids
  Digitalis
  Sedatives, hypnotics
  Tricyclic antidepressants

---

elderly individuals, 28 of 51 persons admitted to the hospital because of acute delirium were found to have an underlying dementia (Rahkonen et al. 2000).

Amnestic Disorder, Alcoholic Dementia, and Wernicke-Korsakoff Syndrome

The primary deficit in amnestic disorder is memory impairment manifested as the inability to learn new information or to recall previously learned information. Although acquired impairment of memory is a central feature of dementia, the diagnosis of amnestic disorder implies a much more discrete deficit that is limited—at least in terms of substantial impairment—to memory function. Of course, careful neuropsychological evaluation often reveals deficits in other cognitive domains in persons who meet criteria for amnestic disorder.

The etiology of an amnestic disorder is usually damage to diencephalic and medial temporal lobe structures, which are important in memory function. Such damage can occur from head trauma, hypoxia, posterior cerebral artery distribution infarction, and herpes simplex encephalitis. However, the most common cause of amnestic disorder is alcoholism. The amnestic disorder caused by alcohol would be diagnosed, according to DSM-IV-TR criteria, as alcohol-induced persisting amnestic disorder. A synonymous term is *Korsakoff's psychosis*. The etiology of this disorder is often generally considered to be multiple episodes of Wernicke's encephalopathy caused by thiamine deficiency in the context of severe binge alcoholism, but direct neurotoxic effects of ethanol and its metabolite acetaldehyde (Charness 1993; Riley and Walker 1978) likely contribute to the pathogenesis of Wernicke-Korsakoff syndrome in many cases.

The diagnosis and definition of alcoholic dementia is a subject of continuing debate and controversy because there are no widely accepted standardized diagnostic or neuropathological criteria (Victor

1994). It is estimated that 10% of alcoholic individuals demonstrate permanent cognitive dysfunction (Charness 1993). Brains of alcoholic individuals exhibit atrophy of the cerebral and cerebellar cortex, corpus callosum, and deeper brain structures, including the mamillary bodies and hippocampus. Chronic alcohol users may have a number of cognitive deficits, depending on the affected brain regions. The common frontal lobe dysfunction in chronic alcohol users appears to be secondary to frontal cortical synapse loss (Brun and Andersson 2001). Presence of the ε4 allele of apoE may lower the threshold for alcoholic dementia (Muramatsu et al. 1997), particularly when cognitive deficits are broader than isolated memory loss.

The acute thiamine deficiency encephalopathy described by Wernicke is manifested by confusion, lateral gaze palsy, nystagmus, and ataxia. These clinical signs and symptoms reflect damage to brain areas adjacent to the third and fourth ventricles and in the medial temporal lobes. Thiamine is specifically therapeutic if administered promptly. This treatable cause of eventual amnestic disorder may be underdiagnosed. Of 51 patients showing the neuropathological stigmata of Wernicke's encephalopathy at postmortem examination, only 7 had received such a diagnosis antemortem (Harper 1979).

Although it is widely believed that alcohol-induced amnestic disorder produces permanent cognitive deficits, the actual prognosis may not be so poor. Victor and Adams (1971) reported complete recovery in 21% of 104 patients, and some degree of recovery of cognitive function occurred in an additional 53% of patients who refrained from alcohol. This classic study suggests that alcohol-induced amnestic disorder is one of the most treatable of the cognitive disorders.

References

Adams RD, Fisher CM, Hakim S: Symptomatic occult hydrocephalus with normal cerebrospinal fluid pressure: a treatable syndrome. N Engl J Med 273:117–126, 1965

Aisen PS, Davis KL, Berg JD, et al: A randomized controlled trial of prednisone in Alzheimer's disease. Neurology 54:588–593, 2000

Alzheimer A: About a peculiar disease of the cerebral cortex (1907). Translated by Jarvik L, Greenson H. Alzheimer Dis Assoc Disord 1:7–8, 1987

American Psychiatric Association: Diagnostic and Statistical Manual of Mental Disorders, 3rd Edition, Revised. Washington, DC, American Psychiatric Association, 1987

American Psychiatric Association: Diagnostic and Statistical Manual of Mental Disorders, 4th Edition, Text Revision. Washington, DC, American Psychiatric Association, 2000

Arai H, Kosaka K, Iizuka R: Changes of biogenic amines and their metabolites in postmortem brains from patients with Alzheimer-type dementia. J Neurochem 43:388–393, 1984

Asthana S, Craft S, Baker LD, et al: Cognitive and neuroendocrine response to transdermal estrogen in postmenopausal women with Alzheimer's disease: results of a placebo-controlled, double-blind, pilot study. Psychoneuroendocrinology 24:657–677, 1999

Avery TL: Seven cases of frontal tumour with psychiatric presentation. Br J Psychiatry 119:19–23, 1971

Balldin J, Gottfries CG, Karlsson I, et al: Dexamethasone suppression test and serum prolactin in dementia disorders. Br J Psychiatry 143:277–281, 1983

Blennow KAH, Wallin A, Gottfries CG, et al: Significance of decreased lumbar CSF levels of HVA and 5-HIAA in Alzheimer's disease. Neurobiol Aging 13:107–113, 1991

Blessed G, Tomlinson BE, Roth M: The association between quantitative measures of dementia and of senile change in the cerebral gray matter of elderly subjects. Br J Psychiatry 114:797–811, 1968

Bondareff W, Mountjoy CQ, Roth M: Loss of neurons of origin of the adrenergic projection to cerebral cortex (nucleus locus ceruleus) in senile dementia. Neurology 32: 164–168, 1982

Boon AJ, Tans JT, Delwel EJ, et al: The Dutch normal-pressure hydrocephalus study: the role of cerebrovascular disease. J Neurosurg 90:221–226, 1999

Breitner JC, Zandi PP: Do nonsteroidal anti-inflammatory drugs reduce the risk of Alzheimer's disease? N Engl J Med 345:1567–1568, 2001

Brown RG, Marsden CD: How common is dementia in Parkinson's disease? (editorial) Lancet 2:1262–1265, 1984

Brun A, Andersson J: Frontal dysfunction and frontal cortical synapse loss in alcoholism—main cause of alcohol dementia? Dement Geriatr Cogn Disord 12:289–294, 2001

Carroll BJ, Feinberg M, Greden JF, et al: A specific laboratory test for the diagnosis of melancholia: standardization, validity, and clinical utility. Arch Gen Psychiatry 38: 15–22, 1981

Charness ME: Brain lesions in alcoholics. Alcohol Clin Exp Res 17:2–11, 1993

Chui HC, Victoroff JI, Margolin D, et al: Criteria for diagnosis of ischemic vascular dementia proposed by the State of California Alzheimer's Disease Diagnostic and Treatment Centers. Neurology 42:473–480, 1992

Clarfield AM: Normal-pressure hydrocephalus: saga or swamp? JAMA 262:2592–2593, 1989

Clarnette RM, Patterson CJ: Hypothyroidism: does treatment cure dementia? J Geriatr Psychiatry Neurol 7:23–27, 1994

Corder EH, Saunders AM, Strittmatter W, et al: Gene dose of apolipoprotein E type 4 allele and the risk of Alzheimer's disease in late onset families. Science 261:921–923, 1993

Corey-Bloom J, Anand R, Veach J: A randomized trial evaluating the efficacy and safety of ENA 713 (rivastigmine tartrate), a new acetylcholinesterase inhibitor, in patients with mild to moderately severe Alzheimer's disease. The ENA 713 B352 Study Group. International Journal of Geriatric Psychopharmacology 1:55–65, 1998

Cross AJ, Crow TJ, Ferrier IN, et al: Serotonin receptor changes in dementia of the Alzheimer type. J Neurochem 43:1574–1581, 1984

Cummings JL, Duchen LW: Kluver-Bucy syndrome in Pick's disease: clinical and pathologic correlations. Neurology 31:1415–1422, 1981

D'Amato RJ, Zweig RM, Whitehouse PJ, et al: Aminergic systems in Alzheimer's disease and Parkinson's disease. Ann Neurol 22: 229–236, 1987

Davies P, Maloney AJ: Selective loss of central cholinergic neurons in Alzheimer's disease (letter). Lancet 2:1403, 1976

Davis KL, Davis BM, Greenwald BS, et al: Cortisol and Alzheimer's disease, I: basal studies. Am J Psychiatry 143:300–305, 1986

Doody RS, Geldmacher DS, Gordon B, et al: Open-label, multicenter, phase III extension study of the safety and efficacy of donepezil in patients with Alzheimer's disease. Arch Neurol 58:427–433, 2001

Erkinjuntti T, Kurz A, Gauthier S, et al: Efficacy of galantamine in probable vascular dementia and Alzheimer's disease combined with cerebrovascular disease: a randomised trial. Lancet 359:1283–1290, 2002

Evans IA, Funkenstein H, Albert MS, et al: Prevalence of Alzheimer's disease in a community population of older persons: higher than previously reported. JAMA 262:2551–2556, 1989

Farlow M, Gracon SI, Hershey LA, et al: A controlled trial of tacrine in Alzheimer's disease. The Tacrine Study Group. JAMA 268:2523–2529, 1992

Farlow M, Anand R, Messina J Jr, et al: A 52-week study of the efficacy of rivastigmine in patients with mild to moderately severe Alzheimer's disease. Eur Neurol 44:236–241, 2000

Feldman H, Gauthier S, Hecker J, et al: A 24-week, randomized, double-blind study of donepezil in moderate to severe Alzheimer's disease. Neurology 57:613–620, 2001

Folstein MF, Folstein SE, McHugh PR: "Mini-mental state": a practical method for grading the cognitive state of patients for the clinician. J Psychiatr Res 12:189–198, 1975

Fox JH, Topel JL, Huckman MS: Dementia in the elderly: a search for treatable illnesses. J Gerontol 30:557–564, 1975

Francis PT, Palmer AM, Sims NR, et al: Neurochemical studies of early-onset Alzheimer's disease. Possible influence on treatment. N Engl J Med 313:7–11, 1985

Freeman FR: Evaluation of patients with progressive intellectual deterioration. Arch Neurol 33:658–659, 1976

Friedland RP: "Normal"-pressure hydrocephalus and the saga of the treatable dementias. JAMA 262:2577–2581, 1989

Gibson CJ, Logue M, Growdon JH: CSF monoamine metabolite levels in Alzheimer's and Parkinson's disease. Arch Neurol 42:489–492, 1985

Glenner GG, Wong CW: Alzheimer's disease: initial report of the purification and characterization of a novel cerebrovascular amyloid protein. Biochem Biophys Res Commun 120:885–890, 1984

Golomb J, Wisoff J, Miller DC, et al: Alzheimer's disease comorbidity in normal pressure hydrocephalus: prevalence and shunt response. J Neurol Neurosurg Psychiatry 68:778–781, 2000

Graham JM, Sussman JD, Ford KS, et al: Olanzapine in the treatment of hallucinosis in idiopathic Parkinson's disease: a cautionary note. J Neurol Neurosurg Psychiatry 65:774–777, 1998

Gross JS, Weintraub NT, Neufeld RR, et al: Pernicious anemia in the demented patient without anemia or macrocytosis: a case for early recognition. J Am Geriatr Soc 34:612–614, 1986

Harper C: Wernicke's encephalopathy: a more common disease than realized. J Neurol Neurosurg Psychiatry 42:226–231, 1979

Hebb AO, Cusimano MD: Idiopathic normal pressure hydrocephalus: a systematic review of diagnosis and outcome. Neurosurgery 49:1166–1184, 2001

Henderson VW, Paganini-Hill A, Miller BL, et al: Estrogen for Alzheimer's disease in women: randomized, double-blind, placebo-controlled trial. Neurology 54:295–301, 2000

Heston LL, White JA, Mastri AR: Pick's disease: clinical genetics and natural history. Arch Gen Psychiatry 44:409–411, 1987

Hoogendijk WJ, Feenstra MG, Botterblom MH, et al: Increased activity of surviving locus ceruleus neurons in Alzheimer's disease. Ann Neurol 45:82–91, 1999

Hutton M, Lendon CL, Rizzu P: Association of missense and 5'-splice-site mutations in tau with the inherited dementia FTDP-17. Nature 393:702–705, 1998

in t' Veld BA, Ruitenberg A, Hofman A, et al: Nonsteroidal antiinflammatory drugs and the risk of Alzheimer's disease. N Engl J Med 345:1515–1521, 2001

Iqbal K, Alonso ADC, Gondal JA, et al: Inhibition of neurofibrillary degeneration: a rational and promising therapeutic target, in Alzheimer's Disease and Related Disorders: Etiology, Pathogenesis and Therapeutics. Edited by Iqbal K, Swaab DG, Winblad B, et al. Chichester, England, Wiley, 1999, pp 269–280

Ishikawa E, Yanaka K, Sugimoto K, et al: Reversible dementia in patients with chronic subdural hematomas. J Neurosurg 96:680–683, 2002

Joachim CL, Morris JH, Selkoe DJ: Clinically diagnosed Alzheimer's disease: autopsy results in 150 cases. Ann Neurol 24:50–56, 1988

Katzman R: The prevalence and malignancy of Alzheimer disease: a major killer (editorial). Arch Neurol 33:217–218, 1976

Katzman R: Alzheimer's disease. N Engl J Med 314:964–973, 1986

Khachaturian ZS: Diagnosis of Alzheimer's disease. Arch Neurol 42:1097–1105, 1985

Kiloh LG: Pseudo-dementia. Acta Psychiatr Scand 37:336–351, 1961

Knapp MJ, Knopman DS, Solomon PR, et al: A 30-week randomized controlled trial of high-dose tacrine in patients with Alzheimer's disease. The Tacrine Study Group. JAMA 271:985–991, 1994

Kosaka K, Tsuchiya K, Yoshimura M: Lewy body disease with and without dementia: a clinicopathological study of 35 cases. Clin Neuropathol 7:299–305, 1988

Kotzbauer PT, Trojanowski JQ, Lee VM: Lewy body pathology in Alzheimer's disease. J Mol Neurosci 17:225–232, 2001

Larson EB, Reifler BV, Featherstone HJ, et al: Dementia in elderly outpatients: a prospective study. Ann Intern Med 100:417–423, 1984

Larson EB, Reifler BV, Sumi SM, et al: Diagnostic tests in the evaluation of dementia: a prospective study of 200 elderly outpatients. Arch Intern Med 146:1917–1922, 1986

Le Bars PL, Katz MM, Berman N, et al: A placebo-controlled, double-blind, randomized trial of an extract of Ginkgo biloba for dementia. North American EGb Study Group. JAMA 278:1327–1332, 1997

Leverenz J, Sumi SM: Parkinson's disease in patients with Alzheimer's disease. Arch Neurol 43:662–664, 1986

Levkoff SE, Evans DA, Liptzin B, et al: Delirium: the occurrence and persistence of symptoms among elderly hospitalized patients. Arch Intern Med 152:334–340, 1992

Levy-Lahad E, Wasco W, Poorkaj P, et al: Candidate gene for the chromosome 1 familial Alzheimer's disease locus. Science 269: 973–976, 1995

Lim A, Tsuang D, Kukull W, et al: Clinico-neuropathological correlation of Alzheimer's disease in a community-based case series. J Am Geriatr Soc 47:564–569, 1999

Lindenbaum J, Healton EB, Savage DG, et al: Neuropsychiatric disorders caused by cobalamin deficiency in the absence of anemia or macrocytosis. N Engl J Med 318: 1720–1728, 1988

Lyketsos CG, Sheppard JM, Steele CD, et al: Randomized, placebo-controlled, double-blind, clinical trial of sertraline in the treatment of depression complicating Alzheimer's disease: initial results from the Depression in Alzheimer's Disease study. Am J Psychiatry 157:1686–1689, 2000

Maelicke A, Samochocki M, Jostock R: Allosteric sensitization of nicotinic receptors by galantamine: a new treatment strategy for Alzheimer's disease. Biol Psychiatry 49:279–288, 2001

Mahley RW, Huang Y: Apolipoprotein E: from atherosclerosis to Alzheimer's disease and beyond. Curr Opin Lipidol 10:207–217, 1999

Mann DMA, Yates PO: Serotonin nerve cells in Alzheimer's disease. J Neurol Neurosurg Psychiatry 46:96–98, 1983

Mann DMA, Lincoln J, Yates PO, et al: Changes in the monoamine-containing neurones of the human CNS in senile dementia. Br J Psychiatry 136:533–541, 1980

Marcantonio ER, Flacker J, Michaels M, et al: Delirium is independently associated with poor functional recovery after hip fracture. J Am Geriatr Soc 48:618–624, 2000

Martin DC, Francis J, Protech J, et al: Time dependence of cognitive recovery with cobalamin replacement: report of a pilot study. J Am Geriatr Soc 40:168–172, 1992

Mattis S: Mental status examination for organic mental syndrome in the elderly patient, in Geriatric Psychiatry: A Handbook for Psychiatrists and Primary Care Physicians. Edited by Bellack L, Karasu TB. New York, Grune & Stratton, 1976, pp 77–121

Mayeux R, Stern Y, Spanton S: Heterogeneity in dementia of the Alzheimer type: evidence of subgroups. Neurology 35:453–461, 1985

Mayeux R, Stern Y, Rosenstein R, et al: An estimate of the prevalence of dementia in idiopathic Parkinson's disease. Arch Neurol 45:260–262, 1988

McAllister TW, Ferrell RB, Price TRP, et al: The dexamethasone suppression test in two patients with severe depressive pseudodementia. Am J Psychiatry 139:479–481, 1982

McGeer EG, McGeer PL: Brain inflammation in Alzheimer disease and the therapeutic implications. Curr Pharm Des 5:821–836, 1999

McGeer PL, Shulzer M, McGeer EG: Arthritis and anti-inflammatory agents as possible protective factors for Alzheimer's disease: a review of 17 epidemiologic studies. Neurology 47:425–432, 1996

McKeith IG, Galasko D, Kosaka K, et al: Consensus guidelines for the clinical and pathologic diagnosis of dementia with Lewy bodies (DLB): report of the consortium on DLB international workshop. Neurology 47:1113–1124, 1996

McKeith I[G], Del Ser T, Spano P, et al: Efficacy of rivastigmine in dementia with Lewy bodies: a randomised, double-blind, placebo-controlled international study. Lancet 356:2031–2036, 2000

McKeith IG, Dickson DW, Lowe J, et al; Consortium on DLB: Diagnosis and management of dementia with Lewy bodies: third report of the DLB Consortium. Neurology 65(12):1863–1872, 2005

McKhann G, Drachman D, Folstein M, et al: Clinical diagnosis of Alzheimer's disease: report of the NINCDS-ADRDA Work Group under the auspices of Department of Health and Human Services Task Force on Alzheimer's disease. Neurology 34:939–944, 1984

Mesulam M-M, Guillozet A, Shaw P, et al: Acetylcholinesterase knockouts establish central cholinergic pathways and can use butyrylcholinesterase to hydrolyze acetylcholine. Neuroscience 110:627–639, 2002

Mitchell TW, Mufson EJ, Schneider JA, et al: Parahippocampal tau pathology in healthy aging, mild cognitive impairment, and early Alzheimer's disease. Ann Neurol 51: 182–189, 2002

Mohs RC, Doody RS, Morris JC, et al: A 1-year, placebo-controlled preservation of function survival study of donepezil in AD patients. Neurology 57:481–488, 2001

Morris JC, McKeel DW, Fulling K, et al: Validation of clinical diagnostic criteria for Alzheimer's disease. Ann Neurol 24:17–22, 1988

Mortimer JA: Alzheimer's disease and senile dementia: prevalence and incidence, in Alzheimer's Disease: The Standard Reference. Edited by Reisberg B. New York, Free Press, 1983, pp 141–148

Mullan M, Crawford F, Axelman K, et al: A pathogenic mutation for probable Alzheimer's disease in the *APP* gene at the N-terminus of beta-amyloid. Nat Genet 1:345–347, 1992

Mulnard RA, Cotman CW, Kawas C, et al: Estrogen replacement therapy for treatment of mild to moderate Alzheimer disease: a randomized controlled trial. Alzheimer's Disease Cooperative Study. JAMA 283: 1007–1015, 2000

Muramatsu T, Kato M, Matsui T, et al: Apolipoprotein E epsilon 4 allele distribution in Wernicke-Korsakoff syndrome with or without global intellectual deficits. J Neural Transm 104:913–920, 1997

Neary D, Snowden J: Fronto-temporal dementia: nosology, neuropsychology, and neuropathology. Brain Cogn 31:176–187, 1996

Nilsson K, Warkentin S, Hultberg B, et al: Treatment of cobalamin deficiency in dementia, evaluated clinically and with cerebral blood flow measurements. Aging (Milano) 12:199–207, 2000

Nyth AL, Gottfries CG, Lyby K, et al: Controlled multicenter clinical study of citalopram and placebo in elderly depressed patients with and without concomitant dementia. Acta Psychiatr Scand 86:138–145, 1992

Palmer AM, Francis PT, Bowen DE, et al: Catecholaminergic neurones assessed antemortem in Alzheimer's disease. Brain Res 414:365–375, 1987

Parkinson Study Group: Low-dose clozapine for the treatment of drug-induced psychosis in Parkinson's disease. N Engl J Med 340:757–763, 1999

Perry EK, Tomlinson BE, Blessed G, et al: Correlation of cholinergic abnormalities with senile plaques and mental test scores in senile dementia. Br Med J 2:1457–1459, 1978

Perry EK, Curtis M, Dick DJ, et al: Cholinergic correlates of cognitive impairment in Parkinson's disease: comparisons with Alzheimer's disease. J Neurol Neurosurg Psychiatry 48:413–421, 1985

Perry EK, Haroutunian V, Davis KL: Neocortical cholinergic activities differentiate Lewy body dementia from classical Alzheimer's disease. Neuroreport 5:747–749, 1994

Perry RH, Irving D, Blessed G, et al: Senile dementia of Lewy body type. A clinically and neuropathologically distinct form of Lewy body dementia in the elderly. J Neurol Sci 95:119–139, 1990

Peskind ER, Wingerson D, Murray S, et al: Effects of Alzheimer's disease and normal aging on cerebrospinal fluid norepinephrine responses to yohimbine and clonidine. Arch Gen Psychiatry 52:774–782, 1995

Peskind ER, Wilkinson CW, Petrie EC, et al: Increased CSF cortisol in AD is a function of *APOE* genotype. Neurology 56:1094–1098, 2001

Poorkaj P, Bird TD, Wijsman E, et al: Tau is a candidate gene for chromosome 17 frontotemporal dementia. Ann Neurol 43:815–825, 1998

Pratt RD, Perdomo CA: Patient populations in clinical trials of the efficacy and tolerability of donepezil in patients with dementia and cerebrovascular disease ("vascular dementia"). The 308 Study Group. Paper presented at the 7th International Geneva/Springfield Symposium on Advances in Alzheimer Therapy, Geneva, Switzerland, April 4, 2002

Prusiner SB, DeArmond SJ: Prion diseases of the central nervous system. Monogr Pathol 32:86–122, 1990

Raber J, Akana SF, Bhatnagar S, et al: Hypothalamic-pituitary-adrenal dysfunction in *APOE*(−/−) mice: possible role in behavioral and metabolic alterations. J Neurosci 20:2064–2071, 2000

Rahkonen T, Luukkainen-Markkula R, Paanila S, et al: Delirium episode as a sign of undetected dementia among community dwelling elderly subjects: a 2 year follow up study. J Neurol Neurosurg Psychiatry 69:519–521, 2000

Rajan S, Wallace JI, Beresford SAA, et al: Screening for cobalamin deficiency in geriatric outpatients: prevalence and influence of synthetic cobalamin intake. J Am Geriatr Soc 50:624–630, 2002

Rajput AH, Offord K, Beard CM, et al: A case-control study of smoking habits, dementia, and other illnesses in idiopathic Parkinson's disease. Neurology 37:226–232, 1987

Raskind MA, Peskind E, Rivard MR, et al: Dexamethasone suppression test and cortisol circadian rhythm in primary degenerative dementia. Am J Psychiatry 139:1468–1471, 1982

Raskind MA, Peskind ER, Halter JB, et al: Norepinephrine and MHPG levels in CSF and plasma in Alzheimer's disease. Arch Gen Psychiatry 41:343–346, 1984

Raskind MA, Peskind ER, Wilkinson CW: Hypothalamic-pituitary-adrenal axis regulation and human aging. Ann N Y Acad Sci 746:327–335, 1994

Raskind MA, Peskind ER, Wessel T, et al: Galantamine in AD: a 6-month randomized, placebo-controlled trial with a 6-month extension. The Galantamine USA-1 Study Group. Neurology 54:2261–2268, 2000

Reifler BV: Arguments for abandoning the term *pseudodementia*. J Am Geriatr Soc 30:665–668, 1982

Reisberg B, Doody R, Söffler A, et al: Memantine in moderate-to-severe Alzheimer's disease. N Engl J Med 348:1333-1341, 2003

Riley JN, Walker DW: Morphological alterations in hippocampus after long-term alcohol consumption in mice. Science 201:646–648, 1978

Risse SC, Lampe TH, Bird TD, et al: Myoclonus, seizures and rigidity in Alzheimer's disease. Alzheimer Dis Assoc Disord 4:217–225, 1990a

Risse SC, Raskind MA, Nochlin D, et al: Neuropathological findings in patients with clinical diagnoses of probable Alzheimer's disease. Am J Psychiatry 147:168–172, 1990b

Rogers SL, Friedhoff LT: The efficacy and safety of donepezil in patients with Alzheimer's disease: results of a US multicenter, randomized, double-blind, placebo-controlled trial. The Donepezil Study Group. Dementia 7:293–303, 1996

Rogers SL, Farlow MR, Doody RS, et al: A 24-week, double-blind, placebo-controlled trial of donepezil in patients with Alzheimer's disease. The Donepezil Study Group. Neurology 50:136–145, 1998

Rosen WG, Mohs RC, Davis KL: A new rating scale for Alzheimer's disease. Am J Psychiatry 141:1356–1364, 1984

Rosenberg RN: A causal role for amyloid in Alzheimer's disease: the end of the beginning. Neurology 43:851–856, 1993

Rösler M, Anand R, Cicin-Sain A, et al: Efficacy and safety of rivastigmine in patients with Alzheimer's disease: international randomised controlled trial. The B303 Exelon Study Group. BMJ 318:633–640, 1999

Rudorfer MV, Clayton PV: Depression, dementia and dexamethasone suppression (letter). Am J Psychiatry 138:701, 1981

Russo-Neustadt A, Cotman CW: Adrenergic receptors in Alzheimer's disease brain: selective increases in the cerebella of aggressive patients. J Neurosci 17:5573–5580, 1997

Sano M, Ernesto C, Thomas RG, et al: A controlled trial of selegiline, alpha-tocopherol, or both as treatment for Alzheimer's disease. The Alzheimer's Disease Cooperative Study. N Engl J Med 336:1216–1222, 1997

Sapolsky R, Armanini M, Packan D, et al: Stress and glucocorticoids in aging. Endocrinol Metab Clin North Am 16:965–980, 1987

Schellenberg GD, Bird T, Wijsman E, et al: Genetic linkage evidence for a familial Alzheimer's disease locus on chromosome 14. Science 258:668–671, 1992

Selkoe DJ: The origins of Alzheimer's disease: a is for amyloid. JAMA 283:1571–1577, 2000

Sherrington R, Rogaev EI, Liang Y, et al: Cloning of a gene bearing missense mutations in early onset familial Alzheimer's disease. Nature 375:754–760, 1995

Sjogren T, Sjogren H, Lindgren AGH: Morbus Alzheimer and Morbus Pick; a genetic, clinical and patho-anatomical study. Acta Psychiatr Neurol Scand 82:1–152, 1952

Skoog I, Nilsson L, Palmertz B, et al: A population-based study of dementia in 85-year-olds. N Engl J Med 328:153–158, 1994

Snowdon DA, Greiner LH, Mortimer JA, et al: Brain infarction and the clinical expression of Alzheimer disease. The Nun Study. JAMA 277:813–817, 1997

Spar JE, Gerner R: Does the dexamethasone suppression test distinguish dementia from depression? Am J Psychiatry 139:238–240, 1982

Strachan RW, Henderson JG: Psychiatric syndromes due to avitaminosis B_{12} with normal blood and bone marrow. Q J Med 34:303–317, 1965

Sumi SM, Bird TD, Nochlin D, et al: Familial presenile dementia with psychosis associated with cortical neurofibrillary tangles and degeneration of the amygdala. Neurology 42:120–127, 1992

Szot P, Leverenz JB, Peskind ER, et al: Tyrosine hydroxylase and norepinephrine transporter mRNA expression in the locus coeruleus in Alzheimer's disease. Brain Res Mol Brain Res 84:135–140, 2000

Tariot PN, Farlow MR, Grossberg GT: Memantine treatment in patients with moderate to severe Alzheimer disease already receiving donepezil: a randomized controlled trial. JAMA 291:317–324, 2004

Tariot PN, Solomon PR, Morris JC, et al: A 5-month, randomized, placebo-controlled trial of galantamine in AD. The Galantamine USA-10 Study Group. Neurology 54:2269–2276, 2000

Teri L: Behavioral treatment of depression in patients with dementia. Alzheimer Dis Assoc Disord 8 (suppl 3):66–74, 1994

Thal L: No differences between rofecoxib, naproxen and placebo on clinical progression in Alzheimer's disease. Paper presented at the American Academy of Neurology annual meeting, Denver, CO, April 2002

Thomasen AM, Borgesen SE, Bruhn P, et al: Prognosis of dementia in normal-pressure hydrocephalus after a shunt operation. Ann Neurol 20:304–310, 1986

Tierney MC, Fisher RH, Lewis AJ, et al: The NINCDS-ADRDA Work Group criteria for the clinical diagnosis of probable Alzheimer's disease: a clinicopathologic study of 57 cases. Neurology 38:359–364, 1988

Tomlinson BE, Blessed G, Roth M: Observations on the brains of demented old people. J Neurol Sci 11:205–242, 1970

Tomlinson BE, Irving D, Blessed G: Cell loss in the locus coeruleus in senile dementia of Alzheimer type. J Neurol Sci 49:419–428, 1981

Trojanowski JQ, Lee VM: Phosphorylation of paired helical filament tau in Alzheimer's disease neurofibrillary lesions: focusing on phosphates. FASEB J 15:1570–1576, 1995

Victor M: Alcoholic dementia. Can J Neurol Sci 21:88–99, 1994

Victor M, Adams RD: The Wernicke-Korsakoff Syndrome. Philadelphia, PA, FA Davis, 1971

Victoratos GC, Lonman JAR, Herzberg L: Neurological investigation of dementia. Br J Psychiatry 130:131–133, 1977

Vitaliano PP, Breen AR, Russo J, et al: The clinical utility of the dementia rating scale for assessing Alzheimer patients. J Chronic Dis 37:743–753, 1984

Volicer L, Direnfeld LK, Freedman M, et al: Serotonin and 5-hydroxyindoleacetic acid in CSF: differences in Parkinson's disease and dementia of the Alzheimer's type. Arch Neurol 42:127–129, 1985

Wang HX, Wahlin A, Basun H, et al: Vitamin B(12) and folate in relation to the development of Alzheimer's disease. Neurology 56:1188–1194, 2001

Weggen S, Eriksen JL, Das P, et al: A subset of NSAIDs lower amyloidogenic Aβ42 independently of cyclooxygenase activity. Nature 414:212–216, 2001

Whitehouse PJ, Price DL, Struble RG, et al: Alzheimer's disease and senile dementia: loss of neurons in the basal forebrain. Science 215:1237–1239, 1982

Whybrow PC, Prange AJ Jr, Treadway CR: Mental changes accompanying thyroid gland dysfunction. Arch Gen Psychiatry 20:48–63, 1969

Wieland RG: Vitamin B_{12} deficiency in the nonanemic elderly. J Am Geriatr Soc 34: 618–619, 1986

Wikkelso C, Anderson H, Blomstrand C, et al: The clinical effect of lumbar puncture in normal-pressure hydrocephalus. J Neurol Neurosurg Psychiatry 45:64–69, 1982

Wilcock GK, Lilienfeld S, Gaens E: Efficacy and safety of galantamine in patients with mild to moderate Alzheimer's disease: multicentre randomised controlled trial. Galantamine International-1 Study Group. BMJ 321:1445–1449, 2000

Wilhelmsen KC, Clark LN, Miller BL, et al: Tau mutations in frontotemporal dementia. Dement Geriatr Cogn Disord 10:88–92, 1999

Wilner E, Brody JA: Prognosis of general paresis after treatment. Lancet 2:1370–1371, 1968

Winblad B, Adolfsson R, Carlsson A, et al: Biogenic amines in brains of patients with Alzheimer's disease, in Alzheimer's Disease: A Report of Progress. Edited by Corkin S. New York, Raven, 1982, pp 25–33

Winblad B, Engedal K, Soininen H: A 1-year, randomized, placebo-controlled study of donepezil in patients with mild to moderate AD. Neurology 57:489–495, 2001

Wood PL, Nair NP, Etienne P, et al: Lack of cholinergic deficit in the neocortex in Pick's disease. Prog Neuropsychopharmacol Biol Psychiatry 7:725–727, 1983

Wyss-Coray T, Mucke L: Ibuprofen, inflammation and Alzheimer disease. Nat Med 6: 973–974, 2000

Yamamoto T, Hirano A: Nucleus raphe dorsalis in Alzheimer's disease: neurofibrillary tangles and loss of large neurons. Ann Neurol 17:573–577, 1985

Zubenko GS: Progression of illness in the differential diagnosis of primary depression. Am J Psychiatry 147:435–438, 1990

Zubenko GS, Moossy J: Major depression in primary dementia. Arch Neurol 45:1182–1186, 1988

Study Questions

Select the single best response for each question.

1. Cognitive deficits of Alzheimer's disease correlate

   A. With density of neurofibrillary tangles.
   B. With hyperphosphorylated tau.
   C. With density of neuritic plaques.
   D. A and B.
   E. A and C.

2. Serotonin abnormalities of Alzheimer's disease include

   A. Loss of serotonergic neurons in brain stem raphe nuclei.
   B. Decreased concentration of serotonin in brain tissue.
   C. Decreased concentration of serotonin in CSF.
   D. Decreased serotonin receptor concentrations.
   E. All of the above.

3. Brain presynaptic cholinergic deficit has been demonstrated in which of the following?

   A. Alzheimer's disease.
   B. Vascular dementia.
   C. Lewy body dementia.
   D. All of the above.
   E. None of the above.

4. Cholinesterase inhibitors are best conceptualized as drugs

   A. That stabilize cognition, activities of daily living, and behavioral function.
   B. That improve cognitive function greatly.
   C. Only indicated for mild to moderate stages of Alzheimer's disease.
   D. Contraindicated in the treatment of Lewy body dementia.
   E. Predominately associated with the side effect of sedation.

5. Vitamin E and selegiline have *not* been shown to

   A. Have beneficial effects on cognitive function per se.
   B. Delay nursing home placement.
   C. Delay progression to severe dementia.
   D. Be more effective in combination than either agent alone.
   E. Delay loss of basic activities of daily living.

6. Dementia with a cerebrovascular contribution

    A. Is as common as Alzheimer's disease.
    B. Is most frequently seen as pure vascular dementia.
    C. Lowers the threshold for and increases the magnitude of dementia caused by Alzheimer's disease.
    D. Is associated with an especially high prevalence and severity of dementia with infarcts in the basal ganglia, thalamus, or deep white matter.
    E. C and D.

7. Most forms of frontotemporal dementia involve

    A. Neuronal cell loss.
    B. Gliosis.
    C. Pick bodies.
    D. Abnormal function of tau protein.
    E. Amyloidopathy.

8. Hypothyroidism

    A. Can produce a dementia accompanied by irritability, paranoid ideation, and depression.
    B. Can produce a dementia for which aggressive thyroid replacement results in the patient's return to previous level of functioning.
    C. Is similar to vitamin B12 deficiency dementia in that B12 replacement leads to remission of dementia.
    D. A and B.
    E. A, B, and C.

9. Delirium in the elderly

    A. Usually persists for months in those hospitalized for medical or surgical reasons.
    B. Rarely results in full resolution of symptoms in a short time.
    C. Is often the initial presentation of an underlying dementia.
    D. Could have an insidious onset.
    E. All of the above.

Movement Disorders

Burton L. Scott, Ph.D., M.D.

As people age, a variety of movement disorders can either appear for the first time or progress after onset earlier in life. Arthritis, bursitis, tendonitis, and other non–central nervous system conditions can in some ways mimic neurological conditions by producing stooped posture and overall slowing of movement. In this chapter, I discuss central nervous system–based movement disorders that occur in elderly individuals and result in impaired or abnormal movement.

Movement disorders in the elderly population can be divided into *hypokinetic movement disorders* (in which the ability to move is decreased or impaired because of a neurological condition) and *hyperkinetic movement disorders* (in which there is excessive abnormal movement). Hypokinetic movement disorders encompass a variety of parkinsonian disorders, in which there is some combination of the following signs and symptoms: tremor at rest, rigidity, slowness of movement (bradykinesia), and balance difficulty (postural instability). These disorders include Parkinson's disease (PD) and several "Parkinson's plus" syndromes. Other gait disorders, such as normal-pressure hydrocephalus (NPH), are also included among the hypokinetic movement disorders. Hyperkinetic movement

disorders include tremors, tics, dystonia, myoclonus, chorea, stereotypies, and other dyskinesias, including tardive dyskinesia and tardive dystonia. Tremor disorders are represented in both groups of movement disorders: tremor at rest is a cardinal feature of parkinsonism (a hypokinetic condition), and postural and kinetic tremor are features of essential tremor (ET; a hyperkinetic movement disorder).

Hypokinetic Movement Disorders

Parkinsonism

The term *parkinsonism* refers to a clinical condition that is characterized by some combination of resting tremor, rigidity, bradykinesia, and postural instability, but no specific etiology is inferred by the term (Weiner 2005). *Parkinson's disease* refers to levodopa-responsive, idiopathic parkinsonism associated with Lewy bodies and neuronal degeneration in the substantia nigra pars compacta. Secondary parkinsonism is parkinsonism due to other lesions of the basal ganglia, such as tumors, strokes (vascular parkinsonism), encephalitis, hypoxic or ischemic insult, and toxins (such as manganese, carbon monoxide, or carbon disulfide). NPH can cause a parkinsonian-like gait disorder, urinary incontinence, and dementia.

Parkinsonism is well known to be associated with use of dopamine receptor–blocking agents, including antipsychotic medications and antiemetics. Patients who take these medications for prolonged periods can also develop tardive movement disorders, including tardive dyskinesia and tardive dystonia.

Parkinson's Disease

PD is a chronic, progressive, neurodegenerative illness that produces rigidity, slowness of movement (bradykinesia), postural instability, and, often, tremor at rest (Nutt and Wooten 2005). It affects up to 1 million individuals in North America and is newly diagnosed in 20,000–50,000 patients each year. The prevalence of PD increases with age, with estimates of 1% at age 60 and up to 2.6% at age 85 or older (Mutch et al. 1986; Sutcliffe et al. 1985). PD results from progressive loss of dopamine-containing neurons in the substantia nigra pars compacta of the midbrain and is characterized pathologically by abnormal collections of proteins, called Lewy bodies, in the cytoplasm of degenerating neurons (Forno 1996; Golbe 1999).

Other common clinical features of PD include hypomimia (masked facies or facial masking), micrographia (small handwriting), stooped posture, retropulsion, and shuffling and festinating gait. Symptoms typically begin gradually on one side of the body, and patients may ignore the initial symptoms when the nondominant arm is the arm affected first, particularly in the absence of tremor. The typical resting tremor in PD has a frequency of 4–6 Hz. When tremor occurs in the hand, it may have the classic pill-rolling appearance—that is, a combination of flexion-extension tremor of the fingers and thumb, giving the appearance of rolling a marble or pill be-

tween the thumb and fingertips. The resting tremor of PD typically attenuates at least transiently during voluntary movement of the affected extremity, such as when the patient picks up an object, and is to be distinguished from the postural, antigravity tremor observed in ET. Usually, treatment with levodopa, a precursor of the neurotransmitter dopamine, results in significant clinical benefit in PD.

PD can be divided into two clinical forms: 1) tremor-dominant PD, in which tremor at rest is a prominent feature, and 2) postural instability and gait disorder, or akinetic-rigid PD, in which resting tremor is minimal, if present at all, and patients exhibit earlier balance difficulty. Both forms respond to levodopa treatment, at least initially; however, tremor-dominant PD tends to progress more slowly and thus has a more favorable prognosis than does akinetic-rigid PD.

The stiffness or rigidity of PD is detected clinically by testing for involuntary resistance to passive movement of the extremities. This resistance can manifest as lead-pipe rigidity—that is, a steady resistance to passive movement. In patients with resting tremor, the combination of rigidity and tremor results in cogwheel rigidity—that is, a jerky resistance to passive movement. In addition, active, voluntary movement of the contralateral extremity (synkinetic movement) can bring out subtle rigidity in an ipsilateral limb. For example, rapid, repetitive opening and closing of the contralateral hand in early PD may result in slightly increased tone in the ipsilateral arm; similarly, repetitive flexion-extension at the contralateral elbow can bring out abnormally increased tone in the ipsilateral leg in early PD.

Slowed movement, or bradykinesia, is tested in the clinic by observing the ease with which the patient performs repetitive movements such as tapping the index finger and thumb together, opening and closing the hand, twisting the hand clockwise and counterclockwise (as if turning a doorknob), and tapping the heel on the ground. Micrographia can be a manifestation of bradykinesia. Early in PD, handwriting might be of normal size at the beginning of a sentence and then become progressively smaller by the end of the sentence.

Postural instability usually occurs later than the other clinical signs of PD and can be very disabling. Patients fall because of an inability to keep their feet under their center of gravity, and these patients exhibit retropulsion (inability to maintain balance when suddenly displaced backward) and anteropulsion (inability to maintain balance when suddenly displaced forward). Festination occurs in an upright, walking PD patient whose feet are lagging behind his or her center of gravity. This clinical sign manifests as rapid, tiny steps taken to keep from falling.

Onset of PD symptoms is usually recognized earlier in individuals with tremor-dominant PD, because even mild tremor is likely to bring a patient into clinic earlier. In patients with resting tremor, the tremor often increases with walking. In addition, patients with early PD often exhibit decreased arm swing when walking. A reduction or absence of arm swing noticed by others may be the first indication of PD in a patient who does not have much resting tremor. Other patients may present with gradual loss of fine coordination of an extremity. The posture in a PD patient is often stooped, with flexion at the neck, upper back, shoulders, hips, and knees. The gait is typically narrow based and shuffling. Symptom onset is usually noticed earlier in patients affected first on the dominant side (i.e., the right hand in a right hand–dominant individual). By several years after onset of symptoms, it is expected that both sides of the body will be affected, although one side is often more affected than the other, even in chronic PD.

Medications for treatment of PD can be divided into putative neuroprotective agents, drugs for treating symptoms (levodopa, dopamine agonists, others), and possible restorative agents (growth factors, neuroimmunophilins). At present, there are no medications that have been proven to slow progression of PD and provide neuroprotection.

PD results from a deficiency of the neurotransmitter dopamine in the brain, and administration of levodopa (L-dopa), a precursor of dopamine, is the most effective treatment for PD symptoms. Dopamine agonists, monoamine oxidase B inhibitors, catechol-O-methyltransferase inhibitors, amantadine, and anticholinergic agents are also used for medical treatment. In addition to anticholinergic side effects (dry mouth, constipation, cognitive difficulty), potential side effects of PD treatments, such as dopamine agonists, are similar to those of levodopa and include hallucinations, dyskinesias (head bobbing and involuntary writhing or twisting movements of the extremities), and dystonia (muscle spasms). Patients may also experience unexpected sleep episodes, even when driving; pathological gambling, hypersexuality, and punding (purposeless repetitive behaviors) from exposure to dopamine agonists.

The most common surgical treatment of PD is deep brain stimulation (DBS), in which a thin stimulating electrode is surgically implanted in basal ganglia targets, usually the subthalamic nucleus (STN) or globus pallidus–inner part (GP_i) (Benabid et al. 2005; Lang and Lozano 1998a, 1998b). The electrode is connected to an implantable pulse generator that can be adjusted to provide electrical pulses of sufficient energy and frequency to alter output from the targeted nuclei, thereby reducing contralateral PD symptoms.

The differential diagnosis of PD includes a host of disorders that can mimic aspects of PD, including ET, drug-induced parkinsonism (see "Parkinsonism" at the beginning of this chapter), and other secondary parkinsonian syndromes (tumors and other mass lesions of the basal ganglia, vascular parkinsonism). Other disorders that can have parkinsonian features are NPH; primary gait ignition failure, which may represent early parkinsonism; and other atypical parkinsonian syndromes, such as progressive supranuclear palsy (PSP), multiple system atrophy, and cortical-basal ganglionic degeneration (or corticobasal degeneration); see "'Parkinson's Plus' Syndromes" below.

Normal-Pressure Hydrocephalus (Communicating Hydrocephalus)

NPH, also known as communicating hydrocephalus, is more common in elderly persons and can be a cause of a progressive gait disorder in addition to urinary incontinence and memory decline. It is associated with a decrease in the rate of removal of cerebrospinal fluid (CSF) at the level of the arachnoid villi in the superior sagittal sinus. NPH can develop after an episode of meningitis or a subarachnoid bleed, but it usually develops in the absence of these relatively rare conditions.

Affected individuals may take small steps and exhibit a "magnetic gait," in which there is difficulty lifting the feet to walk because of a sense that they are stuck to the ground. The triad of gait disorder, urinary incontinence, and memory loss suggests a diagnosis of NPH. Brain imaging demonstrates enlarged intraventricular spaces that are out of proportion to the size of the sulci. The diagnosis is supported by clinical improvement after a large-volume lumbar puncture or by observation of reversed CSF flow, identified by introducing a tracer into the CSF and performing cisternography to visualize the flow of tracer in the brain. Reduction of

CSF during a single diagnostic lumbar puncture may not result in immediate clinical benefit. Surgical placement of a lumbar drain for several days may help determine whether the patient could benefit from shunting surgery to treat NPH.

"Parkinson's Plus" Syndromes

Progressive Supranuclear Palsy

PSP, or Steele-Richardson-Olszewski syndrome (Steele et al. 1964), features parkinsonism without prominent tremor, vertical gaze palsy, axial (midline) more than appendicular (arm and leg) rigidity, early postural instability, and poor response to levodopa (reviewed in Litvan 2004). The syndrome affects an estimated 20,000 people in the United States.

PSP is often associated with frequent falling, lack of eye contact, monotonous speech, sloppy eating, and slowed mentation. Patients may have a surprised or worried facial expression, with raised eyebrows resulting from bradykinesia and increased tone in facial musculature, and have difficulty opening their eyes (eyelidopening apraxia). There is early suppression of vertical optokinetic nystagmus and voluntary vertical saccades. Later in the illness, horizontal saccades and horizontal optokinetic nystagmus become suppressed. Impairment of voluntary downgaze is more specific to PSP, whereas impairment of voluntary upgaze is nonspecific in elderly individuals. As is expected with a supranuclear lesion, passive movement of the head can overcome the compromised voluntary eye movements in PSP.

PSP has an insidious onset, and often the first symptom is a decrease in postural stability, resulting in falls. The usual age at symptom onset is 55–70 years, with a mean in the early 60s (late 50s in PD). In PSP, the posture is upright and rigid, not stooped as in PD, and the gait is typically stiff, with the legs extended at the knees, not flexed as in PD. In addition, PSP patients tend to pivot when turning, rather than exhibiting en bloc turning and shuffling as in PD.

Cognitive decline can begin in the first year of symptoms and may manifest as apathy, impaired abstract thinking, decreased verbal fluency, utilization or imitative behavior, and frontal release signs. Visual symptoms, including diplopia, blurry vision, burning eyes, and light sensitivity, appear in about 60% of cases during the first year, dysarthria in about 40% of cases, and bradykinesia in 20%.

Supranuclear gaze palsy has also been observed in other neurodegenerative disorders including diffuse Lewy body disease [dementia with Lewy bodies] (de Bruin et al. 1992), cortical-basal ganglionic degeneration (Gibb et al. 1990), and other parkinsonian syndromes. Atypical parkinsonian syndromes other than PSP may be suggested by a recent history of encephalitis, alien hand syndrome, cortical sensory deficits, focal frontal or temporoparietal atrophy, early cerebellar signs, early dysautonomia, severely asymmetric parkinsonism, or a relevant structural injury visualized by an imaging study.

Early in the course of PSP, visual pursuit eye movements may become saccadic (jerky), and voluntary saccades may become slow despite preserved range of extraocular movements. Saccades may become smaller or hypometric, and there may be decreased convergence of the eyes when they follow a target brought in toward the patient's nose. The ability to voluntarily suppress the vestibulo-ocular reflex during passive head movement decreases or disappears. Later, there is slowing of eyelid opening and closing, and patients often lose the ability to suppress blinks in response to a bright light.

Another finding that supports a diagnosis of PSP is the presence of symmetric akinesia or rigidity, usually more in the proximal than distal portions of limbs. In contrast, akinesia or rigidity in PD is typically asymmetric at first, occurring initially on one side of the body, with the other side expected to become affected within a few years. Abnormal neck posture, especially retrocollis, is commonly seen in PSP, as are early dysphagia and dysarthria.

Unlike PD, PSP has shown little or no response to levodopa therapy because of degeneration of secondary neurons downstream from primary dopamine-releasing substantia nigra pars compacta neurons. Response to other medical treatment is usually poor as well; however, some patients have at least a transient response to treatment with amantadine, carbidopa/levodopa (Sinemet), or dopamine agonists. There is no known effective neurosurgical intervention for PSP.

After symptom onset, the course of PSP is typically 5–10 years, and death may result from infections such as aspiration pneumonia or from complications of falls.

Neuropathology is the standard for certain diagnosis of PSP, which can be confused clinically with PD, cortical-basal ganglionic degeneration, multiple system atrophy (MSA), Alzheimer's disease, and dementia with Lewy bodies. Pathological changes in PSP include the development of neurofibrillary tangles and neuropil threads (filamentous structures in neuronal cytoplasm). Pathology is primarily found in the pallidum, subthalamic nucleus, substantia nigra, and pons. Abnormalities in tau protein, an important component of intracellular microtubules, have been implicated in some cases of PSP, and tau-positive astrocytes or astrocytic processes have been found in affected areas of the brain.

Multiple System Atrophy

MSA encompasses several "Parkinson's plus" conditions characterized by bilateral, symmetric parkinsonism that is poorly responsive to levodopa therapy, as well as absence or near absence of tremor (Geser et al. 2006). MSA can be subdivided into three types: 1) MSA-parkinsonism (MSA-P) (formerly striatonigral degeneration), in which parkinsonism is the main clinical feature; 2) MSA-cerebellar type (MSA-C) (formerly sporadic olivopontocerebellar atrophy, or OPCA), in which cerebellar ataxia is the main clinical feature; and 3) MSA-autonomic dysfunction (MSA-A) (formerly Shy-Drager syndrome), in which severe orthostatic hypotension and bowel and bladder dysfunction may appear early.

Clinical features that can help distinguish MSA-P from other forms of parkinsonism include falls early in the illness, severe dysarthria and dysphonia, sleep apnea and excessive snoring, anterocollis, respiratory stridor, and pyramidal signs (brisk reflexes and extensor plantar responses). MSA-A is distinguished clinically by early autonomic impairment including orthostatic hypotension or syncope, impotence in males, and bowel and bladder dysfunction (Shy and Drager 1960). In MSA-P, medically refractory parkinsonism and gait disturbance develop early. In addition to neuronal degeneration in substantia nigra, putamen, and other nuclei, neuronal loss usually occurs in the intermediolateral columns of the spinal cord. Treatment of orthostatic symptoms includes liberalizing dietary salt, elevation of the head of the bed, and use of fludrocortisone, midodrine, and sometimes indomethacin and yohimbine. Although the clinical response to treatment is usually poor, trials of levodopa (up to 1,500 mg/day in divided doses) with or without a dopamine agonist (pramipexole, ropinirole) are sometimes beneficial. The clinical course is approximately 10 years. Brain magnetic resonance imaging (MRI) may demonstrate decreased (dark) T2 signal laterally in the putamen of the basal ganglia and a ribbon of increased T2 signal farther laterally outside of the putamen (Kraft et al. 1999).

MSA-C, or sporadic olivopontocerebellar atrophy, often presents with gait ataxia. Other features that may develop are limb ataxia, breakdown of visual smooth pursuit, and cerebellar dysarthria (ataxic dysarthria). Autonomic dysfunction, parkinsonism, and pyramidal signs can also occur, but the cerebellar findings are usually most prominent. Brain MRI can demonstrate cerebellar and brain stem atrophy, particularly in the pons and medulla.

The neuropathology of MSA is significant for degeneration of the substantia nigra and putamen (striatum), with neuronal loss and iron deposition. Glial cytoplasmic inclusions, particularly in oligodendrocytes, are characteristic of all forms of MSA, and cell loss and gliosis can be found in the striatum, substantia nigra, locus coeruleus, pontine nuclei, middle cerebellar peduncles, Purkinje cells of the cerebellum, inferior olives, and the intermediolateral columns of the spinal cord. Lewy bodies and neurofibrillary tangles are not common in MSA.

Cortical-Basal Ganglionic Degeneration

Cortical-basal ganglionic degeneration (CBGD), also referred to as corticobasal degeneration, produces marked, asymmetric parkinsonism and dystonia (Litvan et al. 1997; Riley and Lang 2000; Schneider et al. 1997). Resting tremor is uncommon in this condition. CBGD can result in jerky (myoclonic), apraxic, rigid, akinetic movements and alien hand syndrome, in which one hand seems to have a "mind of its own." There may be early dementia, cortical sensory findings (such as hemineglect to double simultaneous tactile stimulation), or unilateral agraphesthesia (manifested as the inability to identify a number written on the palm of the hand). Stimulus-sensitive myoclonus and action tremor may also be present. Response to levodopa therapy is poor, but administration of up to 1,500 mg/day in divided doses is sometimes of initial benefit. The disease course is typically 5–10 years from the time of symptom onset.

Neuropathological changes include swollen (ballooned) neurons, degeneration of substantia nigra and basal ganglia, and tau-positive inclusion bodies. Brain MRI often demonstrates asymmetric atrophy in posterior frontal and parietal cortex contralateral to the more affected side of the body (Savoiardo et al. 2000).

Frontotemporal Dementia and Parkinsonism Linked to Chromosome 17

In the degenerative condition called frontotemporal dementia and parkinsonism linked to chromosome 17 (FTDP-17), an insidious onset of behavioral or motor changes occurs. Typically in this disease, cognitive impairment leads to dementia, parkinsonism, nonfluent aphasia, a change in personality, and/or psychosis (Foster et al. 1997; Lund and Manchester Groups 1994). Onset is generally in the fifth decade of life and can be as late as the sixth decade. Duration usually is longer than 10 years but can be as short as 3 years.

Behavioral changes range from aggressiveness to apathy and may include hyperorality, hyperphagia, obsessive stereotyped behavior, psychosis, delusions, and muteness. Motor findings can include parkinsonism, particularly rigidity, bradykinesia, and postural instability, but not resting tremor. Hyperreflexia, clonus, and extensor plantar responses may occur. Levodopa treatment produces no significant response. Autonomic function is spared early in the course until dementia becomes severe.

Neuropsychological testing demonstrates disturbed executive functioning, with relative preservation of visual-spatial functioning, orientation, and memory until late in the disease course. Electroencephalographic findings are often normal until late in the disease, and functional imaging suggests frontal and anterior temporal hypoperfusion or hypometabolism.

Hyperkinetic Movement Disorders

Essential Tremor

Tremor is defined as a rhythmic oscillation across a joint resulting from involuntary, alternating activation of agonist and antagonist muscles. For example, tremor at the wrist results from alternating activation of forearm flexor and extensor muscles.

ET is the most prevalent movement disorder among adults and the elderly, affecting up to 2% of the general population. The prevalence of ET increases with age, and in individuals older than 70 years, estimates range up to more than 10%. Also called benign essential tremor and familial tremor, ET may not be benign and can result in severe impairment of activities of daily living. ET manifests as postural and kinetic tremor of the arms and hands; the head and voice are often involved as well (reviewed in Jankovic 2000; Louis 2005).

Postural tremor is tremor that appears when a body part is held against gravity. This tremor should be distinguished from the tremor at rest that is characteristic of tremor-dominant PD. Kinetic tremor is tremor that occurs with action or when approximating a target, such as during finger-to-nose testing. Kinetic tremor can interfere with eating and drinking such that patients may need to use two hands in order to hold a cup or write. The tremor may interfere with bringing food to the mouth, holding a soup spoon, or carrying a tray.

The frequency of hand tremor in ET is typically 6–8 Hz; however, the tremor frequency may decrease with age (Bain et al. 2000). Progression may be more rapid in patients with age at onset of more than

60 years and in patients without head tremor. The tremor in ET is commonly symmetric in both upper extremities; however, one arm may be more involved than the other, and even unilateral tremor may occur. Patients may exhibit "yes-yes," "no-no," or mixed head titubation, and they may have a tremulous voice as well. A key feature of ET, at least early on, is that tremor is absent at rest, only occurring during action or when holding a posture. Later in the course, some resting tremor may appear, but it is always less prominent than the postural or kinetic tremor present. There is usually a clear family history of tremor, and often the tremor attenuates with alcohol use, a phenomenon that can contribute to development of alcoholism in susceptible individuals.

The mainstays of medical treatment for ET are propranolol therapy and primidone therapy. Deep brain stimulation targeting the ventral intermediate nucleus of the contralateral thalamus is sometimes helpful in medically refractory cases.

Other tremor-related disorders seen in the elderly population include enhanced physiologic tremor (characterized by postural or kinetic tremor that is more prominent than normal physiologic tremor) and orthostatic tremor (a high-frequency, low-amplitude leg tremor that develops while the patient is standing still and often responds to clonazepam therapy; Myers and Scott 2003).

Dystonia

Dystonia is a fairly common movement disorder that usually begins by middle age and may persist in elderly individuals (Scott 2000). In dystonia, involuntary muscle spasms result in bizarre, sustained postures. These postures initially occur during attempted voluntary movement and may persist at rest. Dystonia can be idiopathic (associated with no identifiable structural abnormality) or secondary (associated with a known structural lesion demonstrated by an imaging study) and can have a delayed onset, appearing after a previous injury (Scott and Jankovic 1996). Dystonia may be focal (affecting one body part), segmental (affecting two or more adjacent body parts), multifocal (affecting two or more nonadjacent body parts), generalized (affecting most of the body, including at least one leg), or hemi- (affecting one side of the body). Common examples of focal dystonia include writer's cramp (involuntary, sometimes painful cramping during attempted writing), blepharospasm (spasms resulting in increased, forceful blinking), spasmodic torticollis or cervical dystonia (a disorder in which there is sustained, involuntary twisting or turning of the neck), and oromandibular dystonia (muscle contractions producing involuntary grinding of the teeth or opening of the jaws during attempts to eat or talk). An example of segmental dystonia is craniofacial dystonia, in which both blepharospasm and jaw-closing spasms may occur. Hemidystonia most commonly results from a stroke or structural lesion, such as a mass in the contralateral basal ganglia, often the putamen.

When dystonia onset occurs in an adult or an elderly person, the dystonia tends to stay localized to the part of the body first affected, and it is less likely to affect other body parts than when onset occurs during childhood. Medical treatments include administration of anticholinergic agents such as trihexyphenidyl; however, these medications are poorly tolerated by elderly patients. Other medications used are muscle relaxants such as baclofen, and benzodiazepines such as clonazepam. The most effective treatment is often botulinum toxin injections. Dystonia can also be a tardive condition (tardive dystonia; see subsection below on tardive movement disorders) in individuals exposed to dopamine receptor–blocking medications.

Tardive Movement Disorders

The term *tardive movement disorder* refers to hyperkinetic movements that develop in individuals with prolonged exposure to dopamine receptor–blocking medications such as phenothiazine-containing antiemetics and antipsychotic medications (Skidmore and Reich 2005). Elderly women taking these medications appear to be most susceptible to tardive movement disorders. Tardive dyskinesia typically manifests as semivoluntary, repetitive oro-buccolingual movements. The movements often attenuate temporarily with concentration and typically disappear during sleep. The movements can also involve the head, face, and limbs, and may appear choreiform, although they are often more stereotypic and repetitive than the more random movements of classic chorea. Tardive dyskinesia can affect muscles involved in breathing, resulting in respiratory dyskinesia.

The term *tardive dystonia* refers to difficult-to-treat dystonic movements that are associated with chronic use of dopamine receptor–blocking agents. The sustained abnormal posturing of tardive dystonia can affect the neck in the form of retrocollis (backward displacement of the neck) and limb dystonia. *Akathisia* refers to inner restlessness in an individual treated with dopamine receptor–blocking agents. It manifests as constant squirming and fidgeting, for example, when sitting in a chair.

Whenever possible, treatment for tardive movement disorders involves tapering and stopping the offending medication when possible. Tetrabenazine, a dopamine-depleting agent available outside the United States, is often helpful in suppressing tardive movement disorders, particularly tardive dyskinesia. It is currently only available

in the United States under a compassionate use protocol. A newer, atypical antipsychotic medication such as quetiapine can be tried if tetrabenazine is not an option. Botulinum toxin injections are helpful in some patients with bothersome focal dyskinesias.

Chorea

The term *chorea* refers to involuntary, dancelike movements that have a continuous, random, unpredictable, often twitch-like appearance and flow from one body part to another. Chorea can be hard to distinguish from tardive dyskinesia in the absence of a complete history; however, movements in chorea are more random, and movements in tardive dyskinesia tend to be repetitive and stereotyped. Chorea can occur in elderly individuals in association with Huntington's disease, neuroacanthocytosis, overdose of drugs such as amphetamines or stimulants, alcohol intoxication, and metabolic abnormalities such as hyperthyroidism, hypo- or hypernatremia, hypo- or hyperglycemia, hypocalcemia, and hypomagnesemia. The term *hemiballismus* is applied to choreiform throwing or flinging movements affecting one side of the body, and this condition is often associated with a lesion of the contralateral subthalamic nucleus, most commonly due to a stroke. Therapy consists of treating any underlying toxic or metabolic condition and using tetrabenazine or an atypical antipsychotic such as quetiapine.

Tics

Tics are brief, repetitive, semivoluntary, jerklike movements. Vocal tics consist of audible vocalizations, and motor tics consist of rapid movements of the head, face, limbs, or other body parts. Tics can be simple or complex. They can usually be suppressed for a short time, but the patient often builds up an unpleasant sensation in the involved body part and experiences transient relief of the unpleasant sensation by performing the tic once again. The tic disorder—Gilles de la Tourette's syndrome, or Tourette's syndrome—begins in childhood but can persist in adults and the elderly (Singer 2005). Tourette's syndrome is often associated with obsessive-compulsive disorder, which can be more disabling than the tics themselves. Other causes of tic disorders in elderly individuals include use of stimulants or other drugs, encephalitis, carbon monoxide poisoning, head trauma, and stroke. Treatments include administration of antipsychotic medications; however, the clinician must be aware of the associated risk of producing a tardive movement disorder, especially in elderly patients. Treatment with tetrabenazine or clonazepam is also helpful in some patients.

Myoclonus

The word *myoclonus* refers to sudden, jerk-like or shocklike movements due to activation of affected muscles (positive myoclonus) or to sudden loss of activation of affected muscles (negative myoclonus) (Caviness and Brown 2004). The movements are involuntary and can occur randomly or regularly. Myoclonus can arise from dysfunction at multiple levels of the central nervous system, from the cortex to the brain stem to the spinal cord. For example, spinal inflammation from a dermatomal herpes infection (shingles) can result in focal myoclonus in the same dermatome. Negative myoclonus can manifest as asterixis (flapping movements of the hands when the arms are held outstretched with the wrists extended "like stopping traffic"), as seen in hepatic or renal failure. Also, disabling negative myoclonus affecting the legs and trunk upon standing can be a consequence of hypoxic or ischemic brain stem injury in elderly patients. Benzodiazepines such as clonaz-

epam, anticonvulsants such as levetiracetam, and piracetam are sometimes beneficial in the treatment of this condition.

Hemifacial Spasm

Hemifacial spasm is another movement disorder that occurs in the elderly population. The disorder consists of simultaneous, involuntary, rapid, jerklike movements of facial muscles on one side of the face. These movements are not painful. Typically, the patient experiences blinking of one eye and synchronous drawing up of the same side of the face. No sensory deficit on the affected side of the face should be present, because this disorder affects only the facial nerve (cranial nerve VII), which provides motor and not sensory innervation to the face.

Hemifacial spasm appears to be caused by irritation of the facial nerve. The disorder is sometimes associated with an ectatic, tortuous basilar artery at the level of the pons in the brain stem. Physical contact between the basilar artery and the facial nerve at the point where the nerve emerges from the pons is thought to produce aberrant, ephaptic nerve transmission in the facial nerve, resulting in transient activation of facial muscles on one side of the face. An ectatic basilar artery can be identified by brain MRI and magnetic resonance angiography (MRA). Anticonvulsants such as carbamazepine and phenytoin are sometimes helpful, and botulinum toxin injections are often effective. If medical treatment is insufficient, a neurosurgical procedure to insulate the facial nerve from the basilar artery can be considered.

Psychogenic Movement Disorders

Psychogenic movement disorders are diagnoses of exclusion and most commonly take the form of waxing and waning tremor, dystonia, or myoclonus that attenuates with distraction (Schrag and Lang 2005). The onset of these conditions is often abrupt, and it is often possible to identify periods of normal function between periods of dysfunction. Psychogenic tremor is characterized by tremor that speeds up or slows down in synchrony with forced repetitive movements of the opposite limb. The movements may respond to positive or negative suggestion, and successful treatment may involve intensive psychiatric or psychological intervention by professionals who are interested in these complex conditions.

Restless Legs Syndrome

Restless legs syndrome, which can occur in elderly persons, is characterized by unpleasant sensations in the legs when the affected individual is sitting or lying down, particularly when tired. The patient experiences creeping, crawling sensations under the skin of the calves, and these sensations attenuate only when the patient stands up and walks. No visible abnormal movement need be present, but the unpleasant leg sensations interfere with sleep and can be disabling. The condition sometimes results from renal failure or from iron deficiency anemia, in which case symptoms improve with successful treatment of the underlying medical condition. A sleep study (polysomnography) may identify periodic leg movements in sleep, which are commonly associated with restless legs syndrome. Use near bedtime of a dopamine agonist, clonazepam, levodopa, or, sometimes, a narcotic such as codeine may be beneficial. Prolonged use of levodopa, however, has been associated with eventual worsening of symptoms.

Conclusion

Movement disorders in the elderly are to be distinguished from changes associated with normal aging, in which mobility may become more limited because of a life-time of wear and tear on muscles, ligaments, bones, and joints. Normal aging includes some slowing of movement, aches and pains, and perhaps stooping. However, clinical experience permits distinguishing these phenomena of aging from neurodegenerative movement disorders. Excessive poverty of movement is indicative of a hypokinetic movement disorder such as PD or another parkinsonian condition. Development of a hyperkinetic movement disorder such as tremor, tics, chorea, or myoclonus cannot be attributed to normal aging and is worthy of further evaluation to identify whether there is an underlying, treatable condition.

References

Bain P, Brin M, Deuschl G, et al: Criteria for the diagnosis of essential tremor. Neurology 54:S7, 2000

Benabid AL, Chabardes S, Seigneuret E: Deep-brain stimulation in Parkinson's disease: long-term efficacy and safety—what happened this year? Curr Opin Neurol 18(6): 623–630, 2005

Caviness JN, Brown P: Myoclonus: current concepts and recent advances. Lancet Neurol 3:598–607, 2004

de Bruin VMS, Lees AJ, Daniel S: Diffuse Lewy body disease presenting with supranuclear gaze palsy, parkinsonism, and dementia: case report. Mov Disord 7:355–358, 1992

Forno LS: Neuropathology of Parkinson's disease. J Neuropathol Exp Neurol 55:259–272, 1996

Foster NL, Wilhelmsen K, Sima AAF, et al: Frontotemporal dementia and parkinsonism linked to chromosome 17: a consensus conference. Participants of the Chromosome 17–Related Dementia Conference. Ann Neurol 41:706–715, 1997

Geser F, Wenning GK, Seppi K, et al: Progression of multiple system atrophy (MSA): a prospective natural history study by the European MSA Study Group (EMSA SG). Mov Disord 21(2):179–186, 2006

Gibb WRG, Luthert PJ, Marsden CD: Clinical and pathological features of corticobasal degeneration. Adv Neurol 53:51–54, 1990

Golbe LI: Alpha-synuclein and Parkinson's disease. Mov Disord 14:6–9, 1999

Jankovic J: Essential tremor: clinical characteristics. Neurology 54:S21–S25, 2000

Kraft E, Schwarz J, Trenkwalder C, et al: The combination of hypointense and hyperintense signal changes on T2-weighted magnetic resonance sequences: a specific marker for multiple system atrophy? Arch Neurol 56:225–228, 1999

Lang AE, Lozano AM: Parkinson's disease. First of two parts. N Engl J Med 339:1044–1053, 1998a

Lang AE, Lozano AM: Parkinson's disease. Second of two parts. N Engl J Med 339:1130–1143, 1998b

Litvan I: Update on progressive supranuclear palsy. Curr Neurol Neurosci Rep 4:296–302, 2004

Litvan I, Agid Y, Goetz C, et al: Accuracy of the clinical diagnosis of corticobasal degeneration: a clinicopathologic study. Neurology 48:119–125, 1997

Louis ED: Essential tremor. Lancet Neurol 4:100–110, 2005

Lund and Manchester Groups: Clinical and neuropathological criteria for frontotemporal dementia. J Neurol Neurosurg Psychiatry 57:416–418, 1994

Mutch WJ, Dingwall-Fordyce I, Downie AW, et al: Parkinson's disease in a Scottish city. Br Med J (Clin Res Ed) 292:534–536, 1986

Myers BH, Scott BL: A case of combined orthostatic tremor and primary gait ignition failure. Clin Neurol Neurosurg 105:277–280, 2003

Nutt JG, Wooten GF: Clinical practice. Diagnosis and initial management of Parkinson's disease. N Engl J Med 353:1021–1027, 2005

Riley DE, Lang AE: Clinical diagnostic criteria, in Corticobasal Degeneration (Advances in Neurology, Vol 82). Edited by Litvan I, Goetz CG, Lang AE. Philadelphia, PA, Lippincott Williams & Wilkins, 2000, pp 29–34

Savoiardo M, Grisoli M, Girotti F: Magnetic resonance imaging in CBD, related atypical parkinsonian disorders, and dementias, in Corticobasal Degeneration (Advances in Neurology, Vol 82). Edited by Litvan I, Goetz CG, Lang AE. Philadelphia, PA, Lippincott Williams & Wilkins, 2000, pp 197–208

Schneider JA, Watts RL, Gearing M, et al: Corticobasal degeneration: neuropathologic and clinical heterogeneity. Neurology 48:959–969, 1997

Schrag A, Lang AE: Psychogenic movement disorders. Curr Opin Neurol 18:399–404, 2005

Scott BL: Evaluation and treatment of dystonia. South Med J 93:746–751, 2000

Scott BL, Jankovic J: Delayed-onset progressive movement disorders after static brain lesions. Neurology 46:68–74, 1996

Shy GM, Drager GA: A neurological syndrome associated with orthostatic hypotension. Arch Neurol 2:511–527, 1960

Singer HS: Tourette's syndrome: from behavior to biology. Lancet Neurol 4:149–159, 2005

Skidmore F, Reich SG: Tardive dystonia. Curr Treat Options Neurol 7:231–236, 2005

Steele JC, Richardson JC, Olszewski J: Progressive supranuclear palsy: a heterogeneous degeneration involving the brain stem, basal ganglia and cerebellum, with vertical gaze and pseudobulbar palsy, nuchal dystonia and dementia. Arch Neurol 10:333–359, 1964

Sutcliffe RL, Prior R, Mawby B, et al: Parkinson's disease in the district of the Northampton Health Authority, United Kingdom: a study of prevalence and disability. Acta Neurol Scand 72:363–379, 1985

Weiner WJ: A differential diagnosis of parkinsonism. Rev Neurol Dis 2:124–131, 2005

Study Questions

Select the single best response for each question.

1. All of the following are features of Parkinson's disease *except*

   A. Postural instability.
   B. Prevalence increasing with age.
   C. Lewy bodies in the cytoplasm of degenerating neurons.
   D. Resting tremor attenuating at least transiently during voluntary movement, much like that of essential tremor.
   E. Presentation with an akinetic form in which resting tremor is minimal.

2. Synkinetic movement refers to

   A. Resting tremor.
   B. Cogwheel rigidity.
   C. Involuntary resistance to passive movement of the extremities.
   D. Voluntary movement of contralateral extremity bringing out rigidity in ipsilateral limb.
   E. None of the above.

3. Side effects of dopamine agonists include which of the following?

   A. Hallucinations.
   B. Dyskinesias.
   C. Dystonia.
   D. A and B.
   E. A, B, and C.

4. All of the following are features of progressive supranuclear palsy (PSP) *except*

   A. Vertical gaze palsy.
   B. Early postural instability.
   C. Axial rigidity greater than appendicular rigidity.
   D. Good response to levodopa.
   E. Sloppy eating.

5. Which of the following is *not* true of essential tremor?

   A. It is the most prevalent movement disorder among the elderly.
   B. Prevalence increases with age.
   C. Frequency may decrease with age.
   D. Early on, tremor is absent at rest.
   E. Usually it is not associated with a family history of tremor.

6. Which of the following attenuates essential tremor?

   A. Propranolol.
   B. Primidone.
   C. Alcohol.
   D. Deep brain stimulation of the ventral intermediate nucleus of the contralateral thalamus.
   E. All of the above.

CHAPTER 8

Mood Disorders

Harold G. Koenig, M.D., M.H.Sc.

Dan G. Blazer, M.D., Ph.D.

The themes of aging and depression often coalesce. Frequent questions surrounding these themes include the following (Blazer 2003): Do persons become more depressed as they grow older? Does depression become more difficult to treat with increased age? Is depression more difficult to identify in the older adult? The answers to these questions rest in part with the definition of late-life depression. Depression in late life is not a unitary construct. Depending on how depression is defined, the answers to questions regarding late-life depression vary.

Depression can be construed in at least three ways, each of which has clinical relevance for older adults. First, depression can be viewed as a unitary phenomenon, with the various manifestations of depression forming a continuum. Sir Aubrey Lewis (1934) noted that the various classifications of depression are "nothing more than attempts to distinguish between acute and chronic, mild and severe" (p. 1). Although the extremes of the continuum are different, precise boundaries can be found between these extremes. Depression symptom checklists, such as the Center for Epidemiologic Studies Depression Scale

(CES-D; Radloff 1977), the Geriatric Depression Scale (Yesavage et al. 1983), and the Brief Depression Scale (Koenig et al. 1995), are therefore useful in determining the degree to which an individual suffers from depression in late life.

Most modern investigators, however, find it difficult to conceive of depression as phenomenologically homogeneous. A categorical approach, as exemplified in DSM-IV-TR (American Psychiatric Association 2000), has been of more interest to modern clinicians. If one views the affective disorders as a group of distinct entities or independent syndromes, with each of the categories being mutually exclusive, diagnosis and management of depression are allied with the traditional medical model. Given the availability of excellent, but potentially dangerous, biological therapies, the categorical approach has been adopted by most geriatric psychiatrists. A radical overhaul has been suggested for the fifth edition of DSM, which is projected to be available in 2007 (McHugh 2001). In the new system, psychiatric disorders would be divided into four broad categories (disease, dimension, behavior, life story), and the focus would be more on the psychological or biological essence of disorders than on clinical appearance.

The third approach to the conceptualization of the depressed elder is a functional approach: when depressive symptoms become so severe that functioning is impaired, the case is considered worthy of clinical attention. Social functioning, especially the performance of role responsibilities, has been targeted as a critical variable in monitoring treatment. Functioning is a critical element for family members, who do not view symptom remission alone as an essential marker of improvement but, rather, consider a return to social involvement and improved life satisfaction as critical signs.

The categorical approach to diagnosis—that is, a focus on Axis I of DSM-IV-TR—is adopted, for the most part, through the remainder of this chapter. Nevertheless, the reader should recognize that other constructs of depression must complement the categorical approach if it is to be effective in the diagnosis and treatment of older adults. Social and physical functioning, both during and after therapy, are at least as important in assessing the success of therapeutic intervention as is the remission of a series of symptoms.

There have been few changes in the categorization of major depression and other affective disorders in the transition from DSM-III-R to DSM-IV (and its text revision, DSM-IV-TR); where changes are relevant, we point them out.

Epidemiology of Late-Life Depression

Prevalence

General comments on the epidemiology of psychiatric disorders in late life are reported in Chapter 1, "Demography and Epidemiology of Psychiatric Disorders in Late Life." Using a community survey, investigators at

Duke University Medical Center attempted to untangle the different subtypes of depression in late life (Blazer et al. 1987). More than 1,300 older adults in urban and rural communities who were age 60 or older were screened for depressive symptomatology. Of the 27% reporting depressive symptoms, 19% had mild dysphoria only. Persons with symptomatic depression—that is, subjects with more severe depressive symptoms—made up 4% of the population. These individuals were primarily experiencing stressors, such as physical illness and stressful life events. Only 2% had a dysthymic disorder, and 0.8% were experiencing a current major depressive episode. No cases of current manic episode were identified. Finally, 1.2% had a mixed depression and anxiety syndrome. These data suggest that the traditional DSM-III-R depression categories do not apply to most depressed older adults in the community.

Depression in late life remains a generic term that captures many constructs, some of which are well defined and others of which are ill defined. The burden of depression in the elderly, as indicated by the just-described frequency of significant depressive symptoms in community populations, is unquestioned. Many older persons with atypical presentations of depression do not meet criteria for major depression. Nevertheless, the usual reasons given for not identifying severe depression in an older adult in the clinical setting—pseudodementia, somatization, denial of depressive symptomatology, poor response to antidepressant medication, or masked depression—do not apply to most severely depressed elders, such as melancholic older adults. DSM-IV-TR and similar nomenclatures may therefore apply to some, but not all, depressive syndromes in late life.

Because of the association between medical illness and depression, many depressed elders may be either in acute-care settings or in nursing homes and thus be unavailable for (or be unable to participate in) community surveys. In contrast to low rates (1%) of major depression among older adults in the community, it has been estimated that, depending on the diagnostic scheme, up to 21% of hospitalized elders fulfill criteria for a major depressive episode, and an additional 20%–25% have a minor depression (Koenig et al. 1997). Likewise, rates of major depression among elderly nursing home patients are even higher, exceeding 25% in some studies (Gerety et al. 1994).

Manic episodes in late life are uncommon but not unseen. In a study of 6-month prevalence of psychiatric disorders in three communities, no person older than 65 years, of more than 3,000 elders interviewed, was found to have a current manic episode (Myers et al. 1984). One reason for the very low prevalence in community populations may be the inability of structured instruments to identify the atypical presentation of manic episodes in elderly patients. When mania does occur, the syndrome may be so severe that the elder is hospitalized and therefore would not be located during a community inquiry. Alternatively, manic episodes in later life may present with a mixture of manic, dysphoric, and cognitive symptoms, with euphoria being less common (Post 1978). When mania is associated with significant changes in cognitive function—so-called manic delirium—it may be difficult to distinguish it from organic conditions or schizophrenia (Shulman 1986).

Thus, manic episodes may present in an atypical manner that does not allow easy categorization, especially when they have been diagnosed using structured psychiatric interviews administered by lay interviewers, as in the Epidemiologic Catchment Area (ECA) surveys. Despite such considerations, however, the ECA surveys did diagnose bipolar disorder in 9.7% of nursing home patients, which suggests that this setting may have become a dumping ground for such patients (Weissman et al. 1991). In clinical settings, about 10%–25% of geriatric patients with mood disorder have bipolar disorder, and 3%–10% of all older psychiatric patients have this disorder (Wylie et al. 1999; Young and Klerman 1992). About 5% of all individuals admitted as geropsychiatry inpatients present with mania (Yassa et al. 1988).

Snapshot prevalence studies do not adequately represent late-life depression within the context of historical trends. The 20-year follow-up of the Midtown Manhattan Longitudinal Study illustrates the importance of cohort analysis (Srole and Fischer 1980). Nearly 700 of the original 1,660 adults, who were between ages 20 and 59 years at the time of the original study, were reinterviewed 20 years later using an identical instrument. Although in the assessments in both 1954 and 1974, the highest rates of mental health impairment were found among the elderly subjects (22% for the 50- to 59-year-olds, compared with 7% for the 20- to 29-year-olds in 1954), the prevalence of mental health impairment did not increase longitudinally with age. How can these findings be explained? Cohort effects may influence the distribution of depressive symptoms across the life cycle more than may the effects of aging. The burden of depressive symptoms within a birth cohort may remain relatively constant throughout the life cycle.

Mortality

An additional parameter of late-life affective disorders is outcome. The epidemiology of suicide is discussed in Chapter 1, "Demography and Epidemiology of Psychiatric Disorders in Late Life." Examination of the association between depressive symptoms and all-cause mortality among older participants in the ECA study in North Carolina did not reveal a relationship between depressive symptoms and mortality when other known causes of mortality were included in a logistic analysis (Fredman et al. 1989). When age, activities of daily living, gender, and cognitive impairment were controlled, neither the diagnosis of major depression nor the accumulation of significant depressive symptoms at baseline predicted mortality 2 years after the initial interview in more than 1,600 community respondents at least 60 years old. However, in a more recent, 6-year follow-up of 764 community-dwelling women older than 65 years who were living in the Baltimore, Maryland, area, Fredman et al. (1999) found that the risk of death was 14.5% among women with CES-D scores of 0 or 1, 24%–28% among women with scores of 2 to 24, and 47% among those with scores greater than 24. When factors jointly associated with depression and mortality are controlled, however, the risk of mortality among depressed elders decreases significantly (Blazer et al. 2001).

In clinical populations, the findings have been more consistent. Murphy and colleagues (1988) examined all-cause mortality in a 4-year follow-up study involving 120 depressed elderly psychiatric inpatients, comparing them with 197 age- and gender-matched control subjects. Among the depressed women, mortality was twice the expected rate; among the men, it was three times the expected rate. Older men with physical health problems and depression were significantly more likely to die than were similarly aged, physically ill, nondepressed men. Rovner and colleagues (1991) also found greater death rates among elderly nursing home patients with depression. Several subsequent studies involving medically ill elderly patients likewise found

greater mortality among those with depression (Arfken et al. 1999; Covinsky et al. 1999; Black and Markides 1999).

These studies indicate higher rates of mortality for depressed elderly patients (men in particular) with concurrent physical health problems. The association between late-life depression and mortality is intuitively attractive, because older persons are thought to experience loss of meaningful roles and emotional support through retirement, death of friends or a spouse, decreased economic and material well-being, and increased isolation and loneliness (Atchley 1972; Fassler and Gavira 1978). When poor physical health compounds these age-related changes, depression may be particularly prone to affect health outcomes.

Health Care Costs

Health care costs are increased among depressed older adults. In a study that involved more than 9,000 patients age 60 years and older in primary care settings, Katon and colleagues (2003) found that ambulatory and inpatient health care costs were 40%–50% higher in depressed compared with nondepressed elderly patients after adjustment for chronic medical illness. No differences in costs were noted between patients with subthreshold depressive syndromes and those with DSM-IV depressive disorders (diagnoses based on the Structured Clinical Interview for DSM-IV).

Prognosis

Until recently, long-term psychiatric follow-up investigations involving survivors of severe episodes of late-life depression were relatively scarce, given the frequency and clinical importance of the disorder. The typical course of major depression throughout the life cycle is remission and relapse. In patients with a history of recurrent episodes, new episodes tend to be associated with similar symptoms and to last about as long as prior episodes. Classic studies of depression suggest that the duration of major depression throughout the life cycle is approximately 9 months if untreated (Dunner 1985). As individuals age, however, they may experience episodes more frequently, and these episodes can merge into a chronic condition.

Baldwin and Jolley (1986) followed 100 elderly psychiatric inpatients with severe unipolar depression for 3–8 years. Of these patients, 60% remained well throughout or had relapses with complete recovery, and only 7% had continuous depression. Likewise, in a direct comparison of middle-aged and elderly patients hospitalized for major depression, little difference was found between middle-aged and older adults in recovery (Blazer et al. 1992). Of the 44 older adults (at least 60 years old), 48% had not recovered from the depressive episode leading to hospitalization, 27% had recovered completely from the index episode but experienced a recurrence of another episode of major depression, and 25% had recovered completely without a recurrence. Of the 35 middle-aged patients, 46% had not recovered from the index episode, 45% had recovered completely but experienced a recurrence of another episode, and 9% had recovered completely and remained recovered. Significant depressive symptoms at the time of follow-up (a score of 16 or higher on the CES-D) were reported by 59% of the elderly subjects but only 43% of the middle-aged subjects. These 1- to 2-year follow-up findings suggest that in terms of recovery and remission, older adults do not differ from their middle-aged counterparts. If they do recover, however, elders appear to experience residual depressive symptoms.

Most clinicians and clinical investigators report that more than 70% of elderly pa-tients with major depression who are treated with antidepressant medication (at an adequate dose for a sufficient time) recover from the index episode of depression. Reynolds and colleagues (1992) reported that treatment of physically healthy depressed elders with combined interpersonal psychotherapy and nortriptyline was associated with response rates nearing 80%. The combination of psychotherapy and medication, coordinated by a case manager, has been found effective in primary care practice (Hunkeler et al. 2006). In a long-term outcome study of treatment-resistant depression in older adults, 47% of patients were clinically improved 15 months after treatment with an antidepressant or electroconvulsive therapy (ECT); at 4 years of follow-up, that percentage had increased to 71% (Stoudemire et al. 1993). These optimistic results are tempered by the fact that physical illness and impaired cognition may complicate both the course of depression and response to treatment (Baldwin and Jolley 1986; Cole 1983; Koenig et al. 1997; Murphy et al. 1988). Once an older patient has experienced one or more moderate to severe episodes of major depression, he or she may need to continue antidepressant therapy permanently, to minimize the risk of relapse (Greden 1993; Old Age Depression Interest Group 1993).

Factors associated with improved outcome in late-life depression include a history of recovery from previous episodes, a family history of depression, female gender, extroverted personality, current or recent employment, absence of substance abuse, no history of major psychiatric disorder, less severe depressive symptomatology, and absence of major life events and serious medical illness (Baldwin and Jolley 1986; Cole et al. 1999; Post 1972). The results of a number of studies suggest a relationship between social support during an index episode and outcome in psychological distress and depression. Intuition suggests that adequate support should enhance recovery from a severe or moderately severe psychiatric disorder such as major depression. In a study involving 493 community respondents, Holahan and Moos (1981) found that decreases in social support of family and in work environments were related to increases in psychological maladjustment over a 1-year follow-up period.

Coping behavior may also affect prognosis of late-life depression. One of the coping behaviors most commonly used by this generation of older adults is religious involvement. In a study involving 100 middle-aged or elderly adults, one-third of men and nearly two-thirds of women used religious cognitions or behaviors to help them cope with a stressful period (Koenig et al. 1988). A number of investigators have reported inverse associations between religious coping and depressive symptoms in older adults with or without medical illness (Braam et al. 1997b; Idler 1987; Koenig et al. 1992; Pressman et al. 1990). A study involving 850 hospitalized medically ill elders found that those using religion to cope were less likely to be depressed and more likely to experience improvement in depressive symptoms over time (Koenig et al. 1992). Religious involvement also appears to be a predictor of faster recovery from depression in both community-dwelling and clinical samples of older adults (Braam et al. 1997a; Koenig et al. 1998).

The outcome of bipolar disorder in elderly patients remains virtually unknown. In a long-term follow-up study involving 500 patients in Iowa, Winokur (1975) found a tendency for bipolar disorder to occur in clusters over time and speculated that early-onset bipolar illness may "burn itself out" in time. Shulman and Post (1980) studied elderly patients with bipolar disorder and found that only 8% had their first episode of mania before age 40. In a review of records of a small number of untreated patients with severe and prolonged bipolar disorder, Cutler and Post (1982) found a tendency toward more rapid recurrences late in the illness, with decreasing periods of normality. In other words, if bipolar disorder reemerges in the later years, the episodes of mania—or mania mixed with depression—may once again cluster, just as the disorder typically clusters at earlier periods of life. Most clinicians who have worked with patients with bipolar disorder in late life recognize the tendency of these disorders to recur frequently for a time, only to remit for an extended period.

Ameblas (1987) emphasized a relationship between life events and onset of mania, noting that stressful events were more likely to precede early-onset mania than late-onset mania. Likewise, Shulman (1989) stressed that increased cerebral vulnerability due to organic insults (stroke, head trauma, other brain insults) played a stronger role than life events in precipitating late-onset mania (a factor that may also play a role in treatment resistance). Young and Klerman (1992) emphasized the low rates of familial affective disorder and the increased frequency of certain diseases and drug use associated with late age at onset.

Controversy exists over whether age affects response to treatment. Eastham et al. (1998) suggested that elderly patients with bipolar disorder often require lithium doses that are 25%–50% lower than those used in younger patients. Data on the use of valproic acid in elderly patients with this disorder are limited but encouraging. There is almost no information on the use of carbamazepine or other drugs in late-life bipolar disorder. ECT has been reported to be well tolerated and effective in the treatment of these patients (Eastham et al. 1998).

Risk Factors

The etiology of late-life affective disorders is undoubtedly multifactorial. Twin and family studies, along with studies focusing on molecular genetics, provide strong evidence for a heritable contribution to the etiology of major depression and bipolar disorder (Egeland et al. 1987; Slater and Cowie 1971). Evidence that these genetic factors weigh heavily in the etiology of bipolar disorders in late life is virtually nonexistent, although the biological nature of this disorder would suggest some genetic contribution. Evidence from studies of unipolar depression in late life suggests that the genetic contribution is weaker in late-life depression than in depression at earlier stages of the life cycle (Hopkinson 1964; Mendlewicz 1976; Schulz 1951).

Associated with the genetic predisposition for depression is the fact that major depression is more common in women (Myers et al. 1984). Most studies that consider the distribution of major depression across the life span confirm the persistence of the 2:1 ratio of women to men into late life. However, there is no evidence for a genetic predisposition—that is, a sex-linked mode of inheritance—that would favor women in the onset of major depression. Nevertheless, even in the best-controlled studies, the gender difference in the prevalence of the more severe depressions persists. The operable factor or factors persist into the later years. It is possible, however, that women are more likely to admit and complain about their dysphoric feelings than are men, who are more likely to deny feelings and instead act them out (such as through alcoholism or suicide).

Dysregulation of the hypothalamic-pituitary-adrenal (HPA) axis is also thought to contribute to a predisposition for depression. An association between increased cortisol concentrations and depression has been recognized for many years: there is an increase throughout the 24-hour circadian excretion of cortisol in depressed patients (Sachar 1975). This finding led Carroll et al. (1981) to propose the dexamethasone suppression test (DST) as a laboratory test for melancholic depression. In a large study involving men and women ages 20–78 years, Rosenbaum et al. (1984) found that 18% of persons older than 65 years were nonsuppressors of cortisol after administration of dexamethasone, compared with 9.1% of younger subjects. Whether this higher prevalence of nonsuppression reflects an increased propensity of older persons for dysregulation of the HPA axis, or whether it may result from difficulty in absorbing or metabolizing dexamethasone, remains to be discovered.

Dysregulation of the thyroid axis and of growth hormone release has also been implicated in the etiology of depression in later life. Blunted responses of thyroid-stimulating hormone (TSH) to thyrotropin-releasing hormone (TRH) are found in many healthy elderly subjects (Snyder and Utiger 1972) and in depressed patients (Targum et al. 1982). Secretion of growth hormone in elderly persons occurs only during sleep and may cease altogether (Finkelstein et al. 1972). Drugs known to stimulate α-adrenoreceptors, such as clonidine, also affect the release of growth hormone, a response that has been shown to be blunted in patients with endogenous depression (Checkley et al. 1981).

Structural brain changes have also been found in geriatric patients with depression and in those with bipolar disorder. Alexopoulos and colleagues (1997) and Hickie and Scott (1998) reviewed the literature on vascular changes associated with geriatric depression and suggested that preventing these changes may help prevent this disorder. Disruption of prefrontal systems or their modulating pathways by single lesions or by an accumulation of lesions exceeding a threshold is hypothesized to be the central mechanism.

With regard to bipolar disorder, Young et al. (1999) completed brain computed tomography scans in 30 geriatric patients with mania and in 18 age-matched control subjects. Manic patients had significantly greater cortical sulcal widening and lateral ventricle–brain ratio scores compared with control subjects. Cortical sulcal widening was associated with age at illness onset and age at first manic episode.

A relatively new putative contributor to the etiology of depressive disorders is desynchronization of circadian rhythms. The cyclicity of depressive disorders suggests an underlying disruption of the normal biochemical and physiological circadian rhythms. Vogel et al. (1980) noted that the clinical features of depression, especially insomnia and diurnal variation of mood, suggest abnormalities in biological rhythms. The disruption of the sleep cycle with age (though this is the only circadian rhythm known to be dramatically affected by age) suggests the possibility that circadian problems contribute to the etiology of depression in late life. As age increases, total sleep time gradually diminishes and sleep continuity decreases (Kupfer 1984; Ulrich et al. 1980). Endocrine secretion patterns, also associated with depression, are known to be less affected by the aging process (Lakatua et al. 1984).

Finally, social factors must be considered in the development of a risk model for depression in late life. Pfifer and Murrell (1986) examined the additive and interactive roles of six sociodemographic factors—three being from the domain of social resources and three being categories of life events—in the development of depressive symptoms. In a probability sample of more than 1,200 persons age 55 or older, 66 developed significant depressive symptoms (as measured by the CES-D) 6 months after an initial evaluation. Health and social support played both an additive and an interactive role in the onset of depressive symptoms, life events had weak effects, and sociodemographic factors did not contribute to depression onset.

The interaction between social support and depression is more complex. Social support may contribute to the onset of major depression, it may contribute to the outcome of major depression, or it may be affected by depressive symptoms. By studying 331 community subjects selected at random, Blazer (1983) tested the hypothesis that a major depressive disorder contributes to a decline in social support. Impaired support was associated with the presence of major depressive disorder at baseline. Thirty months later, however, the surviving subjects whose social supports had improved were nearly three times more likely to have been depressed earlier than were subjects whose social supports did not improve. In other words, major depressive disorder was a significant predictor of improvement in supports at follow-up.

Diagnosis and Differential Diagnosis of Late-Life Affective Disorders

Four clinical entities listed under the mood disorders in DSM-IV-TR are relevant to depression in elderly patients: 1) bipolar I disorder (manic, depressed, and mixed) and bipolar II disorder; 2) major depressive disorder (single episode, recurrent, with or without melancholia, and with or without psychotic features); 3) dysthymic disorder; and 4) depressive disorder not otherwise specified (NOS), formerly called atypical depression. Depressive symptoms are likewise present in other DSM-IV-TR disorders, such as bereavement, adjustment disorder with depressed mood, substance-induced mood disorder, and mood disorder due to a general medical condition. In still other psychiatric disorders, such as organic psychiatric disorders, paranoid disorders, sleep disorders, and hypochondriasis, depressive symptomatology is a central component of the clinical picture on occasion.

Bipolar Disorder

For a diagnosis of bipolar I disorder to be made, the patient must have experienced at least one manic episode. Bipolar II disorder involves recurrent episodes of major depression and at least one hypomanic episode (that does not meet the full criteria for a manic episode). For a diagnosis of manic episode to be made, at least three classic manic symptoms—such as overactivity, pressure of speech, distractibility, decreased sleep (without feeling a need for sleep), overspending, and grandiosity—must be present. Mood, however, can be either elevated or irritable and may be labile or mixed in the affective presentation (four of the aforementioned symptoms are required, however, if mood is only irritable).

Post (1978) found that most elderly patients with a bipolar disorder exhibited a depressive admixture with manic symptomatology. Spar et al. (1979) reported that manic elders are atypical in presentation, with dysphoric mood and denial of classic manic symptoms. As noted earlier, Shulman (1986) described the special problem of manic delirium. When an individual is experiencing a full-blown manic episode, cognitive function is difficult to test, yet perseverative behavior, catatonia-like symptoms, and even negativistic symptoms may emerge. Differentiating a manic episode from an agitated depressive episode is often not possible without a thorough examination of the longitudinal course and therapeutic response to medications. In fact, more and more evidence suggests that mixed episodes (with both manic and depressive symptoms) may be the rule rather than the exception (American Psychiatric Association 2000, p. 363).

Major Depressive Disorder

First-onset episodes of major depression in late life are common and often go untreated for months or even years. For this reason, many investigators have suggested that late-life depression is masked (Davies 1965; Lesse 1974; Salzman and Shader 1972). Some studies, however, suggest that older persons admit many feelings of sadness on self-rating scales for depression (Epstein 1976; Zung and Green 1972). However, considerable effort at symptom elicitation may be required to obtain an accurate assessment.

Seasonal Affective Disorder

Variants of classic major depression also occur in elderly individuals. One such variant is seasonal affective disorder (Jacobsen et al. 1987). Diagnostic criteria for seasonal affective disorder include a history of depression fulfilling DSM-IV-TR criteria for major depression (as part of either major depressive disorder or bipolar disorder); a history of at least 2 consecutive years of fall or winter depressive episodes remitting in the spring or summer; and the absence of other major psychiatric disorders or psychosocial explanations for the seasonal mood changes.

Light therapy, in which high-intensity light (10,000 lux) is used to approximate the visual experience of a sunny day (usually in the morning), and regular exposure to sunlight through walks in the late afternoon have proved to be of some value in the treatment of patients with these disorders. Recent studies suggest that institutionalized older adults with depression may be particularly responsive to light therapy (Sumaya et al. 2001).

Major Depression With Psychotic Features

Late-onset psychotic depression deserves special attention. Meyers et al. (1984) studied the prevalence of delusions in 50 patients hospitalized for endogenous major depression. Depressed patients with illness onset at age 60 or later had delusions more frequently than did those with earlier onset. Individuals with delusional depression tended to be older and to respond to ECT, as opposed to tricyclic antidepressants (TCAs). Focus on the abdomen is common in an elderly patient with a delusional or psychotic depression. Hallucinations are uncommon, however.

Dysthymic Disorder

Every clinician who has worked with elderly patients has observed significant and unremitting depressive symptoms associated with apparently psychosocial causes. Verwoerdt (1976) suggested that "reactive depressions" become more frequent with age (such as the depression associated with bereavement), whereas dysthymic disorder seems to be less frequent in the later part of the life cycle. However, community data suggest that the prevalence of dysthymic disorder in elderly persons is lower (but not dramatically lower) than the prevalence of major depression in this age group (Myers et al. 1984).

The psychological mechanisms of late-life dysthymic disorder usually do not include the classic mechanism of dysthymia—that is, self-reproach, guilt, and the turning inward of hostile feelings toward loss. Cath (1965) noted that manifest guilt in older persons is less prevalent, although reaction to loss is a common factor. Busse et al. (1954) suggested that in elderly individuals, introjection is seldom a mechanism for developing depression. Instead, late-life depression is associated with a loss of self-esteem that results from the older adult's inability to satisfy needs and drives or to defend himself or herself against threats to security. Levin (1965) noted the role of restraint as a mechanism in the neurotic depressions of later life. Although sexual satisfaction and interest in sexuality continue to be important for the older adult, sexual drive, though persistent, may not at times be as easily mobilized into behavior. Restraint may derive from either physical problems or lack of an available partner.

Other investigators have emphasized the cultural factors that may contribute to a dysthymic disorder in late life. Wigdor (1980) noted that the major resources in today's culture lead to the development of habit patterns that emphasize activity and productivity—that is, Western society is an achievement-oriented society. With retirement from the workforce and cessation of parenting responsibilities, many older adults find that recognition, self-esteem, and confidence are withdrawn. These needs are not easily substituted. Erikson (1950) suggested that the primary developmental task for late life is the acquisition of integrity and that the means for achieving integrity is to resolve developmental crises that have persisted throughout the life cycle. In other words, striving for industry and generativity may continue to be important for the older adult. If the opportunities for realizing these productive urges are unavailable, or if the elder cannot reconcile previous generative disappointments, despair ensues.

In summary, although dysthymic disorders are no more common in late life than at other stages of the life cycle, late-life dysthymic disorders are to be expected, given the psychological tasks that older adults face and a social environment that may restrain and devalue elders. That elderly individuals maintain a sense of satisfaction and fulfillment despite these inevitable losses and responses from others is a testimony to the resilience of older adults and to the psychological integration that permits a mature completion of life's developmental tasks.

Depressive Disorder Not Otherwise Specified

Another subtype of depression in elderly individuals is codified in DSM-IV-TR as depressive disorder NOS. This subtype of depression (called atypical depression in DSM-III [American Psychiatric Association 1980]) is more often intermittent and unexplained by psychosocial or clear biological factors.

Two subcategories of depressive disorder NOS empirically capture the symptom pattern frequently seen by clinicians who work with depressed elders. First, the syndrome may fulfill the criteria for dysthymic disorder; however, there are intermittent periods of normal mood lasting more than a few months. The dysphoric older adult reports prolonged periods of depression, usually lasting for months but not extending for the entire 2 years required for a DSM-IV-TR diagnosis of dysthymic disorder. Other elders meet the second criterion for depressive disorder NOS: a brief episode of depression that does not meet the criteria for major depression and is apparently not a reaction to psychosocial stress (and therefore cannot be classified as an adjustment disorder). These episodes do not last the full 2 weeks required for a DSM-IV-TR diagnosis of major depressive disorder. Nevertheless, the symptoms can be moderately severe and most troubling to the older adult.

DSM-IV-TR includes the category "minor depressive disorder" in its appendix of criteria sets provided for further study (American Psychiatric Association 2000, pp. 775–777). Minor depression is identical to major depressive disorder except that there are fewer symptoms (one or more but fewer than four additional symptoms besides depressed mood or anhedonia).

Bereavement

Bereavement is a universal human experience and therefore cannot properly be classified as a psychiatric disorder. Primary care physicians are likely to encounter the normal symptoms of grief, but these symptoms may be poorly recognized as such by the bereaved elder. Lindemann (1944), for example, suggested that the normal symptoms of bereavement include sensations of somatic distress such as tightness in the throat, shortness of breath, sighing respirations, lassitude, and loss of appetite. The bereaved are preoccupied with the image of the deceased and frequently can identify events about which they report guilt (often guilt at not having met the needs of the deceased). The grieving are often irritable and hostile and change their usual patterns of conduct. These behavior changes are disturbing to the family and include a pressure of speech, restlessness, an inability to sit still, and an inability to initiate and maintain usual activities. Pathological grief, in contrast, is delayed (an apparent denial of the loss) and/or distorted. Overactivity without a sense of loss, acquisition of symptoms of the last illness of the deceased, frank psychosomatic illness, an alteration of relationships with family and friends, hostility toward specific persons (not uncommonly, family members), and persistent loss of patterns of social interaction can be seen.

For additional discussion of bereavement, see Chapter 12, "Bereavement and Adjustment Disorders."

Adjustment Disorder With Depressed Mood

Among the common presentations of depression in late life is depressed mood and expressions of hopelessness as a reaction to an identifiable stressor. The DSM-IV-TR category of adjustment disorder with depressed mood is reserved for those individuals who exhibit a maladaptive reaction to an identifiable stressor. The relationship of the syndrome to the stressful event is clear. Stressors for older adults include life events such as marital problems, difficulty with children, loss of a social role, and an ill-advised change of residence. Retirement is usually not a source of excessive stress for the older adult. Therefore, the onset of significant depressive symptomatology and withdrawal from activities after retirement may indicate a true adjustment disorder. Of much greater frequency, however, is the development of depressive symptomatology secondary to a physical illness. When an episode of depression accompanies a physical illness, and the level of symptoms dramatically exceeds the expected level, a diagnosis of either adjustment disorder or mood disorder due to a general medical condition is indicated.

Mood Disorder Due to a General Medical Condition

Called organic mood syndrome in DSM-III-R, the essential feature of mood disorder due to a general medical condition is a disturbance in mood resembling a major depressive episode caused by a specific organic factor. If that organic factor is a drug, alcohol, or another intoxicant, the syndrome is called substance-induced mood disorder. The toxic factors that most commonly cause depressive symptoms in older adults are medications. Agents frequently prescribed to older adults that can precipitate depressive symptoms include β-blockers, benzodiazepines, clonidine, reserpine, methyldopa, and even TCAs. Withdrawal of these agents produces a dramatic improvement in symptoms, although both patient and clinician may not associate these medications with the onset of the symptoms. Mild cognitive impairment is often observed in conjunction with the change in mood. Fearfulness, anxiety, irritability, and excessive somatic concerns may accompany the depressive symptoms as well.

Metabolic disorders induce appreciable depressive symptoms, and these are properly classified in the category of mood disorder due to a general medical condition. For example, hyperthyroidism and hypothyroidism are known to be associated with depressive features. These disorders are included in the discussion of physical illnesses that may contribute to a depressive episode (see "Depression and Medical Illness").

Depression and Medical Illness

Included in the category of mood disorder due to a general medical condition are depressive disorders that have been associated with a variety of physical illnesses, among them cardiovascular disease (Glassman and Shapiro 1998; Musselman et al. 1998), endocrine disturbances (Anderson et al. 2001), Parkinson's disease (Zesiewicz et al. 1999), stroke (Dam 2001), cancer (Spiegel 1996), chronic pain (Fifield et al. 1998), chronic fatigue syndrome (Kruesi et al. 1989), and fibromyalgia (Okifuji et al. 2000). As noted previously, depressive symptoms and disorders are common findings in surveys of general medical inpatients (Koenig et al. 1991, 1997; Schwab et al. 1965). Controversy continues over the degree to which acute or chronic medical illnesses cause depression because of direct physiological effects on the brain or because of a psychological reaction to the disability and other life changes evoked by these illnesses (Koenig 1991).

The association between depression and *hypothyroidism* has been well established (Pies 1997). Although the profoundly life-threatening symptoms of myxedema—stupor or coma—are rarely missed in diagnosis, less severe symptoms and signs are common with normal aging and major depression. These include constipation, cold intolerance, psychomotor retardation, decreased exercise tolerance, and cognitive changes, as well as flat affect. Laboratory evaluation will generally reveal decreased thyroxine and increased serum TSH concentrations. If these laboratory findings are obtained, intervention for the thyroid difficulty must precede intervention for the flat affect.

Depressive symptoms have also been associated with both the development and outcome of *cancer*. Early in modern medicine, Guy (1759) published his opinion that women with melancholia were more prone to develop breast cancer. Depression may also result from a direct effect on the brain of neurohumoral substances released from the tumor (pancreatic cancer), or as a reaction to the diagnosis of cancer and the morbidity that ensues.

Physical functioning is highly correlated with depression in cancer patients. In one study (Bukberg et al. 1984), among patients with a Karnofsky score of 40 or less (that is, patients who were most disabled), almost 80% had major depression, whereas only 23% of those who scored 60 or better (that is, had moderate to good function) had major depression. Many studies documenting high rates of depression in patients with cancer are controversial because they often involve patients referred for treatment of cancer, who may have more advanced or complicated illness. It is important that myths about depression and cancer be dispelled. One myth is that all cancer pa-

tients are depressed; another is that physicians should not bother to treat depression, because such patients should be depressed. In fact, when cancer patients become depressed, mortality may increase. With regard to hospitalized elders with cancer, at least one study has shown substantially higher mortality in cancer patients with major depression compared with nondepressed cancer patients (Koenig et al. 1989). Studies have also shown that "desire for hastened death" among terminally ill cancer patients is significantly increased among those who are depressed or feeling hopeless (Breitbart et al. 2000).

With regard to *cardiovascular disease* and depression, Frasure-Smith et al. (1993) followed 222 patients for 6 months after myocardial infarction; depression was a significant predictor of mortality (hazard ratio, 5.7; $P < 0.001$), even after other relevant risk factors were controlled. In an extensive review of this literature, Glassman and Shapiro (1998) reported that 9 of 10 studies found increased cardiovascular mortality in depressed patients. Even when community-dwelling populations are examined and prospectively followed, the relationship between depression and cardiovascular mortality persists (after controlling for smoking and other risk factors).

The effect of physical illness on emotion can be more direct. Evidence is emerging that a neurology of depression exists, as noted in "Risk Factors" earlier in this chapter. The right hemisphere may be uniquely specialized for the perception, experience, and expression of emotion (Coffey 1987). Consistent differences have been observed in the emotional behavior of individuals who have had either left or right hemisphere stroke. A left-sided stroke may be associated with depressive and even catastrophic responses manifested as combinations of dysphoria, episodes of crying, despair, feelings of hopelessness, anger, and self-depreciation (Gainotti 1972;

Robinson et al. 1990; Sackeim et al. 1982). A lesion of the right cerebral hemisphere is more often followed by a neutral, indifferent, or even euphoric response, with denial of deficits and social disinhibition. Although there are exceptions to the findings of these studies, the recognition that selective brain lesions may contribute to specific syndromes closely associated with the depressive disorders implies, in some cases, an anatomy of depression rather than generalized neurochemical abnormalities. Depression itself may also increase the subsequent risk of stroke through some poorly understood biological mechanism, as jas been reported (Jonas and Mussolino 2000).

Depression is a frequent accompaniment of *Parkinson's disease*, with prevalence rates ranging from 20% to 90%; Mayeux (1990) determined a rate of 50% after reviewing the medical records of 339 patients with the disease. In terms of the physical symptoms and signs of paralysis agitans, most older persons differ little from persons observed at earlier ages. The major problems encountered in treating an older adult with Parkinson's disease are secondary to either undue sensitivity to medications or the emotional state of the patient. The older adult with parkinsonism may become disoriented and aggressive and experience ideas of persecution. More commonly, the elder withdraws socially and expresses helplessness and hopelessness regarding the future and considerable anger regarding difficulties in adjusting doses of medication (Carter 1986). Slow movement, weakness, rigidity, and masked and unexpressive facial expressions suggest to the clinician the depressed affect associated with progression of Parkinson's disease. However, the appearance of depression may be more severe than the actual affect indicates. Clinicians must be judicious in determining the necessity of pharmacological intervention in a patient with Parkinson's disease.

Nevertheless, depression in patients with Parkinson's disease seldom disappears spontaneously, and many patients improve with treatment.

Vitamin B$_{12}$ (cobalamin) deficiency has long been associated with depressive symptoms. In a study involving 141 patients with neuropsychiatric abnormalities due to cobalamin deficiency, 28% of subjects had no anemia or macrocytosis at the time of initial evaluation (Lindenbaum et al. 1988). Characteristic features of cobalamin deficiency in these patients included a variety of neurological symptoms (neurosensory loss, ataxia, and memory loss) as well as weakness, fatigue, and depressive symptoms. Most of these patients were older than 65 years, and the distribution between men and women was equal. All but one of the patients in the study responded to cobalamin therapy, exhibiting improvement in neuropsychiatric symptoms, including depressed mood. Anemia and macrocytosis should not be used to predict folate or B$_{12}$ deficiencies or refractoriness to antidepressants (Mischoulon et al. 2000); measurement of folate and B$_{12}$ levels should always be done when evaluating treatment refractoriness or ruling out deficiencies of these vitamins.

The association between *chronic pain* and depression has been established for many years (Blumer and Heilbronn 1982; Kraemlinger et al. 1983). The evidence for this association is based on the increased frequency of depression among patients with chronic pain and the frequent reports of pain by depressed patients, coupled with the high concurrence of biological markers for depression and markers for chronic pain. Krishnan et al. (1985) found that most items on a typical depression rating scale, such as the Hamilton Rating Scale for Depression (Hamilton 1960), did not discriminate patients with major depression from those with chronic low back pain. Nevertheless, the items discriminated well between patients with and those without depression. The clinician must distinguish the patient with chronic pain from the individual with hypochondriasis (in which the relationship with depressive symptoms may be different).

Normal Aging

The differential diagnosis of late-life depression must include not only other psychiatric and physical disorders but also the changes of normal aging. Some investigators associate a depressed mood with aging. However, most longitudinal studies of depression and life satisfaction do not validate this assumption. Although Busse et al. (1954) found that elderly subjects were aware of more frequent and more annoying depressive periods than they had experienced earlier in life, only a small number admitted to severe and protracted periods of depression. Approximately 85% of the subjects in this study were able to trace the onset of these depressive episodes to specific stimuli. Epidemiologic data confirm that the frequency of severe late-life depression (major depression) is lower than at earlier stages of the life cycle (see Chapter 1, "Demography and Epidemiology of Psychiatric Disorders in Late Life").

The normal biological changes of aging may interact with depressive symptomatology. Older persons, for example, spend more time lying in bed at night either without attempting to sleep or unsuccessfully trying to sleep, and therefore complain of decreased sleep efficiency. Rapid eye movement (REM) sleep latency, a marker that has been associated with depression (see "Primary Sleep Disorder" later in this chapter), is also known to decrease slightly throughout life in both genders (Dement et al. 1982). Elderly persons are notorious for complaining of poor appetite and reduced food intake. Munro (1981)

found that caloric intake decreases with aging. Poor dentition may contribute to decreased food intake as well. Taste acuity also lessens with increasing years (Schiffman and Pasternak 1979). Lethargy is another common complaint of older adults.

Organic Psychiatric Disorders

The psychiatric disorders that most commonly confound the differential diagnosis of depression are the organic psychiatric disorders: dementia, delirium, other cognitive disorders, and "mental disorders due to a general medical condition," according to DSM-IV-TR. Pseudodementia is a syndrome in which dementia is mimicked or caricatured by a functional psychiatric illness, most commonly depression (Wells 1979). Patients with pseudodementia respond on the mental status examination similarly to those with true degenerative brain disease. Although the condition is not rare among elderly persons, Wells (1979) distinguished depression presenting as pseudodementia from true dementia by the rapid onset of the cognitive problems in depression, the relatively short duration of symptoms, the consistent depressed mood associated with cognitive difficulties, and the tendency among depressed patients to highlight disabilities as opposed to concealing (or attempting to conceal) them. The depressed older adult is more likely to respond with "I don't know" on the mental status examination, whereas the elder with dementia is more likely to attempt answers or to attempt to deflect the questions. Cognitive impairment in depression fluctuates from one examination to another, whereas cognitive impairment in dementia is relatively stable.

Of greater clinical importance, however, is the frequent overlap of depressive symptoms and symptoms of the organic psychiatric disorders. Grinker et al. (1961)

noted impaired recent memory in 21% and poor remote memory in 14% of subjects of all ages with depressive disorders. Reifler et al. (1982) studied 88 cognitively impaired elderly outpatients and found that depression was superimposed on dementia in 17 (19%). Patients with greater cognitive impairment exhibited fewer symptoms of depression. When treated with an antidepressant, patients responded with a remission of the depressive symptoms, but cognitive dysfunction persisted. The combination of depression and reversible dementia in elderly patients often indicates the presence of an early dementing illness (Alexopoulos et al. 1993).

Work done specifically with Alzheimer's patients has shown a concurrent diagnosis of major depression in 20%–30% (Reifler et al. 1986). Both depressed and nondepressed Alzheimer's patients were treated with the relatively potent anticholinergic antidepressant imipramine; patients improved whether or not they were in the treatment group, and cognitive function did not decline (Reifler et al. 1989). Greenwald and colleagues (1989) reported that treatment of depressed elderly individuals with dementia and those without dementia resulted in an improvement of both depression and cognitive impairment.

There is some evidence that sleep studies can help differentiate normal aging, depression, and Alzheimer's disease. Dykierek and colleagues (1998) examined 35 patients with Alzheimer's disease, 39 depressed elderly patients, and 42 healthy older control subjects for two consecutive nights in the sleep laboratory. They found that nearly all REM sleep measures differentiated significantly between the three groups. REM density, rather than REM sleep latency, was particularly important in separating depressed elders from elders with dementia. Earlier, Brenner and colleagues (1989) reported that waking electroencephalograms (EEGs) could help distinguish de-

pressed elderly patients and those with pseudodementia (with few electroencephalographic abnormalities) from those with dementia (who often had EEGs that showed abnormalities, with approximately one-third of these patients having moderate or severe abnormalities).

Primary Sleep Disorder

Idiopathic sleep problems are often accompanied by depressive symptoms. The normal changes in sleep that mimic depressive sleep problems are reviewed in Chapter 13, "Sleep and Circadian Rhythm Disorders." A number of sleep disorders also contribute to symptoms that mimic major depression. Delayed or advanced sleep phase syndrome—that is, the shift of the normal sleep cycle to later or earlier in the evening—is most disturbing to older persons who previously viewed their sleep as a habitual given. The elder who begins a night's sleep at 8:00 or 9:00 P.M. because of boredom or other conditions will awaken at 2:00 or 3:00 A.M. and thus complain of early-morning awakening. In addition, the anxiety inherent in awakening in a darkened home with no activity exacerbates the discomfort associated with a sleep phase syndrome.

Sleep apnea syndrome, which is more common with aging, may not be recognized by the older adult (especially if he or she lives alone; a spouse or sleeping partner cannot spend many nights with an apneic elder without recognizing that something is abnormal about the sleep pattern). However, the elder with sleep apnea typically only complains of lethargy and has vague concerns regarding sleep, including excessive sleep.

Anxiety

Differentiation of depression from primary anxiety syndromes such as generalized anxiety disorder and adjustment disorder with anxiety is difficult because of the frequent coexistence of anxiety in late-life depression. Blazer and colleagues (1989) determined that early-morning anxiety was a symptom in nearly one-third of the elderly and middle-aged patients surveyed between 12 and 24 months after psychiatric admission for depression. Hopko et al. (2000) examined the coexistence of depressive symptoms (measured using the Beck Depression Inventory) in older patients with generalized anxiety disorder. Of all predictors, depressive symptoms accounted for the largest variance in clinician-rated anxiety symptoms, a finding that underscores the importance of evaluation for both syndromes. Anxiety as a primary disorder can usually be distinguished from primary depression by the time of symptom onset: anxiety precedes depressive symptoms. In addition, the patient with anxiety usually has a less depressed mood and more motor tension, autonomic hyperactivity, feelings of apprehension or worry, and hypervigilance.

Alcoholism

Alcoholism peaks in middle age and becomes less frequent in late life. Nevertheless, results of a recent study involving more than 10,000 older persons indicate that between 10% and 15% of elders fulfill criteria for definite or questionable alcohol abuse (Thomas and Rockwood 2001). Symptoms of alcoholism that may mimic depression include cognitive changes, disturbed sleep, chronic fatigue, weight loss, and suicidal thoughts. Alcohol abuse or dependence may also coexist with depression, and many elders with late-onset alcoholism may actually use alcohol as a form of self-medication for their depressive symptoms. However, a diagnosis of depression in an alcoholic patient should not be made until the patient has been sober

for at least 2 weeks, because alcohol withdrawal may include dysphoria and other depressive symptoms.

Diagnostic Workup of the Depressed Older Adult

Of special importance in evaluating the depressed elder is assessment of the duration of the current depressive episode; the history of previous episodes; the history of drug and alcohol abuse; response to previous therapeutic interventions for the depressive illness; a family history of depression, suicide, and/or alcohol abuse; and the severity of the depressive symptoms. Establishing some indication of the risk of suicide is essential, for suicidal risk may determine the location of treatment. The physical examination must include a thorough neurological examination to determine whether soft neurological signs (e.g., frontal release signs) or laterality is present. Weight loss and psychomotor retardation in the depressed older adult may lead to a peroneal palsy, documented by electromyography and nerve conduction studies (Massey and Bullock 1978). Because the older adult is less occupied with physical activities and therefore tends to be sedentary, the peroneal nerve is subject to chronic trauma.

The laboratory workup of the depressed older adult should include a thyroid panel (triiodothyronine, thyroxine, and radioactive iodine uptake) and determination of TSH levels. If a supersensitive test is used, measurement of TSH levels can be relied on to detect both hypothyroidism and hyperthyroidism. TSH values between 5 and 10 μU/mL are suggestive of hypothyroidism, and those above 10 μU/mL are nearly diagnostic. TSH values below 1.0 μU/mL, and especially below 0.5 μU/mL, are suggestive of hyperthyroidism.

A blood screen enables the clinician to detect the presence of an anemia. However, at least one study has shown that red blood cell enlargement and abnormalities are not good predictors of deficits in vitamin B_{12} or folate (Mischoulon et al. 2000). Because both depressive and cognitive symptoms can result from deficits in vitamin B_{12} or folate, it is important to obtain levels of these vitamins.

Psychological testing can assist the clinician in distinguishing permanent from temporary cognitive deficits, as well as in identifying potential laterality of cognitive abnormalities. Nevertheless, in the midst of severe depressive illness, psychological testing may be of less value. Therefore, timing the use of psychological testing is essential to maximize the value of test results in clinical decision making.

Laboratory evaluation of depression has entered a new era. Depressive disorders that were once identified exclusively by clinical signs and symptoms can now be delineated by a combination of these signs and symptoms and biological markers. Although no true laboratory test is available for the diagnosis of major depression (or even the subtypes of major depression), use of the laboratory by clinicians as well as clinical investigators has increased dramatically.

An approach that has received increased attention is the use of sleep EEGs to identify depression. Generally, 2 nights of sleep recording are performed after patients have been drug free for 14 days, and mean data from the 2 nights are used for the study. REM density and REM sleep latency have both been proposed as potential markers for depression (Kupfer et al. 1978). Compared with control subjects, endogenously depressed patients appear to have increased sleep discontinuity (disruption of sleep architecture), reduced slow-wave sleep (Stages III and IV), shortened REM sleep latency (the time between the onset of sleep and the first REM period), and increased REM density (the ratio of the sum of eye movements to the duration of REM sleep). Trends in the sleep EEG that appear to mark endogenous depression are trends that often accompany normal aging. However, using sleep EEGs to study REM density and REM sleep latency in combination with other markers may help to increase the probability of identifying the more biologically derived depressive disorders.

A more thoroughly studied marker that may have both diagnostic and therapeutic implications is blunted TSH response to TRH. TRH stimulates release of TSH from the anterior pituitary gland. The TRH test (measurement of serum TSH concentration after administration of TRH) has become a standard test in endocrinology. Administration of synthetic TRH challenges the anterior pituitary to respond. Differential response in the serum TSH levels may characterize disorders of the HPA axis. Although blunting of TSH response is not specific to depression, a number of studies have shown that TSH response is blunted in patients with depression (Gregoire et al. 1977; Loosen and Prange 1982). However, increasing age is also known to be associated with a blunted TSH response to TRH (Snyder and Utiger 1972).

Because of this abnormality, supplemental thyroid has been prescribed to depressed persons, with occasional beneficial response. For example, liothyronine sodium, 25 g/day, could augment the therapeutic effects of traditional TCAs. This augmentation may be valuable in the treatment of some elders, because subclinical hypothyroidism occasionally contributes to depression in older adults. The first step, however, is a more thorough workup and the use of thyroid agents alone to determine whether the depressive symptoms are solely determined by hypothyroidism.

The marker that has received the most attention in recent years is the presence of subcortical hyperintensities on magnetic resonance imaging scanning. Though these imaging findings provide an excellent opportunity to explore etiologic factors, imaging is not recommended for routine evaluation of the depressed older adult.

Given the ever-increasing list of potential markers—some that are to be investigated further, some that will be dropped from the list because they are not clinically useful—what is the best way for the clinician to integrate these markers into clinical practice? First, clinicians should recognize that the primary utility of such markers is in probing the biological contribution to depressive disorders of late life. None of these biochemical, neuroendocrinological, or circadian abnormalities yet qualifies as a biological marker for testing for a psychiatric disorder. They may never reach this status, because the etiology of late-life depression is multidetermined, with no clear evidence that one factor is necessary for symptoms to emerge. Nevertheless, these markers may be considered analogous to symptoms, in that they can be included in the data collected to increase the probability of delineating a real psychopathological entity that can be effectively treated and whose outcome can be predicted.

Treatment

Treatment of depression in late life is four-pronged, involving psychotherapy, pharmacotherapy, ECT, and family therapy. Because pharmacotherapy is covered in some detail in Chapter 16, "Psychopharmacology," we emphasize the remaining three therapeutic approaches here.

Psychotherapy

Cognitive-behavioral therapy and its variants (e.g., interpersonal therapy) are the only psychotherapies specifically designed to treat depression (Beck et al. 1979). Even the more recent technique of interpersonal therapy (Klerman et al. 1984) is primarily a cognitive-behavioral orientation to improving interpersonal relationships. The advantage of using cognitive-behavioral therapy in treating the older adult is that it is directive and time limited, usually involving between 10 and 25 sessions. Cognitive-behavioral therapy has been found to be effective in depressed elderly patients (Gallagher and Thompson 1982; Steuer et al. 1984) and in patients with chronic medical illnesses such as Type II diabetes (Lustman et al. 1998), heart disease (Kohn et al. 2000), and irritable bowel syndrome (Boyce et al. 2000). It may be particularly useful in patients who show only a partial response to antidepressant drug therapy (Scott et al. 2000).

The goal of behavioral and cognitive therapies is to change behavior and modes of thinking. This change is accomplished through behavioral interventions such as weekly activity schedules, mastery and pleasure logs, and graded task assignments. Cognitive approaches to restructuring negative cognitions or automatic thoughts include subjecting these cognitions to empirical reality testing, examining distortions (such as overgeneralizations, catastrophizing, and dichotomous thinking), and generating new ways of viewing one's life (Steuer et al. 1984). Depressed patients typically regard themselves and their present and future in somewhat idiosyncratic or negative ways. Such patients believe themselves inadequate or defective and believe that unpleasant experiences are caused by a problem with themselves and that they are therefore worthless, helpless, and hopeless. This cognitive triad leads the older adult to believe that he or she has a never-ending depression and that nothing pleasant will ever happen again. The cognitive model presupposes that these symptoms of depression are consequences of negative thinking patterns.

Results of empirical studies (including the work of Gallagher and Thompson [1982], Steuer et al. [1984], and Thompson et al. [1987]) suggest that compared with control subjects, elders who engage in psychotherapy experience incremental improvement. Not only does the percentage of elders who respond to these treatments compare favorably with the percentage of younger subjects who respond, the degree of improvement appears equal to that obtained with medications, especially with milder forms of depression.

Older adults who have minor depression or adjustment disorders, or who experience dysphoria because of losses of various types, often require less intensive forms of psychotherapy. Active listening and simple support may be sufficient to help distressed elders cope with their situation. Because religion is an important factor in the lives of many older adults, referral to a pastoral counselor may be particularly helpful and acceptable (Koenig and Weaver 1997).

Pharmacotherapy

TCAs may be useful for patients with more severe forms of major depression, though they are not considered the agents of choice. In recent years, nortriptyline and desipramine have become the more popular medications for treating older adults with endogenous or melancholic major depression. It is recommended that elderly patients with potential cardiac problems or those who are among the oldest old and frail have an electrocardiogram (ECG) before initiation of treatment and again after therapeutic blood levels have been achieved. If the ECG shows a second-degree (or higher) block, a bifascicular bundle branch block, a left bundle branch block, or a QTc interval greater than 480 milliseconds, treatment with TCAs should not be initiated—or should be stopped, in patients taking these medications.

Selective serotonin reuptake inhibitors (SSRIs) have become the agents of choice in elderly patients (with or without medical illness). Paroxetine (Bump et al. 2001), fluoxetine (Heiligenstein et al. 1995; Judge et al. 2000), sertraline (Krishnan et al. 2001; Newhouse et al. 2000), and citalopram (Weihs et al. 2000) have been shown to be effective in geriatric depression. SSRIs have also proved effective in depressed older adults with stroke (Cole et al. 2001), vascular disease in general (Krishnan et al. 2001), or Alzheimer's disease (Lyketsos et al. 2000). These agents are clearly the drugs of first choice for mild to moderate forms of depression. Their lack of anticholinergic, orthostatic, and cardiac side effects; lack of sedation; and safety in overdose are important advantages in elderly patients. Nevertheless, for a significant number of older adults, the newer antidepressants cause other unacceptable effects, including excessive activation and disturbance of sleep, tremor, headache, significant gastrointestinal side effects, hyponatremia, and weight loss.

Venlafaxine has been used most frequently as a second-choice agent if SSRIs are not effective. Duloxetine, another combined serotonin-norepinephrine reuptake inhibitor, has been demonstrated to be effective in the treatment of older adults.

There is growing evidence that SSRIs are effective for the treatment of minor depression as well as major depression in late life. Rocca and colleagues (2005) recruited 138 consecutive nondemented outpatients over age 65 years with minor depressive disorder (or subsyndromal depression) as assessed with the Structured Clinical Interview for DSM-IV. Subjects were assigned to either sertraline or citalopram, and their clinical response was followed over 12 months. Rocca et al. found that these drugs were well tolerated and significantly improved both depressive symptoms and cognitive function over time.

Antidepressant doses administered to persons in late life should be case specific but are generally lower than those given to persons in midlife. For example, starting therapeutic daily doses of SSRIs are as follows: sertraline, 12.5–50 mg; fluoxetine, 5–20 mg; paroxetine, 10–30 mg; venlafaxine, 37.5–200 mg (in divided doses); mirtazapine, 7.5–30 mg; and citalopram, 10–40 mg. With regard to tricyclics, 25–50 mg of nortriptyline orally at bedtime or 25 mg of desipramine orally twice a day is frequently adequate for relieving depressive symptoms. Plasma levels of tricyclic medications can be helpful in determining dosing: nortriptyline levels between 50 and 150 ng/mL and desipramine levels greater than 125 ng/mL have been found to be therapeutic.

Monoamine oxidase inhibitors (MAOIs) are an alternative to tricyclics and the newer antidepressants. It should be noted, if MAOIs are being considered because of intolerance of side effects of other antidepressants, that older adults usually do not tolerate MAOIs any better. If treatment with an MAOI is to follow treatment with an SSRI, a minimum of 1 or 2 weeks (for fluoxetine, 2–4 weeks) must elapse after discontinuation of SSRI therapy and before initiation of MAOI therapy, to avoid a serotonergic syndrome. If a patient's depression is severe and ECT is contemplated, use of an MAOI also precludes initiation of ECT until 10 days to 2 weeks after the drug is discontinued. Such a delay may seriously impede clinical management of the suicidal elder.

Some clinicians prescribe low morning doses of stimulant medications, such as 5 mg of methylphenidate, to improve mood in the apathetic older adult. The effectiveness of stimulants has not been conclusively demonstrated. Nevertheless, these agents are generally safe at low doses, and rarely does the clinician encounter an elder with a propensity to abuse stimulants or to become addicted when these drugs are given once daily.

In a systematic review of comparable studies, Mitchell and Subramaniam (2005) compared response to treatment and remission rates in late life depression and middle-age depression. They found that response to pharmacotherapy and ECT did not significantly differ. Patients with late-life depression appeared at higher risk for relapse, suggesting that continuation treatment may be more important for older than middle-aged adults. Because of the greater risk for medical co-morbidity, however, the risk of a poorer response to antidepressants and of more side effects in older adults was increased. Number of previous episodes of depression was a strong risk factor regardless of age.

For further details about psychopharmacological treatment of the older adult, see Chapter 16, "Psychopharmacology."

Electroconvulsive Therapy

ECT continues to be the most effective form of treatment for patients with severe major depressive episodes, especially with psychotic disorders (Scovern and Kilmann 1980). The induction of a seizure appears to be the factor that is effective in reversing a major depression. Despite its effectiveness, ECT is not the first-line treatment of choice for a patient with major depression and should be prescribed only because other therapeutic modalities have been ineffective. Many older adults with severe syndromes either do not respond to antidepressant medications or experience toxicity (usually postural hypotension) when taking antidepressants. The presence of self-destructive behavior, such as a suicide attempt or refusal to eat, increases the necessity for intervening effectively; in such situations, ECT may be the treatment of choice.

The medical workup before ECT includes acquisition of a complete medical history, a physical examination, and consultation with a cardiologist if any cardiac abnormalities are recognized. Knowledge of a family history of a psychiatric disorder, of suicide, or of treatment with ECT is helpful in predicting response to treatment. Laboratory examination includes a complete blood count, a urinalysis, routine chemistries, chest and spinal X rays (the latter to document previous compression fractures), an ECG, and a computed tomography scan or magnetic resonance image (with computed tomography or magnetic resonance imaging [MRI] available, an EEG and a skull X ray are not routinely required). The presence of some abnormalities on magnetic resonance images does not militate against the use of ECT, however. For example, a series of older adults with major depression were found to have subcortical arteriosclerotic encephalopathy, demonstrated by MRI, but promptly improved after undergoing ECT (Coffey et al. 1987).

Before an older adult undergoes ECT, all medications should be withdrawn, if possible. As noted earlier (see "Pharmacotherapy"), any MAOI must be withdrawn 10 days to 2 weeks before the procedure, to prevent any toxic interactions with the anesthetic used during ECT. Reserpine and anticholinesterase drugs should also be withdrawn for at least 1 week. Lithium carbonate, TCAs, antipsychotics, and antianxiety agents (including sedative-hypnotics) are not absolutely contraindicated in patients who are to undergo ECT. Benzodiazepines, however, increase the seizure threshold and should be avoided. Generally, a short-acting barbiturate, such as chloral hydrate (500 mg orally at bedtime), is the most appropriate sedative-hypnotic, although chloral hydrate should not be given on the night preceding administration of ECT, if possible. Use of low-dose haloperidol or thiothixene is probably the most appropriate means of controlling severe agitation or psychotic symptoms.

ECT treatments are generally administered three times per week, and usually 6–12 treatments are necessary for adequate therapeutic response. A clear improvement is often noted after one of the treatments, with the patient reporting a remarkable improvement in mood and functioning. Two or three treatments are generally given after the ECT administration leading to improvement.

The risks and side effects of ECT in elderly patients are similar to those in the general population. Cardiovascular effects are of most concern and include premature ventricular contractions, ventricular arrhythmias, and transient systolic hypertension. Multiple monitoring during treatment decreases the (infrequent) risk of one of these side effects leading to permanent problems. Confusion and amnesia often result after a treatment, but the duration of this confusional episode is brief. Even with the use of unilateral nondominant treatment, however, some patients have prolonged memory difficulties. Headaches are a common symptom with ECT; they usually respond to nonnarcotic analgesics. Status epilepticus and vertebral compression fractures are some of the rare but more serious adverse effects. Compression fractures are a particular risk in older women because of the high incidence of osteoporosis in the postmenopausal population.

In terms of outcome, what can the clinician expect from the use of ECT in older adults? The overall success rate of ECT in patients who have not responded to drug therapy is usually 80% or greater, and there is no evidence that effectiveness is lower in older adults (Avery and Lubrano 1979). Wesner and Winokur (1989) examined the influence of age on the natural history of major depressive disorder and found that ECT reduced the rate of chronicity when it was used in patients age 40 or older but, surprisingly, not in those younger than 40 years.

In a prospective, multisite study, Tew and colleagues (1999) concluded that despite a higher level of physical illness and cognitive impairment, patients age 75 or older who had severe major depression tolerated ECT in a manner similar to the way in which younger patients tolerated the treatment, and the old-old patients demonstrated a similar or even better response. There is also evidence that ECT may be more effective and have fewer side effects than antidepressants when used to treat depression in old-old patients (Manly et al. 2000).

The relapse rate with no prophylactic intervention may exceed 50% in the year after a course of ECT. This relapse rate can be decreased if antidepressants or lithium carbonate is prescribed after the treatment. For some patients who exhibit a high likelihood of recurrence despite use of prophylactic medication, and/or who experience high toxicity and therefore cannot tolerate prophylactic medications, maintenance ECT may be necessary. For such patients, weekly or monthly treatments (usually on an outpatient basis) are prescribed, with careful monitoring of response and side effects. The combination of continuation ECT and antidepressant drug therapy has been shown to have greater efficacy than use of medications alone, following an effective course of ECT (Gagne et al. 2000).

Despite the effectiveness of ECT, few deny that treatment may lead to memory difficulties. In a study by Frith et al. (1983), 70 severely depressed patients were randomly assigned to eight real or sham ECT treatments and were divided according to the degree of recovery from depression afterward. Compared with nondepressed control subjects, the depressed patients were impaired on a wide range of tests of memory and concentration before treatment, but afterward performance on most tests improved. Real ECT induced impairments in concentration, short-term

memory, and learning but significantly facilitated access to remote memories. At 6-month follow-up, all differences between real and sham ECT groups had disappeared.

Price and McAllister (1989) examined the efficacy of ECT in elderly depressed patients with dementia. Overall, the patients achieved an 86% response rate, with only 21% experiencing a significant worsening of cognition; the cognition problems were transient in most cases. Of particular importance is that 49% of the patients treated with ECT showed improvement in memory function after treatment. Likewise, Stoudemire et al. (1995) found that over time, ECT may lead to significant improvement in memory of cognitively impaired older adults with depression.

Although data on the safety and efficacy of ECT in patients with concurrent medical illness derive primarily from retrospective studies involving psychiatric patients with stable disease, these data do support the use of ECT in patients with cardiovascular, neurological, endocrine, or metabolic conditions, as well as a variety of other conditions (Stoudemire et al. 1998). For more information on the efficacy and safety of ECT in patients with late-life depressions, see the comprehensive review by Greenberg (1997).

Family Therapy

The final component of therapy for the depressed elderly patient is work with the family. Not only may family dysfunction contribute to the depressive symptoms experienced by the older adult, but family support is critical to a successful outcome in the treatment of the depressed elder. A clinician must attend to 1) those members of the family who will be available to the elder, 2) the interaction between the older adult and family members and the interactions among other family members (both frequency and quality of interaction), 3) the overall family atmosphere, 4) family values regarding psychiatric disorders, 5) family support and tolerance of symptoms (such as expressions of wishing not to live), and 6) stressors encountered by the family other than the depression experienced by the elder (Blazer 1993).

Most depressed elders do not resist interaction between the clinician and family members. With the permission of the patient, the family should be instructed regarding the nature of the depressive disorder and the potential risks associated with depression in late life, especially suicide. Family members can assist the clinician in observing changes in behavior, such as an increase in discomfort (either physical or emotional), increased withdrawal and decreased verbalization, and preoccupation with medications or weapons. The family can assist by removing possible implements of suicide from places of easy access. The family can also take responsibility for administering medications to an older adult who is unreliable or whose potential for suicide is high.

References

Alexopoulos GS, Meyers BS, Young RC, et al: The course of geriatric depression with "reversible dementia": a controlled study. Am J Psychiatry 150:1693–1699, 1993

Alexopoulos GS, Meyers BS, Young RC, et al: "Vascular depression" hypothesis. Arch Gen Psychiatry 54:915–922, 1997

Ameblas A: Life events and mania. Br J Psychiatry 150:235–240, 1987

American Psychiatric Association: Diagnostic and Statistical Manual of Mental Disorders, 3rd Edition. Washington, DC, American Psychiatric Association, 1980

American Psychiatric Association: Diagnostic and Statistical Manual of Mental Disorders, 4th Edition, Text Revision. Washington, DC, American Psychiatric Association, 2000

Anderson RJ, Freedland KE, Clouse RE, et al: The prevalence of comorbid depression in adults with diabetes: a meta-analysis. Diabetes Care 24:1069–1078, 2001

Arfken CL, Lichtenberg PA, Tancer ME: Cognitive impairment and depression predict mortality in medically ill older adults. J Gerontol A Biol Sci Med Sci 54:M152–M156, 1999

Atchley RC: Social Forces in Later Life. Belmont, CA, Wadsworth, 1972

Avery D, Lubrano A: Depression treated with imipramine and ECT: the DeCarolis study reconsidered. Am J Psychiatry 136:559–562, 1979

Baldwin JC, Jolley DJ: The prognosis of depression in old age. Br J Psychiatry 149:574–583, 1986

Beck AT, Rush AJ, Shaw BF, et al: Cognitive Therapy of Depression. New York, Guilford, 1979

Black SA, Markides KS: Depressive symptoms and mortality in older Mexican Americans. Ann Epidemiol 9:45–52, 1999

Blazer DG: Impact of late-life depression on the social network. Am J Psychiatry 140:162–166, 1983

Blazer DG: Depression in Late Life, 2nd Edition. St. Louis, MO, CV Mosby, 1993

Blazer DG: Depression in late life: review and commentary. J Gerontol A Biol Sci Med Sci 58(3):249–265, 2003

Blazer DG, Hughes DC, George LK: The epidemiology of depression in an elderly community population. Gerontologist 27:281–287, 1987

Blazer DG, Hughes DC, Fowler N: Anxiety as an outcome symptom of depression in elderly and middle-aged adults. Int J Geriatr Psychiatry 27:281–287, 1989

Blazer DG, Hughes DC, George LK: Age and impaired subjective support: predictors of symptoms at one-year follow-up. J Nerv Ment Dis 180:172–178, 1992

Blazer DG, Hybels CF, Pieper CF: The association of depression and mortality in elderly persons: a case for multiple, independent pathways. J Gerontol A Biol Sci Med Sci 56(8):M505–509, 2001

Blumer D, Heilbronn M: Chronic pain as a variant of depressive disease: pain-prone disorder. J Nerv Ment Dis 170:381–394, 1982

Boyce P, Gilchrist J, Talley NJ, et al: Cognitive-behaviour therapy as a treatment for irritable bowel syndrome: a pilot study. Aust N Z J Psychiatry 34:300–309, 2000

Braam AW, Beekman ATF, Deeg DJH, et al: Religiosity as a protective or prognostic factor of depression in later life: results from a community survey in the Netherlands. Acta Psychiatr Scand 96:199–205, 1997a

Braam AW, Beekman ATF, van Tilburg TG, et al: Religious involvement and depression in older Dutch citizens. Soc Psychiatry Psychiatr Epidemiol 32:284–291, 1997b

Breitbart W, Rosenfeld B, Pessin H, et al: Depression, hopelessness, and desire for hastened death in terminally ill patients with cancer. JAMA 284:2907–2911, 2000

Brenner RP, Reynolds CF 3rd, Ulrich RF: EEG findings in depressive pseudodementia and dementia with secondary depression. Electroencephalogr Clin Neurophysiol 72:298–304, 1989

Bukberg J, Penman D, Holland JC: Depression in hospitalized cancer patients. Psychosom Med 46:199–210, 1984

Bump GM, Mulsant BH, Pollock BG, et al: Paroxetine versus nortriptyline in the continuation and maintenance treatment of depression in the elderly. Depress Anxiety 13:38–44, 2001

Busse EW, Barnes RH, Silverman AJ, et al: Studies of the processes of aging, VI: factors that influence the psyche of elderly persons. Am J Psychiatry 110:897–903, 1954

Carroll BJ, Feinberg M, Greden JF, et al: A specific laboratory test for the diagnosis of melancholia: standardization, validation, and clinical utility. Arch Gen Psychiatry 38:15–22, 1981

Carter AB: The neurologic aspects of aging, in Clinical Geriatrics, 3rd Edition. Edited by Rossman I. Philadelphia, PA, JB Lippincott, 1986, pp 326–351

Cath SH: Some dynamics of middle and later years: a study in depletion and restitution, in Geriatric Psychiatry: Grief, Loss, and Emotional Disorders in the Aging Process. Edited by Berezin MA, Cath SH. New York, International Universities Press, 1965, pp 21–72

Checkley SA, Slade AP, Schur E: Growth hormone and other responses to clonidine in patients with endogenous depression. Br J Psychiatry 138:51–55, 1981

Coffey CE: Cerebral laterality and emotion: the neurology of depression. Compr Psychiatry 28:197–219, 1987

Coffey CE, Hinkle PE, Weiner RD, et al: Electroconvulsive therapy of depression in patients with white matter hyperintensity. Biol Psychiatry 22:626–629, 1987

Cole MG: Age, age of onset and course of primary depressive illness in the elderly. Can J Psychiatry 28:102–104, 1983

Cole MG, Bellavance F, Mansour A: Prognosis of depression in elderly community and primary care populations: a systematic review and meta-analysis. Am J Psychiatry 156:1182–1189, 1999

Cole MG, Elie LM, McCusker J, et al: Feasibility and effectiveness of treatments for post-stroke depression in elderly inpatients: systematic review. J Geriatr Psychiatry Neurol 14:37–41, 2001

Covinsky KE, Kahana E, Chin MH, et al: Depressive symptoms and 3-year mortality in older hospitalized medical patients. Ann Intern Med 130:563–569, 1999

Cutler NR, Post RM: Life course of illness in untreated manic-depressive patients. Compr Psychiatry 23:101–115, 1982

Dam H: Depression in stroke patients 7 years following stroke. Acta Psychiatr Scand 103:287–293, 2001

Davies BM: Depressive illness in the elderly patient. Postgrad Med 38:314–320, 1965

Dement WC, Miles LE, Carskadon MA: "White paper" on sleep and aging. J Am Geriatr Soc 30:25–50, 1982

Dunner DL: Affective disorder: clinical features, in Psychiatry, Vol 1. Edited by Michels R, Cavenar JO. Philadelphia, PA, JB Lippincott, 1985, pp 59–60

Dykierek P, Stadtmuller G, Schramm P, et al: The value of REM sleep parameters in differentiating Alzheimer's disease from old-age depression and normal aging. J Psychiatr Res 32:1–9, 1998

Eastham JH, Jeste DV, Young RC: Assessment and treatment of bipolar disorder in the elderly. Drugs Aging 12:205–224, 1998

Egeland JA, Gerhard DS, Pauls DL, et al: Bipolar affective disorders linked to DNA markers on chromosome 11. Nature 325:783–787, 1987

Epstein LJ: Depression in the elderly. J Gerontol 3:278–282, 1976

Erikson EH: Childhood and Society. New York, WW Norton, 1950

Fassler LB, Gavira M: Depression in old age. J Am Geriatr Soc 26:471–475, 1978

Fifield J, Tennen H, Reisine S, et al: Depression and long-term risk of pain, fatigue, and disability in patients with rheumatoid arthritis. Arthritis Rheum 41:1851–1857, 1998

Finkelstein JW, Roffwarg HP, Boyar RM, et al: Age-related change in the twenty-four-hour spontaneous secretion of growth hormone. J Clin Endocrinol Metab 35:665–670, 1972

Frasure-Smith N, Lesperance F, Talajic M: Depression following myocardial infarction: impact on 6-month survival. JAMA 270:1819–1825, 1993

Fredman L, Schoenbach VJ, Kaplan BH, et al: The association between depressive symptoms and mortality among older participants in the Epidemiologic Catchment Area–Piedmont Health Survey. J Gerontol 44:S149–S156, 1989

Fredman L, Magaziner J, Hebel JR, et al: Depressive symptoms and 6-year mortality among elderly community-dwelling women. Epidemiology 10:54–59, 1999

Frith CD, Stevens M, Johnstone EC, et al: Effects of ECT and depression on various aspects of memory. Br J Psychiatry 142:610–617, 1983

Gagne GG Jr, Furman MJ, Carpenter LL, et al: Efficacy of continuation ECT and antidepressant drugs compared to long-term antidepressants alone in depressed patients. Am J Psychiatry 157:1960–1965, 2000

Gainotti G: Emotional behavior and hemispheric side of the lesion. Cortex 8:41–55, 1972

Gallagher D, Thompson LW: Differential effectiveness of psychotherapies for the treatment of major depressive disorder in older adult patients. Psychotherapy: Theory, Research and Practice 19:42–49, 1982

Gerety MB, Williams JW Jr, Mulrow CD, et al: Performance of case-finding tools for depression in the nursing home: influence of clinical and functional characteristics and selection of optimal threshold scores. J Am Geriatr Soc 42:1103–1109, 1994

Glassman AH, Shapiro PA: Depression and the course of coronary artery disease. Am J Psychiatry 155:4–11, 1998

Greden JF: Antidepressant maintenance medications: when to discontinue and how to stop. J Clin Psychiatry 54 (suppl 8):39–45, 1993

Greenberg RM: ECT in the elderly. New Dir Ment Health Serv 76:85–96, 1997

Greenwald BS, Kramer-Binsberg E, Marin DB, et al: Dementia with coexistent major depression. Am J Psychiatry 146:1472–1477, 1989

Gregoire F, Brauman H, de Buck R, et al: Hormone release in depressed patients before and after recovery. Psychoneuroendocrinology 2:303–312, 1977

Grinker RR, Miller J, Sabshin M, et al: The Phenomena of Depressions. New York, Harper & Row, 1961

Guy R: An Essay on Scirrhous Tumors and Cancer. London, J & A Churchill, 1759

Hamilton M: A rating scale for depression. J Neurol Neurosurg Psychiatry 23:56–62, 1960

Heiligenstein JH, Ware JE Jr, Beusterien KM, et al: Acute effects of fluoxetine versus placebo on functional health and well-being in late-life depression. International Psychogeriatrics 7 (suppl):125–137, 1995

Hickie I, Scott E: Late-onset depressive disorders: a preventable variant of cerebrovascular disease? Psychol Med 28:1007–1013, 1998

Holahan CJ, Moos RH: Social support and psychological distress: a longitudinal analysis. J Abnorm Psychol 90:365–370, 1981

Hopkinson G: A genetic study of affective illness in patients over 50. Br J Psychiatry 110:244–254, 1964

Hopko DR, Bourland SL, Stanley MA, et al: Generalized anxiety disorder in older adults: examining the relation between clinician severity ratings and patient self-report measures. Depress Anxiety 12:217–225, 2000

Hunkeler EM, Katon WJ, Tang I, et al: Long-term outcomes from the IMPACT randomized trial for depressed elderly patients in primary care. BMJ 332(7536):249–250, 2006

Idler EL: Religious involvement and the health of the elderly: some hypotheses and an initial test. Social Forces 66:226–238, 1987

Jacobsen FM, Wehr TA, Sack DA, et al: Seasonal affective disorder: a review of the syndrome and its public health implications. Am J Public Health 77:57–60, 1987

Jonas BS, Mussolino ME: Symptoms of depression as a prospective risk factor for stroke. Psychosom Med 62:463–471, 2000

Judge R, Plewes JM, Kumar V, et al: Changes in energy during treatment of depression: an analysis of fluoxetine in double-blind, placebo-controlled trials. J Clin Psychopharmacol 20:666–672, 2000

Katon WJ, Lin E, Russo J, et al: Increased medical costs of a population-based sample of depressed elderly patients. Arch Gen Psychiatry 60(9):897–903, 2003

Klerman GL, Weissman MM, Rounsaville BJ, et al: Interpersonal Psychotherapy of Depression. New York, Basic Books, 1984

Koenig HG: Treatment considerations for the depressed geriatric medical patient. Drugs Aging 1:266–278, 1991

Koenig HG, Weaver AJ: Counseling Troubled Older Adults: A Handbook for Pastors and Religious Caregivers. Nashville, TN, Abingdon, 1997

Koenig HG, George LK, Siegler IC: The use of religion and other emotion-regulating coping strategies among older adults. Gerontologist 28:303–310, 1988

Koenig HG, Shelp F, Goli V, et al: Survival and healthcare utilization in elderly medical inpatients with major depression. J Am Geriatr Soc 37:599–607, 1989

Koenig HG, Meador KG, Shelp F, et al: Depressive disorders in hospitalized medically ill patients: a comparison of young and elderly men. J Am Geriatr Soc 39:881–890, 1991

Koenig HG, Cohen HJ, Blazer DG, et al: Religious coping and depression in hospitalized medically ill older men. Am J Psychiatry 149:1693–1700, 1992

Koenig HG, Blumenthal J, Moore K: New version of brief depression scale (letter). J Am Geriatr Soc 43:1447, 1995

Koenig HG, George LK, Peterson BL, et al: Depression in medically ill hospitalized older adults: prevalence, correlates, and course of symptoms based on six diagnostic schemes. Am J Psychiatry 154:1376–1383, 1997

Koenig HG, George LK, Peterson BL: Religiosity and remission from depression in medically ill older patients. Am J Psychiatry 155:536–542, 1998

Kohn CS, Petrucci RJ, Baessler C, et al: The effect of psychological intervention on patients' long-term adjustment to the ICD: a prospective study. Pacing Clin Electrophysiol 23:450–456, 2000

Kraemlinger KG, Swanson DW, Maruta T: Are patients with chronic pain depressed? Am J Psychiatry 140:747–749, 1983

Krishnan KR, France RD, Pelton S, et al: Chronic pain and depression, I: classification of depression in chronic low back pain patients. Pain 22:279–287, 1985

Krishnan KR, Doraiswamy PM, Clary CM: Clinical and treatment response characteristics of late-life depression associated with vascular disease: a pooled analysis of two multicenter trials with sertraline. Prog Neuropsychopharmacol Biol Psychiatry 25:347–361, 2001

Kruesi MJ, Dale J, Straus S: Psychiatric diagnoses in patients who have chronic fatigue syndrome. J Clin Psychiatry 40:53–56, 1989

Kupfer DJ: Neurophysiological "markers": EEG sleep measures. J Psychiatr Res 18:467–495, 1984

Kupfer DJ, Foster FG, Coble P, et al: The application of EEG sleep for the differential diagnosis of affective disorders. Am J Psychiatry 135:69–74, 1978

Lakatua DJ, Nicolau GY, Bogdan C, et al: Circadian endocrine time structure in humans above 80 years of age. J Gerontol 39:648–654, 1984

Lesse S: Masked Depression. New York, Jason Aronson, 1974

Levin S: Depression in the aged, in Geriatric Psychiatry: Grief, Loss, and Emotional Disorders in the Aging Process. Edited by Berezin MA, Cath SH. New York, International Universities Press, 1965, pp 203–225

Lewis AJ: Melancholia: a historical review. J Ment Sci 80:1–42, 1934

Lindemann E: Symptomatology and management of acute grief. Am J Psychiatry 101: 141–148, 1944

Lindenbaum J, Healton EB, Savage DG, et al: Neuropsychiatric disorders caused by co-balamin deficiency in the absence of anemia or macrocytosis. N Engl J Med 318: 1720–1728, 1988

Loosen PT, Prange AJ: Serum thyrotropin response to thyrotropin-releasing hormone in psychiatric patients: a review. Am J Psychiatry 139:405–416, 1982

Lustman PJ, Griffith LS, Freedland KE, et al: Cognitive behavior therapy for depression in type 2 diabetes mellitus. A randomized, controlled trial. Ann Intern Med 129:613–621, 1998

Lyketsos CG, Sheppard JM, Steele CD, et al: Randomized, placebo-controlled, double-blind clinical trial of sertraline in the treatment of depression complicating Alzheimer's disease: initial results from the Depression in Alzheimer's Disease study. Am J Psychiatry 157:1686–1689, 2000

Massey EW, Bullock R: Peroneal palsy in depression. J Clin Psychiatry 39:287, 291–292, 1978

Mayeux R: Depression in the patient with Parkinson's disease. J Clin Psychiatry 51 (suppl):20–23, 1990

McHugh PR: Beyond DSM-IV: from appearances to essences. Paper presented at the 154th annual meeting of the American Psychiatric Association, New Orleans, May 7, 2001

Mendlewicz J: The age factor in depressive illness: some genetic considerations. J Gerontol 31:300–303, 1976

Meyers BS, Kalayam B, Mei-Tal V: Late-onset delusional depression: a distinct clinical entity? J Clin Psychiatry 45:347–349, 1984

Mischoulon D, Burger JK, Spillmann MK, et al: Anemia and macrocytosis in the prediction of serum folate and vitamin B_{12} status, and treatment outcome in major depression. J Psychosom Res 49:183–187, 2000

Mitchell AJ, Subramaniam H: Prognosis of depression in old age compared to middle age: a systematic review of comparative studies. Am J Psychiatry 162(9):1588–1601, 2005

Munro HN: Nutrition and aging. Br Med Bull 37:83–88, 1981

Murphy E, Smith R, Lindsay J, et al: Increased mortality rates in late-life depression. Br J Psychiatry 152:347–353, 1988

Musselman DL, Evans DL, Nemeroff CB: Relationship of depression to cardiovascular disease: epidemiology, biology, and treatment. Arch Gen Psychiatry 55:580–592, 1998

Myers JK, Weissman MM, Tischler GL, et al: Six-month prevalence of psychiatric disorders in three communities, 1980–1982. Arch Gen Psychiatry 41:959–967, 1984

Newhouse PA, Krishnan KR, Doraiswamy PM, et al: A double-blind comparison of sertraline and fluoxetine in depressed elderly outpatients. J Clin Psychiatry 61:559–568, 2000

Okifuji A, Turk DC, Sherman JJ: Evaluation of the relationship between depression and fibromyalgia syndrome: why aren't all patients depressed? J Rheumatol 27:212–219, 2000

Old Age Depression Interest Group: How long should the elderly take antidepressants? A double-blind placebo-controlled study of continuation/prophylaxis therapy with dothiepin. Br J Psychiatry 162:175–182, 1993

Pfifer JF, Murrell SA: Etiologic factors in the onset of depressive symptoms in older adults. J Abnorm Psychol 95:282–291, 1986

Pies RW: Diagnosis and treatment of subclinical hypothyroid states in depressed patients. Gen Hosp Psychiatry 19:344–354, 1997

Post F: The management and nature of depressive illnesses in late life: a follow-through study. Br J Psychiatry 121:393–404, 1972

Post F: The functional psychoses, in Studies in Geriatric Psychiatry. Edited by Isaacs AD, Post F. New York, Wiley, 1978, pp 77–98

Pressman P, Lyons JS, Larson DB, et al: Religious belief, depression, and ambulation status in elderly women with broken hips. Am J Psychiatry 147:758–760, 1990

Price TRP, McAllister TW: Safety and efficacy of ECT in depressed patients with dementia: a review of clinical experience. Convulsive Therapy 5:61–74, 1989

Radloff LS: The CES-D scale: a self-report depression scale for research in the general population. Applied Psychological Measurement 1:385–401, 1977

Reifler BV, Larson E, Henley R: Coexistence of cognitive impairment and depression in geriatric outpatients. Am J Psychiatry 39:623–626, 1982

Reifler BV, Larson E, Teri L, et al: Dementia of the Alzheimer's type and depression. J Am Geriatr Soc 34:855–859, 1986

Reifler BV, Teri L, Raskind M, et al: Double-blind trial of imipramine in Alzheimer's disease patients with and without depression. Am J Psychiatry 146:45–49, 1989

Reynolds CF 3rd, Frank E, Perel JM, et al: Combined pharmacotherapy and psychotherapy in the acute and continuation treatment of elderly patients with recurrent major depression: a preliminary report. Am J Psychiatry 149:1687–1692, 1992

Robinson RG, Morris PLP, Fedoroff P: Depression and cerebrovascular disease. J Clin Psychiatry 51 (suppl 7):26–31, 1990

Rocca P, Calvarese P, Faggiano F, et al: Citalopram versus sertraline in late-life non-major clinically significant depression: a 1-year follow-up clinical trial. J Clin Psychiatry 66(3):360–369, 2005

Rosenbaum AH, Schatzberg AF, MacLaughlin MS, et al: The dexamethasone suppression test in normal control subjects: comparison of two assays and effect of age. Am J Psychiatry 141:1550–1555, 1984

Rovner BW, German PS, Brant LJ, et al: Depression and mortality in nursing homes. JAMA 265:993–996, 1991

Sachar EJ: Neuroendocrine abnormalities in depressive illness, in Topics in Psychoendocrinology. Edited by Sachar EJ. New York, Grune & Stratton, 1975, pp 135–156

Sackeim HA, Greenberg MS, Weiman AL, et al: Hemispheric asymmetry in expression of positive and negative emotions. Neurologic evidence. Arch Neurol 39:210–218, 1982

Salzman C, Shader RI: Responses to psychotropic drugs in the normal elderly, in Psychopharmacology in Aging. Edited by Eisdorfer C, Fann WE. New York, Plenum, 1972, pp 159–168

Schiffman S, Pasternak M: Decreased discrimination of food odors in the elderly. J Gerontol 34:73–79, 1979

Schulz B: Auszählungen in der Verwandtschaft von nach Erkrankungsalter und Geschlecht gruppierten Manisch-Depressiven. Arch Psychiatr Nervenkr 186:560–576, 1951

Schwab JJ, Clemmons RS, Bialow M, et al: A study of the somatic symptomatology of depression in medical inpatients. Psychosomatics 6:273–276, 1965

Scott J, Teasdale JD, Paykel ES, et al: Effects of cognitive therapy on psychological symptoms and social functioning in residual depression. Br J Psychiatry 177:440–446, 2000

Scovern AW, Kilmann PR: Status of electroconvulsive therapy: review of the outcome literature. Psychol Bull 87:260–303, 1980

Shulman KI: Mania in old age, in Affective Disorders in the Elderly. Edited by Murphy E. Edinburgh, Churchill Livingstone, 1986, pp 203–216

Shulman KI: The influence of age and aging on manic disorder. Int J Geriatr Psychiatry 4:63–65, 1989

Shulman KI, Post F: Bipolar affective disorder in old age. Br J Psychiatry 136:26–32, 1980

Slater E, Cowie V: The Genetics of Mental Disorder. London, Oxford University Press, 1971

Snyder PJ, Utiger RD: Response to thyrotropin releasing hormone (TRH) in normal man. J Clin Endocrinol Metab 34:380–385, 1972

Spar JE, Ford CV, Liston EH: Bipolar affective disorder in aged patients. J Clin Psychiatry 40:504–507, 1979

Spiegel D: Cancer and depression. Br J Psychiatry 169 (suppl):109–116, 1996

Srole L, Fischer AK: The Midtown Manhattan Longitudinal Study vs "The Mental Paradise Lost" doctrine: a controversy joined. Arch Gen Psychiatry 37:209–221, 1980

Steuer JL, Mintz J, Hammen CL, et al: Cognitive-behavioral and psychodynamic group psychotherapy in treatment of geriatric depression. J Consult Clin Psychol 52:180–189, 1984

Stoudemire A, Hill CD, Morris R, et al: Long-term outcome of treatment-resistant depression in older adults. Am J Psychiatry 150:1539–1540, 1993

Stoudemire A, Hill CD, Morris R, et al: Improvement in depression-related cognitive dysfunction following ECT. J Neuropsychiatry Clin Neurosci 7:31–34, 1995

Stoudemire A, Hill CD, Marquardt M, et al: Recovery and relapse in geriatric depression after treatment with antidepressants and ECT in a medical-psychiatric population. Gen Hosp Psychiatry 20:170–174, 1998

Sumaya IC, Rienzi BM, Deegan JF 2nd, et al: Bright light treatment decreases depression in institutionalized older adults: a placebo-controlled crossover study. J Gerontol 56:M356–M360, 2001

Targum SD, Sullivan AC, Byrnes SM: Neuroendocrine relationships in major depressive disorder. Am J Psychiatry 139:282–286, 1982

Thomas VS, Rockwood KJ: Alcohol abuse, cognitive impairment, and mortality among older people. J Am Geriatr Soc 49:415–420, 2001

Thompson LW, Gallagher D, Steinmetz-Breckenridge J: Comparative effectiveness of psychotherapies for depressed elders. J Consult Clin Psychol 55:385–390, 1987

Ulrich RF, Shaw DH, Kupfer DJ: Effects of aging on EEG sleep in depression. Sleep 3:31–40, 1980

Verwoerdt A: Clinical Geropsychiatry. Baltimore, MD, Williams & Wilkins, 1976

Vogel GW, Vogel F, McAbee RS, et al: Improvement of depression by REM sleep deprivation: new findings and a theory. Arch Gen Psychiatry 37:247–253, 1980

Weihs KL, Settle EC Jr, Batey SR, et al: Bupropion sustained release versus paroxetine for the treatment of depression in the elderly. J Clin Psychiatry 61:196–202, 2000

Weissman MM, Bruce ML, Leaf PJ, et al: Affective disorders, in Psychiatric Disorders in America: The Epidemiologic Catchment Area Study. Edited by Robins LN, Regier DA. New York, Free Press, 1991, pp 53–80

Wells CE: Pseudodementia. Am J Psychiatry 136:895–900, 1979

Wesner RB, Winokur G: The influence of age on the natural history of unipolar depression when treated with electroconvulsive therapy. Eur Arch Psychiatry Neurol Sci 238:149–154, 1989

Wigdor BT: Drives and motivations with aging, in The Handbook of Aging and Mental Health. Edited by Birren JE, Sloane RB. Englewood Cliffs, NJ, Prentice-Hall, 1980, pp 245–261

Winokur G: The Iowa 500: heterogeneity and course in manic-depressive illness (bipolar). Compr Psychiatry 16:125–131, 1975

Wylie ME, Mulsant BH, Pollock BG: Age of onset in geriatric bipolar disorder: effects on clinical presentation and treatment outcomes in an inpatient sample. Am J Geriatr Psychiatry 7:77–83, 1999

Yassa R, Nair V, Nastase C, et al: Prevalence of bipolar disorder in a psychogeriatric population. J Affect Disord 14:197–201, 1988

Yesavage JA, Brink TL, Rose TL, et al: Development and validation of a geriatric depression screening scale: a preliminary report. J Psychiatr Res 17:37–49, 1983

Young RC, Klerman GL: Mania in late life: focus on age at onset. Am J Psychiatry 149:867–876, 1992

Young RC, Nambudiri DE, Jain H, et al: Brain computed tomography in geriatric manic disorder. Biol Psychiatry 45:1063–1065, 1999

Zesiewicz TA, Gold M, Chari G, et al: Current issues in depression in Parkinson's disease. Am J Geriatr Psychiatry 7:110–118, 1999

Zung WWK, Green RL: Detection of affective disorders in the aged, in Psychopharmacology in Aging. Edited by Eisdorfer C, Fann WE. New York, Plenum, 1972, pp 213–224

Study Questions

Select the single best response for each question.

1. In contrast to low rates of major depression among older adults in the community, it has been estimated that up to what percentage of hospitalized elders fulfill criteria for a major depressive episode?

   A. 6%.
   B. 11%.
   C. 16%.
   D. 21%.
   E. 31%.

2. Mortality among elderly patients is

   A. Increased in older men with physical health problems and depression.
   B. Increased among nursing home patients with depression.
   C. Increased in previously hospitalized depressed women.
   D. A and B.
   E. A, B, and C.

3. Studies of prognosis of late-life depression show all of the following *except*

   A. Older adults differ from their middle-age counterparts in terms of recovery and remission.
   B. Elders who have recovered appear to experience residual depressive symptoms.
   C. Seventy percent of elderly patients with major depression treated with adequate antidepressant regimens recover from the index episode.
   D. Older patients who have experienced one or more moderate to severe episodes of major depression may need to continue antidepressant therapy permanently to minimize relapse.
   E. Physical illness and cognitive impairment are associated with a worse outcome.

4. Bipolar disorder in the elderly may have all of the following characteristics *except*

   A. Tendency toward more rapid recurrences late in the illness.
   B. Stressful events more likely to precede early-onset mania than late-onset mania.
   C. Increased cerebral vulnerability playing a stronger role than life events in precipitating late-onset mania.
   D. Association with low rates of familial affective disorder.
   E. Genetic factors weighing heavily in the etiology.

5. Reversible dementia due to depression

    A. Predicts poor response to treatment of the depression.
    B. Is associated with patients attempting to conceal disabilities rather than high-lighting them on formal mental status exam.
    C. Cannot be differentiated from that of bona fide dementia by way of REM sleep measures.
    D. Often indicates the presence of an early dementing illness.
    E. Should not be treated with a potent anticholinergic antidepressant such as imipramine.

6. According to a recent study, what percentage of elders fulfill criteria for definite or questionable alcohol abuse?

    A. Between 2% and 4%.
    B. Between 3% and 6%.
    C. Between 10% and 15%.
    D. Between 20% and 30%.
    E. Between 30% and 40%.

7. ECT

    A. Is less effective in older adults than in younger ones.
    B. Is no more effective than and has more side effects than antidepressants when used in the old-old populace.
    C. Has a relapse rate that may exceed 50% in the year after a course of ECT, without prophylaxis.
    D. Leads to a significant worsening of cognition in the majority of elderly depressed patients with dementia.
    E. Should be avoided in patients with cardiovascular, neurological, endocrine, or metabolic conditions.

Schizophrenia and Paranoid Disorders

Dilip V. Jeste, M.D.

Christian R. Dolder, Pharm.D., B.C.P.S.

Delusions, hallucinations, and other psychotic symptoms can accompany a number of conditions in late life. These symptoms may be more common than previously thought; a recent Swedish investigation found that the prevalence of any psychotic symptom in a population-based sample of 85-year-old individuals without dementia was 10.1%, with 6.9% experiencing hallucinations, 5.5% having delusions, and 6.9% experiencing paranoid ideation (Ostling and Skoog 2002).

Some conditions that cause psychotic symptoms, such as delirium and substance-induced psychosis, are acute and tend to resolve when the underlying condition is treated. These conditions are discussed elsewhere in this volume.

In this chapter, we review the epidemiology, presentation, and treatment of chronic late-life psychotic disorders not secondary to a mood disorder or a general medical condition other than dementia. Thus, we discuss early-onset schizophrenia, late-onset schizophrenia, very late onset schizophrenia-like psychosis (with onset after 60), delusional disorder, and psycho-

sis of Alzheimer's disease (AD). We also address the risk factors for and the prevalence, course, prevention, and treatment of tardive dyskinesia (TD) in older patients.

Schizophrenia

Early-Onset Schizophrenia

Most individuals with schizophrenia develop the disease in the second or third decade of life (American Psychiatric Association 2000). Although mortality rates in general, and suicide and homicide rates in particular, are higher among individuals with schizophrenia than in the general population (Hannerz et al. 2001; Hiroeh et al. 2001; Joukamaa et al. 2001), many patients with early-onset schizophrenia now live into older adulthood. Thus, approximately 80% of the older adults with schizophrenia typically have had an early onset of the disease and have a chronic course spanning several decades. The prevalence of schizophrenia among individuals ages 45–64 is approximately 0.6%, and prevalence estimates for elderly individuals range from

0.1% to 0.5% (Castle and Murray 1993; Copeland et al. 1998; Keith et al. 1991).

Longitudinal follow-up of schizophrenia patients indicates considerable heterogeneity of outcome. Approximately 20% of patients experience remission of both positive and negative symptoms (Ciompi 1980; Harding et al. 1987; Huber 1997). Another 20% experience worsening of symptoms, and the course in the remaining 60% remains largely unchanged (Belitsky and McGlashan 1993; Cohen 1990; Harvey et al. 1999). Initial deterioration usually occurs shortly after disease onset and is often limited to the first 5–10 years, followed by stability or even improvement of symptoms with aging. Factors associated with poorer prognosis for early-onset schizophrenia include chronicity, insidious onset, premorbid psychosocial or functional deficits, and prominent negative symptoms (Ram et al. 1992).

The course of schizophrenia appears stable, and most older adults with schizophrenia remain symptomatic, although positive symptoms seem to decrease with age (Jeste et al. 2003b).

Cognitive performance tends to remain stable, although it tends to be worse in patients with schizophrenia than in healthy older adults (Heaton et al. 2001; Palmer et al. 2003). Heaton and colleagues (2001) followed a large number of schizophrenia outpatients longitudinally for 6 months to 10 years and compared them with healthy subjects, using a comprehensive battery of neuropsychological measures. Schizophrenia patients had deficits relative to healthy subjects, particularly in the areas of learning, abstraction, and cognitive flexibility, but there was no evidence of cognitive deterioration over time. Harvey and colleagues (1999) followed a group of chronically institutionalized older patients with schizophrenia longitudinally for 30 months and found a subset of approximately 30% who experienced a decline in cognitive and functional status; however, this sample was not representative of most community-dwelling elderly patients.

Level of functional impairment varies considerably among older adults with schizophrenia. Palmer and colleagues (2003) found that 30% of a group of older outpatients with schizophrenia had been employed at least part-time since the onset of psychosis, 43% were current drivers, and 73% were living independently. In general, worse neuropsychological test performance, lower educational level, and negative symptoms, but not positive symptoms or depressed mood, are associated with poorer functional capacity in older outpatients with schizophrenia (Evans et al. 2003).

Late-Onset Schizophrenia

Historically, schizophrenia has been considered a disease of younger adulthood. Kraepelin (1919/1971) denoted schizophrenia *dementia praecox* to distinguish it from organic disorders arising in late life and to indicate a poor prognosis with progressive deterioration. However, a literature review found that approximately 23% of patients with schizophrenia reportedly had an onset of illness after age 40, with 3% being older than 60 years (Harris and Jeste 1988). Interestingly, DSM-III-R (American Psychiatric Association 1987) included a late-onset specifier for patients with schizophrenia of onset at age 45 or later, although in DSM-IV (American Psychiatric Association 1994) and its text revision, DSM-IV-TR (American Psychiatric Association 2000), age at onset is not specified.

The consensus statement by the International Late-Onset Schizophrenia Group suggested that schizophrenia with an onset after age 40 should be called late-onset schizophrenia and considered a subtype of schizophrenia rather than a related disorder (Howard et al. 2000). This decision was primarily based on evidence suggesting that schizophrenia with an onset in middle age is a neurodevelopmental disorder, rather than a neurodegenerative disorder, that shares more similarities than differences with schizophrenia with an earlier onset (Palmer et al. 2001).

Risk factors for and clinical presentation (including positive symptoms such as hallucinations, delusions, bizarre behavior, and thought disorder) of early-onset schizophrenia are similar to those associated with late-onset schizophrenia (Brodaty et al. 1999; Jeste et al. 1995b). The self-reported proportion of individuals with a family history of schizophrenia is similar among patients with early-onset schizophrenia and those with late-onset schizophrenia (10%–15%), and no consistent relationship has been found between age at onset and genetic risk of schizophrenia (Jeste et al. 1997b; Kendler et al. 1987).

Neuroimaging studies of patients with late-onset schizophrenia do not suggest the presence of strokes, tumors, or other abnormalities that could account for the development of schizophrenia in late life (Rivkin et al. 2000; Symonds et al. 1997), although nonspecific structural abnormalities such as enlarged ventricles and increased white matter hyperintensities may be more common in late- than in early-onset schizophrenia (Sachdev et al. 1999).

Long-term neuropsychological follow-up of a group of late-onset schizophrenia patients revealed no evidence of cognitive decline, again suggesting a neurodevelopmental rather than a neurodegenerative process (Palmer et al. 2003). In a long-term follow-up study of patients with a variety of late-life psychiatric illnesses, patients with late-onset schizophrenia had a unique set of outcomes and symptoms (Rabins and Lavrisha 2003).

Early- and late-onset schizophrenia differ with regard to gender ratio, preponderance of the paranoid subtype, prevalence of negative symptoms, cognitive performance, and premorbid functioning. Individuals with an onset of schizophrenia in mid- to late life are predominantly women (Hafner et al. 1998; Jeste et al. 1997b). Estrogen may serve as an endogenous antipsychotic, masking schizophrenic symptoms in vulnerable women until after menopause (Seeman 1996).

There appears to be a higher prevalence of the paranoid subtype of schizophrenia among patients with late-onset schizophrenia relative to patients with early-onset schizophrenia (Jeste et al. 1997b). Patients with late-onset schizophrenia tend to have more auditory hallucinations or hallucinations with a running commentary, persecutory delusions with or without hallucinations, and organized delusions (Howard et al. 2000). Patients with late-onset schizophrenia have lower levels of negative symptoms on average (including affective blunting, alogia, avolition, and inattention) than patients with early-onset schizophrenia; however, late-onset schizophrenia patients have higher levels of negative symptoms than normal subjects (Jeste et al. 1988, 1997b; Palmer et al. 2001).

On neuropsychological tests (after correction for age, education, and gender), patients with late-onset schizophrenia tend to demonstrate less impairment in learning, abstraction, and flexibility in thinking than patients with early-onset schizophrenia (Jeste et al. 1997b). A greater proportion of patients with late-onset schizophrenia have successful occupational and marital histories and generally higher premorbid functioning than do patients with early-onset schizophrenia.

Finally, patients with late-onset schizophrenia typically require lower daily doses of antipsychotic medications compared with age-comparable patients with early-onset schizophrenia, although the general

TABLE 9–1. Comparison of early-onset schizophrenia, late-onset schizophrenia, and very-late-onset schizophrenia-like psychosis

	Early-onset schizophrenia	Late-onset schizophrenia	Very late onset schizophrenia-like psychosis
Age at onset (years)	< 40	~ 40–60 (middle age)	≥60 (late life)
Female preponderance	–	+	+ +
Negative symptoms	+ +	+	–
Minor physical anomalies	+	+	–
Neuropsychological impairment			
Learning	+ +	+	?+ +
Retention	–	–	?+ +
Progressive cognitive deterioration	–	–	+ +
Brain structure abnormalities (e.g., strokes, tumors)	–	–	+ +
Family history of schizophrenia	+	+	–
Early childhood maladjustment	+	+	–
Daily antipsychotic dose	Higher	Lower	Lower
Risk of tardive dyskinesia	+	+	+ +

Note.   + = mildly present; + + = strongly present; ?+ + = probably strongly present, but few data exist; – = absent.

Source.   Adapted from Palmer et al. 2001.

response to such medications is similar in both groups (Jeste et al. 1993, 1997b).

Very Late Onset Schizophrenia-Like Psychosis

In its consensus statement, the International Late-Onset Schizophrenia Group proposed the diagnostic term *very late onset schizophrenia-like psychosis* for patients whose psychosis began after age 60 (Howard et al. 2000). Risk factors for and clinical features of early-onset schizophrenia, late-onset schizophrenia, and very late onset schizophrenia-like psychosis are compared in Table 9–1. Factors distinguishing patients with very late onset schizophrenia from "true" schizophrenia patients in-

clude a lower genetic load, less evidence of early childhood maladjustment, a relative lack of thought disorder and negative symptoms (including blunted affect), greater risk of TD, and evidence of a neurodegenerative rather than a neurodevelopmental process (Andreasen 1999; Howard et al. 1997).

Very late onset schizophrenia-like psychosis is a heterogeneous entity that includes conditions with etiologies as diverse as strokes, tumors, and other neurodegenerative changes. Clinical and research attention should be devoted to the presentation, cause, and course of illness in patients who develop psychotic symptoms for the first time in old age.

Delusional Disorder

At least 6% of older adults have paranoid symptoms such as persecutory delusions, but most of these individuals have dementia (Christenson and Blazer 1984; Forsell and Henderson 1998; Henderson et al. 1998). The essential feature of a delusional disorder is a nonbizarre delusion (e.g., a persecutory, somatic, erotomanic, grandiose, or jealous delusion) without prominent auditory or visual hallucinations. Symptoms must be present for at least 1 month. When delusional disorder arises in late life, basic personality features are typically intact, and functioning outside the delusional sphere is preserved. Intellectual performance and occupational functioning are preserved, but social functioning is compromised. To make a diagnosis of delusional disorder, the clinician must rule out delirium, dementia, psychotic disorders due to general medical conditions or the use of a substance, schizophrenia, and mood disorders with psychotic features. The course of persecutory delusional disorder is typically chronic, but patients with other types of delusions may have partial remissions and relapses.

According to DSM-IV-TR, the prevalence of delusional disorder is 0.03% and is slightly higher among women than among men. The disorder typically first appears in middle to late adulthood; the average age at onset is 40–49 years for men and 60–69 years for women.

Risk factors for delusional disorder include a family history of schizophrenia or avoidant, paranoid, or schizoid personality disorder (Kendler and Davis 1981). Evidence supporting hearing loss as a risk factor for paranoia is mixed (Cooper and Curry 1976; Moore 1981). Finally, immigration and low socioeconomic status may be risk factors for delusional disorder (American Psychiatric Association 1994).

Psychosis of Alzheimer's Disease

Psychotic symptoms in elderly individuals may arise secondary to AD or other dementias. Systematic studies of psychosis in dementia have focused on AD because AD is the most common type of dementia in the elderly population, representing approximately 65%–70% of dementia cases (Cummings and Benson 1992). Approximately 35%–50% of AD patients manifest psychotic symptoms, typically in the middle stages of the disease (Ropacki and Jeste 2005). In a large sample of patients with probable AD, the cumulative incidence of psychotic symptoms was 20% at 1 year, 36% at 2 years, 50% at 3 years, and 51% at 4 years (Paulsen et al. 2000). Delusions, especially of a persecutory nature, tend to be more common than hallucinations, the latter being more common in nursing homes and other institutional settings. Devanand and colleagues (1997) found that hallucinations and paranoid delusions were more persistent than depressive symptoms but less prevalent and less persistent than behavioral disturbances, particularly agitation.

In Table 9–2, characteristics associated with psychosis of AD are compared with characteristics of schizophrenia in elderly patients (Jeste and Finkel 2000). The most common psychotic symptoms in AD are delusions (which tend to be paranoid, concrete, simple, and nonbizarre) and hallucinations (which are more frequently visual than auditory). Misidentification of caregivers is frequent, whereas schneiderian first rank symptoms, such as hearing a running commentary on one's actions or hearing multiple voices talking to one another, are rare (Burns et al. 1990). Delusions or hallucinations may need to be inferred from the patient's behavior because the patient may be unable to verbal-

TABLE 9–2. Comparison of psychosis of Alzheimer's disease with schizophrenia in older patients

	Psychosis of AD	Schizophrenia
Prevalence	35%–50% of AD patients	<1% of general population
Bizarre or complex delusions	Rare	Frequent
Misidentification of caregivers	Frequent	Rare
Common form of hallucinations	Visual	Auditory
Schneiderian first rank symptoms	Rare	Frequent
Active suicidal ideation	Rare	Frequent
Past history of psychosis	Rare	Very common
Eventual remission of psychosis	Frequent	Uncommon
Need for years of maintenance antipsychotic therapy	Uncommon	Very common
Usual optimal daily doses of commonly used atypical antipsychotics		
Risperidone	0.75–1.5 mg	1.5–2.5 mg
Olanzapine	2.5–7.5 mg	7.5–12.5 mg
Recommended adjunctive psychosocial treatment	Sensory enhancement, structured activities, social contact, behavior therapy[a]	Cognitive-behavioral therapy, social skills training[b]

Note. AD = Alzheimer's disease.
[a]Cohen-Mansfield 2001. [b]Granholm et al. 2005; McQuaid et al. 2000.
Source. Adapted from Jeste and Finkel 2000.

ize thoughts or perceptions owing to cognitive impairment, particularly in the later stages of the disease. Because psychotic symptoms in patients with dementia tend to remit in the late stages of the disease, very long term maintenance therapy with antipsychotics is typically unnecessary. Finally, antipsychotic medication doses are lower for AD patients than for older adults with schizophrenia, and much lower than for younger adults.

AD patients with psychosis and those without psychosis differ in several important ways. Neuropsychologically, AD patients with psychosis show greater impairment in executive functioning and a more rapid cognitive decline (Jeste et al. 1992;

Stern et al. 1994). Psychosis is associated with a greater prevalence of extrapyramidal signs in AD (Stern et al. 1994). Neuropathologically, dementia patients with psychosis have shown increased neurodegenerative changes in the cortex, increased norepinephrine levels in subcortical regions, and reduced serotonin levels in both cortical and subcortical areas (Zubenko et al. 1991).

Jeste and Finkel (2000) recommended specific diagnostic criteria for psychosis of AD in order to facilitate epidemiologic, clinical, and therapeutic research. These criteria include the presence of visual or auditory hallucinations or delusions, a primary diagnosis of AD, a chronology indicating that psychotic symptoms followed the onset of dementia, a duration of 1 month or longer, and severity significant enough to disrupt the patient's functioning. Criteria for schizophrenia, schizoaffective disorder, delusional disorder, or mood disorder with psychotic features should never have been met, the disturbance must not occur exclusively during the course of delirium, and the disturbance must not be better accounted for by another general medical condition or by physiological effects of a substance. Associated symptoms may include agitation; negative symptoms such as apathy, flattening of affect, avolition, or motor retardation; and depression (with depressed mood, insomnia or hypersomnia, feelings of worthlessness or excessive or inappropriate guilt, or recurrent thoughts of death).

Treatment

The modern era of pharmacological treatment for schizophrenia and related disorders began with the introduction of chlorpromazine in the early 1950s. Although this and other conventional agents were able to substantially improve the positive symptoms of schizophrenia (e.g., hallucinations and delusions), a number of treatment liabilities have been recognized over the years, such as movement disorders, sedation, orthostatic hypotension, and increased prolactin concentrations. Furthermore, these medications generally do not improve the negative symptoms of schizophrenia (e.g., amotivation, social withdrawal, blunted affect, and alogia) that also play an important role in the daily lives of patients with schizophrenia.

Atypical antipsychotic agents such as clozapine, risperidone, olanzapine, quetiapine, ziprasidone, and aripiprazole are the drugs of choice for older adults with psychotic symptoms and disorders. Because older adults are more susceptible to extrapyramidal symptoms, toxicity, and sedation, the saying "start low and go slow" applies to the use of these medications in older patients. In general, these drugs have fewer extrapyramidal side effects and may be somewhat more effective against negative symptoms than conventional antipsychotics.

Treatment of Schizophrenia and Delusional Disorder

Patients with late-onset schizophrenia respond well to low-dose antipsychotic medication, requiring approximately one-half the dose typically taken by older patients with early-onset schizophrenia and 25%–33% of the dose used in younger schizophrenic patients. Patients with psychosis secondary to dementia typically require even lower doses, approximately 15%–25% of the dose used by younger patients with psychosis. Maintenance pharmacotherapy is usually required for older schizophrenia patients because of the risk of relapse. Because psychosis of dementia frequently remits, it may be possible to taper medications after the psychotic episode has been resolved.

Risperidone and olanzapine are the most studied medications in the treatment of schizophrenia in older adults. The efficacy of risperidone and olanzapine was demonstrated in an 8-week randomized, double-blind trial involving 175 stable elderly patients with chronic schizophrenia (Jeste et al. 2003a). Patients received 2 mg/day of risperidone or 10 mg/day of olanzapine. Both treatment groups experienced significant improvement in positive and negative symptoms. Extrapyramidal side effects were reported by 9% and 16% of patients in the risperidone and olanzapine groups, respectively. In a randomized investigation of olanzapine and haloperidol in older adults with schizophrenia, use of olanzapine was associated with significant improvement in psychiatric symptoms compared with haloperidol (Kennedy et al. 2003). Long-acting injectable risperidone was reported to be efficacious in and generally well tolerated by elderly patients with schizophrenia who were enrolled as part of a 50-week open trial involving symptomatically stable patients (Lasser et al. 2004). Risperidone and olanzapine were found to produce modest cognitive improvement in elderly patients with schizophrenia (Harvey et al. 2003).

Risperidone and olanzapine are not without side effects. Risperidone in higher doses appears to carry a greater risk of extrapyramidal side effects. Other side effects, especially with olanzapine, include orthostatic hypotension, sedation, weight gain, and the risk of developing hyperglycemia and type 2 diabetes (Allison et al. 1999; Jin et al. 2002; Wirshing et al. 1998). In a small open-label trial of hospitalized older adults with schizophrenia, aripiprazole showed promise in reducing positive and negative symptoms with a lack of extrapyramidal symptoms or TD (Madhusoodanan et al. 2004).

Recent results from the Clinical Antipsychotic Trials of Intervention Effectiveness (CATIE) in young and middle-aged adults with schizophrenia have interesting implications for the treatment of schizophrenia. The investigators found that regardless of antipsychotic (risperidone, olanzapine, quetiapine, ziprasidone, perphenazine), the majority of patients discontinued therapy because of perceived lack of efficacy or intolerability. Additionally, the efficacy of perphenazine was similar to that of risperidone, quetiapine, and ziprasidone (Lieberman et al. 2005).

Although antipsychotic medications can be efficacious in older patients with delusional disorder, some patients do not respond to treatment, and others have difficulty with adherence because of their delusional belief system.

Treatment of Psychosis of Alzheimer's Disease

Atypical antipsychotics such as clozapine, risperidone, olanzapine, and quetiapine show promise as agents for treatment of patients with psychosis of dementia (Katz et al. 1999; Street et al. 2000). In a nursing home sample, 1- and 2-mg daily doses of risperidone were more effective than placebo in reducing psychotic symptoms and aggressive behavior, but the 2-mg dose was associated with a greater risk of extrapyramidal symptoms (Katz et al. 1999). Also in a nursing home setting, a placebo-controlled trial of olanzapine found that 5 mg/day was preferable to larger doses in treating AD-related psychosis and behavioral disturbances (Street et al. 2000).

More recently, additional placebo-controlled trials have reported the efficacy of risperidone and olanzapine for the treatment of psychosis and behavioral disturbances in dementia (Brodaty et al. 2003; De Deyn et al. 2004). In a 10-week randomized, double-blind, placebo-controlled investigation of aripiprazole for the treatment of psychosis of Alzheimer's disease, aripiprazole did not differentiate itself from placebo on the Neuropsychiatric Inventory Psychosis subscale but did so on the Brief Psychiatric Rating Scale (De Deyn et al. 2005). There is debate regarding beneficial effects of cholinesterase inhibitors for the neuropsychiatric symptoms of AD (Finkel 2004).

The need for careful patient selection when prescribing antipsychotics in patients with dementia (an off-label use) has been highlighted because of safety concerns. Recently, the U.S. Food and Drug Administration issued a public health advisory concerning increased mortality associated with the use of atypical antipsychotics in elderly patients with dementia. All of the current atypical antipsychotics carry this warning because the increase in mortality was noted after pooling of results from a number of trials involving a variety of atypical antipsychotics (U.S. Food and Drug Administration 2005). The use of conventional antipsychotics instead of atypical agents does not appear to avoid the mortality risk. In a large cohort of elderly patients who received antipsychotic medications, the risk of death within 180 days of patients being prescribed a conventional antipsychotic was significantly higher than that of patients being prescribed an atypical agent (relative risk = 1.37 [95% confidence interval = 1.27–1.49]) (Wang et al. 2005).

Although conventional antipsychotics are reasonably effective in the treatment of psychosis of dementia, their side-effect profiles make them less desirable. The risk of extrapyramidal symptoms is higher among older patients than among younger patients (Jeste et al. 1999c). Moreover, the incidence of TD is higher among patients who begin taking conventional antipsychotics in old age than among similarly aged patients who began taking these medications at younger ages (Jeste et al. 1995b). Other side effects of antipsychotics include sedation, anticholinergic effects, cardiovascular effects (including orthostatic hypotension), parkinsonian reactions, and neuroleptic malignant syndrome. Careful monitoring for these side effects, as well as for involuntary abnormal movements, is recommended when working with psychotic dementia patients.

Psychosocial Treatment

Psychosocial treatment is a useful adjunct to pharmacological therapy. A supportive relationship with the treating physician can improve medication adherence and facilitate monitoring of symptoms, making hospitalization and other crises less likely. Enlisting the help of caregivers, family, neighbors, friends, and other community members may also facilitate the patient's care. Although research has not focused on older patients, a recent randomized, controlled study of cognitive-behavioral social skills training in middle-age and older outpatients with chronic schizophrenia showed the ability of such training to significantly improve coping skills, cognitive insight, and social functioning (Granholm et al. 2005).

Tardive Dyskinesia in Older Adults

TD is one of the most serious adverse effects of treatment with antipsychotics. This disorder, consisting of abnormal, involuntary movements, is generally caused by long-term treatment with antipsychotic medication. The movements are typically choreoathetoid in nature and principally involve the mouth, face, limbs, and trunk.

Incidence and Prevalence

TD is a side effect experienced by some patients receiving long-term treatment with antipsychotics. Yassa and Jeste (1992) reviewed 76 studies (published between 1960 and 1990) of the prevalence of TD. In a total population of roughly 40,000 patients, the overall prevalence of TD was 24.2%, although the prevalence was much higher in studies involving elderly patients treated with antipsychotics. Jeste and colleagues (1999c) evaluated 439 psychiatric patients (mean age, 65 years) and found that 28.8% met criteria for TD during the first 12 months of treatment with antipsychotics, 50.1% had TD by the end of 24 months of treatment, and 63.1% by the end of 36 months of treatment.

Risk Factors

Aging appears to be the most important risk factor for TD (American Psychiatric Association 2000; Yassa and Jeste 1992). Although the mechanism of this increase is unclear, it may be due to pharmacokinetic changes in elderly individuals and to the tendency of the nigrostriatal system to degenerate with age (Jeste and Caligiuri 1993). Previous investigators found TD to be associated with early extrapyramidal symptoms (Chouinard et al. 1979; Saltz et al. 1991), diabetes (Caligiuri and Jeste 2004), alcohol abuse or dependence (Dixon et al. 1992; Olivera et al. 1990), and certain ethnicities (Glazer et al. 1994; Jeste et al. 1996; Lawson 1986). The presence of subtle, subclinical movement disorders at the beginning of antipsychotic treatment, assessed by sensitive instrumental procedures, also increases the risk of TD (Jeste et al. 1999b). Longer total exposure to typical antipsychotic agents has been associated with greater TD risk (Casey 1997), and within the elderly population, the cumulative amount of high-potency typical antipsychotics has been associated with higher TD risk (Jeste et al. 1995a).

Lower risk of extrapyramidal symptoms with the use of atypical agents has led to the expectation that there is a reduced risk of TD during treatment with an atypical antipsychotic. The low risk of TD among clozapine-treated individuals has been reported (Kane et al. 1993), and a lower incidence of TD has also been reported in patients treated with other atypical agents (Chouinard et al. 1993; Dolder and Jeste 2003; Jeste et al. 1999a, 1999b; Tollefson et al. 1997).

Course and Outcome

TD may occur during exposure to antipsychotic medication or within 4 weeks of withdrawal from an oral antipsychotic. Symptoms of TD can also increase transiently when a conventional antipsychotic is replaced by an atypical antipsychotic.

The most common features of TD are involuntary movements of the tongue, face, and neck muscles. The movements of TD are choreiform (rapid, jerky), athetoid (slow, sinuous), or rhythmic (stereotypical) (American Psychiatric Association 2000). The earliest symptoms typically involve buccolingual-masticatory movements. Less common are movements of the upper and lower extremities and trunk (Brandon et al. 1971; Edwards 1970; Guy et al. 1986).

One-third of TD patients experience remission within 3 months of discontinuation of antipsychotic medication, and approximately one-half have remission within 12–18 months of antipsychotic discontinuation (American Psychiatric Association 2000). In studies that followed patients for more than 5 years, TD seems to improve in one-half of the patients, with or without antipsychotic treatment (Kane et al. 1992). Elderly patients are reported to have lower rates of remission, especially if treatment with antipsychotics is continued.

Severe TD may lead to a number of physical and psychosocial problems.

Treatment

Unfortunately, there are no consistently proven therapies for TD. Therefore, clinicians should focus on prevention of the disorder while regularly assessing patients for TD. Use of atypical antipsychotics, especially in elderly patients, is recommended because of the lower risk of TD associated with these drugs. In addition to initiating therapy with an atypical agent and switching to an atypical antipsychotic when feasible, clinicians should minimize antipsychotic use in all patients (Rosenbaum et al. 2005).

Patients who develop TD while taking a conventional antipsychotic should take an atypical antipsychotic instead, because studies have shown that such a switch in medications can lead to improvements of TD symptoms. Clozapine has been shown to be effective in reducing TD in patients with existing TD (Kane et al. 1993; Lieberman et al. 1991; Simpson et al. 1978; Small et al. 1987); however, side effects such as agranulocytosis and anticholinergic effects limit its use. A beneficial effect of other atypical agents (i.e., risperidone and olanzapine) on preexisting TD has also been reported (Bai et al. 2005; Dolder and Jeste 2003; Jeste 2004; Jeste et al. 1997a; Littrell et al. 1998; Street et al. 2000). The reduced risk of TD associated with all atypical agents (when used at appropriate doses), and the possibility of improvement of existing TD symptoms when a typical antipsychotic is replaced by an atypical antipsychotic, supports the use of atypical agents as a preventive measure and as a therapeutic option for those who develop TD while taking a conventional antipsychotic.

The dosing of antipsychotics in elderly patients is an important consideration. Compared with younger patients, older adults often respond to lower doses of antipsychotics. Patients with dementia usually respond to a lower dose than do individuals with schizophrenia or other psychotic disorders.

Numerous studies of various designs, though mostly small trials, have investigated many potential treatments for TD. Taken together, the study results are inconclusive. Nonetheless, vitamin E may be a reasonably safe treatment option for patients with TD, especially in the early stages of the disorder.

Other agents have been studied, including calcium-channel blockers (i.e., diltiazem, verapamil, and nifedipine), clonazepam, and pyridoxine, but more studies are warranted (Gupta et al. 1999; Lerner et al. 2001).

References

Allison DB, Mentore JL, Heo M, et al: Antipsychotic-induced weight gain: a comprehensive research synthesis. Am J Psychiatry 156:1686–1696, 1999

American Psychiatric Association: Diagnostic and Statistical Manual of Mental Disorders, 3rd Edition, Revised. Washington, DC, American Psychiatric Association, 1987

American Psychiatric Association: Diagnostic and Statistical Manual of Mental Disorders, 4th Edition. Washington, DC, American Psychiatric Association, 1994

American Psychiatric Association: Diagnostic and Statistical Manual of Mental Disorders, 4th Edition, Text Revision. Washington, DC, American Psychiatric Association, 2000

Andreasen NC: I don't believe in late onset schizophrenia, in Late-Onset Schizophrenia. Edited by Howard R, Rabins PV, Castle DJ. Philadelphia, PA, Wrightson Biomedical, 1999, pp 111–123

Bai YM, Yu SC, Chen JY, et al: Risperidone for preexisting severe tardive dyskinesia: a 48-week prospective follow-up study. Int Clin Psychopharmacol 20:79–85, 2005

Belitsky R, McGlashan TH: The manifestations of schizophrenia in late life: a dearth of data. Schizophr Bull 19:683–685, 1993

Brandon S, McClelland HA, Protheroe C: A study of facial dyskinesia in a mental hospital population. Br J Psychiatry 118:171–184, 1971

Brodaty H, Sachdev P, Rose N, et al: Schizophrenia with onset after age 50 years, 1: phenomenology and risk factors. Br J Psychiatry 175:410–415, 1999

Brodaty H, Ames D, Snowden J, et al: A randomized placebo-controlled trial of risperidone for the treatment of aggression, agitation, and psychosis of dementia. J Clin Psychiatry 64:134–143, 2003

Burns A, Jacoby R, Levy R: Psychiatric phenomena in Alzheimer's disease, I: disorders of thought content. Br J Psychiatry 157:72–76, 1990

Caligiuri MP, Jeste DV: Association of diabetes with dyskinesia in older psychosis patients. Psychopharmacology (Berl) 176:281–286, 2004

Casey DE: Will the new antipsychotics bring hope of reducing the risk of developing extrapyramidal syndromes and tardive dyskinesia? Int Clin Psychopharmacol 12:S19–S27, 1997

Castle DJ, Murray RM: The epidemiology of late-onset schizophrenia. Schizophr Bull 19:691–700, 1993

Chouinard G, Annable L, Ross-Chouinard A, et al: Factors related to tardive dyskinesia. Am J Psychiatry 136:79–82, 1979

Chouinard G, Jones B, Remington G, et al: A Canadian multicenter placebo-controlled study of fixed doses of risperidone and haloperidol in the treatment of chronic schizophrenic patients. J Clin Psychopharmacol 13:25–40, 1993

Christenson R, Blazer D: Epidemiology of persecutory ideation in an elderly population in the community. Am J Psychiatry 141:1088–1091, 1984

Ciompi L: Catamnestic long-term study on the course of life and aging of schizophrenics. Schizophr Bull 6:606–618, 1980

Cohen CI: Outcome of schizophrenia into later life. Gerontologist 30:790–797, 1990

Cohen-Mansfield J: Nonpharmacologic interventions for inappropriate behaviors in dementia: a review and critique. Am J Geriatr Psychiatry 9:361–381, 2001

Cooper AF, Curry AR: The pathology of deafness in the paranoid and affective psychoses of later life. J Psychosom Res 20:97–105, 1976

Copeland JRM, Dewey ME, Scott A, et al: Schizophrenia and delusional disorder in older age: community prevalence, incidence, comorbidity and outcome. Schizophr Bull 19:153–161, 1998

Cummings JL, Benson DF: Dementia: A Clinical Approach, 2nd Edition. Boston, MA, Butterworth-Heinemann, 1992

De Deyn P, Carrasco MM, Deberdt W, et al: Olanzapine versus placebo in the treatment of psychosis with or without associated behavioral disturbances in patients with Alzheimer's disease. Int J Geriatr Psychiatry 19:115–126, 2004

De Deyn P, Jeste DV, Swanink R, et al: Aripiprazole for the treatment of psychosis in patients with Alzheimer's disease: a randomized, placebo-controlled study. J Clin Psychopharmacol 25:463–467, 2005

Dixon L, Weiden PJ, Haas G, et al: Increased tardive dyskinesia in alcohol-abusing schizophrenic patients. Compr Psychiatry 33:121–122, 1992

Dolder CR, Jeste DV: Incidence of tardive dyskinesia with typical versus atypical antipsychotics in very high risk patients. Biol Psychiatry 53:1142–1145, 2003

Edwards H: The significance of brain damage in persistent oral dyskinesia. Br J Psychiatry 116:271–275, 1970

Evans JD, Heaton RK, Paulsen JS, et al: The relationship of neuropsychological abilities to specific domains of functional capacity in older schizophrenia patients. Biol Psychiatry 53:422–430, 2003

Finkel SI: Effect of rivastigmine on behavioral and psychological symptoms of dementia in Alzheimer's disease. Clin Ther 26:980–990, 2004

Forsell Y, Henderson AS: Epidemiology of paranoid symptoms in an elderly population. Br J Psychiatry 172:429–432, 1998

Glazer WM, Morgenstern H, Doucette J: Race and tardive dyskinesia among outpatients at a CMHC. Hosp Community Psychiatry 45:38–42, 1994

Granholm E, McQuaid JR, McClure FS, et al: A randomized, controlled trial of cognitive behavioral social skills training for middle-aged and older outpatients with chronic schizophrenia. Am J Psychiatry 162:520–529, 2005

Gupta S, Mosnik D, Black DW, et al: Tardive dyskinesia: review of treatments past, present, and future. Ann Clin Psychiatry 11:257–266, 1999

Guy W, Ban TA, Wilson WH: The prevalence of abnormal involuntary movements among chronic schizophrenics. Int Clin Psychopharmacol 1:134–144, 1986

Hafner H, an der Heiden W, Behrens S, et al: Causes and consequences of the gender differences in age at onset of schizophrenia. Schizophr Bull 24:99–113, 1998

Hannerz H, Borga P, Borritz M: Life expectancies for individuals with psychiatric diagnoses. Public Health 115:328–337, 2001

Harding CM, Brooks GW, Ashikaga T, et al: Aging and social functioning in once-chronic schizophrenic patients 22–62 years after first admission: the Vermont story, in Schizophrenia and Aging. Edited by Miller NE, Cohen GD. New York, Guilford, 1987, pp 74–82

Harris MJ, Jeste DV: Late-onset schizophrenia: an overview. Schizophr Bull 14:39–55, 1988

Harvey PD, Silverman JM, Mohs RC, et al: Cognitive decline in late-life schizophrenia: a longitudinal study of geriatric chronically hospitalized patients. Biol Psychiatry 45:32–40, 1999

Harvey PD, Napolitano JA, Mao L, et al: Comparative effects of risperidone and olanzapine on cognition in elderly patients with schizophrenia or schizoaffective disorder. Int J Geriatr Psychiatry 18:820–829, 2003

Heaton RK, Gladsjo JA, Palmer BW, et al: Stability and course of neuropsychological deficits in schizophrenia. Arch Gen Psychiatry 58:24–32, 2001

Henderson AS, Korten AE, Levings C, et al: Psychotic symptoms in the elderly: a prospective study in a population sample. Int J Geriatr Psychiatry 13:484–492, 1998

Hiroeh U, Appleby L, Mortensen PB, et al: Death by homicide, suicide, and other unnatural causes in people with mental illness: a population-based study. Lancet 358:2110–2112, 2001

Howard R, Graham C, Sham P, et al: A controlled family study of late-onset nonaffective psychosis (late paraphrenia). Br J Psychiatry 170:511–514, 1997

Howard R, Rabins PV, Seeman MV, et al: Late-onset schizophrenia and very-late-onset schizophrenia-like psychosis: an international consensus. Am J Psychiatry 157:172–178, 2000

Huber G: The heterogeneous course of schizophrenia. Schizophr Res 28:177–185, 1997

Jeste DV: Tardive dykinesia rates with atypical antipsychotics in older adults. J Clin Psychiatry 65 (suppl 9):21–24, 2004

Jeste DV, Caligiuri MP: Tardive dyskinesia. Schizophr Bull 19:303–315, 1993

Jeste DV, Finkel SI: Psychosis of Alzheimer's disease and related dementias: diagnostic criteria for a distinct syndrome. Am J Geriatr Psychiatry 8:29–34, 2000

Jeste DV, Harris MJ, Pearlson GD, et al: Late-onset schizophrenia. Studying clinical validity. Psychiatr Clin North Am 11:1–13, 1988

Jeste DV, Wragg RE, Salmon DP, et al: Cognitive deficits of patients with Alzheimer's disease with and without delusions. Am J Psychiatry 149:184–189, 1992

Jeste DV, Lacro JP, Gilbert PL, et al: Treatment of late-life schizophrenia with neuroleptics. Schizophr Bull 19:817–830, 1993

Jeste DV, Caligiuri MP, Paulsen JS, et al: Risk of tardive dyskinesia in older patients: a prospective longitudinal study of 266 patients. Arch Gen Psychiatry 52:756–765, 1995a

Jeste DV, Harris MJ, Krull A, et al: Clinical and neuropsychological characteristics of patients with late-onset schizophrenia. Am J Psychiatry 152:722–730, 1995b

Jeste DV, Lindamer LA, Evans J, et al: Relationship of ethnicity and gender to schizophrenia and pharmacology of neuroleptics. Psychopharmacol Bull 32:243–251, 1996

Jeste DV, Klausner M, Brecher M, et al: A clinical evaluation of risperidone in the treatment of schizophrenia: a 10-week, open-label, multicenter trial involving 945 patients. Psychopharmacology (Berl) 131:239–247, 1997a

Jeste DV, Symonds LL, Harris MJ, et al: Nondementia nonpraecox dementia praecox? late-onset schizophrenia. Am J Geriatr Psychiatry 5:302–317, 1997b

Jeste DV, Lacro JP, Bailey A, et al: Lower incidence of tardive dyskinesia with risperidone compared with haloperidol in older patients. J Am Geriatr Soc 47:716–719, 1999a

Jeste DV, Lacro JP, Palmer B, et al: Incidence of tardive dyskinesia in early stages of low-dose treatment with typical neuroleptics in older patients. Am J Psychiatry 156:309–311, 1999b

Jeste DV, Rockwell E, Harris MJ, et al: Conventional vs. newer antipsychotics in elderly patients. Am J Geriatr Psychiatry 7:70–76, 1999c

Jeste DV, Barak Y, Madhusoodanan S, et al: International multisite double-blind trial of the atypical antipsychotics risperidone and olanzapine in 175 elderly patients with chronic schizophrenia. Am J Geriatr Psychiatry 11:638–647, 2003a

Jeste DV, Twamley EW, Eyler Zorrilla LT, et al: Aging and outcome in schizophrenia. Acta Psychiatr Scand 107:336–343, 2003b

Jin H, Meyer JM, Jeste DV: Phenomenology of and risk factors for new-onset diabetes mellitus and diabetic ketoacidosis associated with atypical antipsychotics: an analysis of 45 published cases. Ann Clin Psychiatry 14:59–64, 2002

Joukamaa M, Heliovaara M, Knekt P, et al: Mental disorders and cause-specific mortality. Br J Psychiatry 179:498–502, 2001

Kane JM, Jeste DV, Barnes TRE, et al: Tardive Dyskinesia: A Task Force Report of the American Psychiatric Association. Washington, DC, American Psychiatric Association, 1992

Kane JM, Woerner MG, Pollack S, et al: Does clozapine cause tardive dyskinesia? J Clin Psychiatry 54:327–330, 1993

Katz IR, Jeste DV, Mintzer JE, et al: Comparison of risperidone and placebo for psychosis and behavioral disturbances associated with dementia: a randomized, double-blind trial. J Clin Psychiatry 60:107–115, 1999

Keith SJ, Regier DA, Rae DS: Schizophrenic disorders, in Psychiatric Disorders in America: The Epidemiologic Catchment Area Study. Edited by Robins LN, Regier DA. New York, Free Press, 1991, pp 33–52

Kendler KS, Davis KL: The genetics and biochemistry of paranoid schizophrenia and other paranoid psychoses. Schizophr Bull 7:689–709, 1981

Kendler KS, Tsuang MT, Hays P: Age at onset in schizophrenia: a familial perspective. Arch Gen Psychiatry 44:881–890, 1987

Kennedy JS, Jeste D, Kaiser CJ, et al: Olanzapine vs haloperidol in geriatric schizophrenia: analysis of data from a double-blind controlled trial. Int J Geriatr Psychiatry 18:1013–1020, 2003

Kraepelin E: Dementia Praecox and Paraphrenia (1919). Translated by Barclay RM. Huntington, NY, Krieger, 1971

Lasser RA, Bossie CA, Zhu Y, et al: Efficacy and safety of long-acting risperidone in elderly patients with schizophrenia and schizoaffective disorder. Int J Geriatr Psychiatry 19:898–905, 2004

Lawson WB: Racial and ethnic factors in psychiatric research. Hosp Community Psychiatry 37:50–54, 1986

Lerner V, Miodownik C, Kaptsan A, et al: Vitamin B_6 in the treatment of tardive dyskinesia: a double-blind, placebo-controlled, crossover study. Am J Psychiatry 158:1511–1514, 2001

Lieberman JA, Saltz BL, Johns CA, et al: The effects of clozapine on tardive dyskinesia. Br J Psychiatry 158:503–510, 1991

Lieberman JA, Stroup TS, McEvoy JP, et al; The Clinical Antipsychotic Trials of Intervention Effectiveness (CATIE) Investigators: Effectiveness of antipsychotic drugs in patients with chronic schizophrenia. N Engl J Med 353:1209–1223, 2005

Littrell KH, Johnson CG, Littrell S, et al: Marked reduction of tardive dyskinesia with olanzapine (letter). Arch Gen Psychiatry 55:279–280, 1998

Madhusoodanan S, Brenner R, Gupta S, et al: Clinical experience with aripiprazole in ten elderly patients with schizophrenia or schizoaffective disorder: retrospective case studies. CNS Spectr 9:862–867, 2004

McQuaid JR, Granholm E, McClure FS, et al: Development of an integrated cognitive-behavioral and social skills training intervention for older patients with schizophrenia. J Psychother Pract Res 9:149–156, 2000

Moore NC: Is paranoid illness associated with sensory defects in the elderly? J Psychosom Res 25:69–74, 1981

Olivera AA, Kiefer MW, Manley NK: Tardive dyskinesia in psychiatric patients with substance use disorders. Am J Drug Alcohol Abuse 16:57–66, 1990

Ostling S, Skoog I: Psychotic symptoms and paranoid ideation in a nondemented population-based sample of the very old. Arch Gen Psychiatry 59:53–59, 2002

Palmer BW, McClure F, Jeste DV: Schizophrenia in late-life: findings challenge traditional concepts. Harv Rev Psychiatry 9:51–58, 2001

Palmer BW, Bondi M, Twamley E, et al: Are late-onset schizophrenia spectrum disorders neurodegenerative conditions? Annual rates of change on two dementia measures. J Neuropsychiatry Clin Neurosci 15:45–52, 2003

Paulsen JS, Salmon DP, Thal LJ, et al: Incidence of and risk factors for hallucinations and delusions in patients with probable AD. Neurology 54:1965–1971, 2000

Rabins PV, Lavrisha M: Long-term follow-up and phenomenologic differences distinguish among late-onset schizophrenia, late-life depression, and progressive dementia. Am J Geriatr Psychiatry 11:589–594, 2003

Ram R, Bromet EJ, Eaton WW, et al: The natural course of schizophrenia: a review of first-admission studies. Schizophr Bull 18:185–207, 1992

Rivkin P, Kraut M, Barta P, et al: White matter hyperintensity volume in late-onset and early onset schizophrenia. Int J Geriatr Psychiatry 15:1085–1089, 2000

Ropacki S, Jeste DV: Epidemiology of and risk factors for psychosis of Alzheimer disease: a review of 55 studies published from 1990 to 2003. Am J Psychiatry 162:2022–2030, 2005

Rosenbaum JF, Arana GW, Hyman SE (eds): Handbook of Psychiatric Drug Therapy, 5th Edition. Philadelphia, PA, Lippincott Williams & Wilkins, 2005

Sachdev P, Brodaty H, Rose N, et al: Schizophrenia with onset after age 50 years, 2: neurological, neuropsychological and MRI investigation. Br J Psychiatry 175:416–421, 1999

Saltz BL, Woerner MG, Kane JM, et al: Prospective study of tardive dyskinesia incidence in the elderly. JAMA 266:2402–2406, 1991

Seeman MV: The role of estrogen in schizophrenia. J Psychiatry Neurosci 21:123–127, 1996

Simpson GM, Lee JM, Shrivastava RK: Clozapine in tardive dyskinesia. Psychopharmacology (Berl) 56:75–80, 1978

Small JG, Milstein V, Marhenke JD, et al: Treatment outcome with clozapine in tardive dyskinesia, neuroleptic sensitivity, and treatment-resistant psychosis. J Clin Psychiatry 48:263–267, 1987

Stern Y, Albert M, Brandt J, et al: Utility of extrapyramidal signs and psychosis as predictors of cognitive and functional decline, nursing home admission, and death in Alzheimer's disease: prospective analyses from the Predictors Study. Neurology 44:2300–2307, 1994

Street JS, Tollefson GD, Tohen M, et al: Olanzapine for psychotic conditions in the elderly. Psychiatric Annals 30:191–196, 2000

Symonds LL, Olichney JM, Jernigan TL, et al: Lack of clinically significant gross structural abnormalities in MRIs of older patients with schizophrenia and related psychoses. J Neuropsychiatry Clin Neurosci 9:251–258, 1997

Tollefson GD, Beasley CM, Tran PV, et al: Olanzapine versus haloperidol in the treatment of schizophrenia and schizoaffective and schizophreniform disorders: results of an international collaborative trial. Am J Psychiatry 154:457–465, 1997

U.S. Food and Drug Administration: FDA issues public health advisory for antipsychotic drugs used for the treatment of behavioral disorders in elderly patients. FDA Talk Paper. Available at: http://www.fda.gov/bbs/topics/ANSWERS/2005/ANS01350.html. Accessed April 11, 2005.

Wang PS, Schneeweiss S, Avorn J, et al: Risk of death in elderly users of conventional vs atypical antipsychotic medications. N Engl J Med 353:2335–2341, 2005

Wirshing DA, Spellberg BJ, Erhart SM, et al: Novel antipsychotics and new onset diabetes. Biol Psychiatry 44:778–783, 1998

Yassa R, Jeste DV: Gender differences in tardive dyskinesia: a critical review of the literature. Schizophr Bull 18:701–715, 1992

Zubenko GS, Moossy J, Martinez AJ, et al: Neuropathologic and neurochemical correlates of psychosis in primary dementia. Arch Neurol 48:619–624, 1991

Study Questions

Select the single best response for each question.

1. Factors distinguishing patients with very late onset schizophrenia from "true" schizophrenia of younger patients include all of the following *except*

    A. Lower genetic load.
    B. Less evidence of early childhood maladjustment.
    C. Relative lack of formal thought disorder and negative symptoms.
    D. Lesser risk of tardive dyskinesia.
    E. Evidence of a neurodegenerative rather than a neurodevelopmental process.

2. What approximate percentage of Alzheimer's disease patients manifest psychotic symptoms, typically in the middle stages of the disease?

    A. 10%–20%.
    B. 15%–25%.
    C. 25%–30%.
    D. 35%–50%.
    E. 55%–65%.

3. Alzheimer's disease patients with and without psychosis differ in all of the following *except*

    A. Alzheimer's disease patients with psychosis show greater impairment in executive functioning.
    B. Alzheimer's disease patients with psychosis have a greater prevalence of extrapyramidal signs.
    C. Alzheimer's disease patients with psychosis have shown increased norepinephrine levels and reduced serotonin levels in subcortical regions.
    D. Alzheimer's disease patients with psychosis typically warrant very long term maintenance therapy with antipsychotics.
    E. Alzheimer's disease patients with psychosis have more prevalent behavioral disturbances such as agitation than hallucinations and paranoid delusions.

4. The most important risk factor for tardive dyskinesia is

    A. Alcohol abuse.
    B. Early extrapyramidal symptoms.
    C. Certain ethnicities.
    D. Aging.
    E. None of the above.

Anxiety and Panic Disorders

John L. Beyer, M.D.

Many consider anxiety to be a natural response to aging. As aging occurs, so do concerns about changes in physical health, financial security, social support, and cognitive ability (Blazer 1997; Small 1997). Despite these concerns, it is remarkable that anxiety disorders decrease with age rather than progressively increase throughout life. However, the impact of anxiety and anxiety disorders in older adults is often unrecognized and inadequately treated. When present, anxiety disorders may result in higher medical and psychiatric comorbidity and poorer quality of life (Lindesay et al. 1989).

Epidemiology

Anxiety disorders are the most common psychiatric conditions in the elderly (Blazer et al. 1991a). The most extensive estimate of anxiety disorders in the elderly is from results of the Epidemiologic Catchment Area (ECA) studies conducted in the early 1980s. This survey examined more than 20,000 community-dwelling adults at different sites across the United States for psychiatric disorders based on DSM-III (Amer-

ican Psychiatric Association 1980) criteria. The combined prevalence of phobia, panic disorder, and obsessive-compulsive disorder (OCD) (the only anxiety disorders measured at all five sites) in people over 65 years of age was 5.5%. Although anxiety disorders had the highest 1-year prevalence rate in the elderly of any psychiatric diagnosis (Regier et al. 1990) (a finding consistent with that of all age populations sampled), there was a decline from levels experienced in the middle-aged group. Still, the number of elderly persons with anxiety disorders is significant, especially in older women, for whom the prevalence of any anxiety disorder (6.8%) was higher than the prevalence for men of any age.

DSM-IV-TR (American Psychiatric Association 2000) anxiety disorders are listed in Table 10–1.

Diagnostic Classification and Phenomenology

Panic Disorder

Panic attacks are episodes of intense anxiety accompanied by multiple physical symptoms (e.g., palpitations, sweating,

TABLE 10–1. DSM-IV-TR anxiety disorders

Panic disorder

  With agoraphobia

  Without agoraphobia

Agoraphobia without history of panic disorder

Specific phobia

  Animal type

  Natural environment type

  Blood-injection-injury type

  Situational type

  Other type

Social phobia

Obsessive-compulsive disorder

Posttraumatic stress disorder

Acute stress disorder

Generalized anxiety disorder

Anxiety disorder due to a general medical condition

Substance-induced anxiety disorder

tremulousness, shortness of breath, a choking sensation, chest pain, nausea, lightheadedness, chills, or numbness) and cognitive symptoms (e.g., fear of dying or of "going crazy"). The attack may quickly build to a peak intensity in 5–10 minutes and last from 5 to 30 minutes.

Panic attacks occur in a variety of anxiety disorders or may be caused by certain medications or substances (e.g., caffeine) or medical conditions (e.g., hyperthyroidism). However, in panic disorder, panic attacks become recurrent and the focus of the individual's fear. If the anxiety is very intense, a strong desire to flee from the place of the panic attack may lead to a pattern of avoiding places where the attack occurred or where escape would be difficult if an attack recurred. This condition is called *agoraphobia*. Thus, patients may receive a diagnosis of panic disorder *with* or *without* agoraphobia.

Development of panic disorder in late life is relatively uncommon, but it does occur (Luchins and Rose 1989; Sheikh and Cassidy 2000). In the ECA study, the point prevalence among middle-aged subjects was 1.1%, whereas among those age 65 or older, the point prevalence was 0.4% (Regier et al. 1988; see also Bland et al. 1988; Lindesay et al. 1989; Manela et al. 1996). When lifetime prevalence was considered, 2% of persons ages 45–64 years met the criteria for panic disorder, whereas only 0.3% of older persons met the criteria.

When the diagnosis is first made in elderly patients, it is frequently because it had been missed previously (Sheikh et al. 1991). It is not uncommon for elderly adults to ascribe the symptoms to other causes (e.g., having a heart attack), and the frequent waxing and waning of symptoms may make correct diagnosis difficult.

When elderly persons do experience panic attacks, the symptoms are similar to those that occur in younger people. However, elderly individuals with late-onset panic attacks may have fewer symptoms and may do less to avoid the attacks (Sheikh et al. 1991).

Agoraphobia Without History of Panic Disorder

Agoraphobia occurs when the person avoids public places or situations because of fear of having "panic-like" symptoms. Elderly patients may indeed have realistic concerns that certain physical conditions have the potential for embarrassment (e.g., loss of bladder or bowel control) or require assistance (e.g., being unable to get up after a fall) and thus avoid leaving home. Therefore, the diagnosis of agoraphobia should be made only when the avoidance is clearly in excess of what is usually associated with that medical condition.

Specific Phobia

Specific phobias are characterized by excessive and persistent fear of an object or situation (American Psychiatric Association 2000). There are four types: fear of *animals* (e.g., dogs or snakes), fear of *natural events* (e.g., storms, heights, or water), fear of *blood-injection-injury* (e.g., fear triggered by seeing blood, experiencing an injury, or receiving medication by injection), and *situational* fear (such as fear of driving, flying, crossing bridges, or being in enclosed spaces). Fears of animals and natural events are common during childhood and diminish with age. Situational phobias appear to be closely related to panic disorder and often persist in old age (Blazer et al. 1991b).

Social Phobia

Social phobia is a persistent fear of social or performance situations in which embarrassment may occur. Examples include making a speech, eating in public, and using public restrooms. For elderly individuals, avoidance of eating, drinking, or writing in public may be due to excessive concern or embarrassment about tremors. Social phobia tends to be a lifelong illness; however, the disorder fluctuates in severity and may even remit. For example, social phobia may diminish after a person with fear of dating marries, only to reemerge after the death of the spouse (see American Psychiatric Association 2000).

Obsessive-Compulsive Disorder

Obsessions are "persistent ideas, thoughts, impulses, or images that are experienced as intrusive and inappropriate" (American Psychiatric Association 2000, p. 457). The most common obsessions are about contamination, doubting, ordering, aggression, and sexual imagery. Attempts to suppress the thoughts often increase the anxiety, and individuals may develop *compulsions* to reduce or prevent the anxiety. Common compulsions are hand washing, checking behaviors, ordering, praying, counting, hoarding, and repeating words or phrases. The OCD patient usually knows that the obsessions or compulsions are excessive but feels unable to stop the behavior.

OCD usually begins in adolescence or early adulthood with a gradual onset and a waxing and waning course. The kind of obsession or compulsive activity present may change over time. About 15% of persons with the disorder have a progressive deterioration, while about 5% have episodic presentations with minimal symptoms between episodes. In elderly patients, OCD is often identified when excessive physical complaints require repeated visits to the doctor for reassurance.

Point prevalence of OCD in elderly patients has varied among studies, ranging from 0% to 1.5% (Bland et al. 1988; Copeland et al. 1987; Regier et al. 1988). Despite the low incidence, a review of cases from OCD clinics showed that approximately 5% of patients are over the age of 60 years (Jenike 1991; Kohn et al. 1997).

Posttraumatic Stress Disorder

Posttraumatic stress disorder (PTSD) may develop after exposure to a traumatic event that is experienced directly (e.g., being the victim of a crime, being involved in a motor vehicle accident, or being diagnosed with a life-threatening illness) or indirectly (e.g., witnessing a traumatic accident or violent event) (American Psychiatric Association 2000). In response to the trauma, individuals with PTSD develop three clusters of symptoms:

1. *Reexperiencing*—recurrent and intrusive memories or dreams (individuals behave as though they were reliving the trauma) or intense distress and/or physiological reactions when exposed to reminders of the trauma.

2. *Avoidance*—avoidance of thoughts, feelings, and conversations about the trauma; avoidance of persons, places, or situations that remind them of the trauma; amnesia for significant parts of the trauma; avoidance of emotions; or a sense of a foreshortened future.
3. *Arousal*—difficulty falling asleep, hypervigilance, decreased concentration, exaggerated startle response, or episodes of irritability or anger outbursts.

PTSD usually occurs within the first 3 months of the trauma, though symptoms may also be delayed years. Symptoms resolve in the first 3 months in 50% of individuals, but many persons will continue to have symptoms throughout life. The intensity and duration of the symptoms are positively correlated with the severity of the trauma (Flint 1999).

PTSD may occur at any age, but elderly individuals may be more likely than younger persons to be victimized or to sustain life-threatening injuries, and thus new-onset PTSD may be more common than reported. However, there are no data on the prevalence of PTSD in the general elderly population (Flint 1999). Most research involving elderly patients has examined the impact of PTSD on survivors of the Holocaust or persons who were prisoners of war during World War II (Kuch and Cox 1992; Robinson et al. 1990; Sutker et al. 1993). Among the elderly Holocaust survivors, nearly half met the criteria for PTSD more than 40 years later (Kuch and Cox 1992). Among former prisoners of war, approximately one-quarter met the criteria for PTSD more than 40 years after their release (Kluznik et al. 1986; Rosen et al. 1989).

Acute Stress Disorder

The symptoms of acute stress disorder are similar to those of PTSD. The diagnosis of acute stress disorder is used when the symptoms of anxiety, dissociation, reexperiencing, avoidance, and hyperarousal occur for at least 2 days during the first month after the trauma. However, if symptoms are still significant after 4 weeks, the diagnosis of PTSD is made.

Generalized Anxiety Disorder

Generalized anxiety disorder (GAD) is an excessive anxiousness or worry that occurs on most days for at least 6 months. Other symptoms include restlessness, easy fatigability, difficulty concentrating, irritability, muscle tension, and disturbed sleep.

GAD is the second most common anxiety disorder in the elderly population (phobias are the most common). Point prevalence ranges from 0.7% to 7.1% (Blazer et al. 1991b; Copeland et al. 1987; Lindesay et al. 1989; Manela et al. 1996; Uhlenhuth et al. 1983). In the ECA study, the rate of GAD in elderly subjects was 2.2% (Blazer et al. 1991b).

Anxiety Disorder Due to a General Medical Condition or Substance

Anxiety symptoms are frequent manifestations of underlying disease or use of a medication or substance. To make this diagnosis, the physician must establish that the patient has a disease or has been exposed to a substance that could cause an anxiety response and, in the latter case, that the response is temporally related to the exposure. This diagnosis must be considered when anxiety occurs unexpectedly or with unusual features (e.g., late age at onset). For example, most late-onset panic attacks are associated with cardiovascular, gastrointestinal, and chronic pulmonary diseases (Hassan and Pollard 1994; Raj et al. 1993).

TABLE 10–2. Medications and substances that can cause anxiety

Over-the-counter medications

Caffeine

Stimulants

Prescription medications

Anticholinergics

Psychostimulants (e.g., methylphenidate, amphetamine)

Sedative-hypnotics (withdrawal)

Steroids

Sympathomimetics

Substances

Alcohol

Cocaine

Hallucinogens

Narcotics

A variety of medications/drugs and medical conditions can cause anxiety symptoms (see Tables 10–2 and 10–3).

Differential Diagnosis

Medical Illnesses

There is a complex interaction among anxiety, medical illness, and the medications used to treat these conditions (Flint 1999). First, as noted earlier, many medical illnesses may masquerade as anxiety, but also many anxiety symptoms masquerade as medical illness. For example, the list of the most common reasons for primary care office visits by elderly individuals (dizziness, chest pain, shortness of breath, general weakness, tiredness, nervousness, palpitations, nausea, and urinary frequency) may be related to anxiety (White et al. 1986).

Second, the presence of anxiety itself may contribute to medical problems and complications. For example, people with high levels of anxiety are at higher risk for

TABLE 10–3. Medical disorders associated with anxiety

Cardiac

Angina

Cardiac arrhythmias

Congestive heart failure

Hypertension

Mitral valve prolapse

Myocardial infarction

Endocrine

Cushing's syndrome

Hypoglycemia

Hypo- or hyperparathyroidism

Hypo- or hyperthyroidism

Menopause

Premenstrual syndrome

Neurological

Cerebral arteriosclerosis

Complex partial seizures

Delirium

Early dementia

Huntington's disease

Meniere's disease

Migraine

Multiple sclerosis

Postconcussion syndrome

Vestibular dysfunction

Wilson's disease

Neoplastic

Carcinoid syndrome

Cerebral neoplasm

Pheochromocytoma

Pulmonary

Asthma

Chronic obstructive pulmonary disease

Hypoxic states

Pulmonary embolism

Other

Porphyria

hypertension (Jonas et al. 1997), arrhythmias (Moser and Dracup 1996), and death from cardiovascular disease (Kawachi et al. 1994).

Third, there is the realistic worry about the impact of physical illnesses in the elderly.

Finally, anxiety symptoms may be caused by the medications given to elderly persons to treat either physical or mental diseases.

Interestingly, the prevalence of anxiety disorders in the elderly medically ill is lower than for young and middle-aged patients (Cassem 1990; Magni and De Leo 1984), even though minor illnesses may have more consequences in the elderly person's life.

Comorbid Depression and Anxiety

Anxiety disorders and major depression frequently occur together. It is estimated that two-thirds of patients with anxiety disorders also will have a major depressive disorder at some point in their life (Judd et al. 1998). Conversely, 38% of an elderly depressed outpatient population had at least one anxiety disorder (Alexopoulos et al. 1990).

Treatment

Nonpharmacological Treatment

Several cognitive and behavioral therapies have been demonstrated to be effective in treating anxiety disorders in younger adults, though there have been no systematic studies in older adults. Cognitive-behavioral therapy (CBT) has reliably been found to be effective for the panic disorders, GAD, PTSD, and social phobia. Exposure therapy has been found to be very effective for specific phobias and compulsive behaviors.

These treatments can be useful alternative approaches to treatment in the elderly, especially when medications need to be avoided. However, barriers to their use in the elderly, such as severe physical limitations, cognitive impairments, and difficulty in accessing care, are frequently observed.

Pharmacological Treatment

A variety of medications have been used for the treatment of anxiety disorders in the elderly with varying degrees of success; however, choosing appropriate treatment poses several challenges. First, all medications have the potential for unwanted side effects—a problem of special concern in the elderly because of age-related physical changes (see Chapter 2, "Physiological and Clinical Considerations of Geriatric Patient Care," this volume) and potential interactions with medications prescribed for other physical problems (Jenike 1989; Ouslander 1981; Salzman 1990; Thompson et al. 1983). In addition, changes in neurotransmitter and receptor function in the central nervous system may also increase sensitivity to psychotropic drugs (Salzman 1990). Second, there has been limited research on the treatment of elderly patients with anxiety disorders (Krasucki et al. 1998). Therefore, physicians must use their knowledge of the disease, medications, and the physical health of their patients to make the best decisions for treatment.

Antidepressants

Selective serotonin reuptake inhibitors. Selective serotonin reuptake inhibitors (SSRIs) have become the mainstay of anxiety disorder treatment for several reasons. First, various SSRIs have obtained U.S. Food and Drug Administration–approved indications for use in the treatment of panic disorder, GAD, social phobia, and OCD in the general population. Second, anxiety disorders and depressive disorders frequently co-occur, and the use of a single agent to treat both conditions decreases the use of polypharmacy often seen in the elderly. Finally, the side-effect profiles of the SSRIs are much more acceptable than those of many of the older medications. However, common side effects are nausea and diarrhea, sexual dysfunction, and a decrease in appetite and weight.

Newer antidepressants. Other antidepressants are also being increasingly used for the treatment of anxiety in elderly individuals. Nefazodone has been reported to be effective in depressed elderly patients with prominent anxiety symptoms (Small 1997). Venlafaxine, an antidepressant with both noradrenergic and serotonergic activity, has been found effective for the treatment of depression and GAD (Silverstone and Ravindran 1999). Mirtazapine, a noradrenergic and specific serotonergic antidepressant, has been shown to have beneficial effects on symptoms of anxiety and sleep disturbances (Kasper et al. 1997). This drug may be a good choice for anxious elderly patients who are having difficulty sleeping or are losing weight.

Tricyclic antidepressants. Tricyclic antidepressants (TCAs) have been shown to be effective in treating a variety of anxiety states in elderly patients, such as mixed anxiety-depression states, panic disorder, OCD, and GAD (Crook 1982; Hershey and Kim 1988; Hoehn-Saric et al. 1988; Rickels et al. 1993; Rifkin et al. 1981). However, the overall use of TCAs has decreased because of their significant side effects, their potential toxicity, and the emergence of other medications, such as SSRIs.

Common side effects include significant orthostatic hypotension, cardiac conduction irregularities, sedation, weight gain, dry mouth, blurred vision, constipation, urinary retention, and confusion or even psychosis. Confusion or psychosis may be particularly significant in patients with Alzheimer's disease or other disorders that impair memory.

Monoamine oxidase inhibitors. Monoamine oxidase inhibitors have been found to be effective in treating mixed anxiety-depression and panic disorder (Crook 1982; Hershey and Kim 1988), but they are rarely used now because of their potential side effects, the restrictive diet associated with use, and the availability of newer antidepressants. For elderly patients, the two most difficult possible side effects are orthostatic hypotension and acute hypertensive crisis due to drug-diet interactions.

Benzodiazepines

Benzodiazepines are still frequently prescribed to elderly patients (American Psychiatric Association 1990), though primary treatment with SSRIs is becoming more accepted. All benzodiazepines can cause impairment in cognition and motor functioning. The cognitive impairment may be severe enough to present as a pseudodementia, while motor impairment may cause falls and hip fractures (noted to be almost twice as common in patients over the age of 70 compared with patients younger than age 40; Boston Collaborative Drug Surveillance Program 1973). Benzodiazepines may also cause a paradoxical reaction of restlessness, confusion, irritability, and even aggression.

Benzodiazepines with short half-lives are most often used for insomnia, but the short half-life may be associated with confusion, agitation, and hallucinations in elderly persons (Shorr and Robin 1994). Benzodiazepines with long half-lives can significantly increase the risk of falls and hip fractures in elderly patients (Ray et al. 1989). For the most part, benzodiazepines with midrange half-lives and conjugation metabolism (such as lorazepam) are preferred for use in elderly patients because their clearance is unaffected by aging and they are less likely to accumulate and cause toxicity (American Psychiatric Association 1990).

Buspirone

Buspirone is a novel antianxiety agent unrelated to benzodiazepines that has a high affinity for serotonin$_{1A}$ (5-HT$_{1A}$) receptors and enhances brain dopaminergic and noradrenergic activity (Eison and Temple 1986; Goa and Ward 1986). Clinical trials have found buspirone to be effective in the treatment of GAD in elderly patients (Bohm et al. 1990; Napoliello 1986; Robinson et al. 1988; Singh and Beer 1988), but it does not appear to be effective for panic disorder (Sheehan et al. 1990).

Common side effects of buspirone include nausea, headache, nervousness, dizziness, light-headedness, and fatigue. However, unlike benzodiazepines, buspirone does not appear to cause psychomotor impairment, sedation, dependence, withdrawal, or abuse (Banazak 1997). Therefore, it may be of particular value for treating patients who are unable to tolerate the sedative effects of benzodiazepines, patients with respiratory illness (such as chronic obstructive pulmonary disease), or patients with a history of substance abuse (Steinberg 1994).

The efficacy of buspirone may be reduced in patients who have previously been treated with benzodiazepines (Schweizer et al. 1986).

Antipsychotics

Antipsychotics—especially newer agents such as olanzapine and risperidone—are frequently used in the treatment of severe agitation associated with psychosis, delirium, and dementia (Chou and Sussman 1988) and, more recently, with refractory anxiety in dementia. However, the use of antipsychotics in the treatment of subjective anxiety states, especially in elderly patients, has never been demonstrated (Salzman 1991). Furthermore, adverse reactions such as sedation, extrapyramidal reactions, orthostatic hypotension, anticholinergic effects, and tardive dyskinesia can have devastating effects in elderly individuals. Therefore, antipsychotics are used very sparingly in the treatment of anxiety disorders in elderly patients.

Beta-Blockers

Beta-blockers have demonstrated efficacy in younger patients with somatic symptoms associated with GAD or performance (social) anxiety (Peet 1988). They have also been used in the treatment of aggression and agitation in patients with organic brain disease (Greendyke et al. 1986). However, the usefulness of beta-blockers for treatment of anxiety in the elderly is unknown (Sadavoy and LeClair 1997), and beta-blockers as a class should be avoided in patients with chronic obstructive pulmonary disease, congestive heart failure, heart block, insulin-dependent diabetes, severe renal disease, or peripheral vascular disease.

Antihistamines

Sedating antihistamines such as hydroxyzine and diphenhydramine are sometimes useful for treating anxiety or insomnia in elderly patients, but chronic use of these agents is rarely recommended because they are less effective than benzodiazepines and have significant anticholinergic side effects (Barbee and McLaulin 1990). They may be used in patients with mild symptoms, patients with severe chronic obstructive pulmonary disease, patients with addiction-prone personalities, or patients in whom more traditional drugs are not effective (Rickels 1983).

References

Alexopoulos GS: Anxiety-depression syndromes in old age. Int J Geriatr Psychiatry 5:351–353, 1990

American Psychiatric Association: Diagnostic and Statistical Manual of Mental Disorders, 3rd Edition. Washington, DC, American Psychiatric Association, 1980

American Psychiatric Association: Benzodiazepine Dependence, Toxicity, and Abuse. Washington, DC, American Psychiatric Association, 1990

American Psychiatric Association: Diagnostic and Statistical Manual of Mental Disorders, 4th Edition, Text Revision. Washington, DC, American Psychiatric Association, 2000

Banazak DA: Anxiety disorders in elderly patients. J Am Board Fam Pract 10:280–289, 1997

Barbee JG, McLaulin JB: Anxiety disorders: diagnosis and pharmacotherapy in the elderly. Psychiatric Annals 20:439–445, 1990

Bland RC, Newman SC, Orn H: Prevalence of psychiatric disorders in the elderly in Edmonton. Acta Psychiatr Scand Suppl 338: 57–63, 1988

Blazer DG: Generalized anxiety disorder and panic disorder in the elderly: a review. Harv Rev Psychiatry 5:18–27, 1997

Blazer D[G], George LK, Hughes D: The epidemiology of anxiety disorders: an age comparison, in Anxiety in the Elderly: Treatment and Research. Edited by Salzman C, Lebowitz BD. New York, Springer, 1991a, pp 17–30

Blazer DG, Hughes D, George LK, et al: Generalized anxiety disorder, in Psychiatric Disorders in America: The Epidemiologic Catchment Area Study. Edited by Robins LN, Regier DA. New York, Free Press, 1991b, pp 180–203

Bohm C, Robinson DS, Gammans RE, et al: Buspirone therapy in anxious elderly patients: a controlled clinical trial. J Clin Psychopharmacol 10 (suppl 3):47S–51S, 1990

Boston Collaborative Drug Surveillance Program: Clinical depression of the central nervous system due to diazepam and chlordiazepoxide in relation to cigarette smoking and age. N Engl J Med 288:277–280, 1973

Cassem EH: Depression and anxiety secondary to medical illness. Psychiatr Clin North Am 13:597–612, 1990

Chou JCY, Sussman N: Neuroleptics in anxiety. Psychiatric Annals 18:172–175, 1988

Copeland JRM, Davidson IA, Dewey ME: The prevalence and outcome of anxious depression in elderly people aged 65 and over living in the community, in Anxious Depression: Assessment and Treatment. Edited by Racagni G, Smeraldi E. New York, Raven, 1987, pp 43–47

Crook T: Diagnosis and treatment of mixed anxiety-depression in the elderly. J Clin Psychiatry 43:35–43, 1982

Eison AS, Temple DL Jr: Buspirone: review of its pharmacology and current perspectives on its mechanism of action. Am J Med 80:1–9, 1986

Flint AJ: Anxiety disorders in late life. Can Fam Physician 45:2672–2679, 1999

Goa KL, Ward A: Buspirone: a preliminary review of its pharmacologic properties and therapeutic efficacy as an anxiolytic. Drugs 32:114–129, 1986

Greendyke R, Kanter D, Schuster D, et al: Propranolol treatment of assaultive patients with organic brain disease: a double blind cross-over, placebo-controlled study. J Nerv Ment Dis 174:290–294, 1986

Hassan R, Pollard CA: Late-life-onset panic disorder: clinical and demographic characteristics of a patient sample. J Geriatr Psychiatry Neurol 7:86–90, 1994

Hershey LA, Kim KY: Diagnosis and treatment of anxiety in the elderly. Ration Drug Ther 22:1–6, 1988

Hoehn-Saric R, McLeod DR, Zimmerli WD: Differential effects of alprazolam and imipramine in generalized anxiety disorder: somatic vs. psychic symptoms. J Clin Psychiatry 49:293–301, 1988

Jenike MA: Geriatric Psychiatry and Psycho-pharmacology: A Clinical Approach. Chicago, IL, Year Book Medical, 1989, pp 248–271

Jenike MA: Geriatric obsessive-compulsive disorder. J Geriatr Psychiatry Neurol 4:34–39, 1991

Jonas BS, Franks P, Ingram DD: Are symptoms of anxiety and depression risk factors for hypertension? longitudinal evidence from the National Health and Nutrition Examination Survey I Epidemiologic Follow-up Study. Arch Fam Med 6:43–49, 1997

Judd LL, Kessler RC, Paulus MP, et al: Comorbidity as a fundamental feature of generalized anxiety disorders: results from the National Comorbidity Study (NCS). Acta Psychiatr Scand Suppl 393:6–11, 1998

Kasper S, Przschek-Rieder N, Tauscher J, et al: A risk-benefit assessment of mirtazapine in the treatment of depression. Drug Saf 17:251–264, 1997

Kawachi I, Sparrow D, Vokonas PS, et al: Symptoms of anxiety and risk of coronary heart disease. The Normative Aging Study. Circulation 90:2225–2229, 1994

Kluznik JC, Speed N, Van Valkenburg C, et al: Forty-year follow-up of United States prisoners of war. Am J Psychiatry 143:1443–1446, 1986

Kohn R, Westlake RJ, Rasmussen SA, et al: Clinical features of obsessive-compulsive disorder in elderly patients. Am J Geriatr Psychiatry 5:211–215, 1997

Krasucki C, Howard R, Mann A: Anxiety and its treatment in the elderly. Int Psychogeriatr 11:25–45, 1998

Kuch K, Cox BJ: Symptoms of PTSD in 124 survivors of the Holocaust. Am J Psychiatry 149:337–340, 1992

Lindesay J, Briggs K, Murphy E: The Guy's/Age Concern survey. Prevalence rates of cognitive impairment, depression and anxiety in an urban elderly community. Br J Psychiatry 155:317–329, 1989

Luchins DJ, Rose RP: Late-life onset of panic disorder with agoraphobia in three patients. Am J Psychiatry 146:920–921, 1989

Magni G, De Leo D: Anxiety and depression in geriatric and adult medical inpatients: a comparison. Psychol Rep 55:607–612, 1984

Manela M, Katona C, Livingston G: How common are the anxiety disorders in old age? Int J Geriatr Psychiatry 11:65–70, 1996

Moser DK, Dracup K: Is anxiety early after myocardial infarction associated with subsequent ischemic and arrhythmic events? Psychosom Med 58:395–401, 1996

Napoliello MJ: An interim multicentre report on 677 anxious geriatric out-patients treated with buspirone. Br J Clin Pract 40:71–73, 1986

Ouslander JG: Drug therapy in the elderly. Ann Intern Med 95:711–722, 1981

Peet M: The treatment of anxiety with beta-blocking drugs. Postgrad Med J 64 (suppl 2):45–49, 1988

Raj BA, Corvea MH, Dagon EM: The clinical characteristics of panic disorder in the elderly: a retrospective study. J Clin Psychiatry 54:150–155, 1993

Ray WA, Griffin MR, Downey W: Benzodiazepines of long and short elimination half-life and the risk of hip fracture. JAMA 262:3303–3306, 1989

Regier DA, Boyd JH, Burke JD Jr, et al: One-month prevalence of mental disorders in the United States. Based on five Epidemiologic Catchment Area sites. Arch Gen Psychiatry 45:977–986, 1988

Regier DA, Narrow WE, Rae DS: The epidemiology of anxiety disorders: the Epidemiologic Catchment Area (ECA) experience. J Psychiatr Res 24 (suppl 2):3–14, 1990

Rickels K: Nonbenzodiazepine anxiolytics: clinical usefulness. J Clin Psychiatry 44:38–43, 1983

Rickels K, Downing R, Schweizer E, et al: Antidepressants for the treatment of generalized anxiety disorder: a placebo-controlled comparison of imipramine, trazodone, and diazepam. Arch Gen Psychiatry 50:884–895, 1993

Rifkin A, Klein DF, Dillon D, et al: Blockade by imipramine or desipramine of panic induced by sodium lactate. Am J Psychiatry 138:676–677, 1981

Robinson D, Napoliello MJ, Schenk J: The safety and usefulness of buspirone as an anxiolytic drug in elderly versus young patients. Clin Ther 10:740–746, 1988

Robinson S, Rapaport J, Durst R, et al: The late effects of Nazi persecution among elderly Holocaust survivors. Acta Psychiatr Scand 82:311–315, 1990

Rosen J, Fields RB, Hand AM, et al: Concurrent posttraumatic stress disorder in psychogeriatric patients. J Geriatr Psychiatry Neurol 2:65–69, 1989

Sadavoy J, LeClair JK: Treatment of anxiety disorders in late life. Can J Psychiatry 42 (suppl 1):28S–34S, 1997

Salzman C: Practical considerations in the pharmacologic treatment of depression and anxiety in the elderly. J Clin Psychiatry 51(suppl):40–43, 1990

Salzman C: Pharmacologic treatment of the anxious elderly patient, in Anxiety in the Elderly: Treatment and Research. Edited by Salzman C, Lebowitz BD. New York, Springer, 1991, pp 149–173

Schweizer E, Rickels K, Lucki I: Resistance to the anti-anxiety effect of buspirone in patients with a history of benzodiazepine use. N Engl J Med 314:719–720, 1986

Sheehan DV, Raj AB, Sheehan KH, et al: Is buspirone effective for panic disorder? J Clin Psychopharmacol 10:3–11, 1990

Sheikh JI, Cassidy EL: Treatment of anxiety disorders in the elderly: issues and strategies. J Anxiety Disord 14:173–190, 2000

Sheikh JI, King RJ, Taylor CB: Comparative phenomenology of early onset versus late-onset panic attacks: a pilot study. Am J Psychiatry 148:1231–1233, 1991

Shorr RI, Robin DW: Rational use of benzodiazepines in the elderly. Drugs Aging 4: 9–20, 1994

Silverstone PH, Ravindran A: Once-daily venlafaxine extended release (XR) compared with fluoxetine in outpatients with depression and anxiety. Venlafaxine XR 360 Study Group. J Clin Psychiatry 60:22–28, 1999

Singh AN, Beer M: A dose range–finding study of buspirone in geriatric patients with symptoms of anxiety (letter). J Clin Psychopharmacol 8:67–68, 1988

Small GW: Recognizing and treating anxiety in the elderly. J Clin Psychiatry 58 (suppl 3): 41–47, 1997

Steinberg JR: Anxiety in elderly patients: a comparison of azapirones and benzodiazepines. Drugs Aging 5:335–345, 1994

Sutker PB, Allain AN Jr, Winstead DK: Psychopathology and psychiatric diagnoses of World War II Pacific theater prisoner of war survivors and combat veterans. Am J Psychiatry 150:240–245, 1993

Thompson TL II, Moran MG, Nies AS: Psychotropic drug use in the elderly. N Engl J Med 308:134–138, 1983

Uhlenhuth EH, Balter MB, Mellinger GD, et al: Symptom checklist syndromes in the general population. Correlations with psychotherapeutic drug use. Arch Gen Psychiatry 40:1167–1173, 1983

White LR, Cartwright WS, Cornoni-Huntley J: Geriatric epidemiology. Annu Rev Gerontol Geriatr 6:215–311, 1986

Study Questions

Select the single best response for each question.

1. According to the Epidemiologic Catchment Area (ECA) study of the 1980s, the combined prevalence of phobia, panic disorder, and obsessive-compulsive disorder in people over age 65 is approximately what percentage?

    A. 2.5%.
    B. 3.5%.
    C. 5.5%.
    D. 6.5%.
    E. 7%.

2. Panic disorder in those older than 65

    A. Has a point prevalence of 0.4%.
    B. Is not uncommonly ascribed to other causes by the elderly.
    C. May present with fewer symptoms.
    D. Is a relatively uncommon development in late life.
    E. All of the above.

3. In at least one study, what percentage of elderly Holocaust survivors met criteria for posttraumatic stress disorder more than 40 years after the war?

    A. 10%.
    B. 20%.
    C. 30%.
    D. 40%.
    E. 50%.

4. The most common anxiety disorder of the elderly population is

    A. Generalized anxiety disorder.
    B. Posttraumatic stress disorder.
    C. Social phobia.
    D. Specific phobia.
    E. Obsessive-compulsive disorder.

5. Which of the following factors could pertain to medical illnesses and anxiety among the elderly?

    A. The older adult may worry about the effect and meaning of physical illness.
    B. Anxiety may contribute to medical problems and complications.
    C. Many anxiety symptoms may masquerade as medical illness.
    D. Anxiety symptoms may be caused by medications given to elderly persons.
    E. All of the above.

6. Which of the following pharmacological agents has become the mainstay treatment of anxiety disorder in the elderly?

    A. Tricyclic antidepressants (TCAs).
    B. Monoamine oxidase inhibitors (MAOIs).
    C. Selective serotonin reuptake inhibitors (SSRIs).
    D. Benzodiazepines.
    E. Buspirone.

Somatoform Disorders

Marc E. Agronin, M.D.

Somatoform disorders comprise a heterogeneous group of disorders in which physical symptoms or complaints without objective organic causes are present and in which there are strongly associated psychological factors. The seven somatoform disorders listed in DSM-IV-TR (American Psychiatric Association 2000) are somatization disorder, undifferentiated somatoform disorder, hypochondriasis, conversion disorder, pain disorder, body dysmorphic disorder (BDD), and somatoform disorder not otherwise specified.

Older individuals with somatoform disorders are seen in all health care settings, where they frequently overuse medical services (Barsky 1979) and overburden general practitioners (Reid et al. 2001). They often come to the attention of a geriatric psychiatrist after another clinician has attempted unsuccessfully to resolve their physical symptoms.

Somatoform disorders have not been well studied in late life, in part because many of the disorders tend to begin in early adulthood. In addition, somatoform symptoms in late life are often obscured by comorbid physical and psychiatric illnesses.

Clinical Features

Somatoform symptoms are experienced by the affected individual as real physical sensations, pain, or discomfort, usually indistinguishable from symptoms of actual medical disorders and frequently coexisting with them. However, by definition, these symptoms do not have an established organic basis, despite the fact that they can lead to significant emotional distress and functional impairment. Associated psychological factors are presumed but not always apparent, and patients vary in their degree of insight into such factors.

In general, transient somatoform symptoms may be seen in 30%–50% of patients presenting to medical settings (Barsky et al. 1990; Busse 1993; Kellner 1985). When symptoms shift from representing transient expressions of somatic concern to representing more serious bodily preoccupation and impairment, and no organic cause emerges, a somatoform disorder becomes a more likely diagnosis. Somatoform disorders do not represent intentional, conscious attempts by patients to present factitious physical symptoms. Neither do they represent delusional thinking as found in psychotic states.

Patients are generally able to accept that their symptoms may be functional and have psychological roots (Martin and Yutzy 1994). Somatoform disorders differ from psychosomatic disorders, which are characterized by actual disease states with presumed psychological triggers. Instead, somatoform disorders involve a complex interaction between brain and body, in which the affected individual is unknowingly expressing psychological stress or conflict through the body. Not surprisingly, increased somatic symptoms and preoccupation with illness are often associated with anxiety and depression. It is possible that the underpinnings of these disorders, especially in late life, may be related to frontal lobe dysfunction (Flor-Henry et al. 1981).

Specific Disorders

Somatization Disorder

Somatization disorder is characterized by multiple physical complaints, in excess of what would be expected given the patient's history and examination findings. These complaints cannot be fully explained by medical workup and must include pain at four or more sites, as well as two gastrointestinal symptoms, one sexual symptom, and one pseudoneurological symptom (other than pain). Another term used in the literature for this disorder is *Briquet's syndrome* (Liskow et al. 1986; Orenstein 1989). Symptoms typically appear before age 30 and have usually persisted for years by the time of diagnosis.

Somatization disorder is seen almost exclusively in women and may have a prevalence rate ranging from less than 1% to 3% (Faravelli et al. 1997; Martin and Yutzy 1994). Associated problems include drug abuse and dependence, depression and suicidality, and multiple and unnecessary medical treatments, including surgeries (Goodwin and Guze 1989).

Somatization disorder is a chronic psychiatric disorder, with the majority of individuals demonstrating consistent symptom patterns as they age (Cloninger et al. 1986; Pribor et al. 1994). The most difficult diagnostic feature to establish in elderly patients is the onset of symptoms before age 30, because such history can rarely be accurately determined. In addition, the presence of multiple physical symptoms in excess of what would be expected is a relative factor in late life, given the high incidence of comorbid illnesses.

Undifferentiated Somatoform Disorder

In most elderly patients with somatoform symptoms, a diagnosis of undifferentiated somatoform disorder can be more easily made than a diagnosis of somatization disorder. Undifferentiated somatoform disorder is defined by the presence of one of more physical complaints, lasting at least 6 months, that cannot be fully explained by appropriate medical workup, and that result in considerable social, occupational, or functional impairment. Again, diagnosis is complicated in late life by the frequency of comorbid medical disorders. Prevalence rates for undifferentiated somatoform disorder have not been well established for any age group, although one community study in Italy found a rate of 13.8%—significantly higher than rates for every other somatoform disorder (Faravelli et al. 1997). Patients with chronic pain have been found to have quite high rates of undifferentiated somatoform disorder (Aigner and Bach 1999).

Hypochondriasis

Hypochondriasis is characterized by a preoccupation with fears of having a serious illness. These fears arise from misinterpretation of bodily symptoms, and the individual's preoccupation is resistant to medical evaluation and reassurance. Varying degrees of hypochondriacal symptoms are more common among individuals who are under stress due to medical illness in themselves or a relative or who have a history of serious illness, especially in childhood (Kellner 1987). Physical complaints tend to be based on common but transient symptoms that are viewed as portending a serious illness.

The line between normal somatic concern and hypochondriasis can be difficult to draw but depends on a pattern of dysfunctional behaviors that ultimately serve to increase anxiety and constrain medical treatment. Barsky (1979) suggested that underlying this pattern is a psychological state that tends to amplify bodily perceptions. In the person with hypochondriasis, it is the resultant conviction of having a disease that leads to a pattern of 1) anxious ruminations that one has a terrible illness and 2) repetitive medical consultations.

The prevalence of hypochondriasis in medical outpatients is around 5% (Barsky 2001; Faravelli et al. 1997), and there is some debate regarding whether factors such as low education level, low socioeconomic status, and old age increase this rate (Barsky et al. 1991; Brink et al. 1981; Kellner 1986; Rief et al. 2001). Comorbid psychiatric disorders are common, especially major depression, panic disorder, and obsessive-compulsive disorder (Barsky et al. 1992).

Conversion Disorder

Conversion disorder is characterized by one or more motor or sensory deficits that cannot be fully explained by appropriate medical workup and that appear to be causally related to psychological factors. The diagnosis should specify whether the symptom or deficit is a motor or sensory one, involves a seizure, or entails a mixed

presentation. As with other somatoform symptoms, however, the presence of true medical comorbidity can cloud the picture. The key to diagnosis of conversion symptoms is identification of the psychological conflict that seems to be prompting the symptom, but this approach may require in-depth psychotherapeutic investigation, which is not always feasible in older individuals.

Although conversion disorder has been reported in the elderly population (Weddington 1979), it is more common in young women. The prevalence rate in the community is less than 1% (Cloninger 1986; Faravelli et al. 1997), although much higher rates are seen in psychiatric inpatient consultations. Psychogenic nonepileptic seizures, sometimes referred to as pseudoseizures, represent one subtype of conversion symptoms. They are characterized by behavioral spells that mimic various forms of seizures but are not associated with electroencephalographic findings and have a presumed emotional etiology (Volow 1986). Nonepileptic seizures are more frequent in young women and are seen in 5%–20% of outpatients with epilepsy, often in combination with an actual seizure disorder (Chabolla et al. 1996).

Risk factors for conversion disorder include sexual abuse (Martin 1994), personality disorder, and other neurological illnesses (Ford and Folks 1985; Slater and Glithero 1965). Conversion disorder in late life is likely associated with an actual comorbid neurological disorder. The prognosis is limited: in one sample, persistent symptoms were present in nearly 40% of subjects at 10-year follow-up (Mace and Trimble 1996).

Pain Disorder

Pain is the most common medical complaint in elderly persons, with pain due to musculoskeletal disease being the most common type of pain (Leveille et al. 2001). Close to 50% of elderly individuals have chronic pain, and the percentage approaches 70% for those in long-term care (Otis and McGeeney 2000). Persistent pain is associated with significant functional and social impairment (Scudds and Ostbye 2001), as well as comorbid psychiatric symptoms including depression, insomnia, and substance abuse. Pain assessment is often limited because of its dependence on subjective patient reports, which can be influenced by numerous confounding factors in late life, including dementia.

In pain disorder, pain is the major focus of the clinical presentation, and psychological factors are believed to play critical roles in the onset, severity, exacerbation, or continuation of the pain. Diagnostic variants of pain disorder in DSM-IV-TR include pain disorder associated with psychological factors, a general medical condition, or both. Even when there are specific causes of pain, diagnosis hinges on identifying an overwhelming preoccupation with pain—a preoccupation sometimes involving a pattern of treatment resistance. The determination of such psychological factors is difficult, especially in late life, and the ensuing divisions between the relative roles of mind and body raise questions about diagnostic validity (Boland 2002).

Body Dysmorphic Disorder

BDD is characterized by a preoccupation with an imagined or small defect in appearance. Common body parts that become the object of focus include facial features (e.g., the nose), breasts, and genitals. If there is an actual physical defect, this preoccupation greatly exceeds what would be expected. Affected individuals often spend considerable time engaging in repetitive behaviors such as looking at the body part in the mirror, touching or picking at it, and

seeking reassurance from others regarding their concern (Phillips 1996). Symptoms tend to be chronic and often lead patients to make extraordinary attempts to deal with the imagined or slight defect, including unnecessary plastic surgery (Martin and Yutzy 1994). For this reason, BDD often presents to plastic surgeons long before coming to the attention of a psychiatrist. The disorder is commonly diagnosed in young adults and in women around the time of menopause, and it is often associated with comorbid depression, obsessive-compulsive behaviors, personality disorders, and even suicidality (Phillips 1998).

The estimated prevalence of BDD in women in the community is 0.7% (Faravelli et al. 1997; Otto et al. 2001). In a study involving 74 individuals with BDD, Phillips and McElroy (2000) found comorbid personality disorders in 57% of the sample. In up to 50% of individuals with BDD, the somatic preoccupation may be delusional (Phillips 1998; Phillips et al. 1998). Although no prevalence figures for BDD in late life are available, such specific complaints are less common in older patients.

Somatoform Disorder Not Otherwise Specified

The diagnosis of somatoform disorder not otherwise specified is used when the patient has somatoform symptoms that do not meet the criteria for other somatoform disorders but that result in similar degrees of social, occupational, and functional impairment. Some somatoform presentations that fit this category are hypochondriacal symptoms of less than 6 months' duration; unexplained physical symptoms of less than 6 months' duration; and pseudocyesis, in which the false belief that one is pregnant is associated with objective (albeit false) symptoms of pregnancy.

Etiology

The causes of somatoform disorders are usually multifactorial and are often rooted in early developmental experiences and personality traits. For example, somatization and all somatoform disorders have been associated with the experience of serious illness early in life (Stuart and Noyes 1999), childhood abuse (Martin 1994; Walker et al. 1992), significant psychological stress (Hollifield et al. 1999; Ritsner et al. 2000), and the personality trait neuroticism (Affleck et al. 1992; Chaturvedi 1986; Costa and McCrae 1980; Phillips and McElroy 2000), which presents as a tendency to experience more negative emotions. As noted throughout the chapter, somatoform disorders are also highly associated with comorbid depression, anxiety and panic disorders, substance abuse, and personality disorders (Noyes et al. 2001). Somatization may be more common in women and in older individuals, although the prevalence of actual somatoform disorders has not been associated with increased age (with the exception of hypochondriasis). When present in late life (especially when onset was recent), somatoform disorders may be associated with neuropsychological impairment and/or comorbid neurological illness (Sheehan and Banerjee 1999).

Psychodynamic approaches suggest that somatoform disorders result from unconscious conflict in which intolerable impulses or affects are expressed through more tolerable somatic symptoms or complaints. The classic example of this phenomenon is found in conversion disorder, in which intolerable, unconscious impulses are converted into motor or sensory dysfunction. Freud first wrote about such a mechanism on the basis of his studies involving women who had what was then termed *hysteria* (Breuer and Freud 1893–

1895/1955). Specifically, psychodynamic theory suggests that excessive and intolerable guilt or hostility are psychological sources of somatization—in particular, hypochondriasis (Barsky and Klerman 1983). In such cases, physical symptoms serve as a means of self-punishment for unacceptable unconscious impulses. Anger directed toward caregivers is indirectly expressed through distrust of and dissatisfaction with multiple physicians. Some researchers have suggested that underlying and complicating this psychodynamic rechannelization of anger or guilt is alexithymia, in which an individual has a relative inability to identify and express emotional states (Cox et al. 1994; Sriram et al. 1987). The experiencing and reporting of bodily sensations thus becomes a mode of emotional expression. Although alexithymia has long been postulated to play a role in both somatoform and psychosomatic illness, not all empirical research has supported the correlation of alexithymia with somatic complaints (Lundh and Simonsson-Sarnecki 2001).

In late life, somatoform disorders may represent a dysfunctional attempt to cope with accumulating physical and psychosocial losses, especially when these losses are associated with functional disability, anxiety, and depression. These include loss of or isolation from family, friends, and caregivers; loss of beauty and strength; financial setbacks; loss of independence; and loss of social role (e.g., as a result of retirement, the loss of a spouse, or occupational disability). The psychological distress and anxiety over such losses may be less threatening and more controllable when it is shifted to somatic complaints or symptoms. In turn, a sick role might be reinforced by increased social contacts and support. The presence of comorbid medical problems and the use of multiple medications may provide somatic symptoms around which psychological conflict can center. In long-term care, older individuals are faced with many additional over-whelming losses, and their own bodies often serve as the last bastion of control. Somatic preoccupation thus serves as a means of coping with stress, even though it is maladaptive and can result in excessive and unnecessary disability. It may also serve to mobilize and control resources and staff attention within the long-term-care environment.

Treatment

By definition, persons with somatoform disorders present to clinicians with what appear to be legitimate somatic complaints of unknown physical etiology. It is only after repeated but fruitless workups, multiple and persistent complaints and requests, and sometimes angry and inappropriate reactions to treatment that clinicians begin to suspect a somatoform disorder. In some cases, the manner of presentation and the symptom complex are more immediately suggestive of a particular somatoform disorder.

In any event, it is important for the clinician to remember that to the patient, the symptoms and complaints are quite real and disturbing. Even after workups have made it obvious that there are psychological factors involved, it is never wise to challenge the patient or suggest that the symptoms are "all in your mind." The typical response to such a suggestion is for the patient to seek additional opinions and medical tests, which in turn can perpetuate a cycle of somatization, in which underlying issues are never addressed.

Instead, the role of the physician must be to foster a supportive, consistent, and professional relationship with the affected individual. Such a relationship will provide reassurance as well as protect the patient from excessive and unnecessary medical visits and procedures. The clinician should

focus on responding to individual complaints, perhaps with periodic but regularly scheduled appointments (Smith et al. 1986), and setting limits on workup and treatment, in a firm but empathic manner. This can be difficult to do when patients become demanding and attempt to consume excessive clinic time, but the clinician must endeavor to remain professional and to not personalize the situation or feel as though he or she were failing the patient. The clinician should focus on symptom reduction and rehabilitation and not attempt to force the patient to gain insight into the potential psychological nature of his or her symptoms (Kellner 1987).

It would obviously be hazardous for a clinician to diagnose a somatoform disorder prematurely, because underlying organic pathology might have eluded diagnosis. For example, multiple sclerosis, systemic lupus erythematosus, and acute intermittent porphyria often have complex presentations that elude initial diagnostic workup (Kellner 1987). Somatoform disorders may coexist with actual disease states; for example, many individuals with pseudoseizures also have a seizure disorder (Desai et al. 1982; Luther et al. 1982). Moene et al. (2000) found that slightly more than 10% of patients who received an initial diagnosis of conversion disorder actually had a true neurological disorder. This study finding is consistent with findings of other investigations (Mace and Trimble 1996).

It is important for the clinician to set limits on what he or she can offer and to make appropriate referrals to specialists and/or mental health clinicians. The geriatric psychiatrist, in particular, will play a more active role in addressing the somatoform disorder rather than simply the physical complaints.

Unfortunately, most disorders tend to be lifelong. Therefore, the goal of treatment is not to cure the patient but to control symptoms. The clinician must form a therapeutic alliance through empathic listening and acknowledging of physical discomfort, without trivializing the somatic complaints. Sometimes an offer to review all available medical records can be a tangible way of conveying one's seriousness to the patient. Educating the patient about various symptom complexes and involving him or her in part of the decision making can be empowering for the patient, especially a patient with chronic pain (McDonald 1993).

Individual therapy that takes a psychodynamic approach will focus on helping the patient identify and then discuss psychological conflict and associated emotion. Cognitive-behavioral therapy will focus on identifying distorted thought patterns and anxiety triggers and replacing them with more realistic and adaptive strategies. In conversion disorder, hypnosis is sometimes used as both a diagnostic and therapeutic tool.

Pharmacotherapy is a central component of treatment for somatoform disorders. It can be targeted at a specific disorder or at underlying anxiety, depression, or thought patterns that appear delusional. Somatization disorder has been treated successfully with both antidepressants (Menza et al. 2001) and anticonvulsants or mood stabilizers (Garcia-Campayo and Sanz-Carrillo 2001). Hypochondriacal symptoms have responded to a variety of antidepressant medications—in particular, selective serotonin reuptake inhibitors—as well as to anxiolytics (Barsky 2001; Fallon et al. 1996; Oosterbaan et al. 2001). A meta-analysis of antidepressant therapy in pain disorder found that pharmacotherapy decreased pain intensity significantly more than placebo (Fishbain et al. 1998). Anticonvulsants have also been found to be useful in treating pain disorder, especially when the disorder is associated with

a comorbid mood disorder (Maurer et al. 1999). BDD has responded well to antidepressant treatment (Phillips 1996; Phillips et al. 2002) and has also been treated with antipsychotics (Grant 2001; Phillips 1996). A study by Phillips et al. (2001) demonstrated a 60% response rate with selective serotonin reuptake inhibitors, a high relapse rate when medications were discontinued, and increased response with antidepressant augmentation.

The tendency of many psychiatrists to focus more on pharmacotherapy can become a trap with somatoform disorders, because the therapeutic relationship is such a key element. Given the chronic nature of somatoform symptoms, it is unlikely that pharmacotherapy will be a quick fix. When this narrow focus on treatment with medications fails to result in rapid control of symptoms, the patient may abandon the therapist for alternative treatment. Other patients may welcome such a focus because it keeps them from having to face underlying psychological issues. Instead, clinicians must be in it for the long haul and strike a balance between reasonable pharmacotherapy that targets specific symptoms of anxiety or depression and a supportive alliance in which the most appropriate therapy for the patient is used. If another clinician serves as the therapist, frequent communication between psychiatrist and therapist is necessary to coordinate treatment.

References

Affleck G, Tennen H, Urrows S, et al: Neuroticism and the pain-mood relation in rheumatoid arthritis: insights from a prospective daily study. J Consult Clin Psychol 60:119–126, 1992

Aigner M, Bach M: Clinical utility of DSM-IV pain disorder. Compr Psychiatry 40:353–357, 1999

American Psychiatric Association: Diagnostic and Statistical Manual of Mental Disorders, 4th Edition, Text Revision. Washington, DC, American Psychiatric Association, 2000

Barsky AJ: Patients who amplify bodily sensations. Ann Intern Med 91:63–70, 1979

Barsky AJ: The patient with hypochondriasis. N Engl J Med 345:1395–1399, 2001

Barsky AJ, Klerman GL: Overview: hypochondriasis, bodily complaints, and somatic styles. Am J Psychiatry 149:273–283, 1983

Barsky AJ, Wyshak G, Klerman G: Transient hypochondriasis. Arch Gen Psychiatry 47:746–752, 1990

Barsky AJ, Frank C, Cleary P, et al: The relation between hypochondriasis and age. Am J Psychiatry 148:923–928, 1991

Barsky AJ, Wyshak G, Klerman G: Psychiatric comorbidity in DSM-III-R hypochondriasis. Arch Gen Psychiatry 49:101–108, 1992

Boland RJ: How could the validity of the DSM-IV pain disorder be improved in reference to the concept that it is supposed to identify? Curr Pain Headache Rep 6:23–29, 2002

Breuer J, Freud S: Studies on hysteria (1893–1895), in The Standard Edition of the Complete Psychological Works of Sigmund Freud, Vol 2. Translated and edited by Strachey J. London, Hogarth Press, 1955, pp 1–319

Brink T, Janakes C, Martinez N: Geriatric hypochondriasis: situational factors. J Am Geriatr Soc 29:37–39, 1981

Busse EW: Duke University Longitudinal Studies of Aging. J Gerontol 26:123–128, 1993

Chabolla DR, Krahn LE, So EL, et al: Psychogenic nonepileptic seizures. Mayo Clin Proc 71:493–500, 1996

Chaturvedi SK: Chronic idiopathic pain disorder. J Psychosom Res 30:199–203, 1986

Cloninger CR: Somatoform and dissociative disorders, in The Medical Basis of Psychiatry. Edited by Winokur G, Clayton PJ. Philadelphia, PA, WB Saunders, 1986, pp 123–151

Cloninger CR, Martin RL, Guze SB, et al: A prospective follow-up and family study of somatization in men and women. Am J Psychiatry 143:873–878, 1986

Costa PT Jr, McCrae RR: Somatic complaints in males as a function of age and neuroticism: a longitudinal analysis. J Behav Med 3:245–257, 1980

Cox BJ, Kuch K, Parker JD, et al: Alexithymia in somatoform disorder patients with chronic pain. J Psychosom Res 38:523–527, 1994

Desai BT, Porter RJ, Penry JK: Psychogenic seizures. A study of 42 attacks in six patients, with intensive monitoring. Arch Neurol 39:202–209, 1982

Fallon BA, Schneier FR, Marshall R, et al: The pharmacotherapy of hypochondriasis. Psychopharmacol Bull 32:607–611, 1996

Faravelli C, Salvatori S, Galassi F, et al: Epidemiology of somatoform disorders: a community survey in Florence. Soc Psychiatry Psychiatr Epidemiol 32:24–29, 1997

Fishbain DA, Cutler RB, Rosomoff HL, et al: Do antidepressants have an analgesic effect in psychogenic pain and somatoform pain disorder? a meta-analysis. Psychosom Med 60:503–509, 1998

Flor-Henry P, Fromm-Auch D, Tapper M, et al: A neuropsychological study of the stable syndrome of hysteria. Biol Psychiatry 16:601–626, 1981

Ford CV, Folks DG: Conversion disorders: an overview. Psychosomatics 26:371–383, 1985

Garcia-Campayo J, Sanz-Carrillo C: Gabapentin for the treatment of patients with somatization disorder (letter). J Clin Psychiatry 62:474, 2001

Goodwin DW, Guze SB: Psychiatric Diagnosis, 4th Edition. New York, Oxford University Press, 1989

Grant JE: Successful treatment of nondelusional body dysmorphic disorder with olanzapine: a case report. J Clin Psychiatry 62:297–298, 2001

Hollifield M, Tuttle L, Paine S, et al: Hypochondriasis and somatization related to personality and attitudes towards self. Psychosomatics 40:387–395, 1999

Kellner R: Functional somatic symptoms and hypochondriasis: a survey of empirical studies. Arch Gen Psychiatry 42:821–833, 1985

Kellner R: Somatization and Hypochondriasis. New York, Praeger, 1986

Kellner R: Hypochondriasis and somatization. JAMA 258:2718–2722, 1987

Leveille SG, Ling S, Hochberg MC, et al: Widespread musculoskeletal pain and the progression of disability in older disabled women. Ann Intern Med 135:1038–1046, 2001

Liskow B, Othmer E, Penick EC, et al: Is Briquet's syndrome a heterogeneous disorder? Am J Psychiatry 143:626–629, 1986

Lundh LG, Simonsson-Sarnecki M: Alexithymia, emotion, and somatic complaints. J Pers 69:483–510, 2001

Luther JS, McNamara JO, Carwile S, et al: Pseudoepileptic seizures: methods and video analysis to aid diagnosis. Ann Neurol 12:458–462, 1982

Mace CJ, Trimble MR: Ten-year prognosis of conversion disorder. Br J Psychiatry 169:282–288, 1996

Martin RL: Conversion disorder, proposed autonomic arousal disorder, and pseudocyesis, in DSM-IV Sourcebook, Vol 2. Edited by Widiger TA, Frances AJ, Pincus HA, et al. Washington, DC, American Psychiatric Association, 1994, pp 893–914

Martin RL, Yutzy SH: Somatoform disorders, in The American Psychiatric Press Textbook of Psychiatry, 2nd Edition. Edited by Hales RE, Yudofsky SC, Talbott JA. Washington, DC, American Psychiatric Press, 1994, pp 591–622

Maurer I, Volz HP, Sauer H: Gabapentin leads to remission of somatoform pain disorder with major depression. Pharmacopsychiatry 32:255–257, 1999

McDonald JS: Management of chronic pelvic pain. Obstet Gynecol Clin North Am 20:817–838, 1993

Menza M, Lauritano M, Allen L, et al: Treatment of somatization disorder with nefazodone: a prospective, open-label study. Ann Clin Psychiatry 13:153–158, 2001

Moene FC, Landberg EH, Hoogduin KA, et al: Organic syndromes diagnosed as conversion disorder: identification and frequency in a study of 85 patients. J Psychosom Res 49:7–12, 2000

Noyes R Jr, Langbehn DR, Happel RL, et al: Personality dysfunction among somatizing patients. Psychosomatics 42:320–329, 2001

Oosterbaan DB, van Balkom AJ, van Boeijen CA, et al: An open study of paroxetine in hypochondriasis. Prog Neuropsychopharmacol Biol Psychiatry 25:1023–1033, 2001

Orenstein H: Briquet's syndrome in association with depression and panic: a reconceptualization of Briquet's syndrome. Am J Psychiatry 146:334–338, 1989

Otis JAD, McGeeney B: Managing pain in the elderly. Clinical Geriatrics 8:48–62, 2000

Otto MW, Cohen WS, Harlow BL: Prevalence of body dysmorphic disorder in a community sample of women. Am J Psychiatry 158:2061–2063, 2001

Phillips KA: Body dysmorphic disorder: diagnosis and treatment of imagined ugliness. J Clin Psychiatry 57 (suppl 8):61–64, 1996

Phillips KA: Body dysmorphic disorder: clinical aspects and treatment strategies. Bull Menninger Clin 62:A33–A48, 1998

Phillips KA, McElroy SL: Personality disorders and traits in patients with body dysmorphic disorder. Compr Psychiatry 41:229–236, 2000

Phillips KA, Dwight MM, McElroy SL: Efficacy and safety of fluvoxamine in body dysmorphic disorder. J Clin Psychiatry 59:165–171, 1998

Phillips KA, Albertini RS, Siniscalchi JM, et al: Effectiveness of pharmacotherapy for body dysmorphic disorder: a chart-review study. J Clin Psychiatry 62:721–727, 2001

Phillips KA, Albertini RS, Rasmussen SA: A randomized placebo-controlled trial of fluoxetine in body dysmorphic disorder. Arch Gen Psychiatry 59:381–388, 2002

Pribor EF, Smith DS, Yutzy SH: Somatization disorder in elderly patients. J Geriatr Psychiatry 2:109–117, 1994

Reid S, Whooley D, Crayford T, et al: Medically unexplained symptoms—GPs' attitudes towards their cause and management. Fam Pract 18:519–523, 2001

Rief W, Hessel A, Braehler E: Somatization symptoms and hypochondriacal features in the general population. Psychosom Med 63:595–602, 2001

Ritsner M, Ponizovsky A, Kurs R, et al: Somatization in an immigrant population in Israel: a community survey of prevalence, risk factors, and help-seeking behavior. Am J Psychiatry 157:385–392, 2000

Scudds RJ, Ostbye T: Pain and pain-related interference with function in older Canadians: the Canadian Study of Health and Aging. Disabil Rehabil 23:654–664, 2001

Sheehan B, Banerjee S: Review: somatization in the elderly. Int J Geriatr Psychiatry 14: 1044–1049, 1999

Slater ETO, Glithero E: A follow-up of patients diagnosed as suffering from "hysteria." J Psychosom Res 9:9–13, 1965

Smith GR Jr, Monson RA, Ray DC: Psychiatric consultation in somatization disorder: a randomized controlled study. N Engl J Med 314:1407–1413, 1986

Sriram TG, Chaturvedi SK, Gopinath PS, et al: Controlled study of alexithymia characteristics in patients with psychogenic pain disorder. Psychother Psychosom 47:11–17, 1987

Stuart S, Noyes R Jr: Attachment and interpersonal communication in somatization. Psychosomatics 40:34–43, 1999

Volow MR: Pseudoseizures: an overview. South Med J 79:600–607, 1986

Walker EA, Katon WJ, Hansom J, et al: Medical and psychiatric symptoms in women with childhood sexual abuse. Psychosom Med 54:658–664, 1992

Weddington WW: Conversion reaction in an 82 year old man. J Nerv Ment Dis 167:368–369, 1979

Study Questions

Select the single best response for each question.

1. Somatization disorder is a psychiatric illness characterized by numerous physical complaints that are in excess of examination findings. This may be an especially challenging problem in the older patient with other chronic medical conditions. Which of the following is also true regarding somatization disorder?

    A. Patients with somatization disorder have pain localized to one site.
    B. Somatization disorder is seen almost exclusively in women.
    C. As somatization disorder patients age, their reported symptoms tend to change.
    D. The prevalence rate has been estimated to be 8%–10%.
    E. Another term for somatization disorder is Munchausen syndrome.

2. Undifferentiated somatoform disorder and hypochondriasis may present in the geriatric psychiatric patient. Distinguishing between these two conditions may be difficult in the clinical setting. Which of the following statements is true?

    A. Undifferentiated somatoform disorder requires the presence of persistent physical complaints for at least 12 months.
    B. Patients with chronic pain rarely also qualify for a diagnosis of undifferentiated somatoform disorder.
    C. The psychological preoccupation in hypochondriasis relates to the symptoms experienced, rather than the possible disease "represented" by the symptoms.
    D. It has been clearly established that high educational level and high socioeconomic status lead to a predisposition to hypochondriasis, because individuals with these factors may be more aware of medical conditions and have greater access to information.
    E. Comorbid depressive and anxiety disorders are common in hypochondriasis.

3. Conversion disorder is characterized by motor and/or sensory deficits that suggest neurological illness(es) but that cannot be elucidated by the appropriate neurological and neuroimaging evaluations. Which of the following is true regarding this syndrome?

    A. Conversion disorder is more common in elderly than in young patients.
    B. Conversion disorder is seen almost exclusively in women.
    C. A risk factor for conversion disorder is sexual abuse.
    D. Although nonepileptic seizures (often referred to as pseudoseizures) are a subtype of conversion disorder, they are rarely seen in patients with a bona fide seizure disorder.
    E. Conversion disorder in late life is rarely associated with a comorbid neurological disorder.

4. The etiology of somatoform disorders has been subject to much theoretical speculation. Which of the following is true?

   A. The prevalence of all definitively diagnosed somatoform disorders increases with age.
   B. When somatoform disorders present in the older patient, comorbid neurological illness may be associated with them, but neuropsychological (cognitive) impairment is not.
   C. Somatoform disorders are associated with a history of serious illness of a parent, but not in the patient, early in life.
   D. Comorbid panic disorder is common in somatoform disorders, but other anxiety disorders are not.
   E. The personality trait of neuroticism, wherein the subject experiences more negative emotions, is associated with the development of somatoform disorders.

5. Treatment of somatoform disorders calls for an integrative biopsychosocial approach by the physician. Which of the following approaches is recommended?

   A. The physician should arrange appointments on an as-needed basis.
   B. A focus on obtaining insight into the psychological context of somatoform symptoms should be the first priority for intervention.
   C. The physician should not offer to review all prior medical records, as this merely reinforces maladaptive somatization behavior.
   D. Hypochondriasis has been shown to respond to antidepressants and anxiolytics.
   E. The clinician should avoid forming a therapeutic alliance, since doing so would reinforce preexisting systems.

Bereavement and Adjustment Disorders

Larry W. Thompson, Ph.D.

Paulette C.Y. Tang, Ph.D.

John Di Mario, B.S.

Marty Cusing, M.A.

Dolores Gallagher-Thompson, Ph.D., A.B.P.P.

In this chapter, we discuss late-life bereavement in some depth, because the amount of conceptual and empirical research on this topic has substantially increased in the recent past. More is known about late-life bereavement than about the second topic covered in this chapter, adjustment disorders in the elderly population. A brief description of "normal grief" is presented along with issues such as what constitutes "abnormal grief," how grief manifests in older adults, and how it changes over time, as well as risk factors related to grief intensity. We also review several interventions that are helpful for treatment of complex grief reactions.

In the section on adjustment disorders, we briefly review research and clinical data, focusing on information about how elderly persons tend to cope with stressful life events that are less threatening than the death of a loved one. Adjustment disorder is an important but often overlooked diagnosis in geriatric psychiatry, and it is hoped that continued focus on this topic will encourage relevant research and clinical investigation.

Late-Life Bereavement

In the United States, among persons age 65 or older, about 45% of women and 15%

This work was supported in part by grant R01-AG01959 from the National Institute on Aging and grants R01-MH36834 and R01-MH37196 from the National Institute of Mental Health.

of men have experienced spousal bereavement (Federal Interagency Forum on Aging Related Statistics 2000). Widowhood has long been regarded as a "woman's issue" because men die younger: the mean age at loss of spouse is 66 years for women compared with 69 years for men. Given that the average life expectancy for men who are now age 70 is 13.2 years, whereas for women at age 70 it is 15.8 years, there is clearly a longer duration of widowhood for women than for men (Centers for Disease Control and Prevention 2002). Rates of bereavement are similar for whites and Hispanics and are slightly higher for African Americans (U.S. Census Bureau 1998). Given that the population of ethnically diverse elders will increase markedly over the next 20 years (Federal Interagency Forum on Aging Related Statistics 2000), there is a clear need to understand not only the bereavement process itself but also how it is mediated by cultural factors.

Bereavement has been characterized by many as a highly charged emotional state that creates significant risk factors for certain negative outcomes, including mortality and major physical and mental health disturbances (Stroebe et al. 2005). However, with respect to the elderly, some clinicians and researchers emphasize that many survive and cope quite well following their spouse's death. For example, the Changing Lives of Older Couples (CLOC) Study (Bonnano et al. 2002, 2004) found that over 45% of that sample of older widowed persons displayed little depression prior to their spouse's death and continued to report remarkably few symptoms of distress 6 and 18 months after the death, which the researchers interpreted as indicating an adaptive pattern of coping with the loss. In addition, depressive symptoms (when present initially) tended to abate over time.

These results are similar to those reported earlier by McCrae and Costa (1993),

who found that the majority of older bereaved persons in their 10-year follow-up study showed considerable resilience in adapting to this major life stress. However, not all older adults respond so well. In the CLOC Study, for example, about 16% of the participants were labeled "chronic grievers" because they failed to return to preloss levels of positive adjustment at any point in the 18-month follow-up (Bonnano et al. 2004). These findings are in agreement with other estimates of chronic grief across several studies in which 15%–20% of bereaved adults evidence serious long-term difficulties (Prigerson and Jacobs 2001). Given this range of emotional response to spousal loss, it is important to identify elders at risk for negative outcomes who could benefit from psychiatric care. This determination seems to be dependent in large part on whether the bereavement is "complicated" or "uncomplicated."

"Uncomplicated" Versus "Complicated" Bereavement

In DSM-IV-TR (American Psychiatric Association 2000a), bereavement is in the V Code section, meaning it is a condition that may be the focus of attention or treatment but that is not, in itself, a psychiatric disorder. Uncomplicated bereavement is defined in DSM-IV-TR as follows:

> This category can be used when the focus of clinical attention is a reaction to the death of a loved one. As part of their reaction to the loss, some grieving individuals present with symptoms characteristic of a Major Depressive Episode (e.g., feelings of sadness and associated symptoms such as insomnia, poor appetite, and weight loss). The bereaved individual typically regards the depressed mood as "normal," although the person may seek professional help for relief of associated symptoms such as insomnia or anorexia. The duration and expression of "normal" bereavement vary consider-

ably among different cultural groups. The diagnosis of Major Depressive Disorder is generally not given unless the symptoms are still present 2 months after the loss. (American Psychiatric Association 2000a, pp. 740–741)

Several specific symptoms that are not considered to be characteristic of a normal grief reaction are also listed in DSM-IV-TR. These include

1) guilt about things other than actions taken or not taken by the survivor at the time of the death; 2) thoughts of death other than the survivor feeling that he or she would be better off dead or should have died with the deceased person; 3) morbid preoccupation with worthlessness; 4) marked psychomotor retardation; 5) prolonged and marked functional impairment; and 6) hallucinatory experiences other than thinking that he or she hears the voice of, or transiently sees the image of, the deceased person. (American Psychiatric Association 2000a, p. 741)

If such symptoms are evident as well, the likelihood of complications during bereavement is increased, and interventions may be called for.

The lack of consensus regarding the differences among abnormal or complicated grief, normal grief, major depression, and other stress disorders has posed challenges for clinicians and researchers alike (Shuchter and Zisook 1993). Two sets of criteria have been proposed for identifying individuals undergoing a complicated or traumatic bereavement. Horowitz et al. (1997) proposed criteria for "complicated grief disorder" that focus on two major areas: 1) *intrusive symptoms* (e.g., unbidden memories, strong spells of severe emotion related to the lost relationship, distressingly strong yearnings for the deceased) and 2) *signs of avoidance and failure to adapt* (e.g., feelings of emptiness or of being very much alone; avoidance of people,

places, or activities that remind one of the deceased person; unusual levels of sleep disturbance; loss of interest in social, occupational, or recreational activities). These symptoms and signs need to be present for at least 14 months after the loss.

Prigerson et al. (1999) proposed criteria for "traumatic grief" that focus on *separation distress* (e.g., yearning and searching for the deceased person, loneliness, intrusive thoughts about the deceased person) and *traumatic distress* (e.g., purposelessness; numbness or detachment; disbelief; feelings of meaninglessness; loss of a sense of trust, security, or control; excessive irritability, bitterness, or anger related to the death). These features must be present for at least 2 months. In addition to the time-frame difference (i.e., 2 months' duration versus presence at 14 months or thereafter), the criteria proposed by Prigerson et al. (1999) do not include symptoms of avoidance.

At present, it is not possible to state that one or the other set of criteria is superior or more valid in determining whether abnormal grief is present, but the development of such definitions will aid researchers in establishing constructs relevant for clinical and research purposes. As evidence accumulates, we are likely to see continued changes in the criteria for complicated bereavement. For example, few compelling arguments remain that it is really necessary to reduce substantially one's sense of attachment to a deceased individual in order to resolve one's grief. Nor that it is reasonable to expect an elder bereaved person to be free of grief within a span of 2 years, the duration most often used to demarcate a chronic grief reaction. Until data are accumulated to address this problem, it seems appropriate to continue to use currently available (and evolving) diagnostic criteria, which clearly affirm that normal grief is not equivalent to a clinical syndrome and which indicate specific symptoms to be evaluated to determine whether their presence and/or severity level suggests that a differential diagnosis is warranted.

Theories About Adjustment to Permanent Losses

A number of theoretical perspectives have been developed to explain how people (of any age) respond to significant loss. These are covered in detail in several comprehensive reviews (Bonnano and Kaltman 1999; Regehr and Sussman 2004; Stroebe and Schut 1999; Stroebe et al. 2001, 2005).

From the classic work of Freud (1917 [1915]/1957) ("Mourning and Melancholia") and Lindemann's (1944) early study of acute grief, a major theory evolved in which the prime task of mourning was the gradual surrender of psychological attachment to the deceased individual so that new relationships could be formed. The mourning process was thought to involve specific tasks over a limited time, and if these tasks were not completed properly, psychopathology might result. In contrast, Bowlby (1961, 1980), in his attachment theory, emphasized that bereavement, as an involuntary separation from a loved one, gives rise to many forms of attachment behavior (such as separation anxiety and pining), the functions of which are not withdrawal from the lost object but reunion with it. The desire to reunite with or regain proximity to the deceased person, Bowlby (1961, 1980) predicted, would gradually dissipate through a series of stages, including shock, protest, despair, and, finally, breakage of the bond and adjustment to a new sense of self.

Many of these early models depicted grief as a process involving phases or stages of reaction (Horowitz 1976; Parkes 1972, 1998), with the first phase beginning at the time of the death and persisting for several weeks. Shock and disbelief, combined with emotional numbness, characterize this period, along with intense free-floating anxiety and sharp mood fluctuations. Specific somatic symptoms include sleeplessness, loss of appetite, and vague muscular aches and pains, which lead to increased contact with primary care physicians and, commonly, requests for medication.

The second phase was described as beginning when numbness and anxiety started to decrease—usually in about 4–6 weeks—and often lasting for the better part of a year. Specific symptoms such as frequent crying, chronic sleep disturbance, blue mood, poor appetite, low energy, feelings of fatigue, loss of interest in daily living, and problems with attention and concentration are common. Nevertheless, most individuals do not develop major depression, despite the fact that certain symptoms of grief and depression overlap.

Parkes (1972, 1998) referred to this second phase as a time of "yearning and protest," characterized by actual searching for the deceased individual in both behavioral and cognitive ways (e.g., going to places frequented by the deceased person). Such endeavors bring momentary comfort and also, paradoxically, intensify feelings of grief. Often, someone so similar to the lost loved one is seen that, for a moment, the survivor is certain it must be the deceased person. Auditory and visual hallucination and "sense-of-presence" experiences are a common part of grieving. Bereaved persons may see the deceased individual sitting in his or her favorite chair, hear their names being called, or receive a message that all is well. These vivid experiences appear to be a normal part of grieving and have been documented in the clinical literature for more than 25 years (Grimby 1993; Rees 1971). Other cognitive components include frequent searching for the meaning of the death and for an explana-tion of why it occurred the way it did.

The third phase focuses on identity re-construction (Lopata 1975), which is the gradual disengagement of some or most of the psychic energy that has been bound up with the deceased person and reinvest-ment of that energy into other relation-ships and activities. The length of this pro-cess is thought to depend on the centrality of roles that were lost as a result of the death and on the amount and kind of learning that is needed to develop a new sense of self. Lopata (1975) estimated this process takes at least a year, during which time many of the troublesome somatic, cogni-tive, and behavioral symptoms abate.

Although stage theories have been widely accepted by health care profes-sionals, little empirical evidence exists to support them. Many argue that bereave-ment is a dynamic process that may con-tinue for a number of years and even pos-sibly for the remainder of one's life (Bierhals et al. 1995; Rosenblatt 1996; Stroebe et al. 2001). Furthermore, bereaved individuals do not proceed from one clearly identifi-able phase to another in an orderly fash-ion, a fact particularly true of older adults (Kastenbaum 1981).

In brief, one might best view these stages or phases of adaptation to loss in descriptive terms, which may be helpful for individuals to understand and deal with this complicated phenomenon.

Other theories of grief hold that expe-riencing a *continuing bond* with the de-ceased individual is an essential part of the process of adaptation (Bowlby 1980; Glick et al. 1974; Parkes 1972, 1998)—in con-trast to the "disengagement" view. For ex-ample, Stroebe and Stroebe (1989) found that not only did widows and widowers maintain ties with their deceased spouses through sensing their presence and search-ing for them, but they also actively re-flected on past actions of those persons and

used these actions as models for decision making and problem solving. Such data have led to a widespread consensus that psychologically healthy bereaved persons do maintain an active, dynamic connec-tion with the deceased and that a rela-tively continuous sense of grief does not necessarily reflect poor adjustment (Klass 1996; Reisman 2001; Rosenblatt 1996; Rosenblatt and Elde 1990; Silverman and Klass 1996). However, a useful distinction can still be made between adaptive and maladaptive continuing attachment, on the basis of whether the attachment is ab-stract or concrete: maintaining abstract ties with the deceased seems suggestive of healthier adaptation (Field et al. 1999; Pincus 1974).

Recent theorists have also focused at-tention more on the cognitive and social processes involved in grieving. Many now regard grieving as an ongoing effort of the person to adapt to and construct a *mean-ing* for the loss (e.g., Neimeyer 1998). Ac-cording to this theory, the meaning of loss of one's spouse (or other major loss of old age) is determined by one's construction of its significance rather than the "brute facts" themselves. Neimeyer (2001) writes that "like a novel that loses a central char-acter in the middle chapters, the life story disrupted by loss must be reorganized... to find a new strand of continuity that bridges the past with the future..." (p. 263).

Neimeyer relates this process of mean-ing reconstruction to the "dual-process model" of Stroebe and Schut (1999, 2001) that describes the value of identifying two distinct types of bereavement-related stres-sors and coping styles. *Loss-oriented stres-sors and coping* are associated with the na-ture of the loss itself and are manifested as emotional, behavioral, physiological, and cognitive symptoms. *Restoration-oriented stressors and coping* refer to what an indi-vidual needs to deal with to adapt to the larger, objective environment, such as facing changes in social and household roles, learning skills to perform tasks that the deceased used to do, and developing a new sense of self. During the course of bereavement, the individual's focus of attention oscillates as he or she attempts to deal with the management of these two related, but distinct, types of stressors (Stroebe and Schut 2001). It seems essential for the "dosage" of these stressors to be reasonably balanced. Psychological mechanisms (e.g., denial, suppression of negative emotions, inhibition of thoughts about the deceased individual) often associated with psychopathology can be useful, according to these theories, provided they are not persistent and overwhelming. As oscillation between the stressors occurs more often, the likelihood of engaging relentlessly in mourning tasks is decreased, thus allowing for more opportunities to address other important interpersonal and environmental issues in a timely manner. As meaning is created and one's "self-narrative" is rewritten (Neimeyer 2001, 2005), the bereaved individual can develop a richer, more elaborate sense of identity as well.

Anticipatory Bereavement

Hospice and other end-of-life settings are becoming increasingly common in the care of many elderly patients facing terminal illnesses (Hospice Foundation of America 2003).

Bereavement counseling is often an integral part of hospice care, both before and after a patient's death. Although little research has been completed in this area, a recent survey of patients, family members, and physicians found that at least 90% believed that being free from anxiety, having someone who will listen, and saying goodbye to important people were very important at the end of life (Steinhauser et al. 2000). Despite the lack of replicated findings concerning effectiveness (Seale and Kelly 1997; Wrenn et al. 2001), bereave-

ment counseling is advocated by leading hospice organizations and is legislated as a standard component of the Medicare hospice benefit (Hospice Care 2001).

A number of studies suggest that a period of forewarning can have positive effects on the bereavement process (Kramer 1997; O'Bryant 1990–1991; Stroebe et al. 2005). In contrast, other studies suggest that anticipatory work focusing on the impending death of a loved one has negative effects or no effects on outcomes after bereavement (Clayton et al. 1973; Lindemann 1944). More work in this area is needed to develop useful models for implementing constructive interventions during the time of anticipatory bereavement.

Cultural Variations in Bereavement Responses

Some theorists view death, loss, and grief as social constructs that are shaped by one's sociocultural environment (Bowman and Singer 2001; Braun and Nichols 1997; Corwin 1995). In the United States, the proportion of older adults of nonEuropean ancestry is steadily increasing. Because reactions to death and the perceived meaning of death are different among different ethnic and cultural groups, care providers must become aware of their clients' specific cultural assumptions and biases about how grief should be experienced and managed. To begin to understand this, one should inquire about their 1) normative ways of expressing psychological pain resulting from death, 2) mourning practices and rituals, 3) beliefs regarding the degree of influence the deceased person continues to have on the bereaved person, and 4) how these beliefs potentially facilitate or hinder the process of coming to terms with the loss (Braun and Nichols 1997).

The belief and meaning systems of a culture may have major implications for how individuals react to death and cope with bereavement. For many culturally mainstream Americans, death means the end of the relationship with the person, and a time for public and private expressions of grief follows (Shuchter and Zisook 1988). In other cultures, active ongoing interaction with a deceased family member (such as ancestor rituals like *sosen suhai* in Japan) may be the norm rather than the exception (Goss and Klass 1997). Similarly, outward emotional expressions of grief are believed to be effective in helping bereaved individuals adjust in the mainstream culture, but many other cultures and religions view such expressions differently (Ablon 1971; al-Adawi et al. 1997; Goss and Klass 1997; al-Issa 1995; Janof-Bulman and Timko 1987; Wikan 1988).

For persons from more collectivistic cultures in which extensive familial networking and familial support exist, mourning may not be so much an individual process as a grieving event for the entire extended family and even the community, such as among recent Mexican immigrants (Block 1998) and in the Rauto culture in Australia (Wisocki and Skowron 2000). In this context, helpful interventions may be those designed to increase familial involvement so that grieving becomes a collaborative process for all family members (Nadeau 2001).

In summary, it is clear that culture plays an important role in reactions to loss, the course of grieving, and outcomes of bereavement. Therefore, it is important to understand the cultural idioms of distress that are specific to a given cultural or ethnic group and to consider how individuals from that group may communicate distress idiosyncratically.

Longitudinal Studies of Late-Life Bereavement

Results from early longitudinal studies on bereavement in the elderly have been summarized in edited books (Lund 1989; Stroebe et al. 2001). Findings have been fairly consistent with regard to the kinds of symptoms that change over time, the rate of change expected to occur, and the presence or absence of gender differences. The most significant differences between bereaved and nonbereaved adults on standard measures of mood, anxiety, and well-being were found to occur 2–6 months after the spouse's death, with the bereaved reporting more distress than the nonbereaved. By 12 months postloss, levels of distress were generally no longer significantly different between the two groups, although women's levels of distress generally remained higher (Harlow et al. 1991; Lund et al. 1989; Thompson et al. 1991).

Expression of grief, on the other hand, was notably different. Thompson and colleagues (1991) found that elderly men and women still had substantially higher mean scores than comparison groups on the Texas Revised Inventory of Grief (TRIG; Faschingbauer 1981) at 12 and 30 months postloss. Also, no gender differences in level of grief were reported, contrary to results on other indices of psychological distress. These authors concluded that the level of grief remains high for at least 30 months after a spouse's death and that this appears to be a part of normal grief.

In a recent reanalysis of these data, the TRIG was found to have three independent factors (thoughts about grief, nonacceptance of the loss, and strong feelings of loss) that reliably discriminated between bereaved and comparison participants, suggesting that grief in older adults may have several dimensions that are worthy of evaluation and that could be helpful to the clinician in guiding the choice of intervention approach (Futterman et al., in review).

At the same time, normal grief can be distinguished from depressed mood and related symptoms. This finding is consistent with earlier work by Zisook and Shuchter (1985, 1986), who also found that grief (as indexed by a continuing sense of attachment to the deceased person) was still strong, at times, even at 4 years postloss. Thus, while symptoms of distress may abate, *recovery* from grief may be an unrealistic goal for older adults.

Risk Factors for Intense and/or "Complicated" Grief

As noted earlier, some individuals do develop complications during bereavement, and it is important to identify elders who may be at risk for these negative outcomes (cf. Sanders 1993 and Stroebe et al. 2001 for comprehensive reviews of studies in this area). Age and gender of the survivor, mode of death, presence of significant depression shortly after the death, evidence of other psychiatric disorders, low self-esteem and poor coping skills, poor marital satisfaction, and inadequate social support are some of the factors frequently found to be related to the development of complicated bereavement. Strength of religious commitment and involvement, participation in culturally appropriate mourning rituals, and redistribution of roles within the family after the death may also have an impact on the grief process, although the literature is not clear on the relative contribution of these factors.

Older bereaved men who have lost their spouses are at higher risk for death than older bereaved women (Bowling 1988–1989; Stroebe and Stroebe 1993; Thompson et al. 1984). Thompson et al. (1984) reported that 16% of the widowers in their longitudinal study died within 18 months, whereas only 1% of the widows and one of the control men died during this time period. Bowling (1988–1989) reported that low social contact in the 500 subjects he followed predicted mortality. Gallagher-Thompson and co-workers (1993) found that widowers who died within the first

year of spousal bereavement had reported more often than survivors that 1) their wife was their main confidant, 2) they had minimal involvement in activities with other persons after their wife's death, and 3) they would have enjoyed increased socialization but did not know how to make this happen. Clinicians should be alerted that older widowers, particularly those who have low socialization and lack the ability to develop adequate social networks, are at high risk for mortality and may require attention to increase socialization and to develop an emotionally supportive network during the first 2 years following loss of the spouse.

Numerous studies have demonstrated that adaptation is more difficult when the death is violent (as in a homicide), stigmatized (as in the case of AIDS), or very unexpected or unanticipated (cf. O'Neil 1989, Parkes and Weiss 1983, and Worden 1991 for detailed discussion of the clinical effects). Within the first month or so following the loss, spouses of individuals who committed suicide showed little difference from spouses whose mates died of natural causes. However, as time passed, spouses of suicide victims continued to have elevated depression and distress during the first and second years of bereavement (Farberow et al. 1992a; Wijngaards-de Meij et al. 2005). In the third year, these differences tended to diminish, but spouses of suicide victims who reported moderate to severe depression initially had higher levels of depression over time (Farberow et al. 1992a) and were at greater risk for development of other psychopathological symptoms (Gilewski et al. 1991).

The presence of clinically significant symptoms of depression within the first 2 months after a spouse's death is a significant risk factor for continued depression and poor coping beyond the first 2 years (Breckenridge et al. 1986; Gilewski et al.

1991; Lund et al. 1993; Wortman and Silver 1989).

Bereaved elderly individuals with low self-esteem and/or inadequate coping skills are also at greater risk for continued high levels of stress in the second year (Johnson and colleagues 1986). Satisfaction with the marital relationship has been widely addressed in the clinical literature (e.g., Parkes and Weiss 1983), but there is little empirical research to support or refute the clinical lore as to how it may operate as a risk factor. Futterman and co-workers (1990) reported that the bereaved elder's retrospective assessment of marital adjustment was positively related to self-reported levels of depression. Itzhar-Nabarro (2004) also found that retrospective assessment of marital satisfaction was positively correlated with depression at 2 months following the loss, but this relationship was no longer evident by the end of the first year of bereavement. Further research is clearly needed on this subject.

Social support has been widely recognized as providing a buffer against the impact of many kinds of life stress (Cobb 1976), including normal bereavement (Dimond et al. 1987) and bereavement resulting from suicide (Farberow et al. 1992b). In the latter study, it was also found that those spouses who had greater difficulty confiding in members of their network were more likely to report dissatisfaction with support from their network, compared with spouses of individuals who died of natural causes (Farberow et al. 1992b).

Taken together, these studies suggest that certain risk factors, either singly or in combination, are associated with a more complicated grief reaction in elderly individuals. However, most of this research involved volunteer subjects, often from relatively advantaged socioeconomic backgrounds, who could see some benefit to themselves from being interviewed. Much

remains to be learned about bereavement among elderly persons who are economically disadvantaged, are in poor health, or who have little or no family to rely on as well as specific risk factors among ethnically and culturally diverse elders.

Interventions for Late-Life Bereavement

The following questions can be helpful in deciding whether a psychiatric intervention is warranted: Does the symptom picture reflect normal grief, or does the grief appear to be complicated by clinical depression or some other psychiatric disorder? What risk factors are present to suggest that the individual may have a difficult grieving process ahead?

Treating Complicated Bereavement

If a clinical level of depression is present, that problem should be treated first, with medication and/or psychotherapy, so that it can resolve sufficiently to permit the grieving process to become the focus of attention when the patient is ready (American Psychiatric Association 2000b; "NIH Consensus Conference" 1992; Raphael et al. 2001; Reynolds 1992). Posttraumatic stress disorder, bereavement-related anxiety disorders, and subsyndromal depression are other common complications that require treatment in themselves (Reynolds et al. 1999; Rosenzweig et al. 1997; Schut et al. 1997).

Differentiation between normal and abnormal bereavement is vital to appropriate intervention choices (Raphael et al. 2001) because there is growing consensus in the literature that "counseling" of various kinds with normal grievers shows little positive effect. On the other hand, in cases of complicated bereavement, a variety of treatments do show reliable positive effects (Neimeyer 2000). Pharmacological treatments combined with psychotherapy appear to be more effective than either intervention alone in reducing depressive symptoms in the context of bereavement (Miller et al. 1997; Reynolds et al. 1999), although this conclusion is based on a small number of studies at present.

Various forms of individual and group psychotherapy have been used to treat patients with complicated bereavement reactions. Offering social support, encouraging emotional disclosure, and helping the bereaved to reinterpret the meaning of their loss experience seem to be the main components of successful grief therapy, regardless of the theoretical perspective underlying the intervention (Neimeyer 2005; Stroebe et al. 2005). However, findings regarding the effectiveness of individual versus small group intervention methods have been mixed (see Schut et al. 2001 for review of clinical efficacy studies of individual and group interventions over the past 20 years).

Raphael and colleagues (1993) describe a variety of methods (including psychodynamic approaches, behavioral therapies, and cognitive therapies) for treating complex grief reactions. Horowitz's (1976) time-limited psychodynamic therapy is an example of a personality-oriented approach to help patients work through their reactions to serious life events in 12 sessions. Techniques such as abreaction, clarification, and interpretation of defenses and affects are used to facilitate realistic appraisals of the implications of a death and to explore the effect of this loss on the bereaved person's self-concept. This approach was empirically studied by Horowitz and colleagues (e.g., Horowitz et al. 1981, 1984; Windholz et al. 1985). Marmar et al. (1988) describes the application of this approach to older bereaved, depressed women.

The effective use of a relatively brief, intensive, structured behavioral program, called *guided mourning*, to facilitate reso-

lution of chronic grief was reported by Mawson and co-workers (1981), and these findings were replicated by Sireling and associates (1988). In this approach, 90-minute sessions are held three times weekly for 2 weeks, with subsequent less intense follow-up for 28 weeks. Patients are helped to repeatedly confront aspects of their loss so that they can relive painful memories and eventually diminish negative effects associated with them.

Several forms of cognitive and cognitive-behavioral therapy have also been successfully used to treat patients with complex bereavement reactions. Viney's (1990) "personal construct" approach focuses on describing core constructs that are disrupted in intense grief and how to reconstruct these core beliefs. Other examples of the use of cognitive-behavioral methods can be found in publications by Abrahms (1981), Fleming and Robinson (1991), Florsheim and Gallagher-Thompson (1990), Gantz et al. (1992), and Malkinson (2001). A recent review of meta-analyses on studies using CBT (Butler et al. 2006) did not specifically cover studies on bereavement but provides data about the efficacy of CBT to treat many of the problems found in complicated bereavement, such as depression and generalized anxiety disorder, and may therefore be of interest to clinical researchers in this field.

Finally, the "meaning reconstruction" approach of Neimeyer (2001, 2005) deserves mention in this section, despite the current lack of empirical research regarding its efficacy. The heart of this treatment is to foster evolution of the "self-narrative" (which is the term Neimeyer uses to describe the sense of identity that is constantly changing in adults in response to significant internal and external events) by reflection and questioning that help the client perform narrative repair and/or revision. It is thought that the therapeutic relationship provides a vital context for validation of the client's changing sense of identity. A variety of cognitive and behavioral interventions are used to facilitate this process, although theoretically the approach is grounded in constructivist views (Neimeyer 2001). For the 15%–20% of bereaved adults whose grief remains chronic and debilitating and who lack adequate social support (Ott 2003), narrative interventions that make use of systematic writing about trauma and loss can help promote expression and integration of such experiences, as meta-analyses of these methods have shown (Pennebaker 1997).

Treating Traumatic Grief

In recent years the construct of traumatic grief has received considerable attention (Prigerson et al. 1999). Criteria include intrusive and distressing preoccupation with the deceased in combination with many symptoms associated with the ex-perience of severe trauma observed in posttraumatic stress disorder. Regehr and Sussman (2004) noted similarities and differences in grief theory and trauma theory and reviewed studies that focused on the treatment of indivduals who were experiencing both. They concluded that although not all people experiencing a traumatic loss require treatment, individuals with unresolved relationship issues with the deceased can benefit from therapies that focus on these issues. Further, cognitive restructuring and behavioral management of symptoms based on cognitive and behavioral principles are also helpful (Malkinson 2001).

Researchers at the Western Pennsylvania Psychiatric Institute (Frank et al. 1997; Shear et al. 2001) developed a treatment for traumatic grief that involves principles similar to those featured in the treatment of posttraumatic stress disorder, including a series of cognitive-behavioral techniques such as imaginal exposure to the death scene; in vivo, graded exposure to avoided death-related circumstances; mindful breathing; and writing good-bye letters to the deceased person. Also integral to the treatment are homework assignments involving listening to tapes of imaginal exposure. The results have been encouraging: complicated grief, anxiety, and depressive symptoms were significantly reduced, and patients who did not respond to interpersonal psychotherapy did respond to traumatic grief therapy.

Worden (1991) described what he termed "grief therapy" for chronic or unresolved grief. This method included reviving memories of the deceased person, facilitating the experiencing of a range of emotions; helping the patient to acknowledge and deal with ambivalent feelings; exploring and defusing "linking objects" (objects a mourner keeps to maintain a relationship with the deceased person); and helping the bereaved individual to say a final good-bye. Worden recommended specific modifications of this approach for patients with particularly difficult losses, such as suicides and other forms of traumatic death.

Facilitating Normal or Typical Grief Reactions

Opinions differ regarding the use of medication to treat the unpleasant depressive symptoms (such as sleep and appetite problems) that typically accompany the first year of bereavement in patients experiencing a normal grief reaction. According to some psychiatrists and other health care providers, medication should be used sparingly and only briefly, if at all, because it is assumed that to recover adequately from grief, it is necessary to experience grief fully (e.g., Parkes 1972, 1998; Worden 1991). However, Regehr and Sussman (2004) concluded (from their review of the literature) that there is only limited empirical evidence supporting the position that *expression* of grief is important to resolution. Wortman and Silver (1987) reached a similar conclusion and therefore argued that pharmacological (and other) treatments for pain and suffering should be available to those who request them. In contrast, Raphael et al. (2001) warned that in the case of bereavement without depression, prescribing antidepressants is not recommended, while others believe that the provider should intervene sooner rather than later, given the tendency of depressive symptoms to persist (Reynolds 1992).

Similarly, mixed opinions exist with regard to the value of providing formal counseling or therapy to individuals who are experiencing normal or typical bereavement. An early writer on this topic (Worden 1991) described grief counseling that included using guided imagery and symbols (e.g., photos of the deceased) to evoke emotional expression. He also described what are referred to as the four "tasks" of normal grieving (e.g., accepting the reality of the loss). Individual or group sessions were used, and the work was seen as adjunctive to the bereaved person's own psychological work on these issues. However, it is clear from data regarding why older adults seek mental health treatment that the majority do not in fact seek professional assistance for their grief.

Self-help groups are much more widely accessed—these are support groups specifically for bereaved persons that have been recommended for and pursued by those experiencing an uncomplicated (but painful and lonely) bereavement. Lieberman (1993) described basic curative factors in such groups, including a family-like atmosphere, encouragement of emotional expression, and sanction of development of a new self-image that reflects one's current status as an "I" rather than a "we." In contrast to the various forms of psychotherapy reviewed above in "Treating Complicated Bereavement," which tend to be relatively brief (or at least time limited), self-help groups encourage long-term in-

volvement; as Lieberman (1993) stated, "[M]embership is indeterminate and may persist far beyond professionally defined recovery" (p. 420). After reviewing the empirical data in support of this approach, Lieberman (1993) concluded that self-help groups for grieving persons (often groups with specific emphases, such as the "Compassionate Friends" self-help network for grieving parents) are effective in facilitating the process. From this, it seems reasonable to assume that bereaved individuals may have their social and psychological needs met sufficiently through this kind of intervention so that they do not require anything more.

Yet there is a specific circumstance in which it may be beneficial to institute a specific form of treatment with elders who are *not* experiencing "complicated bereavement"—that is, with older men whose wives have died and who are at risk for subsequent mortality. This approach proposes to help the widower develop new affectional bonds to replace the major bond that was severed (Stoddard and Henry 1985) and is based on the assumption that most older men have only one strong emotional bond (i.e., with their wife). When that bond ends, the ensuing void must be filled with other affectional or emotional relationships, to protect against increased vulnerability to negative outcomes. This therapy consists of encouragement and support to turn social friendships into relationships that are emotionally fulfilling and not just socially gratifying. Although there is limited empirical support for this method at present, it is a conceptually appealing approach that warrants further investigation.

In summary, current intervention reviews indicate that the effectiveness of grief therapy and counseling is modest, though positive, and is typically observed in those individuals experiencing higher levels of distress—not in older adults experiencing normal grief (Kato and Mann 1999; Neimeyer 2000). Therefore, attention should be paid to selection of patients likely to benefit most from available interventions: as with any patient, a thorough initial assessment and diagnostic formulation are critical to determining which methods of intervention to select.

Adjustment Disorders in Late Life

The diagnostic category of adjustment disorders has been underused in the assessment and treatment of older adults. DSM-IV-TR defines adjustment disorder as "a psychological response to an identifiable stressor or stressors that results in the development of clinically significant emotional or behavioral symptoms. The symptoms must develop within 3 months after the onset of the stressor(s)" (American Psychiatric Association 2000a, p. 679). Evidence of impairment in social or occupational functioning should be apparent during the reaction, or symptoms should be above and beyond what would be expected as a normal reaction to a given stressor. This diagnosis is not applied if the symptom picture meets criteria for another specific disorder or if the reaction appears to be an exacerbation of another psychiatric disorder.

If the stressor has a discrete beginning and end, it is assumed that this reaction will subside within a brief time after the stressor disappears. If the stressor is maintained for a long period, it is assumed that the individual will develop a more adaptive pattern of responding over time. By definition, an adjustment disorder must resolve within 6 months after the termination of the stressor. However, symptoms may persist longer if the stressor is chronic or has enduring consequences.

According to DSM-IV-TR, adjustment disorders are common, with prevalence rates between 2% and 8% in community samples of elderly individuals. In the past, very little attention was focused on these disturbances in the literature. During the past 20 years, however, an increasing number of studies have focused on this disorder, especially in medical populations. Grossberg et al. (1990) determined that of 147 geriatric patients seen by psychiatrists in a 2-year period, 26% were diagnosed as having an adjustment disorder, with only the rate of affective disorder being higher (27%). Adjustment disorders are also common among older patients with multiple sclerosis, cancer, or lupus and among patients receiving cardiac ventricular support or heart transplants (Cullivan et al. 1998; de Walden-Galuszko 1996; Harper et al. 1998; Petrucci et al. 1999; Sullivan et al. 1997).

In more recent epidemiological studies, Blazer et al. (1987) identified a clinical subtype, referred to as *symptomatic depression*, which they suggested may apply to elderly individuals in the community who have adjustment disorder. However, they acknowledged that a definitive diagnosis could not be made on the basis of their data. The symptomatic depression subgroup constituted 4% of their community sample, but it is likely that even this proportion is an underestimate of the prevalence of the disorder.

Further evidence of the high prevalence of adjustment disorders among older patients was offered by Smith and colleagues (1998), who found that 29% of patients referred to a consultation-liaison service for depressive spectrum disorders received an accurate diagnosis of an adjustment disorder. Use of this diagnosis places the focus squarely on external stressors and the psychological and social resources available to the patient for coping with whatever unfortunate events might have occurred. Because age-related changes are likely in all these domains, this classification could be useful in many instances for the assessment and subsequent treatment of elderly patients. However, at the present time, no empirically based intervention studies could be found that focused on the treatment of a specific adjustment disorder in the elderly. Unfortunately, then, there is little empirical data on which to base decision making for what kind of interventions would be most appropriate to use with a given patient. Clearly, this situation needs to be remedied in the future, to better serve our growing population of older adults and address their mental health needs.

References

Ablon J: Bereavement in a Samoan community. Br J Med Psychol 44:329–337, 1971

Abrahms JL: Depression versus normal grief following the death of a significant other, in New Directions in Cognitive Therapy. Edited by Emery G, Hollon S, Bedrosian R. New York, Guilford, 1981, pp 255–270

al-Adawi S, Burjorjee R, al-Issa I: Mu-Ghayeb: a culture-specific response to bereavement in Oman. Int J Soc Psychiatry 43:144–151, 1997

al-Issa I: The illusion of reality or the reality of illusion: hallucinations and culture. Br J Psychiatry 166:368–373, 1995

American Psychiatric Association: Diagnostic and Statistical Manual of Mental Disorders, 4th Edition, Text Revision. Washington, DC, American Psychiatric Association, 2000a

American Psychiatric Association: Practice Guideline for the Treatment of Patients With Major Depressive Disorder, 2nd Edition. Washington, DC, American Psychiatric Association, 2000b

Bierhals AJ, Prigerson HG, Fasiczka A, et al: Gender differences in complicated grief among the elderly. Omega (Westport) 32:303–317, 1995

Blazer DG, Hughes DC, George LK: The epidemiology of depression in an elderly community population. Gerontologist 27:281–287, 1987

Block JB: The meaning of death, in Healing Latinos: The Art of Cultural Competence in Medicine. Edited by Hayes-Bautista D, Chiprut R. Los Angeles, CA, Cedars-Sinai Health System, 1998, pp 79–85

Bonnano GA, Kaltman S: Toward an integrative perspective on bereavement. Psychol Bull 123:760–776, 1999

Bonnano GA, Wortman CB, Lehman DR, et al: Resilience to loss and chronic grief. J Pers Soc Psychol 83:1150–1164, 2002

Bonnano GA, Wortman CB, Nesse RM: Prospective patterns of resilience and maladjustment during widowhood. Psychol Aging 19:260–271, 2004

Bowlby J: Processes of mourning. Int J Psychoanal 42:317–340, 1961

Bowlby J: Attachment and Loss, Vol 3: Loss: Sadness and Depression. London, Hogarth Press, 1980

Bowling A: Who dies after widow(er)hood? a discriminant analysis. Omega (Westport) 19:135–153, 1988–1989

Bowman KW, Singer PA: Chinese seniors' perspectives on end-of-life decisions. Soc Sci Med 53:455–464, 2001

Braun KL, Nichols R: Death and dying in four Asian American cultures: a descriptive study. Death Stud 21:327–359, 1997

Breckenridge J, Gallagher D, Thompson LW, et al: Characteristic depressive symptoms of bereaved elders. J Gerontol 41:163–168, 1986

Butler AC, Chapman JE, Forman EM, et al: Empirical status of cognitive-behavioral therapy: a review of meta-analyses. Clin Psychol Rev 26:17–31, 2006

Centers for Disease Control and Prevention: U.S. life tables, 2002. Hyattsville, MD, National Center for Health Statistics, 2002. Available at http://www.cdc.gov/nchs/data/dvs/life2002.pdf. Accessed March 1, 2006.

Clayton P, Halikas J, Maurice W, et al: Anticipatory grief and widowhood. Br J Psychiatry 122:47–51, 1973

Cobb S: Social support as a moderator of life stress. Psychosom Med 3:300–314, 1976

Corwin MD: Cultural issues in bereavement therapy: the social construction of mourning. In Session: Psychotherapy in Practice 1:23–41, 1995

Cullivan R, Crown J, Walsh N: The use of psychotropic medication in patients referred to a psycho-oncology service. Psychooncology 7:301–306, 1998

de Walden-Galuszko K: Prevalence of psychological comorbidity in terminally ill cancer patients. Psychooncology 5:45–49, 1996

Dimond M, Lund DA, Caserta MS: The role of social support in the first two years of bereavement in an elderly sample. Gerontologist 27:599–604, 1987

Farberow NL, Gallagher-Thompson D, Gilewski M, et al: Changes in grief and mental health of bereaved spouses of older suicides. J Gerontol 47:P357–P366, 1992a

Farberow NL, Gallagher-Thompson D, Gilewski M, et al: The role of social supports in the bereavement process of surviving spouses of suicide and natural deaths. Suicide Life Threat Behav 22:107–124, 1992b

Faschingbauer TR: Texas Inventory of Grief—Revised Manual. Houston, TX, Honeycomb Publishing, 1981

Federal Interagency Forum on Aging Related Statistics: Older Americans 2000: Key Indicators of Well-Being. Washington, DC, Federal Interagency Forum on Aging Related Statistics, 2000

Field NP, Nichols C, Holen A, et al: The relation of continuing attachment to adjustment in conjugal bereavement. J Consult Clin Psychol 67:212–218, 1999

Florsheim M, Gallagher-Thompson D: Cognitive/behavioral treatment of atypical bereavement: a case study. Clin Gerontologist 10:73–76, 1990

Frank E, Prigerson HG, Shear MK, et al: Phenomenology and treatment of bereavement related distress in the elderly. Int Clin Psychopharmacol 12 (suppl 7):S25–S29, 1997

Freud S: Mourning and melancholia (1917 [1915]), in The Standard Edition of the Complete Psychological Works of Sigmund Freud, Vol 14. Translated and edited by Strachey J. London, Hogarth Press, 1957, pp 237–260

Futterman A, Gallagher D, Thompson LW, et al: Retrospective assessment of marital adjustment and depression during the first 2 years of spousal bereavement. Psychol Aging 5:277–283, 1990

Futterman A, Brown P, Gallagher-Thompson D, et al: Factorial validity of the Texas Inventory of Grief—Revised. Psych Assessment (in review)

Gallagher-Thompson D, Futterman A, Farberow N, et al: The impact of spousal bereavement on older widows and widowers, in Handbook of Bereavement. Edited by Stroebe MS, Stroebe W, Hansson R. Cambridge, UK, Cambridge University Press, 1993, pp 227–239

Gantz F, Gallagher D, Rodman J: Cognitive/behavioral facilitation of inhibited grief, in Comprehensive Casebook of Cognitive Therapy. Edited by Freeman A, Dattilio F. New York, Plenum, 1992, pp 201–207

Gilewski MJ, Farberow NL, Gallagher DE, et al: Interaction of depression and bereavement on mental health in the elderly. Psychol Aging 6:67–75, 1991

Glick IO, Weiss, RS, Parkes CM: The First Year of Bereavement. New York, Wiley, 1974

Goss RE, Klass D: Tibetan Buddhism and the resolution of grief: the Bardo-thodol for the dying and the grieving. Death Stud 21:377–395, 1997

Grimby A: Bereavement among elderly people: grief reactions, post-bereavement hallucinations, and quality of life. Acta Psychiatr Scand 87:72–80, 1993

Grossberg GT, Zimny GH, Nakra BR: Geriatric psychiatry consultations in a university hospital. Int Psychogeriatr 2:161–168, 1990

Harlow SD, Goldberg EL, Comstock GW: A longitudinal study of the prevalence of depressive symptomatology in elderly widowed and married women. Arch Gen Psychiatry 48:1065–1068, 1991

Harper RG, Chacko RC, Kotik-Harper D, et al: Detection of a psychiatric diagnosis in heart transplant candidates with MBHI. J Clin Psychol Med Settings 5:187–198, 1998

Horowitz MJ: Stress Response Syndromes. New York, Jason Aronson, 1976

Horowitz MJ, Krupnick J, Kaltreider N, et al: Initial response to parental death. Arch Gen Psychiatry 38:316–323, 1981

Horowitz MJ, Weiss DS, Kaltreider N, et al: Reactions to the death of a parent: results from patients and field subjects. J Nerv Ment Dis 172:383–392, 1984

Horowitz MJ, Siegel B, Holen A, et al: Diagnostic criteria for complicated grief disorder. Am J Psychiatry 154:904–910, 1997

Hospice Care, 42 CFR § 418.88 (2001)

Hospice Foundation of America: What is hospice? Available at http://www.hospicefoundation.org/what_is. Accessed July 21, 2003.

Itzhar-Nabarro Z: The relationship between marital satisfaction and bereavement over 30 month period. Dissertation Abstracts International: Section B: Sciences and Engineering 65(6-B):3132, 2004

Janof-Bulman R, Timko C: Coping with traumatic life events: the role of denial in light of people's assumptive worlds, in Coping With Negative Life Events: Clinical and Social Psychological Perspectives. Edited by Snyder CR, Ford CE. New York, Plenum, 1987, pp 135–159

Johnson RJ, Lund DA, Dimond M: Stress, self-esteem, and coping during bereavement among the elderly. Soc Psychol Q 49:273–279, 1986

Kastenbaum RJ: Death, Society, and Human Experience, 2nd Edition. St. Louis, MO, CV Mosby, 1981

Kato PM, Mann T: A synthesis of psychological interventions for the bereaved. Clin Psychol Rev 19:275–296, 1999

Klass D: Grief as an Eastern culture: Japanese ancestor worship, in Continuing Bonds: New Understandings of Grief (Series in Death Education, Aging, and Health Care, 0275-3510). Edited by Klass D, Silverman PR, Nickman SL. Washington, DC, Taylor & Francis, 1996, pp 59–70

Kramer D: How women relate to terminally ill husbands and their subsequent adjustment to bereavement. Omega (Westport) 34:93–106, 1997

Lieberman MA: Bereavement self-help groups: a review of conceptual and methodological issues, in Handbook of Bereavement. Edited by Stroebe MS, Stroebe W, Hansson R. Cambridge, UK, Cambridge University Press, 1993, pp 411–426

Lindemann E: Symptomatology and management of acute grief. Am J Psychiatry 101:141–148, 1944

Lopata HZ: On widowhood: grief work and identity reconstruction. J Geriatr Psychiatry 8:41–55, 1975

Lund DA, Caserta M, Dimond M: Impact of spousal bereavement on the subjective well-being of older adults, in Older Bereaved Spouses. Edited by Lund DA. New York, Hemisphere, 1989, pp 3–15

Lund DA, Caserta M, Dimond M: Course of spousal bereavement in later life, in Handbook of Bereavement. Edited by Stroebe MS, Stroebe W, Hansson R. Cambridge, UK, Cambridge University Press, 1993, pp 240–254

Malkinson R: Cognitive-behavioral therapy of grief: a review and application. Research on Social Work Practice 11:671–698, 2001

Marmar C, Horowitz MJ, Weiss DS, et al: A controlled trial of brief psychotherapy and mutual-help group treatment of conjugal bereavement. Am J Psychiatry 145:203–212, 1988

Mawson D, Marks IM, Ramm L, et al: Guided mourning for morbid grief: a controlled study. Br J Psychiatry 138:185–193, 1981

McCrae RR, Costa PT: Psychological resilience among widowed men and women: a 10-year follow-up of a national sample, in Handbook of Bereavement. Edited by Stroebe M, Stroebe W, Hansson R. Cambridge, UK, Cambridge University Press, 1993, pp 196–207

Miller MD, Wolfson L, Frank E, et al: Using interpersonal psychotherapy (IPT) in a combined psychotherapy/medication research protocol with depressed elders. A descriptive report with case vignettes. J Psychother Pract Res 7:47–55, 1997

Nadeau JW: Meaning making in family bereavement: a family systems approach, in Handbook of Bereavement Research: Consequences, Coping, and Care. Edited by Stroebe MS, Hansson RO, Stroebe W, et al. Washington, DC, American Psychological Association, 2001, pp 329–347

Neimeyer R: The Lessons of Loss: A Guide to Coping. Raleigh, NC, McGraw-Hill, 1998

Neimeyer RA: Searching for the meaning of meaning: grief therapy and the process of reconstruction. Death Studies 24:541–558, 2000

Neimeyer RA (ed): Meaning Reconstruction and the Experience of Loss. Washington, DC, American Psychological Association, 2001

Neimeyer RA: Widowhood, grief and the quest for meaning: a narrative perspective on resilience, Late Life Widowhood in the United States. Edited by Carr D, Nesse RM, Wortman CB. New York, Springer, 2005, pp 227–252

NIH Consensus Conference. Diagnosis and treatment of depression in late life. JAMA 268:1018–1024, 1992

O'Bryant SL: Forewarning of a husband's death: does it make a difference for older widows? Omega (Westport) 22:227–239, 1990–1991

O'Neil M: Grief and bereavement in AIDS and aging. Generations 13:80–82, 1989

Ott CH: The impact of complicated grief on mental and physical health at various points in the bereavement process. Death Studies 27:249–272, 2003

Parkes CM: Bereavement: Studies of Grief in Adult Life. New York, International Universities Press, 1972

Parkes CM: Bereavement: Studies of Grief in Adult Life, 3rd Edition. New York, International Universities Press, 1998

Parkes CM, Weiss RS: Recovery From Bereavement. New York, Basic Books, 1983

Pennebaker JW: Writing about emotional experiences as a therapeutic process. Psychol Sci 8:162–169, 1997

Petrucci R, Kushon D, Inkles R, et al: Cardiac ventricular support: considerations for psychiatry. Psychosomatics 40:298–303, 1999

Pincus L: Death and the Family. New York, Pantheon, 1974

Prigerson HG, Jacobs SC: Diagnostic criteria for traumatic grief, in Handbook of Bereavement Research. Edited by Stroebe RO, Hansson W, Stroebe W, et al: Washington, DC, American Psychological Association, 2001, pp 614–646

Prigerson HG, Shear MK, Jacobs SC, et al: Consensus criteria for traumatic grief: a preliminary empirical test. Br J Psychiatry 174:67–73, 1999

Raphael B, Middleton W, Martinek N, et al: Counseling and therapy of the bereaved, in Handbook of Bereavement. Edited by Stroebe MS, Stroebe W, Hansson R. Cambridge, UK, Cambridge University Press, 1993, pp 427–453

Raphael B, Minkov C, Dobson M: Psychotherapeutic and pharmacological intervention for bereaved persons, in Handbook of Bereavement Research: Consequences, Coping, and Care. Edited by Stroebe MS, Hansson RO, Stroebe W, et al. Washington, DC, American Psychological Association, 2001, pp 587–612

Rees WD: The hallucinations of widowhood. Br Med J 4:37–41, 1971

Regehr C, Sussman T: Intersections between grief and trauma: toward an empirically based model for treating traumatic grief. Brief Treatment and Crisis Intervention 4:289–309, 2004

Reisman AS: Death of a spouse: illusory basic assumptions and continuation of bonds. Death Stud 25:445–460, 2001

Reynolds CF 3rd: Treatment of depression in special populations. J Clin Psychiatry 53 (suppl):45–53, 1992

Reynolds CF 3rd, Miller MD, Pasternak RE, et al: Treatment of bereavement-related major depressive episodes in later life: a controlled study of acute and continuation treatment with nortriptyline and interpersonal psychotherapy. Am J Psychiatry 156:202–208, 1999

Rosenblatt PC: Grief that does not end, in Continuing Bonds: New Understandings of Grief (Death Education, Aging, and Health Care Series, 0275-3510). Edited by Klass D, Silverman PR, Nickman SL. Washington, DC, Taylor & Francis, 1996, pp 45–58

Rosenblatt PC, Elde C: Shared reminiscence about a deceased parent: implications for grief education and grief counseling. Fam Relat 39:206–210, 1990

Rosenzweig A, Prigerson H, Miller MD, et al: Bereavement and late-life depression: grief and its complications in the elderly. Annu Rev Med 48:421–428, 1997

Sanders CM: Risk factors in bereavement outcome, in Handbook of Bereavement. Edited by Stroebe MS, Stroebe W, Hansson R. Cambridge, UK, Cambridge University Press, 1993, pp 255–267

Schut HA, Stroebe MS, van den Bout J: Intervention for the bereaved: gender differences in the efficacy of two counselling programmes. Br J Clin Psychol 36:63–72, 1997

Schut H[A], Stroebe MS, van den Bout J, et al: The efficacy of bereavement interventions: determining who benefits, in Handbook of Bereavement Research: Consequences, Coping, and Care. Edited by Stroebe MS, Hansson RO, Stroebe W, et al. Washington, DC, American Psychological Association, 2001, pp 705–737

Seale C, Kelly M: A comparison of hospice and hospital care for the spouses of people who die. Palliat Med 11:101–106, 1997

Shear MK, Frank E, Foa E, et al: Traumatic grief treatment: a pilot study. Am J Psychiatry 158:1506–1508, 2001

Shuchter SR, Zisook S: Widowhood. The continuing relationship with the dead spouse. Bull Menninger Clin 52:269–279, 1988

Shuchter SR, Zisook S: The course of normal grief, in Handbook of Bereavement. Edited by Stroebe MS, Stroebe W, Hansson R. Cambridge, UK, Cambridge University Press, 1993, pp 23–43

Silverman PR, Klass D: Introduction: what's the problem? in Continuing Bonds: New Understandings of Grief (Series in Death Education, Aging, and Health Care, 0275-3510). Edited by Klass D, Silverman PR, Nickman SL. Washington, DC, Taylor & Francis, 1996, pp 3–27

Sireling L, Cohen D, Marks I: Guided mourning for morbid grief: a replication. Behav Ther 29:121–132, 1988

Smith GC, Clarke DM, Handrinos D, et al: Consultation-liaison psychiatrists' management of depression. Psychosomatics 39: 244–252, 1998

Steinhauser KE, Christakis NA, Clipp EC, et al: Factors considered important at the end of life by patients, family, physicians, and other care providers. JAMA 284:2476–2482, 2000

Stoddard J, Henry JP: Affectional bonding and the impact of bereavement. Advances 2:19–28, 1985

Stroebe MS: Coping with bereavement: a review of the grief work hypothesis. Omega (Westport) 26:19–42, 1992–1993

Stroebe M[S], Schut H: The dual process model of coping with bereavement: rationale and description. Death Stud 23:197–224, 1999

Stroebe MS, Schut H: Models of coping with bereavement: a review, in Handbook of Bereavement Research: Consequences, Coping, and Care. Edited by Stroebe MS, Hansson RO, Stroebe W, et al. Washington, DC, American Psychological Association, 2001, pp 375–403

Stroebe M, Stroebe W: Who participates in bereavement research? a review and empirical study. Omega (Westport) 20:1–29, 1989

Stroebe MS, Stroebe W: The mortality of bereavement: a review, in Handbook of Bereavement. Edited by Stroebe MS, Stroebe W, Hansson R. Cambridge, UK, Cambridge University Press, 1993, pp 175–195

Stroebe MS, Hansson RO, Stroebe W, et al: Introduction: concepts and issues in contemporary research on bereavement, in Handbook of Bereavement Research: Consequences, Coping, and Care. Edited by Stroebe MS, Hansson RO, Stroebe W, et al. Washington, DC, American Psychological Association, 2001, pp 3–22

Stroebe W, Schut H, Stroebe MS: Grief work, disclosure and counseling: do they help the bereaved? Clin Psychol Rev 25:395–414, 2005

Sullivan MJ, Mikail S, Weinshenker B. Coping with a diagnosis of multiple sclerosis. Can J Behav Sci 29:249–257, 1997

Thompson LW, Breckenridge JN, Gallagher D, et al: Effects of bereavement on self-perceptions of physical health in elderly widows and widowers. J Gerontol 39:309–314, 1984

Thompson LW, Gallagher-Thompson D, Futterman A, et al: The effects of late-life spousal bereavement over a 30-month interval. Psychol Aging 6:434–441, 1991

U.S. Census Bureau: Current Population Survey Report. Marital and Living Arrangements: March 1998 (Update) (P20-514). Available at http://www.census.gov/prod/99pubs/p20-514u.pdf. Accessed November 3, 2003.

Viney L: The construing widow: dislocation and adaptation in bereavement. Psychotherapy Patient 6:207–222, 1990

Wijngaards-de Meij L, Stroebe M, Schut H, et al: Couples at risk following the death of their child: predictors of grief versus depression. J Consult Clin Psychol 73:617–623, 2005

Wikan U: Bereavement and loss in two Muslim communities: Egypt and Bali compared. Soc Sci Med 27:451–460, 1988

Windholz MJ, Weiss DS, Horowitz MJ: An empirical study of the natural history of time-limited psychotherapy for stress response syndromes. Psychotherapy: Theory, Research, Practice, Training 22:547–554, 1985

Wisocki PA, Skowron J: The effects of gender and culture on adjustment to widowhood, in Handbook of Gender, Culture, and Health. Edited by Eisler RM, Hersen M. Mahwah, NJ, Erlbaum, 2000, pp 429–448

Worden JW: Grief Counseling and Grief Therapy, 2nd Edition. New York, Springer, 1991

Wortman C, Silver RC: Coping with irrevocable loss, in Cataclysms, Crises, and Catastrophes: Psychology in Action. Edited by VandenBos G, Bryant B. Washington, DC, American Psychological Association, 1987, pp 185–235

Wortman C, Silver RC: The myths of coping with loss. J Consult Clin Psychol 57:349–357, 1989

Wrenn RL, Zylicz Z, Balk DE: Hospice care and the bereavement process in two countries: experience from the United States and the Netherlands. Illness, Crisis & Loss 9:173–189, 2001

Zisook S, Shuchter SR: Time course of spousal bereavement. Gen Hosp Psychiatry 7:95–100, 1985

Zisook S, Shuchter SR: The first four years of widowhood. Psychiatr Ann 15:288–294, 1986

Study Questions

Select the single best response for each question.

1. Bereavement is a common focus of clinical inquiry in geropsychiatry. The epidemiology of partner loss as a locus for bereavement has led to some conclusions that are of interest to the practicing clinician. Which of the following is true regarding widowhood and widowerhood in the United States?

    A. The mean age of spousal loss is 69 years for women and 66 years for men.
    B. The mean duration of widowhood is longer than the mean duration of widowerhood.
    C. The rates of widowhood among persons older than 65 are much higher for Hispanic and Asian Americans than for Caucasians.
    D. Among those older than 65, about 15% of women have lost a spouse.
    E. None of the above.

2. Stroebe and Schut are notable for their recent work on a dual-process model of bereavement. According to this model, which of the following is considered to be a restoration-oriented rather than a loss-oriented stressor?

    A. Emotional symptoms.
    B. Behavioral symptoms.
    C. New identity development.
    D. Physiological symptoms.
    E. Cognitive symptoms.

3. In clinical classification of cases that present with depressive symptoms in the context of interpersonal loss or grief, the physician often faces the task of deciding when symptoms cross the threshold of becoming complicated bereavement. This distinction is not always simple. To address this, DSM-IV-TR includes several specific symptoms that are not considered to be characteristic of a "normal" grief reaction. Which of the following symptoms would *not* be considered evidence of complicated bereavement?

    A. Guilt about actions not taken at the time of death.
    B. Preoccupation with personal worthlessness.
    C. Marked psychomotor retardation.
    D. Prolonged and marked functional impairment.
    E. Hallucinations not containing imagery of the dead person.

4. Several longitudinal studies of late-life bereavement have revealed some specific findings. Which of the following is true?

    A. Symptoms of anxiety and depression among bereaved subjects differ from controls only in the first 2 months following the loss.
    B. All studies have shown a higher psychological symptom burden among bereaved men than among bereaved women.
    C. When separated operationally from other symptoms such as anxiety and depression, grief has been found to remain for longer time periods.
    D. Women have been found to have higher rates of persistent grief than men.
    E. Older women who have lost their spouses have a higher risk of death than older bereaved men.

5. Which of the following is true regarding clinical interventions for complicated bereavement in older patients?

   A. If depression is present, it should not be treated first. The grieving process must first be addressed.
   B. Even if major depression is present, it should not be treated for at least 6 months.
   C. Since most deaths of elderly patients are due to chronic illness, posttraumatic stress disorder in survivors is rare.
   D. Combined pharmacological and psychotherapeutic treatment has been shown to be more effective than either intervention alone.
   E. Bereavement-related anxiety disorders are rare.

Sleep and Circadian Rhythm Disorders

Andrew D. Krystal, M.D., M.S.

Jack D. Edinger, Ph.D.

William K. Wohlgemuth, Ph.D.

Joseph M. Sharpe, M.D.

Sleep disorders are an important aspect of geriatric psychiatry. In the United States, more than half of noninstitutionalized individuals older than 65 years report chronic sleep difficulties (Foley et al. 1995; "National Institutes of Health Consensus Development Conference Statement" 1991; Prinz et al. 1990). Sleep disturbances affect quality of life, increase the risk of accidents and falls, and, perhaps most importantly, are among the leading reasons for long-term-care placement (Pollack and Perlick 1991; Pollack et al. 1990; Sanford 1975). Working effectively with elderly individuals requires expertise in the diagnosis and treatment of sleep disorders.

Reviewing the basic nomenclature used to describe sleep disorders provides a first step in understanding sleep disorders in the elderly. The major disorders of sleep are typically divided into three groups: 1) difficulties in initiating and maintaining sleep (insomnias); 2) disorders of excessive daytime sleepiness; and 3) disorders of cir-

cadian rhythm. Insomnias are characterized by complaints of sustained difficulty in initiating or maintaining sleep and/or complaints of nonrestorative sleep, along with significant distress or impairment in daytime function (American Psychiatric Association 2000; American Sleep Disorders Association 1997). These disorders are frequently classified as either *primary insomnia* (in which no underlying psychiatric or medical disorder is associated with the condition) or *secondary insomnia* (in which a psychiatric or medical disorder is etiologically related to the sleep disturbance) (American Psychiatric Association 2000).

Disorders of excessive daytime sleepiness are characterized by persistent daytime sleepiness that causes significant distress or impairment in function (American Psychiatric Association 2000; American Sleep Disorders Association 1997). The most important disorders of excessive sleepiness are sleep apnea, periodic limb movement disorder (PLMD), and narco-lepsy.

Circadian rhythm disorders manifest as a misalignment between an individual's sleep-wake cycle and the pattern that is desired or required (American Psychiatric Association 2000; American Sleep Disorders Association 1997). Affected individuals report that they cannot sleep at the times when sleep is desired, needed, or expected and that they fall asleep at times when wakefulness is desired, needed, or expected. The circadian rhythm is important for function because it is a cycle not only of sleep and wakefulness but also of many physiological processes and phenomena, including body temperature, alertness, cognitive performance, and hormone release (Czeisler et al. 1990; Folkard and Totterdell 1994; Minors et al. 1994).

Despite the variety and differing pathophysiologies of sleep disorders, the incidence of nearly all these disorders increases with age. The majority of age-related changes in sleep appear to stem from an increased incidence of sleep disturbances that lead to secondary sleep-related symptoms such as sleep apnea, PLMD, and medical and psychiatric disorders (Bliwise 1993; Foley et al. 1995; Gislason and Almqvist 1987; Prinz 1995; Prinz et al. 1990). Yet evidence shows that in healthy elderly individuals without such disorders, changes in sleep and the circadian rhythm occur (Bliwise 1993; Foley et al. 1995; Gislason and Almqvist 1987; Prinz 1995; Prinz et al. 1990). Given that these changes are not necessarily associated with complaints of sleep disturbance or diminished daytime function, sleep and circadian rhythm disturbances may not be an inevitable consequence of aging. These factors provide some challenges for clinical care. One of these challenges is the need to use a different threshold for normality in elderly patients. Sleep attributes that are considered abnormal in a younger individual may not be as-

sociated with symptoms in an elderly person. Furthermore, clinical care of the elderly population requires a heightened awareness of and expertise in identifying underlying medical and psychiatric disorders.

Although these challenges can be formidable, they are not insurmountable. In this chapter, we first review the changes in sleep and circadian rhythm that occur in individuals without medical and psychiatric disorders. We then review the disorders that can cause disturbances of sleep and chronobiology and whose likelihood increases with age. Finally, we discuss treatment of elderly individuals with a sleep complaint or suspected sleep-related dysfunction.

Influence of Aging on Sleep and Circadian Functions

Since the 1970s, extensive research has shown that marked changes in sleep and circadian rhythm accompany aging. Normative data derived from adults without complaints of sleep disturbance have implied that marked changes in the duration, continuity, and depth of nocturnal sleep accompany normal aging (Hirshkowitz et al. 1992).

Nocturnal sleep time steadily decreases across the life span, and nocturnal wake time increases, because of an increase in arousals. Accompanying these changes are marked reductions in Stage III and IV sleep (these stages are the deeper stages of non–rapid eye movement [REM] sleep). Although the clinical significance of these changes is unknown, they may relate to the reported reduction in subjective sleep quality and lowering of the arousal threshold with age (Riedel and Lichstein 1998; Zepelin et al. 1984).

The sleep-wake cycle appears to change significantly with age as well. The amplitudes of both the sleep-wake cycle and the

24-hour body temperature rhythm appear to decrease with aging (Bliwise 2000; Czeisler et al. 1999). Additionally, compared with younger age groups, older adults tend to awaken at an earlier phase (i.e., closer to the nadir of their 24-hour temperature rhythms), and they show a greater propensity to awaken during the later portions of their sleep episodes (Dijk et al. 1997; Duffy et al. 1998). Furthermore, multiple psychosocial changes that accompany aging may alter or eliminate important zeitgebers or time markers for the circadian system and promote the onset of sleep difficulties among older adults.

Disorders That Cause Sleep and Circadian Rhythm Disturbances

A number of medical and psychiatric conditions cause sleep difficulties and occur more frequently as age increases.

Primary Sleep Disorders

Sleep Apnea

In patients with sleep apnea, breathing ceases for periods of 10 seconds or more (Aldrich 2000), either because no effort is made to breathe (central sleep apnea) or because the oropharynx collapses during attempts to breathe (obstructive sleep apnea). The predominant type of sleep apnea seen in elderly individuals is obstructive sleep apnea (Ancoli-Israel et al. 1987). A number of studies suggest that the frequency of obstructive sleep apnea increases with age (Ancoli-Israel 1989; Ancoli-Israel et al. 1991; Dickel and Mosko 1990; Roehrs et al. 1983). Apnea generally causes excessive sleepiness, although mild to moderate apnea can be associated with insomnia. Referral to a sleep disorders specialist is required for diagnosis and treatment.

Periodic Limb Movement Disorder and Restless Legs Syndrome

In periodic limb movement disorder (PLMD), repetitive muscular contractions occur during sleep; these contractions most commonly involve the legs and often cause sleep disturbances. When these events occur infrequently, they are not considered pathological, because they tend not to be associated with any symptoms (Roehrs et al. 1983). The frequency of these events is characterized in terms of the number of movements associated with arousal that occur per hour of sleep (the movement-arousal index). There is some debate about what movement-arousal index is abnormal. Thresholds ranging from 5 to 15 movements per hour have been suggested (Ancoli-Israel et al. 1991; Dickel and Mosko 1990). Some authors have suggested that a higher threshold for abnormality should be applied to elderly patients, who tend to be symptom free at movement-arousal indices typically associated with significant symptoms in younger individuals (Ancoli-Israel 1989). Perhaps even more relevant for those working with elderly patients is that PLMD, like sleep apnea, is more prevalent in the elderly population (Roehrs et al. 1983). Several studies indicate that clinically significant PLMD is seen in 30%–45% of adults age 60 years or older, compared with 5%–6% of all adults (Ancoli-Israel et al. 1991).

Individuals with PLMD may complain of leg kicks (most commonly noticed by the bed partner), cold feet, excessive daytime sleepiness, and insomnia (Ancoli-Israel 1989; Ancoli-Israel et al. 1991; Roehrs et al. 1983). The insomnia may be characterized by difficulty in falling asleep or staying asleep (Ancoli-Israel 1989). Unfortunately, the presence of this disease is difficult to reliably predict based on the patient's history (Ancoli-Israel 1989; Dickel and Mosko 1990). Furthermore, a high level of confidence in the diagnosis is needed before institution of treatment, because treatment typically involves long-term use of medications that can have significant side effects (see "Pharmacological Treatment" later in this chapter). Therefore, when a history is suggestive of PLMD, standard practice is to make a referral for a polysomnogram for definitive diagnosis (Ancoli-Israel 1989). Polysomnography is also indicated when an individual has significant insomnia or hypersomnia that does not respond to usual treatment. Such a patient may have significant PLMD that was undetected when the patient's history was obtained.

Restless legs syndrome (RLS) is often associated with PLMD and is described as an uncomfortable feeling in the lower extremities that creates an irresistible urge to move. RLS occurs in 6% of the adult population and is present in up to 28% of patients older than 65 years (Clark 2001). Polysomnography is not needed for a diagnosis of RLS, which is made through history taking.

When compared in the general population, RLS is almost twice as prevalent in elderly women as elderly men. RLS, as well as PLMD, has been associated with anemia (O'Keeffe et al. 1994). In elderly patients, ferritin levels less than 45 μg/L have a positive correlation with an increased risk of RLS, and such patients often benefit from administration of supplemental iron (O'Keeffe et al. 1994). Also associated with PLMD and RLS are diabetes mellitus, pregnancy, iron deficiency anemia, and use of certain medications, including antidepressants (Bliwise et al. 1985). Workup to exclude these conditions is typically carried out before initiating medication treatment.

The same medications are effective for both RLS and PLMD. They include anticonvulsants, benzodiazepines, dopaminergic agonists, and opiates. Many practitio-

ners use gabapentin and clonazepam as first-line agents because of the drugs' relatively favorable side-effect profiles; however, dopaminergic agonists appear to be the most effective medications. Opiates are typically reserved for patients who fail to respond to these other drugs.

Neuropsychiatric Disorders

Bereavement

Psychological factors that most commonly affect sleep in elderly persons are reactions to loss, such as loss of health or functional capacity, and reactions to the death of a friend or loved one. Although bereavement is normal, it is often associated with substantial sleep disturbance (American Psychiatric Association 2000). When bereavement is associated with more frequent intrusive thoughts and avoidance behaviors, there appears to be more sleep disturbance, predominantly in the form of difficulty in falling asleep (Hall et al. 1997). Bereavement and depression are closely linked, however. Depression is usually diagnosed only when symptoms have persisted for more than 2 months after a loss or when symptoms are severe, such as suicidal ideation, psychotic symptoms, malnutrition, or dehydration (American Psychiatric Association 2000). Antidepressant medication may be helpful.

Major Depression

Depression is a frequent cause of sleep disruption in individuals older than 60 years. Roughly 10%–15% of individuals older than 65 years experience clinically significant depressive symptoms (Hoch et al. 1989). The most frequent complaints in affected individuals are 1) a decrease in total sleep time and 2) waking earlier than desired. Daytime sleepiness may occur but is usually better characterized as fatigue.

Treatment of insomnia in individuals with major depression should always involve use of antidepressant medication. Administration of a sedating antidepressant is desirable for addressing the insomnia (see "Pharmacological Treatment" later in this chapter), but the drug may not be tolerated because of side effects. Whether to administer sedative-hypnotic medication along with a nonsedating antidepressant is a subject of debate. During treatment, the hope is that the insomnia will be short-lived and it will be possible to taper the sedative-hypnotic medication when other symptoms of depression begin to improve. Antidepressants may themselves cause sleep disturbance (Asnis et al. 1999). One study found that zolpidem 10 mg administered for 4 weeks to a nongeriatric population was highly effective and safe, with only 1 night of rebound insomnia after abrupt discontinuation (Asnis et al. 1999). Longer-term use for treatment of elderly patients has not been studied. In general, it is better to avoid use of sedative-hypnotic medication if possible and to consider behavioral therapy (see "Cognitive-Behavioral Therapy" later in this chapter).

Alzheimer's Disease

Individuals with Alzheimer's disease have been found to experience an increased number of arousals and awakenings, to take more daytime naps, and to have a diminished amount of REM sleep and slow-wave sleep (Prinz et al. 1982). Individuals with dementia often experience evening or nocturnal agitation and confusion. This phenomenon, called *sundowning*, is among the leading reasons that individuals with dementia become institutionalized (Pollack and Perlick 1991; Pollack et al. 1990; Sanford 1975). The pathophysiology of sundowning is poorly understood. A number of features appear to increase the risk of sundowning, including greater dementia severity, pain, fecal impaction, malnutri-

tion, polypharmacy, infections, REM sleep behavior disorder, PLMD, and environmental sleep disruptions (Bliwise 2000).

Treatment of sundowning should begin with an assessment for such conditions. If no causative condition can be found, or if attempts to eliminate the cause are unsuccessful, treatment should be instituted. Nonmedication management includes light therapy, elimination of daytime napping, and a structured activity program (Bliwise 2000). More research is needed to determine the efficacy of these interventions.

Medication management of sundowning is also an area in which more research is needed. Several studies have examined the use of benzodiazepines for the treatment of sleep problems in patients with Alzheimer's disease and sundowning, and these studies suggest that benzodiazepines are ineffective (Bliwise 2000). Atypical benzodiazepines (nonbenzodiazepine omega-1 benzodiazepine receptor agonists) have been prescribed to treat insomnia (see "Pharmacological Treatment" later in this chapter). Of the atypical benzodiazepines currently available in the United States to treat insomnia, zaleplon and zolpidem, only a preliminary study of zolpidem has been carried out, and the study findings suggest that it may have some efficacy (Shaw et al. 1992).

Of all medications prescribed for sundowning, antipsychotic medications have the most evidence of efficacy (Bliwise 2000). Most studies involved older agents. Newer antipsychotics, such as risperidone, olanzapine, and quetiapine, have fewer side effects and are generally recommended (Bliwise 2000); however, studies of these medications are needed. Preliminary data suggest that melatonin may also have some utility. Clearly, more research is needed to address the highly important and difficult-to-treat problem of sleep disorders in patients with Alzheimer's disease.

Parkinson's Disease

Sleep complaints are noted in 60%–90% of individuals with Parkinson's disease (Trenkwalder 1998). The majority of Parkinson's disease patients with affected sleep experience difficulty in initiating and maintaining sleep, daytime fatigue, RLS, and an inability to turn over in bed. The last of these features was rated as the most troublesome symptom of sleep disturbance in a study by Lees et al. (1988). Another sleep problem seen in patients with Parkinson's disease is REM sleep behavior disorder, in which the patient acts out dreams because the paralysis that usually occurs during REM sleep is absent (Clarenbach 2000). Dopaminergic medications used to treat Parkinson's disease, such as carbidopa/levodopa, may contribute to sleep initiation problems and sleep difficulties in the first half of the night and may cause nightmares (Trenkwalder 1998). No study findings indicate how to manage sleep difficulties in patients with Parkinson's disease.

Medical Conditions

Pain

Pain is a central feature of many medical conditions that occur with increased frequency in elderly individuals; these conditions include arthritis, neuropathies, angina, reflux esophagitis, and peptic ulcer disease (Aldrich 2000). Disruption of sleep is frequently noted in persons with significant pain (Pilowsky et al. 1985). Attempts to ameliorate the condition causing the pain should be the first step. When these attempts fail, treatment for the pain should be instituted. Often, combined behavioral and pharmacological treatment is needed. When treatment of the pain does not eliminate the sleeping difficulty, treatment for the insomnia should be instituted (see section "Treatment of Insomnia" later in this chapter).

Chronic Obstructive Pulmonary Disease

Individuals with chronic obstructive pulmonary disease (COPD) have been found to have both subjective and objective evidence of disturbed sleep, but the degree of sleep disruption is unrelated to hypoxemia (Douglas 2000). Also, daytime sleepiness, which is seen in patients with sleep apnea, does not appear to occur. Polysomnography is not routinely indicated for individuals with COPD who have sleep difficulties (Connaughton et al. 1988). Sleep apnea appears to be no more common in persons with COPD than in the general population.

Oral theophyllines, which are frequently used in COPD treatment, are adenosine receptor antagonists and may have a sleep-disruptive effect (Douglas 2000). Also, patients with COPD should be instructed to avoid alcohol, which can exacerbate hypoxemia and promote other complications. Benzodiazepines should be used with great caution because they may increase inhibition of ventilatory responses and may worsen nocturnal hypoxemia (Douglas 2000). The effects of nonbenzodiazepine sedatives on COPD have not been determined, but these drugs should be used cautiously.

Nocturia

The urge to urinate is an often overlooked cause of awakenings in the elderly population (Bliwise 2000). Surprisingly, it has been reported that nocturia (excessive urination at night) is the most common explanation given by elderly individuals for difficulty in maintaining sleep; 63%–72% of elderly persons cite nocturia as a reason for sleep maintenance problems (Middelkoop et al. 1996). Furthermore, several studies have documented the sleep disturbance caused by and daytime adverse effects of nocturia (Bliwise 2000). The most common causes of nocturia are conditions that increase in frequency with age: benign prostatic hypertrophy in men and decreased urethral resistance due to decreased estrogen levels in women (Bliwise 2000). Sleep apnea, which also increases in prevalence in the elderly population, can also lead to nocturia (Bliwise 2000).

Menopause

Despite the enormous number of individuals with menopause-related sleep difficulties, there is a striking lack of research in this area (Krystal et al. 1998). There appears to be evidence that many women experience sleep disruption in association with vasomotor symptoms (night sweats, hot flushes) (Bliwise 2000; Krystal et al. 1998). However, many disorders that cause insomnia are highly prevalent during the period in which women experience menopausal changes. Hormone replacement therapy often does not ameliorate the sleep disturbance (Krystal et al. 1998). It has been suggested that the insomnia is perpetuated by behavioral conditioning (Krystal et al. 1998).

Elderly women with insomnia should be evaluated to determine whether there is an association between changes in menstrual periods, vasomotor symptoms, and insomnia symptoms. If an association between insomnia and menopausal changes appears to exist, a trial of hormone replacement therapy could be considered. If hormone replacement therapy is contraindicated, or use of this treatment is not preferred, other treatments such as pharmacological management of insomnia or cognitive-behavioral sleep therapy should be considered (see discussions in "Pharmacological Treatment" and "Cognitive-Behavioral Therapy" later in this chapter). If hormone replacement therapy ameliorates vasomotor symptoms but insomnia complaints persist, behavioral therapy should be considered.

Loss of Hearing, Vision, and Mobility

Many elderly individuals experience decrements in hearing, vision, and mobility, resulting in attempts to sleep more than needed in order to pass the time. The result is fragmentation of sleep and loss of circadian rhythmicity. Although this problem should be easily solved by increasing activity and developing new activity options, in practice, making these changes is difficult to achieve.

Treatment of Insomnia

Cognitive-Behavioral Therapy

Myriad lifestyle changes that accompany aging increase risks of insomnia among older adults (Morgan 2000). With aging comes the increased incidence of infirmities that lead to reduced activity levels and a general flattening of the sleep-wake activity rhythm. Retirement leads to increased vacant time and a loss of both routine and zeitgebers that regulate and stabilize the sleep-wake cycle. Retirement coupled with loss of a spouse may lead to dramatically reduced social contacts and increased boredom. Many individuals attempt to reduce hours of daytime boredom by daytime napping and by staying in bed longer during their nighttime sleep period. Such practices often lead to increased nocturnal wake time. Dysfunctional beliefs about sleep, such as "everyone should try to get 8 hours a night" and "older adults can do little to improve their sleep," may actually perpetuate sleep difficulties over time (Means and Edinger 2002; Morin et al. 1993). Nonpharmacological interventions that address these misconceptions and the sleep-disruptive habits they sustain are often useful for combating insomnia in older patients.

Currently, a range of behavioral interventions are available for treating these patients, including relaxation therapies, cognitive therapies, and treatments that target disruptive sleep habits. Among the more effective of these interventions is *stimulus control therapy*, which was developed by Bootzin (1972). This treatment is particularly useful for older adults who have fallen out of a normal sleep-wake routine and for those who compromise their nighttime sleep by excessive daytime napping. Stimulus control therapy addresses such problems by curtailing daytime napping and by enforcing a consistent sleep-wake schedule. In addition, this treatment enhances sleep-inducing qualities of the bedroom by eliminating sleep-incompatible behaviors in bed. The patient with insomnia is instructed to go to bed only when sleepy; establish a standard wake-up time; get out of bed whenever he or she is awake for more than 15–20 minutes; avoid reading, watching TV, eating, worrying, and engaging in other sleep-incompatible behaviors in the bed and bedroom; and refrain from daytime napping. This treatment has appeal because it is easily understood and usually can be outlined in one visit. However, follow-up visits are usually needed to assure compliance and achieve optimal success.

Because older adults appear to have a reduced homeostatic sleep drive (Dijk et al. 1997) as well as a propensity to spend excessive time in bed (Carskadon et al. 1982), measures are often needed to reduce the amount of time older patients with insomnia routinely allot for nocturnal sleep. Such a reduction is the aim of *sleep restriction therapy* (Spielman et al. 1987). Typically, this treatment begins with the patient maintaining a sleep log. After 2–3 weeks, the average total sleep time (TST) is calculated. Subsequently, an initial time-in-bed (TIB) prescription may be set either at the average TST or at a value equal to the average TST plus an amount of time that is deemed to represent normal nocturnal wakefulness (e.g., 30 minutes). However, unless evidence suggests that the individual has an unusually low sleep requirement, the initial TIB prescription is seldom set at less than 5 hours per night. The TIB prescription is increased by 15- to 20-minute increments after weeks in which the person with insomnia sleeps more than 85%–90% of the TIB, on average, and continues to report daytime sleepiness. Conversely, TIB is usually reduced by similar increments after weeks in which the individual sleeps less than 80% of the time spent in bed, on average. Because TIB adjustments are usually necessary, sleep restriction therapy typically entails an initial visit, when treatment instructions are given, and follow-up visits, when TIB prescriptions are altered.

Research suggests that stimulus control and sleep restriction therapies are more effective than most other nonpharmacological interventions (Morin et al. 1999; Murtagh and Greenwood 1995). Moreover, a recent meta-analytic comparison suggests that behavioral therapies compare favorably with hypnotic pharmacotherapies in terms of short-term treatment effects and, unlike hypnotics, have enduring benefits and few side effects (Smith et al. 2002). Recent clinical trials have also generally suggested that therapies combining stimulus control, sleep restriction, and cognitive strategies to alter dysfunctional, sleep-related beliefs hold particular promise for treatment of the sleep maintenance difficulties so common in older age groups (Edinger et al. 2001; Morin et al. 1999). Given such findings, behavioral interventions should be included in treatment plans for older patients with insomnia, particularly when improper sleep scheduling and other lifestyle factors contribute to sleep complaints.

TABLE 13–1. Attributes of medications used to treat insomnia

	Half-life (hours)	Principal side effects
Benzodiazepines	2.9–74[a]	Motor and cognitive impairment
Zolpidem	2.6 ± 1	Motor and cognitive impairment (less than with benzodiazepine use)
Zaleplon	1	Motor and cognitive impairment (less than with benzodiazepine use)
Tricyclic antidepressants	12–43	Anticholinergic effects, weight gain, orthostatic hypotension, sexual dysfunction
Trazodone	11 ± 5	Orthostatic hypotension, priapism (rare)
Mirtazapine	20–40	Dry mouth, weight gain
Nefazodone	17 ± 6	Dry mouth, dizziness
Diphenhydramine	4 ± 2	Anticholinergic effects, motor impairment
Chloral hydrate	7 ± 3	Alcohol interaction, gastric irritation, motor and cognitive impairment, respiratory depression at high doses

[a]Benzodiazepine half-lives (hours): flurazepam = 74 ± 24; diazepam = 43 ± 13; quazepam = 39; lorazepam = 14 ± 5; estazolam = 12 ± 12; temazepam = 11 ± 6; triazolam = 2.9 ± 1.
Source. Golden et al. 1998; Hobbs et al. 1996; Physicians' Desk Reference 2002; Potter et al. 1998.

Pharmacological Treatment

The decision to prescribe medications for the treatment of insomnia should involve weighing the risks and benefits associated with medication management versus the risks and benefits of other options.

Once the decision has been made to use medications to treat insomnia, a number of factors should be considered. Different types of medications are used to treat insomnia. These drugs have different mechanisms of action and differ significantly in their attributes. The predominant medications include benzodiazepines, non-benzodiazepine omega-1 receptor agonists (sometimes referred to as *atypical benzodiazepines*, the term used throughout this chapter), antidepressants, antihistamines (most commonly, diphenhydramine), and chloral hydrate.

Nearly all medications approved by the U.S. Food and Drug Administration (FDA)

for the treatment of insomnia are related to benzodiazepine receptors. The efficacy of these medications has been demonstrated in a number of studies (Nowell et al. 1997). Currently, the most commonly prescribed medications are the atypical benzodiazepines. Although not FDA-approved for the treatment of insomnia, sedating antidepressant medications are also frequently used (Walsh and Engelhardt 1992). Factors to be considered when choosing medications include half-life and side effects (see Table 13–1 for comparison of these factors by drug and drug class).

The fact that the most commonly prescribed medications, atypical benzodiazepines, have the shortest half-lives reflects an appreciation that the ideal sedative-hypnotic agent acts during the desired sleep period and has no effect after this period. Nearly all the older drugs have longer half-lives, increasing the risk of daytime impairment. Furthermore, problems with daytime impairment with these long-half-life medications are exacerbated in the elderly, who tend to metabolize drugs more slowly.

Of the medications most frequently used to treat insomnia, zaleplon has the shortest half-life, and therefore this drug is well suited for treating problems falling asleep. Because of its short half-life, zaleplon may also be useful in the middle of the night for individuals who sometimes wake up at that time (Stone et al. 2002). For some individuals, the effects of zaleplon are too short-lived to address their sleep difficulties, and zolpidem, which has a longer half-life, may be helpful. The need for a longer-acting agent may be particularly likely with elderly individuals, who tend to be particularly prone to difficulty in staying asleep (see "Influence of Aging on Sleep and Circadian Functions" earlier in this chapter).

Medication-caused motor impairment is a particular concern in the elderly population. A risk of falls and associated fractures can occur 1) between the time of taking medication and getting into bed; 2) when the individual gets up in the middle of the night to use the bathroom (or for other reasons); and 3) the following day, in the case of long-half-life drugs. For this reason, it is best to avoid prescribing benzodiazepines and any medication that causes motor impairment or, if use of such drugs is absolutely necessary, to prescribe as low a dose as possible, which will decrease the risk of falls. Furthermore, it is important to warn patients of the possibility of being unsteady on their feet when they are taking a medication that may cause this side effect; patients can then take precautions.

Similarly, many elderly individuals with insomnia have coexisting memory impairment that may be exacerbated by sedative-hypnotic medications. As a result, it is best to avoid using medications with memory impairment as a side effect, if possible, and

to use the lowest dose possible in all circumstances. The anticholinergic effects of some antidepressants and diphenhydramine may also exacerbate memory difficulties, and these drugs are not tolerated well by elderly individuals prone to constipation.

In summary, medications may be needed for primary and secondary insomnia when other treatment options are not effective. In elderly patients, it is generally best to use short-half-life drugs; however, drugs with longer half-lives are sometimes needed if difficulty in staying asleep, a particular problem in the elderly population, is not adequately addressed. It is best to avoid using medications that cause motor and cognitive impairment, and it is generally best to start with lower doses than used in nonelderly adults.

Conclusion

Management of sleep disorders in elderly patients is challenging. Although sleep disorders are not an inevitable consequence of aging, elderly persons are more prone to primary sleep disorders and medical and psychiatric conditions that cause sleep difficulties. Therefore, evaluation of a sleep complaint in an elderly individual should include a thorough workup to determine whether primary sleep pathology and associated psychiatric and medical disorders are present. Effective behavioral and medication treatments exist for treating sleep and circadian rhythm disorders in elderly patients, but these treatments have significant limitations. More research is needed to develop and assess nonmedication therapies that are effective in treating insomnia and normalizing the circadian rhythm.

In addition, research to improve medication treatment is needed. Medications are needed that can help elderly individuals stay asleep and that do so without causing next-day sedation. Furthermore, medications are needed that do not cause motor or cognitive impairment or anticholinergic side effects and that are not associated with tolerance, dependence, or withdrawal problems. Controlled studies of the long-term safety and efficacy of the atypical benzodiazepines are needed. Also, few studies of the efficacy and safety of antidepressants as sedative-hypnotics have been carried out; such studies are also needed. New sedative-hypnotic drugs under development include compounds that are unrelated to benzodiazepine receptors. Such compounds may be free of typical benzodiazepine effects, including motor and cognitive impairment, tolerance, dependence, and withdrawal symptoms.

References

Aldrich MS: Cardinal manifestations of sleep disorders, in Principles and Practice of Sleep Medicine, 3rd Edition. Edited by Kryger MH, Roth T, Dement WC. Philadelphia, PA, WB Saunders, 2000, pp 526–534

American Psychiatric Association: Diagnostic and Statistical Manual of Mental Disorders, 4th Edition, Text Revision. Washington, DC, American Psychiatric Association, 2000

American Sleep Disorders Association: The International Classification of Sleep Disorders: Diagnostic and Coding Manual, Revised Edition. Rochester, MN, American Sleep Disorders Association, 1997

Ancoli-Israel S: Epidemiology of sleep disorders. Clin Geriatr Med 5:347–362, 1989

Ancoli-Israel S, Kripke DF, Mason W: Characteristics of obstructive and central sleep apnea in the elderly: an interim report. Biol Psychiatry 22:741–750, 1987

Ancoli-Israel S, Kripke D, Klauber M, et al: Periodic limb movements in sleep in the community-dwelling elderly. Sleep 14:496–500, 1991

Asnis GM, Chakraburtty A, DuBoff EA: Zolpidem for persistent insomnia in SSRI-treated depressed patients. J Clin Psychiatry 60:668–676, 1999

Bliwise DL: Sleep in normal aging and dementia. Sleep 16:40–81, 1993

Bliwise DL: Normal aging, in Principles and Practice of Sleep Medicine, 3rd Edition. Edited by Kryger MH, Roth T, Dement WC. Philadelphia, PA, WB Saunders, 2000, pp 26–42

Bliwise D[L], Petta D, Seidel W, et al: Periodic leg movements during sleep in the elderly. Arch Gerontol Geriatr 4:273–281, 1985

Bootzin RR: A stimulus control treatment for insomnia. Proc Am Psychol Assoc 7:395–396, 1972

Carskadon MA, Brown ED, Dement WC: Sleep fragmentation in the elderly: relationship to daytime sleep tendency. Neurobiol Aging 3:321–327, 1982

Clarenbach P: Parkinson's disease and sleep. J Neurol 247 (suppl 4):IV20–IV23, 2000

Clark MM: Restless legs syndrome. J Am Board Fam Pract 14:368–374, 2001

Connaughton JJ, Catterall JR, Elton RA, et al: Do sleep studies contribute to the management of patients with severe chronic obstructive pulmonary disease? Am Rev Respir Dis 138:341-344, 1988

Czeisler CA, Johnson MP, Duffy JF, et al: Exposure to bright light and darkness to treat physiologic maladaptation to night work. N Engl J Med 322:1253–1259, 1990

Czeisler CA, Duffy JF, Shanahan TL, et al: Stability, precision, and near-24-hour period of the human circadian pacemaker. Science 284:2177–2181, 1999

Dickel MJ, Mosko SS: Morbidity cut-offs for sleep apnea and periodic leg movements in predicting subjective complaints in seniors. Sleep 13:155–166, 1990

Dijk DJ, Duffy JF, Riel E, et al: Altered interaction of circadian and homeostatic aspects of sleep propensity results in awakening at an earlier circadian phase in older people. J Sleep Res 26:710, 1997

Douglas NJ: Chronic obstructive pulmonary disease, in Principles and Practice of Sleep Medicine, 3rd Edition. Edited by Kryger MH, Roth T, Dement WC. Philadelphia, PA, WB Saunders, 2000, pp 965–975

Duffy JF, Dijk DJ, Klerman EB, et al: Later endogenous circadian temperature nadir relative to an earlier wake time in older people. Am J Physiol 275:R1478–R1487, 1998

Edinger JD, Wohlgemuth WK, Radtke RA, et al: Cognitive behavioral therapy for treatment of chronic primary insomnia: a randomized controlled trial. JAMA 285:1856–1864, 2001

Foley DJ, Monjan AA, Brown SL, et al: Sleep complaints among elderly persons: an epidemiologic study of three communities. Sleep 18:425–432, 1995

Folkard S, Totterdell P: "Time since sleep" and "body clock" components of alertness and cognition. Acta Psychiatr Belg 94:73–74, 1994

Gislason T, Almqvist M: Somatic diseases and sleep complaints. An epidemiological study of 3,201 Swedish men. Acta Med Scand 221:475–481, 1987

Golden RN, Dawkins K, Nicholas L, et al: Trazodone, nefazodone, bupropion, and mirtazapine, in Textbook of Psychopharmacology, 2nd Edition. Edited by Schatzberg AF, Nemeroff CB. Washington, DC, American Psychiatric Press, 1998, pp 251–269

Hall M, Buysse DJ, Dew MA, et al: Intrusive thoughts and avoidance behaviors are associated with sleep disturbances in bereavement-related depression. Depress Anxiety 6:106–112, 1997

Hirshkowitz M, Moore CA, Hamilton C, et al: Polysomnography of adults and elderly: sleep architecture, respiration, and leg movement. J Clin Neurophysiol 9:56–62, 1992

Hobbs WR, Rall TW, Verdoorn TA: Hypnotics and sedatives; ethanol, in Goodman & Gilman's The Pharmacological Basis of Therapeutics, 9th Edition. Edited by Hardman JG, Limbird LE. New York, McGraw-Hill, 1996, pp 361–398

Hoch CC, Buysse DJ, Reynolds CF: Sleep and depression in late life. Clin Geriatr Med 5:259–272, 1989

Krystal AD, Edinger J, Wohlgemuth W, et al: Sleep in perimenopausal and postmenopausal women. Sleep Med Rev 2:243–253, 1998

Lees AJ, Blackburn NA, Campbell VL: The nighttime problems of Parkinson's disease. Clin Neuropharmacol 11:512–519, 1988

Means MK, Edinger JD: Behavioral treatment of insomnia. Expert Review of Neurotherapeutics 2:127–137, 2002

Middelkoop HA, Smilde-van den Doel DA, Neven AK, et al: Subjective sleep characteristics of 1,485 males and females aged 50–93: effects of sex and age and factors related to self-evaluated quality of sleep. J Gerontol A Biol Sci Med Sci 51:M108–M115, 1996

Minors DS, Waterhouse JM, Akerstedt T: The effect of the timing, quality, and quantity of sleep upon the depression (masking) of body temperature on an irregular sleep/wake schedule. J Sleep Res 3:45–51, 1994

Morgan K: Sleep and aging, in Treatment of Late-Life Insomnia. Edited by Lichstein KL, Morin CM. Thousand Oaks, CA, Sage, 2000, pp 3–36

Morin CM, Stone J, Trinkle D, et al: Dysfunctional beliefs and attitudes about sleep among older adults with and without insomnia complaints. Psychol Aging 8:463–467, 1993

Morin CM, Colecchi C, Stone J, et al: Behavioral and pharmacological therapies for late-life insomnia: a randomized controlled trial. JAMA 281:991–1035, 1999

Murtagh DR, Greenwood KM: Identifying effective psychological treatments for insomnia: a meta-analysis. J Consult Clin Psychol 63:79–89, 1995

National Institutes of Health Consensus Development Conference Statement: Treatment of sleep disorders in older people. Sleep 14:169–177, 1991

Nowell PD, Mazumdar S, Buysse DJ, et al: Benzodiazepines and zolpidem for chronic insomnia: a meta-analysis of treatment efficacy. JAMA 278:2170–2177, 1997

O'Keeffe ST, Gavin K, Lavan JN: Iron status and restless legs syndrome in the elderly. Age Ageing 23:200–203, 1994

Physicians' Desk Reference, 56th Edition. Montvale, NJ, Medical Economics, 2002

Pilowsky I, Crettenden I, Townley M: Sleep disturbance in pain clinic patients. Pain 23:27–33, 1985

Pollack CP, Perlick D: Sleep problems and institutionalization of the elderly. J Geriatr Psychiatry Neurol 4:204–210, 1991

Pollack CP, Perlick D, Lisner JP, et al: Sleep problems in the community elderly as predictors of death and nursing home placement. J Community Health 15:123–135, 1990

Potter WZ, Manji HK, Rudorfer MV: Tricyclics and tetracyclics, in The American Psychiatric Press Textbook of Psychopharmacology, 2nd Edition. Edited by Schatzberg AF, Nemeroff CB. Washington, DC, American Psychiatric Press, 1998, pp 239–250

Prinz PN: Sleep and sleep disorders in older adults. J Clin Neurophysiol 12:139–146, 1995

Prinz PN, Peskind ER, Vitaliano PP, et al: Changes in the sleep and waking EEGs of nondemented and demented elderly subjects. J Am Geriatr Soc 30:86–93, 1982

Prinz PN, Vitiello MV, Raskind MA, et al: Geriatrics: sleep disorders and aging. N Engl J Med 323:520–526, 1990

Riedel BW, Lichstein KL: Objective sleep measures and subjective sleep satisfaction: how do older adults with insomnia define a good night's sleep? Psychol Aging 13:159–163, 1998

Roehrs T, Zorick F, Sicklesteel J, et al: Age-related sleep-wake disorders at a sleep disorder center. J Am Geriatr Soc 31:364–370, 1983

Sanford JRA: Tolerance of debility in elderly dependants by supporters at home: its significance for hospital practice. Br Med J 3:471–473, 1975

Shaw SH, Curson H, Coquelin JP: A double-blind comparative study of zolpidem and placebo in the treatment of insomnia in elderly psychiatric inpatients. J Int Med Res 20:150–161, 1992

Smith MT, Perlis ML, Park A, et al: Comparative meta-analysis of pharmacotherapy and behavior therapy for persistent insomnia. Am J Psychiatry 159:5–11, 2002

Spielman AJ, Saskin P, Thorpy MJ: Treatment of chronic insomnia by restriction of time in bed. Sleep 10:45–55, 1987

Stone BM, Turner C, Mills SL, et al: Noise-induced sleep maintenance insomnia: hypnotic and residual effects of zaleplon. Br J Clin Pharmacol 53:196–202, 2002

Trenkwalder C: Sleep dysfunction in Parkinson's disease. Clin Neurosci 5:107–114, 1998

Walsh JK, Engelhardt CL: Trends in the pharmacologic treatment of insomnia. J Clin Psychiatry 53:10–17, 1992

Zepelin H, McDonald CS, Zammit GK: Effects of age on auditory awakening thresholds. J Gerontol 39:294–300, 1984

Study Questions

Select the single best response for each question.

1. Sleep disorders are an important and often obscure cause of clinical distress in elderly patients. As such, their full evaluation and thoughtful management may enhance patients' quality of life substantially. Which of the following is true?

   A. One-quarter of noninstitutionalized persons older than 65 report chronic sleep problems.
   B. Despite clinical distress due to sleep disorders, they are an infrequent reason for long-term care placement.
   C. Most age-related sleep disturbances are caused by primary, as opposed to secondary, sleep-related symptoms.
   D. Sleep and circadian rhythm changes in elderly patients are absent unless there is a sleep disorder.
   E. With increasing age, an increased number of arousals is causative in the increased amount of nocturnal wake time.

2. Sleep apnea (SA), periodic limb movement disorder (PLMD), and restless legs syndrome (RLS) are relatively commonly encountered in older patients. Which of the following is true?

   A. The more common form of SA in elderly patients is central rather than obstructive.
   B. SA, even in mild cases, is not associated with insomnia.
   C. Referral to a sleep disorder specialist is not required to diagnose SA.
   D. Clinically significant PLMD is five to six times more common in elderly patients, when compared to younger adults.
   E. Polysomnography is required for the diagnosis of both PLMD and RLS.

3. Alzheimer's disease and Parkinson's disease are associated with many neuropsychiatric complications. Among these is disturbed sleep; when sleep disturbance is associated with behavioral agitation, the term "sundowning" is used. Which of the following is true regarding sleep disorders and their management in these neurodegenerative conditions?

   A. Alzheimer's disease patients have increased arousals and awakenings, and increased amounts of REM and slow-wave sleep.
   B. Benzodiazepines are the treatment of choice for the sundowning in Alzheimer's disease.
   C. Antipsychotics may be helpful for the treatment of Alzheimer's disease patients with sundowning, and the atypical agents are generally well tolerated.
   D. Sleep complaints are notable in less than one-half of Parkinson's disease patients.
   E. Although carbidopa/levodopa combinations may cause initial insomnia, they do not increase risk of nightmares.

4. Comorbid medical conditions are common in older patients with sleep complaints, and the management of the chronic illness may be of great utility in assisting these patients. Which of the following is true for those patients with chronic obstructive pulmonary disease (COPD)?

   A. In COPD, the degree of sleep disruption is correlated with the degree of hypoxemia.
   B. Daytime sleepiness is typical in COPD.
   C. Polysomnography is routinely necessary to evaluate sleep complaints in COPD because sleep apnea is much more common in these patients.
   D. Oral theophyllines are adenosine receptor antagonists and may themselves disrupt sleep in COPD.
   E. Benzodiazepines are the treatment of choice for COPD patients with sleep complaints.

Alcohol and Drug Problems

Dan G. Blazer, M.D., Ph.D.

Paul D. Nagy, M.S.

The problems of alcohol and drug abuse in late life are closely related. Of the two, alcohol abuse is the more publicized but not necessarily the more prevalent. Misuse of both alcohol and drugs in the United States derives from the context of Western society. Primary care physicians and geriatric psychiatrists cannot diagnose or treat these disorders without appreciating the milieu from which they emerge and the factors that reinforce the behaviors.

Both alcohol and drug problems confront clinicians who treat older adults. Occasionally, medication and alcohol misuse or abuse is the primary problem encountered. More often, however, this problem accompanies other disorders and complicates therapy. In this chapter, alcohol and drug problems are reviewed separately because, although these disorders undoubtedly overlap, each has unique characteristics and deserves separate attention.

Alcohol Abuse and Dependence

Investigation of alcohol abuse and dependence among older adults has increased in recent years. The reason for this attention is not a dramatic or even a persistent increase in rates of alcohol problems in the elderly. As reviewed elsewhere in this volume (see Chapter 1, "Demography and Epidemiology of Psychiatric Disorders in Late Life"), the current prevalence of alcohol abuse and dependence for persons ages 65 years and older ranges from 1.9% to 4.6% for men and from 0.1% to 0.7% for women (Myers et al. 1984). In other cultures, rates may be higher. For example, among men age 70 years and older in Sweden, 10% abused alcohol or were heavy drinkers (Mellstrom 1981). Although no differences were found among racial and ethnic groups in the Epidemiologic Catchment Area (ECA) studies (Myers et al. 1984), some studies suggested that rates are higher in older whites than in older African Americans (Ruchlin 1997). In the United States, even the lifetime prevalence of alcohol problems in older adults is lower than for younger persons in the population. This finding may partially be explained by cohort differences in drinking experiences and selective survival of more moderate drinkers. It is anticipated that with the increase of life expectancy rates and the aging of baby boomers, there will be an overall increase in alcohol problems among older adults, given the increase in alcohol problems throughout the population (Liberto et al. 1992).

Another point to consider is the increased probability of alcohol-related problems in later life, even at lower levels of use. Saunders (1994) reported that 15% of men and 12% of women older than age 60 treated in primary care clinics drank in excess of the limits recommended by the National Institute on Alcohol Abuse and Alcoholism (NIAAA). The risk factors for alcohol abuse in elderly persons are similar to those for the general population—male gender, poor education, low income, and a history of other psychiatric disorders, especially depression. The comorbidity of alcohol problems and psychiatric illness in late life is 10%–15% (Finlaysen et al. 1988).

Given the fact that consumption of alcohol appears to be higher for the current midlife group (Blow et al. 2002), that the rate of lifetime illicit drug use among the "baby boom" generation is considerably higher relative to the rate in the existing older adult cohort, and that the population size of the baby boom generation is larger than the previous generation, it is predicted that the number of older adults with substance abuse problems will double from current rates to 4.4 million in 2020. According to Gfroerer and colleagues (2002), 8.8% of persons age 50 or older were classified as at-risk users (having used alcohol and marijuana before age 30); in the group projected to be ages 50–70 in 2020, 49.9% were in the high-risk group. One such indication of growing prevalence of problem drug use among older adults is that the number of individuals seeking treatment for primary drug problems increased by 32% between 1995 and 2002, according to the Substance Abuse and Mental Health Services Administration Treatment Episode Data Set (TEDS) (Office of Applied Studies 2000).

Longitudinal studies of risk factors for alcohol problems in elderly persons are virtually nonexistent. Nevertheless, suggestive data from cross-sectional research may be informative in regard to potential etiological agents. For example, Glatt (1978) identified three precipitating factors in late-onset alcoholism: a habitual drinking pattern before late life, personality factors, and environmental factors. Personality characteristics that predispose to late-life drinking problems include anxiety and worry about one's social environment, such as loss of a loved one and loneliness. Personality factors appear to be less related to late-onset alcoholism than to an onset at earlier stages of the life cycle. Instead, alcohol problems in elderly individuals may precipitate stressful events such as marital discord and social isolation (especially from family).

Risk-factor studies of alcohol intake over time are relatively rare in the literature. Longitudinal studies for drinking patterns, however, are more common and provide insight into changing patterns of alcohol intake through the adult years. For example, more than 1,800 men ages 28–87 were studied for more than 10 years in the Veterans Administration's Normative Study of Aging (Glynn et al. 1984). In this panel there was almost no change in mean alcohol consumption during the follow-up period. In addition, rates of problems with drinking did not decline over time. These data do not support the findings from previous cross-sectional studies that aging modifies drinking behaviors. Men in their 40s and 50s in 1973 were especially persistent in their alcohol intake over time.

In a follow-up of nearly 1,300 adults treated for moderately severe to severe alcohol problems, Helzer and colleagues (1984) found few age differences that predicted outcome. There was some evidence that among the survivors, older alcoholic individuals were less likely to experience persistent, severe problems. At the same time, all-cause mortality was higher for older adults, and alcohol-related mortality was similar for both young and elderly subjects. Among the predictors of continued alcoholism, social isolation was more strongly correlated in the older group than in the younger group. Organic brain syndrome was not associated with outcome for the younger sample, but its absence was associated with a good outcome for the older group. In summary, this sample of treated alcoholic patients followed for 6–10 years revealed a good outcome in a large proportion of the older subjects.

Physical Consequences of Alcoholism in Later Life

When evaluating alcohol intake over time, the clinician must attend to the interaction between alcohol use and chronic or periodic illness in elderly patients. Although alcohol directly affects organ systems—alcohol increases cardiac rate and output secondary to its effect on cardiac muscle—the primary effect is cumulative. To illustrate this cumulative effect, consider the example of a person with chronic alcoholism who develops compromised hepatic functioning. This compromise in liver function may exacerbate osteomalacia secondary to decreased hepatic metabolism of vitamin D_3 to its more active 25-hydroxylated form.

Undernutrition resulting from chronic alcohol intake, especially among those who use large amounts of alcohol over long periods (the "skid-row alcoholics"), commonly leads to cirrhosis. Cirrhosis is one of the eight leading causes of death among persons ages 65 years and older. Alcohol can damage the heart, resulting in alcohol-induced cardiomyopathies. In contrast, however, some investigators reported a reduction in coronary artery disease in subjects who drink moderate quantities of alcohol over time (Yano et al. 1977). This does not mean, however, that older persons should be advised to drink alcohol to prevent coronary heart disease.

Chronic effects of alcohol intake on the gastrointestinal tract are well known to clinicians who work with older adults. In general, persons with chronic alcoholism have a lower gastric basal acid output, a maximal acid output, and an increased likelihood of developing chronic atrophic gastritis. The preexisting atrophic gastritis that is common in elderly alcoholic individuals may facilitate the formation of gastric mucosal lesions, which lead to upper gastrointestinal bleeding. Absorption of both folic acid and vitamin B_{12} declines with chronic alcohol use. Because these substances are essential to cognitive functioning, their loss through malabsorption or through decreased dietary intake among elderly alcoholic persons may lead to cognitive and psychological impairment as well as the resultant anemias. Peripheral neuropathy may occur in as many as 45% of chronic alcoholic patients because of deficiency in thiamine and other B-complex vitamins.

Nutritional requirements do not change dramatically with aging, although older persons may require more protein (Gersovitz et al. 1982). Chronic alcoholism is associated with reduced intake of a number of nutrients, including protein. Protein malnutrition is manifested in individuals with alcoholism as muscle wasting, hypoproteinemia, and edema. Iron deficiency also occurs, but it is generally due to gastrointestinal blood loss rather than to decreased dietary intake or malabsorption. As noted above, older adults may be more subject to gastric lesions, which in turn may lead to chronic occult bleeding.

A concern equal in importance to the medical consequences of late-life alcohol use is the interaction of aging, alcohol, and dementia. Many investigators report chronic alcoholism to be associated with a variety of neuropsychological and cognitive deficits. Although chronic alcoholism does not appear to disrupt cognitive and neuropsychological functioning diffusely, specific clusters of cognitive functions are affected in the older alcoholic individual. Most investigators agree that intelligence remains relatively unaffected, but deficits are known to occur in memory and information processing. These deficits are similar to the impairment seen in patients suffering from alcoholic amnestic dementia (Wernicke-Korsakoff disease). Specifically, deficits most frequently found in alcoholic individuals are impaired performance in tasks involving visuospatial analysis, tactual spatial analysis, nonverbal abstraction, and set flexibility. Although recovery of many of these functions may occur with abstinence from alcohol, recovery rarely leads to complete remission of symptoms.

Alcoholic amnestic dementia, seen in those with long-term alcoholism, is caused by thiamine deficiency as well as by the direct toxic effects of alcohol on brain tissue. Clinically, the end stage of alcoholic dementia is characterized by relatively intact intellectual functioning associated with severe anterograde and retrograde amnesia. In contrast to patients with Alzheimer's disease, those with alcoholic dementia who abstain may exhibit stable or even improved short-term memory and motor performance over time.

To appreciate the scope of alcohol problems in the elderly population, the risk of death from alcohol use should be explored. In the 8-year outcome study described by Helzer et al. (1984), 24% of the 234 alcoholic subjects who were age 60 years or older at enrollment died before the study was completed, compared with 9% of the 1,048 alcoholic subjects younger than age 60. However, the proportion of subjects reported to have died of alcohol-related causes was similar for the younger and older alcoholic groups. Although use of data from death certificates leads to an underestimation of the overall number of deaths due to alcohol, that bias is consistent across age groups.

A number of parallels have been observed between the sleep characteristics in persons experiencing normal aging and in chronic alcoholic individuals who are abstinent. For example, the sleep of chronic alcoholic patients who have withdrawn from alcohol is characterized by decreased slow-wave sleep, interruptions of sleep, and decreased or interrupted periods of rapid eye movement (REM) sleep (Adamson and Burdick 1973). Prolonged abstinence from alcohol in middle life, however, will lead to improved sleep over time. In other words, the central nervous system (CNS) abnormalities produced by alcohol apparently reverse. The older person who uses alcohol as a sedative experiences an additional sleep problem. The relatively rapid metabolism of alcohol, in contrast to most sedative-hypnotics, may produce a rebound awakening at a point 3–4 hours into sleep. Even though the older adult using alcohol may fall asleep without difficulty, his or her sleep is disrupted during the night.

Given the relatively large number of prescription and nonprescription drugs used by older adults, the interaction of alcohol with these drugs is of special importance to elderly persons. The impairments produced by alcohol are augmented by drugs such as sedatives, anticonvulsants, antidepressants, major and minor tranquilizers, and analgesics (especially the opiates). Poor muscle coordination, impaired judgment, and slurred speech are common when these agents are used together. Other side effects are less frequent but can be equally serious. Older adults using oral hypoglycemic agents to treat adult-onset diabetes (type 2 diabetes mellitus) may experience unpleasant symptoms such as nausea and flushing, as do patients who combine disulfiram and alcohol use. Unpredictable fluctuations of plasma glucose concentrations are another potential adverse effect. The efficacy of some drugs, such as coumarin-type anticoagulants, is blocked by alcohol, because alcohol increases the metabolism of these drugs (Ritchie 1981). In contrast, plasma concentrations of alcohol are usually not changed by the use of other medications (Garver 1984).

Addiction, Tolerance, and Withdrawal

The most significant clinical problem faced by the clinician treating the older alcoholic individual is the potential for addiction and tolerance to the agent, with the concomitant problem of alcohol withdrawal. Because alcohol is a readily available addictive agent in Western society, it is usually the drug of choice for individuals who want to block unpleasant emotions with drugs.

Older adults manifest their addiction when placed in a situation in which alcohol is not readily available. They may demonstrate increased anxiety and may pursue alcohol to decrease this anxiety. In addition, they experience sleep disturbance, nausea, and weakness, which are concomitants of a lowered blood alcohol level. Addiction is a unique problem for older adults, for at least two reasons. First, patterns of drinking have continued for many years (often from early or middle life), and lifelong habits are often not associated with problems of recent onset. In addition, the relatively "quiet" use of alcohol over the years desensitizes both the older adult and the family to the problems with alcohol (Pascarelli 1974; Schuckit 1977).

Akin to addiction is the potential for tolerance with chronic use of alcohol. Not only can older adults become tolerant to alcohol, but they may also become cross-tolerant to drugs similar to alcohol. Despite the potential for relatively normal function among alcoholic individuals (even when ethanol blood levels are relatively high), the heavy use of alcohol associated with tolerance continues to create irreversible changes in the liver, the gastrointestinal tract, and the CNS (Bosmann 1984). Cross-tolerance, especially to benzodiazepines, is of major clinical concern. Given that older adults are more likely to take benzodiazepines than are younger persons, the potential for abuse of both agents—separately or in combination—increases dramatically (Mellinger et al. 1978).

Symptoms following alcohol withdrawal are not appreciably different across the life cycle. Nevertheless, the older adult may manifest these symptoms, especially the more severe ones, for a longer period after acute cessation of alcohol intake. Initial symptoms include tremors, anxiety, nausea, vomiting, and perspiration. If the withdrawal syndrome is allowed to continue without intervention—either with a cross-tolerant drug (such as diazepam) or with reinstitution of alcohol—the tremulous state will peak within 1–2 days after the onset of the withdrawal syndrome. This tremulous peak is accompanied by hallucinations and, in severe cases, withdrawal seizures. Confusion, agitation, and disorientation mark the individual's level of consciousness. In the older adult with compromised health, the severity of this withdrawal syndrome is naturally greater (Bosmann 1984; Mello and Mendelson 1977).

Diagnostic Workup

Substance abuse problems in older adults are commonly missed. The Center for Substance Abuse Treatment's (CSAT's) Consensus Panel on Substance Abuse Among Older Adults (1998) recommends that every 60-year-old person should be screened for alcohol and prescription drug abuse as part of any routine physical examination. It is unusual for an older adult or a family member to present alcohol or drug use as a problem, and patient identification of a problem is unlikely to occur without prompting. The clinician is advised to assume that the patient drinks alcohol, and all questions related to the patient's alcohol use should be normalized as a routine and necessary part of every history and physical examination. The NIAAA guideline for older adults should be shared with the patient to help the patient conduct his or her own risk assessment and as a baseline to determine the need for a fuller evaluation. This guideline, as outlined in the *Physician's Guide to Helping Patients with Alcohol Problems* (National Institute on Alcohol Abuse and Alcoholism 1995), recommends no more than one drink per day and a maximum of two drinks on any drinking occasion. Symptoms of substance or alcohol abuse such as memory impairment, falls, or conflicts with family members may be misidentified as symptoms of aging. Presentation of these types of symptoms can be ideal opportunities to evaluate the patient's alcohol use.

The diagnostic workup of the older adult in whom an alcohol problem is suspected hinges on a comprehensive history. Detailed information should first be obtained from the patient on specifics of the drinking behavior. This information must be supplemented by family members, preferably from two generations. Unfortunately, some alcoholic older adults have virtually no family or other social network (the "skid-row alcoholics"), and historical information is therefore limited.

Questions that should be asked include the following: Does the elderly patient drink, and how often does he or she drink? Does he or she drink constantly? Is there a pattern of binge drinking? Elderly persons who suffer from chronic problems with alcohol are usually regular drinkers. Tolerance for binges decreases with age. A lifetime history of alcohol use provides a background for present patterns of use.

The CAGE questions (Ewing 1984) are commonly used for screening for alcohol problems:

Have you…

- **C**—…felt the need to **C**ut down on your drinking?
- **A**—…ever felt **A**nnoyed by criticism of your drinking?
- **G**—…had **G**uilty feelings about drinking?
- **E**—…ever taken a morning "**E**ye-opener"?

The CAGE questions are not as useful in screening older persons as they are in helping to identify alcohol problems among the younger population. Because older alcoholic individuals with a persistent drinking pattern over time tend to have problems with emergent physical and psychological symptoms, personal guilt or concern about drinking is less common. In fact, the older adult may not recognize the connection between new symptoms and drinking habits that have continued for decades. The Michigan Alcoholism Screening Test—Geriatric Version is a screening instrument specific to elderly persons that has particular utility in screening for alcoholism in older adults (Blow et al. 1992).

Additional data to identify drinking problems in the elderly should be derived from the following categories: personal health, family health problems, interpersonal difficulties, and work difficulties (Ewing 1985). Patients should be asked about gastrointestinal symptoms such as nausea, vomiting, diarrhea, abdominal pain, and unexplained gastrointestinal hemor-rhages. Neurological problems should be re-viewed, including episodes of amnesia, headaches, and peripheral neuropathy. Falls, bruises, cuts, sprains, cigarette burns, skin diseases, and lack of attention to personal health often result from excessive alcohol use.

A thorough review of psychiatric symp-toms is essential, including a detailed eval-uation of cognitive status, history of major depression, symptoms of generalized anx-iety, and psychotic symptoms (delusions and hallucinations). Paranoid ideation re-garding relatives or friends is not uncom-mon in the older person who is severely alcoholic. It is critical to document sui-cidal ideation, given the elevated risk for suicide in both elderly and alcoholic pop-ulations.

A genetic predisposition to alcohol prob-lems is less likely to be a contributing eti-ological factor in the elderly alcoholic pa-tient—especially if the onset of significant drinking problems occurs later in life. More-over, a history of alcohol abuse in the fam-ily of the older adult is also prone to bias, because complete historical information from alcoholic elderly patients regarding parents and siblings is usually difficult or impossible to obtain. A documented fam-ily history of psychiatric disorders (espe-cially major depression and schizophrenia) or alcohol abuse or dependence is impor-tant nonetheless, and the clinician should search medical records in addition to in-terviewing the elderly alcoholic patient.

An indicator of emerging alcohol prob-lems among older persons is concomitant problems in interpersonal relations. Al-though such problems occur most often in the marriage, they can also occur between the older adult and children or, occasion-ally, friends. Family problems may be the result of the drinking behavior (such as arguments over an appropriate amount to drink) or may result from symptoms of

the alcohol abuse (such as paranoid ideation or cognitive difficulties).

During the physical examination of the older adult with alcoholism, the clinician should screen for medical problems that may exacerbate alcohol problems—or that may be exacerbated by chronic alcohol use—as well as for evidence of alcohol abuse, such as signs of neglect of personal hygiene. The neurological examination should be performed in detail, with atten-tion directed to the evaluation of periph-eral neuropathy. Traditional signs of chronic alcohol abuse, such as flushing of the face, injected conjunctiva, tremors, and malnu-trition, may merge with normal signs of aging or poor health status.

If evidence of cognitive abnormalities emerges during the mental status exami-nation (and it often does), further cog-nitive workup is indicated. The clinician should make every effort to keep the alco-holic older adult abstinent for 2–3 weeks before a detailed cognitive evaluation. Psychological tests may be threatening to the older adult who fears that deficits will appear that have been previously undetec-ted. Baseline cognitive scores, however, can be especially important in monitoring the longitudinal progress of the patient, as well as in providing additional force to the clinical admonition to abstain from fur-ther alcohol use. For example, Parker et al. (1982) found that alcohol consumption above usual levels significantly increases problems with abstraction in formal test-ing.

Laboratory evaluation of the acutely al-coholic older adult should include thorough liver function evaluation—lactate dehydrog-enase (LDH), serum glutamic-oxaloacetic transaminase (SGOT), serum glutamic-pyruvic transaminase (SGPT), and alka-line phosphatase. Given the potential for an electrolyte imbalance in this popula-tion, a screening chemistry is essential, with special attention to glucose. Low blood magnesium reflects a magnesium deficiency that may occur with alcohol use. Elevated serum and urine amylase suggest chronic pancreatitis. Alcoholic cardiomyopathy may be manifested on an electrocardiogram as frequent arrhythmias, especially atrial fibrillation.

Intervention with the older adult alcoholic can be a challenging predicament. An array of motivational techniques and strategies have been developed and tested with positive results. Fleming et al. (1997) showed that 10%–30% of nondependent problem drinkers modified their drinking behaviors following a brief office-based intervention. Blow and Barry (2000) recently applied this model to adults with success. Prochaska et al. (1992) and Miller and Rollnick (1991) showed that motivational counseling directed toward a patient's readiness for change can lead the patient to accept the need for treatment. Miller and Sanchez (1994) developed the **FRAMES** model of intervention, providing the following schema for talking with patients about their abuse:

- **F**eedback about the person's use
- **R**esponsibility of the patient to address the problem
- **A**dvice with regard to what the patient might reasonably do
- **M**enu of options the patient has for addressing the problem
- **E**mpathy directed to understanding the patient's ambivalence
- **S**elf-efficacy of the patient to do something about the problem

Older adults will typically respond to an intervention approach that addresses substance use in the context of health and related issues. Establishing a controlled-drinking contract when clinically appropriate might be one way of leading patients to their own conclusions about the degree to which they have lost control of their ability to manage their alcohol use behav-

ior. Providing an educational overview of the issue that includes a comparison of the patient's drinking with that of other older adults and with recommended guidelines (e.g., those of NIAAA, discussed earlier in this chapter) may be another useful way of awakening the patient's attention to the need to address the issue further. It is critical that the patient be duly informed of any intervention or treatment that he or she might receive and that an opportunity be given to establish a therapeutic partnership for change. Dictating terms and conditions regarding next steps may compromise the patient's likelihood of compliance. Including others such as family members, peer supports, social workers, and home health personnel in any educational and recommendation communications may prove helpful. It is critical that issues of stigma be addressed by ensuring a clinical presentation of the patient's circumstances. Acknowledging patient ambivalence and the challenges that exist with respect to any recommended behavior change is useful. Cultural issues that reinforce drinking behavior may need to be addressed. A direct and nonjudgmental but serious attitude will better ensure that the patient receives the correct message about the alcohol problem.

Treatment

According to Atkinson and Kofoed (1982), older adults respond to treatment the same as or better than younger adults. Most appropriate are specialized behavioral treatments for substance abuse that employ medical and community-based approaches directed to older adults. The treatment of the older patient with alcohol abuse or dependence must include biological, psychological, and psychotherapeutic interventions within the patient's social milieu, especially the family. The level of care for the older adult should be considered in the context of the patient's motivation, concerns about medical and/or psychiatric risks, and availability of community support.

A useful guide in determining placement options might be *Patient Placement Criteria for the Treatment of Substance Related Disorders*, published by the American Society of Addiction Medicine (1996). Generally, the least intensive treatments should be considered first. However, if the older adult has acute intoxication that leads to a stuporous or comatose state, acute hospitalization must be instituted for withdrawal from alcohol and for institution of the therapeutic program (initially, pharmacological therapy). In milder cases of alcohol dependence, in which withdrawal is the first step, treatment may proceed in the outpatient setting. Outpatient withdrawal is possible only if the patient is highly motivated and is willing to allow open monitoring of the withdrawal program by the family, with frequent (often daily) contact with the clinician. In any case, the initial step in the treatment of alcoholism is to stop alcohol intake. Attempts to work over longer periods of time with the alcoholic individual who continues to drink are doomed to failure.

In the treatment of the older patient who is severely alcoholic, restoration of fluid and electrolyte balance during the initial phase of withdrawal is essential. Complaints of thirst and dry mucous membranes may delude the clinician into accepting a diagnosis of dehydration when, in fact, drying is resulting from alcohol expiration through the lungs. To avoid iatrogenic overhydration, the clinician should begin administration of 500–1,000 mL of a 5% normal saline solution while waiting for the results of the blood chemistry screen. Use of glucose solutions should be avoided; the older alcoholic patient may have subsisted on a diet high in carbohydrates, in

addition to alcohol, which is metabolized almost entirely as a carbohydrate, and glucose solutions can lead to an iatrogenic increase in blood glucose to diabetic levels. Because of poor dietary nutritional intake, fluids should be supplemented with parenteral B vitamins. Individuals with chronic alcoholism, as noted above, may suffer from magnesium deficiency. Adding a deep intramuscular injection of magnesium at a dose of 0.10–0.15 mL/kg to the initial therapeutic regimen is an important adjunct to treatment (Blazer and Siegler 1984).

The next step in treatment is the institution of medications that are cross-tolerant with alcohol. Diazepam has been the drug of choice for managing patients in withdrawal because of its relatively extended half-life and cross-tolerance with alcohol. Initial doses depend on the patient's age and weight and the amount of alcohol consumed during the week before admission. Even with these data, however, doses must be carefully titrated during the first 24–48 hours of withdrawal. The usual starting dosage is between 5 mg and 15 mg every 6–12 hours until the delirium, agitation, and/or hallucinations are sufficiently decreased. If therapy proceeds on an outpatient basis, careful monitoring is necessary in order to ensure that alcohol is not added to the regimen of the benzodiazepine. After the first day, the diazepam dose can usually be decreased at a rate of approximately 20% per day. Other medium- to long-acting benzodiazepines—such as chlorazepate—can be used as well.

When an overt delirium emerges with seizures and hallucinations, diazepam is the anticonvulsant of choice because of its rapid onset of effect. An increase in memory problems, the onset of dysarthria, and the development of ataxia in the elderly patient indicate that drug intoxication has developed secondary to excessive medication or as a result of the synergistic effects of the drug with alcohol. When such intoxication occurs, the drug should be discontinued for 24–36 hours and the patient should be carefully observed for a recurrence of the withdrawal symptoms; the drug can then be reinstituted. If persistent signs and symptoms of withdrawal are seen longer than 3 days after the last known drink, the clinician should suspect dependence on minor tranquilizers or hypnotics as well as alcohol.

Some withdrawal programs in communities encourage withdrawal within a social setting based on social support in the absence of drug use (a detoxification center). Although some rehabilitation centers in hospitals may overuse medication, the severe effects of withdrawal, such as delirium tremens, should dissuade the clinician from routinely using alternative withdrawal settings, especially for the older adult.

Medication-Assisted Treatments

Emerging best practices for addiction treatment now include the application of specific medication-assisted treatments that are increasingly recognized as key to engaging and retaining relapsing populations in treatment and to increasing periods of sustained partial or full remission. In particular, buprenorphine as an opiate replacement therapy for managing higher-functioning patients has shown promising results. Naltrexone, an opioid antagonist, is a useful agent for supporting individuals once they have become opiate free. Naltrexone has also been approved for use in the treatment of alcoholism to reduce craving and block the reinforcing effects of alcohol. Vivitrol, the long-acting injectable form of naltrexone, has received U.S. Food and Drug Administration (FDA) approval for treatment of alcohol dependence "in patients who are able to abstain from alcohol in an outpatient setting" prior to initia-

tion of Vivtrol treatment. Vivitrol should be "part of a comprehensive management program that includes psychosocial support" (www.vivitrol.com).

Acamprosate (calcium acetyl homotaurinate) is the third medication to receive FDA approval for postwithdrawal maintenance of alcohol abstinence. Having been used for over 20 years in Europe, it has been shown to be safe and effective for treating alcohol dependence (Mann et al. 2004). Although patients with liver damage are unable to take either disulfiram or naltrexone, these patients can safely take acamprosate, which is not metabolized in the liver.

Preliminary evidence suggests that acamprosate combined with either naltrexone or disulfiram may lead to improved treatment outcomes compared with use of any of these medications alone (Besson et al. 1998). Combination therapy also has been found to be safe in adult populations.

The NIAAA randomized clinical trial COMBINE (Combining Medications and Behavioral Interventions) provides an informed perspective on the efficacy of medication-assisted treatment for alcohol dependence in combination with medical management and behavioral intervention (Anton et al. 2006). The COMBINE study evaluated eight patient groups that included patients receiving medical management with 16 weeks of naltrexone (100 mg/day) or acamprosate (3 g/day), both, and/or both placebos, with or without a combined behavioral intervention. A ninth group received a behavioral intervention only and did not receive medication or placebo. Patients in this study were also evaluated for up to 1 year following treatment.

The COMBINE researchers concluded that patients receiving medical management with naltrexone and behaviorial treatment made significant improvements with respect to drinking outcomes (Anton et al. 2006). In this study, acamprosate showed no evidence of efficacy, with or without behavioral treatment or naltrexone or both. Additional findings were that 1) no combination produced better efficacy than naltrexone or behavioral intervention alone in the presence of medical management and 2) between-group effects were sustained at 1 year posttreatment but were no longer significant.

As neither the COMBINE study nor other clinical trials of medication-assisted treatment for alcohol dependence have evaluated the use of these medications specifically with older adults, clinicians are encouraged to carefully consider the use of these agents in clinical practice. In consideration of the higher risks of diminished renal function among this population, acamprosate should particularly be used with caution with these patients. As reflected in the COMBINE study, providing medical management and behavioral intervention concurrently may produce the best results when medication-assisted treatments are being applied to alcohol dependence.

Other Therapeutic Considerations

Therapeutic intervention with the family is essential. First, family members should be warned of the severe and potentially irreversible problems, especially memory problems, that alcohol can cause in the older adult. Most families are more concerned with the immediate effects of intoxication. If the older family member drinks silently without overt signs of intoxication, the behavior may be tolerated. The threshold for concern in the family must therefore be lowered through education. Patient, family, and clinician become a team as they seek to correct the problem. Family members may benefit from family education groups, multifamily therapy, and individual family therapy that might be of-

fered through local outpatient substance abuse clinics. Participation in Al-Anon groups could be another place where family members could learn about alcoholism and establish adaptive ways to respond to the patient's recovery efforts or to relapses should they occur. Atkinson et al. (1993) found that married older alcoholics were more likely to comply with treatment if their spouses also became involved in the treatment process.

Specialized substance abuse treatment approaches may be of particular benefit to the older adult. Mainstreaming patients into treatment as usual may present particular challenges. Older adults will probably respond better to a nonconfrontational, informed approach. The key elements of effective treatment for the older adult are the involvement of family, the development of a viable community base of support, and counseling directed to dealing with issues such as depression, isolation, and boredom. Groups for older adults, if available, might be of particular benefit. Some evidence to date supports age-specific treatment approaches with regard to compliance and outcomes (Atkinson et al. 1993; Kashner et al. 1992; Kofoed et al. 1987; Thomas-Knight 1978). Kashner et al. (1992) showed that elderly patients in programs specific to their age group were 2.9 times more likely and 2.1 times more likely at 1 year to report abstinence than were patients in a mixed-age program.

Case management supports may need to be organized to ensure linkage with appropriate community resources. A patient's medical, psychiatric, and social needs must be met, because substance abuse treatment may be of limited benefit if other critical and related issues are not addressed. Patients with coexisting psychiatric disorders will benefit most from an integrated and coordinated approach to the treatment of the comorbidity. Issues related to housing, transportation, and meals may need to be considered for certain patients, who might require a higher level of care (such as a day treatment program) than is normally provided in traditional outpatient treatment. Age-specific settings such as senior centers, faith-based community areas such as houses of worship, and Veterans Affairs clinics may be ideal locations for offering specific group-based programs for the older adult patient. Ideally, these centers will be staffed with persons experienced and interested in working with older adults. It is critical that the specialized care concerns of this patient cohort be taken into account in the treatment planning process.

Self-help groups are essential to the long-term support of the abstinent alcoholic person. The Alcoholics Anonymous (AA) program has proved over many years to be effective in encouraging abstinence for individuals throughout the life cycle. Support groups provide social support coupled with appropriate pressure from peers who have experienced similar problems. AA is complementary to the authority of the clinician and must not be considered a threat to medical authority. AA meetings may be especially beneficial to the older alcoholic individual who is discouraged and lonely because of isolation and feelings of uselessness. Involvement in the group setting, coupled with a sense of helping others and interaction with younger persons, may reintegrate the sober elderly person into society. Ideally, the older adult will establish a relationship with his or her program sponsor, who can help ease the patient's transition into the AA community and serve as an ongoing resource and source of support to the older adult, particularly during the initial challenges of accepting the alcohol use as a problem.

However, many older persons resist the suggestion that they join a self-help group. Some reasons are that elderly persons continue to deny that they have a problem or that they believe themselves perfectly capable of correcting the problem alone. The self-sufficient attitude of the current elderly cohort is one reason that such beliefs are so persistent in the elderly. More commonly, the older adult feels no "fit" with the environment of such self-help groups. Thus, the cohort of elderly alcoholic persons in the latter part of the twentieth century did not experience recovery groups and self-help phenomena, unlike those persons who are reaching old age in the early years of the twenty-first century. Given these groups' frequent success, participation in self-help groups should be encouraged, but clinicians should not force the older adult to participate. In certain communities it is more likely that particular meetings exist that are more attractive to the neophyte older adult AA member: these will be more established, more traditional in structure, and more fully attended by long-standing members of the AA community.

Support from family members and the clinician, as well as integration into more traditional social environments, may accomplish the same purpose as self-help and support groups (Butler and Lewis 1977). In mobilizing coping resources, the social environment (acute and chronic stressors, social network resources), the health care system (availability of health care services such as medical intervention, behavioral therapy, and educational programs), and the coping strategies of the older patient can be woven into a unique matrix for a given elderly person. Such an integrated approach not only makes possible a more comprehensive evaluation of the diagnostic profile but also provides a framework on which successful treatment can be built. Intervention should target for change specific points within the system, but the intervention strategy should also reflect the clinician's continuing recognition that the entire system is interdependent.

Drug Abuse and Dependence

Drug abuse is usually associated with adolescents and young adults. Certainly the abuse of illicit drugs is uncommon in older adults. Nevertheless, the fact that drug abuse occurs among persons in later life must not be overlooked. The propensity of older adults to use prescription drugs inappropriately renders late life a period of high risk for the side effects of this misuse. Glantz (1981) suggested that the motivation for elderly persons to abuse drugs may be similar to the motivation for adolescents. Both must negotiate a period of uncertain and changing roles as well as changes in self-concept. Older persons face step-downs on the economic ladder and disadvantages in the employment market. Friends and relatives may not be as available because of distance, or may be removed by death. Although self-sufficiency continues to be a means of coping (adolescents and the elderly both strive for control), the ability of the impaired older adult to maintain self-reliance and independence is compromised. Drugs are easily available to both groups. The adolescent seeks illegal drugs on the street; the older adult obtains addictive drugs from local physicians. For example, Capel et al. (1972) discovered that the majority of drug-addicted persons who survive to late life continue their drug use via concealed habits, using substitute narcotics such as hydromorphone hydrochloride. Alcohol and barbiturates may be added to enhance the effects of this narcotic.

Even the progress from milder to more powerful drugs, frequently seen in the steps to addiction among adolescents, may have parallels among the elderly (Glantz 1981). Older persons begin taking mild analgesics and sedative-hypnotic agents but fail to obtain the relief they desire. Without realizing the danger of addiction, they progress to the use of narcotic analgesics for chronic pain problems and higher doses of tranquilizing and sedative-hypnotic agents. Once addiction and tolerance are established, older adults exhibit little initiative to reverse the problem. By obtaining medications from multiple physicians and borrowing medicines from family members, they feed their habit over time. Frequently, hospitalization uncovers the addiction, because withdrawal symptoms appear 3–4 days after admission to the hospital.

Problems deriving from excessive and inappropriate use of prescription and over-the-counter drugs are well documented in the geriatric literature. Law and Chalmers (1976) estimated that 85% of older persons living in the community and 95% of those residing in long-term-care facilities receive prescription drugs. In 1976, more than 12 prescriptions were written per person each year for persons ages 65 years and older (Lamy and Vestal 1976). Of drugs prescribed to older adults, 17%–23% are benzodiazepines (D'Archangelo 1993). Undoubtedly, such estimates would be even higher today.

Scope of the Problem

The frequency of excessive drug use in the elderly, especially the use of psychoactive drugs, is well documented. From a household survey of more than 2,000 people, Mellinger et al. (1978) reported that among persons older than age 60 years, 20% of women and 17% of men had regularly used psychoactive drugs during the year preceding the survey—rates higher than those for any other age group. In this age group, 11% of the men and 25% of the women had used a minor tranquilizer and/or a sedative at least once during the year preceding the survey—again, rates higher than those for any other age group. These rates may be declining in community samples, because rates of antianxiety and sedative-hypnotic use have decreased (Hanlon et al. 1992). Heightened public awareness of problems secondary to benzodiazepine use probably contributed to this decline.

A report from the National Medical Care Expenditure Survey (Rossiter 1983) documented that persons age 65 years and older were more likely than middle-age persons to have used pain relievers (25.9%) prescribed by a physician during the past year. Except for cardiovascular medications, analgesic and psychotherapeutic agents were the drugs used the most by older adults. In a review of nursing home prescribing habits, Ray et al. (1980) found that in 173 Tennessee nursing homes, 43% of the patients had received antipsychotic medications during the year preceding the survey, and 9% were chronic recipients—that is, they had received at least one dose daily for 365 days during the preceding year.

Christopher et al. (1978), reporting on 873 hospitalized persons in Dundee, Scotland, concluded that prescribing in this inpatient population was not excessive; an average of three medications was received at any given time. Patients on the geriatric ward were receiving the highest number of drugs. However, certain drug groups, especially the sedative-hypnotics, were prescribed excessively, with few attempts made to reduce the dose with patients' increasing age. The prevalence of hypnotic use ranged from more than 40% among the medical patients to more than 70% on the geriatric wards. In a survey involving 195 hospitalized persons over age 60 years, Salzman and van der Kolk (1980) found that one-third had received at least one psychotropic drug the day of the survey. Hypnotics were the most frequently prescribed drugs, with flurazepam as the drug of choice. The authors noted that each of the psychoactive drugs prescribed had potentially dangerous side effects and that

the dosing did not reflect that the treating clinicians paid attention to the age of patients.

In the community, however, the evidence of significant abuse of illicit drugs in the elderly is remarkably absent. The best data available are those derived from the ECA studies. Myers et al. (1984) found no evidence of drug abuse in the age group 65 years and older at two of the three ECA sites surveyed and a prevalence of just 0.2% at the third site. More than 3,000 persons ages 65 years and older were interviewed for this survey. Regarding the lifetime prevalence of drug abuse or dependence, fewer than 0.1% of the subjects at these three ECA sites reported any such history (Robins et al. 1984). These studies are subject to bias, given the subjects' difficulty in recalling information regarding drug abuse and/or their denial of such use. Nevertheless, denial and selective recall are probably no more a problem for elderly persons than for persons at any other stage of life. What is more likely to contribute to the relatively low prevalence of current and lifetime drug abuse among elderly persons is a cohort effect (persons who were elderly in the 1980s were never heavy users of drugs) and selective mortality (persons from the present generation of older adults who used illicit medications did not survive to late life). However, community surveys that rely on household data may underestimate drug abuse, especially by failure to include homeless and transient persons.

Behavioral and Social Correlates

Many psychosocial factors contribute to the potential toxicity and addictive potential of both prescription and illicit drugs among the elderly population (Blazer 1983). Certain character traits of older adults contribute to increased drug use

(Baldessarini 1977). The more passive older adult may use drugs prescribed by a number of physicians without question. Even "double prescribing," the prescription of the same drug by two or more physicians, can go unchallenged by the dependent elderly person. Addiction accrues over time without being noticed by the patient, family, or physician. Only when such a patient is admitted to the hospital for an unrelated disorder do the symptoms of addiction become apparent. Once hospitalized, passive older adults often fail to report the medications they were taking before hospitalization, expecting the physician to know how to manage their problem. The patients who appear most compliant could be the most prone to drug abuse in an outpatient medical or psychiatric practice.

In addition to character traits, the social setting surrounding the prescription of medications affects the patient's potential for abusing medications. Many psychosocial factors determine abuse of therapeutic drugs. Noncompliance, a most important factor in treating psychiatric disorders, usually does not contribute to drug abuse. Rather, older adults are more inclined not to take prescribed medications on schedule than to use prescribed drugs excessively. Blackwell (1973) estimated that up to 50% of patients do not take prescribed medications. The potential for addiction may be actualized, however, if the milieu for prescribing medications discourages communication between the older adult and the physician (Lamy 1980). Frequently, in the distracting and hurried environment of the physician's office, proper use of a medication is not communicated to older adults. Because older persons are hesitant to ask questions, they leave the office without understanding how a drug is to be used. To please the physician, they take the medication, but not at the dose required. The tendency for older persons to carry all their medications in one container increases the potential for confusion about when a particular drug should be taken. Intoxication from excessive use of the benzodiazepines is not uncommon under these circumstances.

The practice of sharing and swapping medications among older adults is not infrequent as a precipitant of abuse or dependence. Friends, roommates, or spouses can be treated by different physicians for similar problems. Through informal communication with one another regarding the effectiveness of individual drug therapies, the elderly person may mistakenly determine that a friend's physician has prescribed a better treatment than his or her own clinician. Because limited finances preclude obtaining a second opinion (or even an initial consultation), medications are informally shared. Through the additive effects of drugs, such as the sedative-hypnotics, evidence of addiction or abuse appears, often unexplained to the primary care physician. The diagnosis of the problem is further complicated because older adults are hesitant to reveal that they have obtained medications from another source.

Another contributor to problems of abuse is use of over-the-counter drugs. In Western societies, over-the-counter drugs are used even more often than prescription drugs. Chaiton et al. (1976) estimated that more than 50% of elderly persons responding to a community survey had used at least one over-the-counter drug during the 48 hours preceding the survey. Most of these persons had not consulted a physician about the use of the drug or its potential interaction with prescription drugs. The most commonly used over-the-counter drugs are agents to improve sleep, to improve gastrointestinal symptoms such as constipation, and to relieve pain. The misuse of such drugs is likely to be associated with the use of multiple substances, insomnia, chronic pain, and relief from stress. The combination of nonprescription drugs that have anticholinergic effects (such as diphenhydramine) with prescribed antidepressants and/or phenothiazines can lead to anticholinergic toxicity or even a full-blown central anticholinergic syndrome.

"Do-something" prescribing is an iatrogenic contributor to drug abuse in elderly patients. The older adult who pays for a doctor's consultation expects a result—usually a prescription. The physician who writes a prescription also gains some assurance that he or she has upheld the patient–physician contract. Drugs prescribed under these circumstances are often not prescribed for specific target symptoms. Benzodiazepines, sedative-hypnotic agents, tricyclic antidepressants, and even neuroleptics become the drugs of choice because of the mistaken view that the drugs promote the general well-being of the patient. Not only do such prescribing practices reinforce a pattern of medical care that discourages the physician from talking with the older adult, but these practices also increase the likelihood of polypharmacy.

A variation on the theme of do-something prescribing that may contribute to drug addiction and/or abuse in elderly patients is defensive prescribing. Physicians who serve as medical directors of nursing homes or who have large consulting practices in long-term-care facilities are frequently called by nursing staff and even family members about patients' disturbing and uncontrollable physical or behavioral symptoms. Agitation and sleep problems are among those most commonly encountered by a stressed nursing staff. Against his or her better judgment, a physician may prescribe medications, not so much to alleviate a specific symptom in an older adult as to reassure staff and family members. Defensive prescribing is not an indictment of the care given by a physi-

cian, nursing staff, or family. Rather, it is a symptom of a difficult situation—the management of an acutely agitated and cognitively impaired older adult in a facility with limited personnel. Nevertheless, such prescribing practices must be recognized as major contributors to addiction and abuse in older adults.

Diagnostic Workup

The diagnostic workup of the older adult in whom a diagnosis of drug abuse or dependence is suspected is similar to the workup described in this chapter for those with suspected alcohol abuse and dependence. Many of the symptoms described earlier apply to prescription and nonprescription drug abuse as well. Although older adults may be seen after taking an overdose of a sedative, narcotic, or other agent, the most common presentations of drug misuse or abuse are symptoms of toxicity and/or withdrawal.

The benzodiazepines (both anxiolytics and sedative-hypnotics) are the most commonly prescribed drugs and are therefore the most likely to be abused. Symptoms characteristic of benzodiazepine toxicity include sedation, confusional states, "sundowning" (heightened agitation or frank delirium at night), ataxia, and even stupor or coma. The potential for a fatal overdose is low with these agents alone, but when benzodiazepines are combined with other agents, such as alcohol, this potential increases dramatically. Withdrawal symptoms, in contrast, may mimic the psychiatric disorder for which the drugs were originally prescribed. Anxiety and agitation, sleep problems, muscle cramps (especially in the legs), tremors, and perceptual distortions may emerge upon withdrawal. It is important to note the most serious withdrawal symptom: the onset of seizures.

Tricyclic antidepressants are frequently prescribed and may contribute to increased memory problems, confusion, and sedation. Confusion and even fugue states are described as occurring in the morning after an excessive nighttime dose of tricyclic antidepressants; these symptoms are frequently accompanied by postural hypotension and excessive lethargy. In a patient with bipolar disorder, successful use of an antidepressant to reverse depressive symptoms may later trigger an elevation in mood and an increase in activity. Even a frank manic episode with delusions and hallucinations can be precipitated by these drugs.

Lithium carbonate, a most effective drug in the treatment of manic-depressive illness, can be especially problematic for older adults. Symptoms including dizziness, ataxia, drowsiness, and confusion may occur when serum levels are below 1.0 mEq/L. Older persons do not tolerate lithium therapy as well as persons in middle life, and therefore the drug must be prescribed with extreme caution. Self-abuse with lithium is uncommon, but the desire of the clinician to obtain therapeutic effect in a patient who suffers from rapid-cycling bipolar disorder or unipolar recurrent depression augments the potential for lithium toxicity.

When these or other symptoms emerge, obtaining a thorough history from the patient and family (similar to that described earlier in the chapter for alcohol problems) is the next clinical step of importance. If the clinician questions the history provided by the patient, many laboratories provide a drug toxicity screen. Most of these laboratories can return results to the clinician within 6 hours. Specimens can be obtained from either urine or blood. Toxicity screens must be interpreted cautiously, for drugs are often cross-reactive to the probes used in the screen. Other ancillary laboratory procedures, such as electrophysiological tracing, cardiac monitoring, and radiologic examination (for problems deriving from drug use), can be obtained as well but are usually not required.

Treatment

Treatment approaches for drug abuse and dependence in the older adult are similar to those used for patients at other stages of the life cycle. Given that the older adult is frail, however, the clinician must be careful to err on the side of being conservative. Specifically, early hospitalization is indicated when evidence of abuse is present. For example, the older adult who chronically takes benzodiazepines and is found to be excessively lethargic should be hospitalized, despite the clinician's recognition of the cause of the problem and the family's insistence that the problem can be managed at home.

The immediate goal upon hospitalization is to remove the potential for acute toxicity from the medication. If drug ingestion is recent, gastric evacuation is indicated. In elderly patients, however, special care must be taken to avoid aspiration. Activated charcoal (30 g) has been recommended along with the lavage to absorb barbiturates, alcohol, and propoxyphene (Ellinwood et al. 1985). Once the clinician is convinced that the potential for acute toxicity has been removed, the patient should be transferred to a ward where close monitoring is possible. Electrocardiographic monitoring is often indicated for the first 24–48 hours. Monitoring of respiration, however, is of greatest importance, especially if the patient shows evidence of slow, rapid, or shallow breathing. When improvement does not ensue, peritoneal dialysis or hemodialysis may be indicated.

Once the patient has survived the immediate problems of overdose, the next challenge presented to the clinician is to manage withdrawal symptoms. Depending on the half-life of the drug, withdrawal may last from 6 hours to 8–10 days (the half-life of flurazepam, for example, may exceed 200 hours in an older adult). Support with the medication or a substitute drug is indicated during this period. At the same time, the clinician must begin educating the patient and family about the cause of the hospitalization and the need to change the outpatient drug therapy significantly in order to prevent the recurrence of such a problem. With most elderly persons, education and intervention during the course of an acute hospitalization for drug problems are effective. Older adults are often unaware of the potential problems of drug use and, when informed, are most happy to be free of the potential of future addiction or toxic reactions to a medication.

In some cases, however, the older adult will continue to seek medications, especially analgesics and benzodiazepine-like compounds. For these patients, careful outpatient monitoring and work with the family provide the best means of successfully achieving long-term abstinence from potentially abusable drugs. Because elderly persons tend to use the same pharmacy despite having multiple physicians, contact with the pharmacist can be especially helpful in monitoring drug use.

Older adults have a variety of reasons for resisting change, particularly if the addictive behavior has begun to have an instrumental effect on their lives. Brief intervention and motivational interviewing approaches are particularly helpful in engaging older adult patients toward an examination of their alcohol or drug use behaviors through patient-centered styles that emphasize therapeutic elements such as empathy, unconditional regard, and genuineness. These approaches recognize that ambivalence plays a major role in addictive behavior and view the awareness and resolution of such ambivalence as necessary to the change process.

The transtheoretical model of behavior change (Prochaska et al. 1992) provides a useful framework for assessing a patient's readiness to change and for targeting the caregiver's interventions at points of greatest receptivity and need. For example, if an individual is staged at a precontemplation level of readiness, strategies focusing on crisis resolution and engagement are targeted. At a contemplation level of readiness, a patient may be more willing to increase awareness about the impact of his alcohol or drug use behaviors and opportunities for change.

Motivational interviewing is designed to enhance patients' intrinsic motivation by exploring their perspective and ambivalence. This approach directs patients to evaluate their behavior in the context of their values, interests, and concerns. It recognizes that patient motivation is influenced by a positive therapeutic relationship grounded in a person-centered philosophy based on the perspective that when resistance is evoked, change is less likely to occur.

Motivational interviewing is based on the four principles of providing empathy, developing discrepancy, rolling with resistance, and supporting patient self-efficacy. In contrast to traditional approaches that rely on confrontation, education, and authority, motivational interviewing relies on communicating patient responsibility, emphasizing collaboration, and soliciting the patient's ideas regarding how best to change. Techniques of motivational interviewing include open-ended questions, reflective listening, affirmation, use of summary, and eliciting of change talk. Reinforcing change talk, building on a person's strengths, and reinforcing motivation are key strategies for engaging an individual in a change process (Miller and Rollnick 2004; Rollnick and Miller 1995).

References

Adamson J, Burdick JA: Sleep of dry alcoholics. Arch Gen Psychiatry 28:146–149, 1973

American Society of Addiction Medicine: Patient Placement Criteria for the Treatment of Substance-Related Disorders, 2nd Edition. Washington, DC, American Society of Addiction Medicine, 1996

Anton RF, O'Malley SS, Ciraulo DA, et al: Combined pharmacotherapies and behavioral interventions for alcohol dependence: the COMBINE study: a randomized controlled trial. JAMA 295:2003–2017, 2006

Atkinson RM, Kofoed LL: Alcohol and drug abuse in old age: a clinical perspective. Subst Alcohol Actions Misuse 3:353–368, 1982

Atkinson RM, Tolso RL, Turner JA: Factors affecting outpatient treatment compliance of older male problem drinkers. J Stud Alcohol 54:102–106, 1993

Baldessarini RJ: Chemotherapy in Psychiatry. Cambridge, MA, Harvard University Press, 1977

Besson J, Aeby F, Kasas A, et al: Combined efficacy of acamprosate and disulfiram in the treatment of alcoholism: a controlled study. Alcohol Clin Exp Res 22(3):573–579, 1998

Blackwell B: Drug therapy: patient compliance. N Engl J Med 289:249–252, 1973

Blazer D: Drug management in the elderly, in Experimental and Clinical Interventions in Aging. Edited by Walker RF, Cooper RL. New York, Marcel Dekker, 1983, pp 343–354

Blazer D, Siegler IC: A Family Approach to Health Care in the Elderly. Menlo Park, CA, Addison-Wesley, 1984

Blow FC, Barry KL: Older patients with at-risk and problem drinking patterns: new developments in brief interventions. J Geriatr Psychiatry Neurol 13:115–123, 2000

Blow FC, Brower KJ, Schulenberg JE, et al: The Michigan Alcoholism Screening Test—Geriatric Version (MAST-G): a new elderly-specific screening instrument. Alcohol Clin Exp Res 16:372, 1992

Blow FC, Barry KL, Welsh DE, et al: National Longitudinal Alcohol Epidemiologic Survey (NLAES): Alcohol and drug use across age groups, in Substance Use by Older Adults: Estimates of Future Impact on the Treatment System. Edited by Korper SP, Council CL. Rockville, MD, SAMHSA, Office of Applied Studies, Dec 2002. Available at: http://www.oas.samhsa.gov/aging/chap7.htm. Accessed May 12, 2006.

Bosmann HB: Pharmacology of alcoholism in aging, in Alcoholism in the Elderly. Edited by Hartford JT, Samorajski T. New York, Raven, 1984, pp 161–174

Butler RN, Lewis MI: Aging and Mental Health: Positive Psychosocial Approaches, 2nd Edition. St. Louis, MO, CV Mosby, 1977

Capel WC, Goldsmith BM, Waddell KJ, et al: The aging narcotic addict: an increasing problem for the next decades. J Gerontol 27:102–106, 1972

Center for Substance Abuse Treatment: Substance Abuse Among Older Adults. Treatment Improvement Protocol (TIP) Series, No 26 (DHHS Publ No SMA 98-3179). Washington, DC, U.S. Government Printing Office, 1998

Chaiton A, Spitzer WO, Roberts RS, et al: Patterns of medical drug use: a community focus. Can Med Assoc J 114:33–37, 1976

Christopher LJ, Ballinger BR, Shepherd AMM, et al: Drug-prescribing patterns in the elderly: a cross-sectional study of inpatients. Age Ageing 7:74–82, 1978

D'Archangelo E: Substance abuse in later life. Can Fam Physician 39:1986–1993, 1993

Ellinwood EH, Woody G, Krishnan RR: Treatment for drug abuse, in Psychiatry, Vol 2. Edited by Michels R, Cavenar JO. Philadelphia, PA, Lippincott, 1985, pp 1–12

Ewing JA: Detecting alcoholism: CAGE questionnaire. JAMA 252:1905–1907, 1984

Ewing JA: Substance abuse: alcohol, in Psychiatry, Vol 2. Edited by Michels R, Cavenar JO. Philadelphia, PA, Lippincott, 1985

Finlaysen RE, Hunt RD, Davis LJ, et al: Alcoholism in elderly persons: a study of the psychiatric and psychosocial features of 216 inpatients. Mayo Clin Proc 63:761–768, 1988

Fleming MF, Barry KL, Manwell LB, et al: Brief physician advice for problem drinkers: a randomized controlled trial in community-based primary care practices. JAMA 277:1039–1045, 1997

Garver DL: Age effects on alcohol metabolism, in Alcoholism in the Elderly. Edited by Hartford JT, Samorajski T. New York, Raven, 1984, pp 153–160

Gersovitz M, Motio K, Munro HN, et al: Human protein requirements: assessment of the adequacy of the current recommended dietary allowance for dietary protein in elderly men and women. Am J Clin Nutr 35:6–14, 1982

Gfroerer JC, Penne MA, Pemberton MR, et al: The aging baby boom cohort and future prevalence of substance abuse, in Substance Use by Older Adults: Estimates of Future Impact on the Treatment System. Edited by Korper SP, Council CL. Rockville, MD, Substance Abuse and Mental Health Services Administration, Office of Applied Studies, December 2002. Available at: http://www.oas.samhsa.gov/aging/chap5.htm. Accessed May 12, 2006.

Glantz M: Predictions of elderly drug abuse. J Psychoactive Drugs 13:117–126, 1981

Glatt MM: Experiences with elderly alcoholics in England. Alcoholism 2:23–26, 1978

Glynn RJ, Bouchard GR, Locastro JS, et al: Changes in alcohol consumption behaviors among men in the normative aging study, in Nature and Extent of Alcohol Problems Among the Elderly. Research Monograph No 14 (DHHS Publ No ADM 84-1321). Edited by Maddox G, Robins LN, Rosenberg N. Rockville, MD, National Institute on Alcohol Abuse and Alcoholism, 1984, pp 101–116

Hanlon JT, Fillenbaum GG, Burchett B, et al: Drug-use patterns among black and non-black community-dwelling elderly. Annals of Pharmacology 26:679–685, 1992

Helzer JE, Carey KE, Miller RH: Predictors and correlates of recovery in older versus younger alcoholics, in Nature and Extent of Alcohol Problems Among the Elderly. Research Monograph No 14 (DHHS Publ No ADM 84-1321). Edited by Maddox G, Robins LN, Rosenberg N. Rockville, MD, National Institute on Alcohol Abuse and Alcoholism, 1984, pp 83–100

Kashner TM, Rodell DE, Ogden SR, et al: Outcomes and costs of two VA inpatient programs for older alcoholic patients. Hosp Community Psychiatry 43:985–989, 1992

Kofoed LL, Tolson RL, Atkinson RM, et al: Treatment compliance of older alcoholics: an elder-specific approach is superior to "mainstreaming." J Stud Alcohol 48:47–51, 1987

Lamy PP: Prescribing for the Elderly. Littleton, MA, PSG Publishing, 1980

Lamy PP, Vestal RE: Drug prescribing for the elderly. Hosp Pract (Off Ed) 11:111–118, 1976

Law R, Chalmers C: Medicines and elderly people: a general practice survey. Br Med J 1:565–568, 1976

Liberto JG, Oslin DW, Ruskin PE: Alcoholism in older persons: review of the literature. Hosp Community Psychiatry 43:975–984, 1992

Mann K, Lehert P, Morgan MY: The efficacy of acamprosate in the maintenance of abstinence in alcohol-dependent individuals: results of a meta-analysis. Alcohol Clin Exp Res 28(1):51–63, 2004

Mellinger GD, Balter MB, Manheimer DI, et al: Psychic distress, life crisis, and use of psychotherapeutic medications: national household survey data. Arch Gen Psychiatry 35:1045–1052, 1978

Mello NK, Mendelson JH: Clinical aspects of alcohol dependence, in Drug Addiction, Vol 1: Morphine, Sedative/Hypnotic and Alcohol Dependence. Edited by Martin WR. Berlin, Springer, 1977, pp 613–666

Mellstrom D: Previous alcohol consumption and its consequences for aging, morbidity and mortality in men aged 70–75. Age Ageing 10:277–283, 1981

Miller WR, Rollnick S: Motivational Interviewing. New York, Guilford, 1991

Miller WR, Rollnick S: Talking oneself into change: Motivational Interviewing, stages of change and therapeutic process. J Cogn Psychother Int Q 18:299–308, 2004

Miller WR, Sanchez V: Motivating young adults for treatment and lifestyle change, in Alcohol Use and Misuse by Young Adults. Edited by Howard GS, Nathan PE. South Bend, IN, University of Notre Dame Press, 1994

Myers JK, Weissman MM, Tischler GL, et al: Six-month prevalence of psychiatric disorders in three communities: 1980 to 1982. Arch Gen Psychiatry 41:959–967, 1984

National Institute on Alcohol Abuse and Alcoholism: The Physician's Guide to Helping Patients With Alcohol Problems (NIH Publ No 95-3769). Rockville, MD, National Institute on Alcohol Abuse and Alcoholism, 1995

Office of Applied Studies: Treatment Episode Data Set (TEDS): 1993-1998: National admissions to substance abuse treatment services (DHHS Publ No SMA 00-3463, Drug and Alcohol Services Information System Series S-11). Rockville, MD, Substance Abuse and Mental Health Services Administration, 2000. Available at: http://www.dasis.samhsa.gov/teds98/teds98.htm. Accessed August 2, 2006.

Parker ES, Parker DA, Brodie JA, et al: Cognitive patterns resembling premature aging in male social drinkers. Alcoholism 6:46–52, 1982

Pascarelli EF: Drug dependence: an age-old problem compounded by old age. Geriatrics 29:109–110, 1974

Prochaska JO, DiClemente CC, Norcross JC: In search of how people change: applications to addictive behaviors. Am Psychol 47:1102–1114, 1992

Ray WA, Federspiel CF, Schaffner W: A study of antipsychotic drug use in nursing homes: epidemiologic evidence suggesting misuse. Am J Public Health 70:485–491, 1980

Ritchie JN: The aliphatic alcoholics, in The Pharmacological Basis of Therapeutics, 6th Edition. Edited by Gilman AG, Goodman LS, Gilman A. New York, Macmillan, 1981, pp 376–390

Robins LN, Helzer JE, Weissman MM, et al: Lifetime prevalence of specific psychiatric disorders in three sites. Arch Gen Psychiatry 41:949–958, 1984

Rollnick S, Miller WR: What is Motivational Interviewing? Behav Cogn Psychother 23:325–334, 1995

Rossiter LF: Prescribed medicines: findings from the National Medical Care Expenditure Survey. Am J Public Health 73:1312–1315, 1983

Ruchlin HS: Prevalence and correlates of alcohol use among older adults. Prev Med 26 (5 pt 1):651–657, 1997

Salzman C, van der Kolk B: Psychotropic drug prescriptions for elderly patients in a general hospital. J Am Geriatr Soc 28:18–22, 1980

Saunders PA: Epidemiology of alcohol problems and drinking patterns, in Principles and Practice of Geriatric Psychiatry. Edited by Copeland JR, Abou-Saleh MT, Blazer DG. New York, Wiley, 1994, pp. 801–805

Schuckit MA: Geriatric alcoholism and drug abuse. Gerontologist 17:168–174, 1977

Thomas-Knight R: Treating alcoholism among the aged: the effectiveness of a special treatment program for older problem drinkers. Diss Abstr Int 39:3000, 1978

Yano K, Rhoads GG, Kajan A: Coffee, alcohol, and risk of coronary artery disease among Japanese men living in Hawaii. N Engl J Med 297:405–409, 1977

Study Questions

Select the single best response for each question.

1. Substance abuse and dependence problems may cause significant distress for the older patient and need to be evaluated fully by the geropsychiatrist. Which of the following is true regarding substance use disorders in this population?

   A. The prevalence of substance use disorders in patients over 65 ranges from 0.1% to 0.7% for men.
   B. Risk factors for elder substance abuse are similar to those for younger adults (e.g., male gender, lower educational attainment, and comorbid mood disorder).
   C. The comorbidity of alcohol problems and psychiatric illness in late life is 5%–7%.
   D. In the United States, the lifetime prevalence of alcohol problems in older adults is higher than in younger persons.
   E. Some studies suggest that the prevalence of alcohol abuse among older persons is higher in African Americans than in whites.

2. The physician may be consulted to manage some of the chronic effects of alcohol on neurophysiology and cognitive function in the elderly patient. Which of the following is true regarding alcohol's chronic effects?

   A. Peripheral neuropathy in persons with alcoholism, which often follows deficiency states of thiamine and other B-complex vitamins, is seen in 25% of individuals with chronic alcoholism.
   B. The cognitive effects of alcohol typically result in a decreased overall level of intelligence as reflected in the IQ on formal testing.
   C. Focal cognitive deficits with chronic alcoholism include deficits in visuospatial analysis and nonverbal abstraction.
   D. The use of alcohol for sleep may produce prolonged sleep (8–10 hours) in the elderly.
   E. Alcoholic dementia deficits are permanent; abstinence does not reverse deficits in short-term memory.

3. The useful mnemonic **FRAMES** (Miller and Sanchez) can be used to organize clinical interventions for substance abuse in the elderly patient. Which of the following statements is *not* part of the **FRAMES** schema?

   A. Feedback about substance use.
   B. Responsibility to address the problem of substance use.
   C. Abstinence as an early requirement.
   D. Menu of patient options.
   E. Empathy for the patient's ambivalence and challenge.

Agitation and Suspiciousness

Lisa P. Gwyther, M.S.W.

David C. Steffens, M.D., M.H.S.

Suspiciousness and Paranoia

Psychiatrists working with older adults frequently encounter suspicious or paranoid behaviors, especially in patients with agitation. In fact, such ideation is not very uncommon in community populations of elderly adults. In a community study of elderly persons in San Francisco, 17% of the subjects reported that they were highly suspicious and 13% reported delusions (Lowenthal and Berkman 1967). Another study that included elderly persons in both urban and rural areas of North Carolina found that 4% of older adults experienced a sense of persecution by those around them (Christenson and Blazer 1984). Perceptions of a hostile social environment or ideas of persecution lead to greater stress, vigilance, and agitation among elderly persons, resulting in alienation from families and friends. Such individuals represent a challenge for clinicians who care for them.

Among suspicious or paranoid elderly persons, one group has long been recognized, particularly in Europe. The term *late-life paraphrenia* has been used to identify psychosis that has a late age at onset and to distinguish the condition from both chronic schizophrenia and dementia. Kraepelin used *paraphrenia* to classify a small group of patients who exhibited paranoid delusions and yet were able to maintain functioning in their social milieu for months or years. He observed that persons with paraphrenia were typically women, usually living alone. Although current DSM diagnostic nomenclature would classify many of those individuals as having delusional disorder, this late-life syndrome may be more complex. Sometimes paranoid ideation is accompanied by hallucinations. In addition, patients with this condition may have comorbid sensory deficits, especially visual or hearing loss. Thus, although the condition may have features of delusional disorder, it may also have features and comorbidities that point to its being a different entity, perhaps along a continuum with schizophrenia. When the condition is accompanied by agitation, neuroleptics are usually the first-line treatment, although information is lacking on the effectiveness of this class of medications in delusional disorder. Caution with these medications is also warranted, given the increased sensitivity of elderly persons to neuroleptics (Soares and Gershon 1997).

Clearly, chronic paranoid schizophrenia persisting into late life is a major cause of suspiciousness and agitation in elderly persons. Multimodal treatment—including neuroleptic medication, case management, and family education and involvement—is essential for ensuring adequate care. The occurrence of agitation in chronic paranoid schizophrenia patients is common and may indicate a need for an adjustment in neuroleptic dosing. However, new agitation arising in a previously stable older patient with schizophrenia may also indicate another problem, and clinicians need to be particularly attuned to the possibility of an acute medical problem.

Classic delusional disorder may occur at any age and is usually characterized by delusions centered on a single theme or series of connected themes. Agitation may become an issue when such individuals are confronted by family or clinicians about their delusion.

Diagnostic Approach to Patients With New Onset of Suspiciousness and Paranoia

As with most mental disorders, a careful psychiatric evaluation and history are key components of the initial approach to the suspicious or paranoid patient. Interviews of family members may be necessary for establishing a diagnosis, particularly if delusions and agitation are present. Part of the task of the clinician is to determine whether suspicious behavior is warranted. Older adults are occasionally abused or neglected; therefore, confronting family members about a patient's accusations of harm or neglect is often part of the assessment. If after such a confrontation the clinician is not convinced that the accusations are totally explained by the delusion, a social services agency or department should be requested to investigate further.

On the other hand, challenging the delusional patient is usually not recommended. It is important to seek an understanding of the patient's thought processes, so providing an atmosphere of acceptance (although not necessarily agreement) will allow the patient to express his or her beliefs and feelings. Reassurance should be provided in a manner conveying that although the clinician may not fully understand the whole situation, the goal is for the patient to feel better and more secure.

A laboratory workup is usually needed in new cases of paranoia to rule out an organic delusional syndrome. Blood chemistry, a complete blood count, and a thyroid profile should be obtained. If respiratory symptoms are present, a chest X ray may be needed. A computed tomography or magnetic resonance imaging brain scan may be indicated, especially if cognitive impairment or focal neurological findings are present. Because suspiciousness is often associated with sensory impairment, particularly visual and auditory deficits, audiometric and visual testing may identify potential areas for further intervention.

Treatment of paranoia may include neuroleptic medication, depending on the diagnosis, as discussed earlier in this chapter. (For a complete discussion of neuroleptics, please see Chapter 16, "Psychopharmacology.") Regardless of whether neuroleptics are prescribed, key components of management of paranoia include reassurance for the patient, education for the family, and careful monitoring for development of agitation.

Agitation in Elderly Persons

Behavioral manifestations of dementia are common (Lyketsos et al. 2000) and represent major predictors of caregiver depression, burden, and stress across cultures

(Chen et al. 2000; Gallicchio et al. 2002; Teri 1997). Anxiety and agitation, the most commonly cited psychiatric manifestations of dementia, can be as disruptive and painful for the person with dementia as they are for family caregivers. Disruptive or resistive behaviors resulting from anxiety and agitation increase the risk of harm to the affected individual and others (Chow and MacLean 2001; Tractenberg et al. 2001), and caregivers frequently become frightened, upset, or simply exhausted by the demands of caring for a family member with agitation.

Nonpharmacological Approaches

Nonpharmacological strategies are recommended as first-line approaches for the noncognitive manifestations of dementia. These approaches can be taught effectively to family and nonprofessional caregivers (Doody et al. 2001). Nonpharmacological approaches are most effective as adjuncts to pharmacotherapy, when pharmacotherapy is contraindicated, or when behaviors are obviously manifested in response to environmental or interpersonal triggers.

Key Messages for Families About Agitation in Dementia

Families of persons with dementia should be told directly that anxiety, suspiciousness, and restless agitation are common symptoms of brain disorders, even in the context of excellent, well-intentioned family care. At the same time, it is helpful to suggest that disruptive behaviors do not occur in a vacuum. Agitation has a person-specific situational context and meaning that may often, but not always, be understood. Agitated or even aggressive behavior is often beyond a dementia patient's control or intentionality. In fact, he or she may not be aware of agitation or a change in behavior.

Frequent or escalating agitation requires a prompt and multimodal response. Ignoring agitated or disruptive behaviors will not make them go away. Persons with dementia are most likely to be angry at what they perceive as an intolerable situation that no longer makes sense. For this reason it is wise for families not to take attacks or accusations personally. Families should also be reminded that persons with dementia are more likely to take out their frustration on those closest to them while appearing gracious and appropriate with strangers.

Families should be told that people with dementia generally cannot "try harder." A corollary is that reasoning, arguing, coaxing, pleading, confronting, or punishing agitated persons may only escalate the distressing behavior. Families respond effectively if they understand that agitated people with dementia are likely to be scared and overwhelmed by disorientation and that they may forget appropriate public or private behavior. Agitation is frequently accompanied by a loss of impulse control that can result in uncharacteristic cursing, insensitivity, tactlessness, or sexually inappropriate behavior. Although people with dementia may seem insensitive to others' feelings, they are extremely sensitive to and will respond negatively to patronizing, angry, tense, rushed, or demanding nonverbal communication from family members.

Agitated persons with dementia generally respond well to calm, familiar settings with predictable routines and to requests tailored to their capacities, remaining strengths, and energy levels. Although Alzheimer's disease patients may appear to do less as a result of apathy, they can become fatigued from just trying to make sense of what is going on around them. Late-day fatigue or wearing out may explain some agitated behavior associated with "sundowning" (patients' becoming more confused, agitated, or psychotic in the late afternoon or early evening) and extremely exaggerated reactions to minor incidents. Furthermore, patients with mild to moderate Alzheimer's disease may resist activities they perceive as too difficult or too demeaning, in order to limit embarrassment or failure.

Questions to Guide Problem Solving for Agitation in Dementia

Consideration of the following nine questions can help pinpoint and resolve caregivers' problems with a patient's agitated behavior:

1. Which agitated, anxious, or resistive behaviors are most disruptive to family life at this point?
2. Describe the behavior. Is it harmful or does it cause distress to the person with dementia or to others? Can the family change expectations or increase tolerance for this change in the person as they knew him or her?
3. Is there any pattern, trigger, or time of day that sets off the behavior (e.g., a move, travel, hospitalization, or being asked to do a complex task)?
4. Does anything happen afterward that makes it worse (e.g., caregiver anger or abandonment or patient failure)?
5. Is the person uncomfortable (e.g., pain, hunger, thirst, constipation, full bladder, fatigue, infection, cold, fear, misperceived threats, difficult communication)?
6. Is the person looking for something familiar from the past (e.g., rummaging in drawers, searching for an outhouse or an old employer)?
7. Will a change in environment help (e.g., reduce number of people, confusion, stimuli, noise)?
8. Can the caregiver use familiar phrases to calm or reassure the person (e.g., "I'll get right on it"; "Ain't that the truth?"; "Even the Lord rested on Sundays")?
9. Can routines be changed or adapted to prevent future occurrences of the behavior (e.g., exercising early in the day, bathing less frequently, avoiding rush-hour shopping)?

Common Strategies That Reduce Agitation

Nonpharmacological strategies for reducing agitation usually involve redirection of the person's attention away from triggering events or contexts or distraction with offers of pleasant events specific to the person (going out for ice cream or a ride, listening to favorite music, or watching old videotapes). Other strategies include breaking down complex tasks into one-step guided directions, simplifying instructions, and allowing adequate rest or passive observation between stimulating activities.

Environmental strategies include using labels, cues, or pictures; hazard-proofing the environment to reduce dangers of exploration or egress; removing guns or hazardous equipment; and using lighting or security objects to reduce nighttime confusion or daytime fear or uncertainty.

Communication Begins With Understanding

Families begin to communicate effectively when they can understand the experience and perspectives of people with dementia. With the current focus on early diagnosis and treatment of Alzheimer's disease, more individuals with insight who have new diagnoses of Alzheimer's disease are willing to provide direction:

When a person with dementia is agitated, he or she may be thinking along the following lines (Gwyther 2000, p. 998):

How dare you question me? I have always taken care of myself.

I make sense—you and events don't.

Your reality and reasoning wear me out.

I am only protecting what is mine from those people—things keep disappearing.

Can't you see this is not a good time? I'm overwhelmed and scared.

Communication Strategies to Reduce Agitation

First it is necessary to get the person's attention. Make sure vision and hearing are adequate or "tuned up." Use eye contact, call her by name in a clear adult tone, approach slowly from the side or front or crouch down at her level, and offer your hand, palm up. Listen, but do not feel compelled to talk constantly. Words are not as important as a calm tone, pleasant expression, and nondistracting environment (turn off the TV or turn down the radio). Use simple words, speak slowly, and give her time to process and respond. Repeat your words exactly, if necessary (do not paraphrase). Ask questions if you are unsure of her meaning. ("Am I getting closer to what you want?") Be patient—you may need to repeat to reassure her.

If frustration mounts, take a deep breath and suggest a better time to talk or another topic. Avoid popular expressions that may be ambiguous or vague, like "Don't go there," "NOT," or "bottom line." Use concrete subjects, names, and references. Avoid pronouns. Do not test or ask him if he remembers you. Use positive statements like "Let's go," rather than "Do you want to go now?" Explain what happens next, but wait until just before it will happen. Demonstrate or model so he can follow your lead. Use appropriate respectful humor or his favorite phrases ("See ya later, alligator"). It is always appropriate to make fun of yourself, especially if you forget. Smile, nod, gesture, or use photos when words fail.

Summary of Nonpharmacological Approaches

Families often want brief, concrete suggestions for dealing with agitation. The follow-

ing format may be helpful (Alzheimer's Association 2001; Gwyther 2001):

DO—slow down, soothe the person, or structure the situation. Encourage and reinforce positive adaptations that work for the person ("I depend on my husband for brute strength in carrying those grocery bags"). Be extra gracious and polite. Back off and ask permission. Repeatedly reassure. Use visual and verbal cues and add light. Offer guided choices between two options. Avoid complex multistep directions or ambiguity. Distract with a favorite snack or ask for help with raking or another adult repetitive task. Increase time spent in pleasant activities like sitting in a porch glider at sunset. Offer security object, rest, or privacy after an upset. Limit caffeine and alcohol. Use comforting rituals like holding hands during grace, an afternoon tea break, checking the bird feeder, or a hand massage or manicure. Do for her what she can no longer comfortably do on her own. Join her in modified favorite activities—social, creative, or sports. Remove her from confusing, frustrating, or scary experiences like TV shows that she believes are happening to her.

DO NOT—raise your voice, take offense, corner, crowd, restrain, rush, criticize, ignore, confront, argue, reason, shame, blame, demand, lecture, condescend, moralize, force, explain, teach, show alarm, or make a sudden move out of the person's view.

SAY—May I help you? Do you have time to help me? Let's take a break now—we have earned it. You're safe here. I will get right on it. Everything is under control. I apologize (even if you didn't do it!). I'm sorry you are upset. I know it's hard. We're in this together. I will make sure those men can't get in here. Do what you can and I'll finish up. We're doing fine now.

TABLE 15–1. Common medical causes of agitation in elderly persons

Medication

    Drug-drug interaction

    Accidental misuse

    CNS-toxic side effect

    Systemic disturbance (e.g., medication induced electrolyte imbalance)

Urinary tract infection

Poor nutrition, decreased oral intake of food and fluid

Respiratory infection

Recent stroke

Occult head trauma if patient fell recently

Pain

Constipation

Alcohol/substance withdrawal

Chronic obstructive pulmonary disease

Pharmacological/Medical Approaches

There are times when agitation warrants pharmacological intervention. Most clinicians view agitation as a condition manifested by excessive verbal and/or motor behavior. It is distinguished from aggression, which can also be verbal (e.g., cursing or threats) or physical (e.g., hitting, kicking, shoving objects or people). Agitation can escalate to aggression, so it is vital for the clinician to intervene early in approaching agitated patients. First, it becomes essential to determine the cause of agitation. Interventions are then directed at both treating the underlying cause and managing the agitation itself. Medical causes of agitation are shown in Table 15–1.

Agitation in the Context of Delirium

Delirium is a common disorder, with an estimated prevalence of 15%–50% among hospitalized elderly patients (Inouye 1998; Levkoff et al. 1991). Characterized by a disturbance of consciousness and a change in cognition, delirium typically has a rapid onset and runs a short course. DSM-IV-TR categorizes delirium by presumed etiology (including delirium secondary to a medical condition, substance intoxication, and substance withdrawal), mixed or multiple etiologies, and uncertain etiology (American Psychiatric Association 2000).

Delirium typically develops over hours to days and is provoked by certain medical illnesses, metabolic derangements, intoxications, and withdrawal states (Lipowski 1989). A prodromal period of subtle confusion, irritability, or psychomotor behavior change may precede the advent of the full syndrome. Confusion, intermittent clouding of sensorium or consciousness, and alterations in perception commonly occur, as do psychotic symptoms such as paranoia. Marked disturbances of the sleep cycle contribute to sundowning. Autonomic changes such as tachycardia and hypertension can also occur, particularly in the hyperactive form of delirium. Patients with this form often have increased irritability and startle responses and may be acutely sensitive to light and sound. In addition, delirious patients may experience profound shifts in mood and use rambling, illogical language while still having lucid intervals of relatively normal mental functioning. Although short-term memory may be disturbed, long-term memory is typically preserved. The syndrome usually runs a course of several days; however, the duration of illness is largely controlled by the course of the underlying condition that provoked the delirious episode.

Management of delirium is focused mainly on identifying and treating the underlying cause. However, the agitated delirious patient requires immediate attention, because the workup of the delirium may be impeded by agitated behavior, which may also put the patient and others at physical risk. Acute treatment of the agitation will probably require intramuscular or intravenous agents, typically benzodiazepines and neuroleptics. If there is no intravenous access, initial treatment with intramuscular lorazepam or haloperidol, alone or in combination, may be required. When intravenous access is established, these agents can also be used. Alternatives include other short-acting benzodiazepines such as midazolam or more sedating neuroleptics such as thiothixene. Use of intramuscular chlorpromazine should be avoided because of its effects on cardiovascular response, including orthostatic hypotension, which may occur should the patient try to stand up or get out of bed.

Agitation in the Context of Dementia

Agitation is a frequent behavioral symptom in dementia, with 24% of caregivers in one survey reporting agitation and/or aggression (Lyketsos et al. 2000). It occurs at some time in about half of all patients with dementia (Small et al. 1997). A person with dementia may become agitated throughout the day, intermittently through the day, or at specific times of day. For example, sundowning commonly occurs in dementia. One-fourth of inpatients with Alzheimer's disease were found on nursing evaluation to exhibit sundowning behavior (Little et al. 1995). Behaviors associated with agitation in patients who have dementia include aggression, combativeness, disinhibition, and hyperactivity. As with all behavioral problems, the first step in treatment is to identify the precipitants. Evaluation should include assessment for common systemic causes (e.g., infection, dehydration, constipation, and other illnesses) as well as changes in medication.

Pharmacological Treatment

If environmental measures are insufficient to control agitated or aggressive behavior, medication is usually needed. Guidelines for pharmacological treatment of agitation in elderly patients with dementia have been developed (Alexopoulos et al. 1998). High-potency neuroleptics (e.g., haloperidol) are effective for controlling acute agitation, especially when psychotic features are present (Small et al. 1997). Although there is no evidence to suggest that one neuroleptic agent is more effective than another, the atypical antipsychotics—clozapine (Clozaril), risperidone (Risperdal), olanzapine (Zyprexa), quetiapine (Seroquel), and ziprasidone (Geodon)—have a lesser frequency of extrapyramidal side effects (e.g., parkinsonism, tardive dyskinesia). These medications are particularly useful in agitated, psychotic patients with Parkinson's disease because their selective dopaminergic blockade does not interfere with dopamine's therapeutic effect on the basal ganglia. However, atypical antipsychotics are expensive, and most (with the exception of ziprasidone) are not currently available in injectable forms. Benzodiazepines can also be used to treat anxiety or infrequent agitation, but they are less effective than other agents for long-term treatment.

In general, when agitation is a consistent problem and neuroleptic treatment is required, we recommend starting with a low dose (e.g., 0.5 mg of haloperidol or 1 mg of risperidone) and administering it on a regular basis rather than attempting to treat specific episodes of agitation. Trying to treat a patient who is already agitated makes administering medication difficult, requires larger doses, and is likely to cause sedation and further clouding of thought.

The anticonvulsants carbamazepine and divalproex sodium (Depakote) are effective in treating behavioral disturbances in dementia and have a side-effect profile different from that of neuroleptics. In a double-blind study, Tariot and colleagues (1998) found that, compared with the placebo group, patients taking carbamazepine showed significant improvement in agitation and aggression. The drug was well tolerated. The modal daily dose of carbamazepine was 300 mg, achieving a mean serum level of 5.3 μg/mL. One study has shown that carbamazepine may also be effective when added to neuroleptic therapy in patients with refractory agitation (Lemke 1995). Divalproex has also been shown to be an effective treatment for agitation in dementia (Narayan and Nelson 1997). In this study, the mean final divalproex dose was 1,650 mg/day, with a mean blood level of 64 μg/mL. Divalproex was well tolerated in this population except for reversible sedation in eight patients and transient worsening gait and confusion in one patient.

Other classes of drugs are useful for treating agitation. Antidepressants, especially selective serotonin reuptake inhibitors (SSRIs) and trazodone, are effective even in the absence of clear depressive symptoms. There is no established dose range for treatment of agitation with SSRIs, and in our experience the final doses used to achieve successful treatment of agitation have ranged widely. The acetylcholinesterase inhibitors, tacrine (Cognex), donepezil (Aricept), rivastigmine (Exelon), and galantamine (Reminyl), decrease agitation, possibly by stimulating attention and concentration (Levy et al. 1999). The beta-blocker propranolol hydrochloride (Inderal) inhibits impulsive behavior after frontal lobe injury and can be used to decrease agitation and aggressive behavior in dementia, but it may cause bradycardia and hypotension (Shankle et al. 1995).

The need for continued pharmacological treatment of agitation should be regularly reassessed. Generally, medication for agitation should not be viewed as long-term therapy. In one study, neuroleptic treatment was discontinued after agitation was successfully treated in nine patients with dementia (Borson and Raskind 1997). A placebo was then administered, and behavior was monitored for the next 6 weeks. Of the nine patients, eight did not need additional pharmacological treatment. Interestingly, five of the patients were less agitated after drug treatment was stopped.

However, some patients may require chronic medication treatment for agitation. In such cases, antidepressants, especially SSRIs, or anticonvulsants are the preferred treatments. Benzodiazepines and neuroleptics have obvious inherent risks when used chronically in elderly patients with dementia, and close monitoring for side effects (e.g., sedation and extrapyramidal side effects) is required. In the case of neuroleptics, agitated patients without an established psychotic illness must have clear documentation of previous failed trials of other medications and presence of severe agitated behavior. Such patients should have a trial period without the neuroleptic to determine whether ongoing use of the drug is needed.

References

Alexopoulos GS, Silver JM, Kahn DA, et al. (eds): Agitation in Older Persons with Dementia: A Postgraduate Medicine Special Report (The Expert Consensus Guideline Series). New York, McGraw-Hill, 1998

Alzheimer's Association: Fact Sheet: About Agitation and Alzheimer's Disease. Chicago, IL, Alzheimer's Association, 2001. Available at http://www.alz.org/Resource Center/ ByType/FactSheets.htm (click on "Agitation"). Accessed October 7, 2003.

American Psychiatric Association: Diagnostic and Statistical Manual of Mental Disorders, 4th Edition, Text Revision. Washington, DC, American Psychiatric Association, 2000

Borson S, Raskind MA: Clinical features and pharmacologic treatment of behavioral symptoms of Alzheimer's disease. Neurology 48 (suppl 6):S17–S24, 1997

Chen JC, Borson S, Scanlan JM: Stage-specific prevalence of behavioral symptoms in Alzheimer's disease in a multi-ethnic community sample. Am J Geriatr Psychiatry 8: 123–133, 2000

Chow TW, MacLean CH: Quality indicators for dementia in vulnerable community-dwelling and hospitalized elders. Ann Intern Med 135:668–676, 2001

Christenson R, Blazer D: Epidemiology of persecutory ideation in an elderly population in the community. Am J Psychiatry 141: 1088–1091, 1984

Doody RS, Stevens JC, Beck C, et al: Practice Parameter: Management of Dementia (An Evidence-Based Review): Report of the Quality Standards Subcommittee of the American Academy of Neurology. Neurology 56:1154–1166, 2001

Gallicchio L, Siddiqui N, Langenberg P, et al: Gender differences in burden and depression among informal caregivers of demented elders in the community. Int J Geriatr Psychiatry 17:154–163, 2002

Gwyther L: Family issues in dementia: finding a new normal. Neurol Clin 18:993–1010, 2000

Gwyther L: Caring for People with Alzheimer's Disease: A Manual for Facility Staff. Washington, DC, American Health Care Association and Alzheimer's Association, 2001

Inouye SK: Delirium in hospitalized older patients. Clin Geriatr Med 14:745–764, 1998

Lemke MR: Effect of carbamazepine on agitation in Alzheimer's inpatients refractory to neuroleptics. J Clin Psychiatry 56:354–357, 1995

Levkoff S, Cleary P, Liptzin B, et al: Epidemiology of delirium: an overview of research issues and findings. Int Psychogeriatr 3:149–167, 1991

Levy ML, Cummings JL, Kahn-Rose R: Neuropsychiatric symptoms and cholinergic therapy for Alzheimer's disease. Gerontology 45 (suppl 1):15–22, 1999

Lipowski ZJ: Delirium in the elderly patient. N Engl J Med 320:578–582, 1989

Little JT, Satlin A, Sunderland T, et al: Sundown syndrome in severely demented patients with probable Alzheimer's disease. J Geriatr Psychiatry Neurol 8:103–106, 1995

Lowenthal MF, Berkman PL: Aging and Mental Disorders in San Francisco: A Social Psychiatry Study. San Francisco, CA, Jossey-Bass, 1967

Lyketsos CG, Steinberg M, Tschanz JT, et al: Mental and behavioral disturbances in dementia: findings from the Cache County Study on Memory in Aging. Am J Psychiatry 157:708–714, 2000

Narayan M, Nelson JC: Treatment of dementia with behavioral disturbance using divalproex or a combination of divalproex and a neuroleptic. J Clin Psychiatry 58:351–354, 1997

Shankle WR, Nielson KA, Cotman CW: Low-dose propranolol reduces aggression and agitation resembling that associated with orbitofrontal dysfunction in elderly demented patients. Alzheimer Dis Assoc Disord 9:233–237, 1995

Small GW, Rabins PV, Barry PP, et al: Diagnosis and treatment of Alzheimer disease and related disorders: consensus statement of the American Association for Geriatric Psychiatry, the Alzheimer's Association, and the American Geriatrics Society. JAMA 278:1363–1371, 1997

Soares JC, Gershon S: Therapeutic targets in late-life psychoses: review of concepts and critical issues. Schizophr Res 27:227–239, 1997

Tariot PN, Erb R, Podgorski CA, et al: Efficacy and tolerability of carbamazepine for agitation and aggression in dementia. Am J Psychiatry 155:54–61, 1998

Teri L: Behavior and caregiver burden: behavioral problems in patients with Alzheimer disease and its association with caregiver burden. Alzheimer Dis Assoc Disord 11 (suppl 4): S35–S38, 1997

Tractenberg RE, Garmst A, Weiner MF, et al: Frequency of behavioral symptoms characterizes agitation in Alzheimer's disease. Int J Geriatr Psychiatry 16:886–891, 2001

Study Questions

Select the single best response for each question.

1. Which of the following is true regarding the psychotic disorder of late life referred to as late-life paraphrenia?

    A. It is the late-life recurrence of an earlier onset of schizophrenia in a patient who had been symptom-free for many years.
    B. According to Kraepelin's original description, most patients were male.
    C. Psychotic symptoms of the late-life episode typically include delusions, but hallucinations are not experienced.
    D. Patients have been reported to have simultaneous sensory deficits.
    E. Antipsychotics have been shown to be effective for late-life delusional disorder.

2. The clinical evaluation of the suspicious and/or paranoid older patient requires consideration of specific concerns about psychotic disorders in older patients. Which of the following is true?

    A. Because of tendency of patients with schizophrenia to isolate and have a shorter life expectancy, chronic paranoid schizophrenia is an infrequent cause of suspiciousness in elderly patients.
    B. Elderly patients with schizophrenia are best managed with medication alone, rather than comprehensive treatment models.
    C. Agitation in elderly patients with chronic paranoid schizophrenia is rare.
    D. Agitation may follow family members' challenging of the patient's delusions.
    E. None of the above.

3. When the physician evaluates the older patient with suspicious and/or paranoid complaints, which of the following is *not* recommended?

    A. Determine whether suspicious behavior is warranted; for example, consider the possibility of neglect or abuse.
    B. Challenge the delusion to verify that it is indeed fixed in the patient's mind.
    C. Obtain routine laboratory studies, including chemistry and complete blood count.
    D. Consider use of neuroimaging (e.g., CT or MRI of the head).
    E. Consider specialty referrals for vision and hearing examination and correction.

4. Agitation in dementia is a common clinical problem, for both the patient and the family. Which of the following is true regarding behavioral approaches to agitation in dementia?

    A. Pharmacological approaches should precede nonpharmacological ones.
    B. Patients with dementia are more likely to act out frustration with strangers than with family members because strangers are unfamiliar.
    C. Agitation often correlates with other areas of impulsive behavior.
    D. Because of their cognitive impairments, patients with dementia are usually nonresponsive to nonverbal behavior of caregivers.
    E. Excessively calm, familiar surroundings and predictable routines unnecessarily understimulate the patient with dementia and thus should be avoided.

5. Communication strategies in dementia may facilitate the patient's maintenance of behavioral control and avoidance of escalation into agitation. All of the following communication strategies are helpful *except*

    A. Ensuring adequate vision and hearing correction.
    B. Maintaining good eye contact and approaching the patient slowly.
    C. Decreasing "clutter" in the sensory milieu (e.g., turning off noisy electronic equipment).
    D. In assisting understanding, paraphrasing, rather than simply repeating, ideas that are not apparently understood.
    E. Using specific names and references and avoiding pronouns and other nonspecific language devices.

Treatment of Psychiatric Disorders in Late Life

Psychopharmacology

Benoit H. Mulsant, M.D., M.S., FRCPC

Bruce G. Pollock, M.D., Ph.D., FRCPC

Pharmacological intervention in late life requires special care. The elderly are more susceptible to drug-induced adverse events. Particularly troublesome among older persons are peripheral and central anticholinergic effects such as constipation, urinary retention, delirium, and cognitive dysfunction; antihistaminergic effects such as sedation; and antiadrenergic effects such as postural hypotension. In addition to interfering with basic activities, pronounced sedation and orthostatic hypotension pose a significant safety risk to elderly patients because they can lead to falls and fractures. This increased susceptibility to adverse effects is largely due to the pharmacokinetic and pharmacodynamic changes associated with aging (Table 16–1).

In addition, polypharmacy and the associated risk of drug interactions add another level of complexity to the pharmacological treatment of older patients.

Finally, poor adherence to treatment regimens (which can be due to impaired cognitive function, confusing drug regimens, or lack of motivation or insight associated with the psychiatric disorder being treated) is a significant obstacle to effective and safe pharmacological treatment.

Despite these challenges, psychiatric disorders can be successfully treated in late life with psychotropic drugs. In this chapter, we summarize relevant data published in scientific journals as of February 2006 on the efficacy, tolerability, and safety of the major psychotropic drugs.

Antidepressant Medications

Selective Serotonin Reuptake Inhibitors

The selective serotonin reuptake inhibitors (SSRIs) are first-line drugs for treating late-life depression (Alexopoulos et al. 2001) because of their efficacy for both depressive and anxiety syndromes, their ease of use, and their safety and good tolerability.

As with most drugs, few clinical trials of SSRIs have been conducted under "real-life" geriatric situations (e.g., in long-term-care facilities) or in very old patients. However, as of February 2006, more than 30 randomized, controlled trials of SSRIs involving more than 5,000 geriatric patients with depression have been published (Table 16–2). Several controlled and open studies have

TABLE 16–1. Physiological changes in elderly persons associated with altered pharmacokinetics

Organ system	Change	Pharmacokinetic consequence
Circulatory system	Decreased concentration of plasma albumin and increased α_1-acid glycoprotein	Increased or decreased free concentration of drugs in plasma
Gastrointestinal tract	Decreased intestinal and splanchnic blood flow	Decreased rate of drug absorption
Kidney	Decreased glomerular filtration rate	Decreased renal clearance of active metabolites
Liver	Decreased liver size; decreased hepatic blood flow; variable effects on cytochrome P450 isozyme activity	Decreased hepatic clearance
Muscle	Decreased lean body mass and increased adipose tissue	Altered volume of distribution of lipid-soluble drugs leading to increased elimination half-life

Source. Adapted from Pollock BG: "Psychotropic Drugs and the Aging Patient." *Geriatrics* 53 (suppl 1):S20–S24, 1998.

also been conducted in special populations (Solai et al. 2001); reviews of many of these trials concluded that SSRIs are efficacious, safe, and well tolerated in older patients, including those with mild cognitive impairment (Devanand et al. 2003), dementia (Katona et al. 1998; Lyketsos et al. 2003; Nyth and Gottfries 1990; Nyth et al. 1992; Olafsson et al. 1992; Petraca et al. 2001; Taragano et al. 1997), minor depression (Rocca et al. 2005), schizophrenia (Kasckow et al. 2001), cardiovascular disease (Glassman et al. 2002; Serebruany et al. 2003), cerebrovascular disease (Whyte and Mulsant 2002), stroke (Andersen et al. 1994; Murray et al. 2005; Rampello et al. 2004; Rasmussen et al. 2003; Robinson et al. 2000), or other medical conditions (Arranz and Ros 1997; Evans et al. 1997; Goodnick and Hernandez 2000; Karp et al. 2005; Trappler and Cohen 1998).

Available data show that all available SSRIs have similar efficacy and tolerability in the treatment of depression in younger (Kroenke et al. 2001) and in older adults (Schneider and Olin 1995; Solai et al. 2001). However, experts favor the use of citalopram, escitalopram, or sertraline over fluvoxamine, fluoxetine, or paroxetine (Alexopoulos et al. 2001; Mulsant et al. 2001a). This preference is in large part because of their favorable pharmacokinetic profiles (Table 16–3), their lower potential for clinically significant drug interactions (Table 16–4), and data suggesting their superiority in terms of cognitive improvement (Burrows et al. 2002; Doraiswamy et al. 2003; Furlan et al. 2001; Newhouse et al. 2000; Nyth and Gottfries 1990; Nyth et al. 1992).

SSRIs have well-established efficacy for anxiety disorders in younger adults (Nemeroff 2002). However, only one published placebo-controlled trial (Lenze et al. 2005) and two small open studies (Sheikh et al. 2004b; Wylie et al. 2000) support their efficacy in older patients with anxiety disorders. In the absence of such data, the use of SSRIs to treat geriatric anxiety disorders is mostly based on extrapolation from studies in younger adults and expert opinion (Flint 2005; Lenze et al. 2002). By con-

TABLE 16–2. Summary of published randomized controlled trials of SSRIs for acute treatment of geriatric depression

	Number of published trials (cumulative # older participants)	Dosages studied (mg/day)	Comments
Citalopram	7[a] (N = 1,052)	10–40	Citalopram was more efficacious than placebo in one of two trials and as efficacious as amitriptyline and venlafaxine. It was better tolerated than nortriptyline but associated with a lower remission rate. Several trials included patients with stroke and dementia.
Escitalopram	1[b] (N = 517)	10	In this failed study, escitalopram and fluoxetine were well tolerated but not superior to placebo on primary endpoint.
Fluoxetine	12[c] (N = 1,792)	10–80	Fluoxetine was more efficacious than placebo in two of four trials and as efficacious as amitriptyline, doxepin, escitalopram, paroxetine, sertraline, and trimipramine. In patients with dysthymic disorder, fluoxetine was marginally superior to placebo. In patients with dementia of the Alzheimer type, fluoxetine did not differ from placebo.
Fluvoxamine	4[d] (N = 278)	50–200	Fluvoxamine was more efficacious than placebo and as efficacious as dothiepin, imipramine, mianserin, and sertraline.
Paroxetine	8[e] (N = 1,444)	10–40	Paroxetine was more efficacious than placebo and as efficacious as amitriptyline, bupropion, clomipramine, doxepin, fluoxetine, and imipramine. Mirtazapine was marginally superior to paroxetine. In very old long-term-care patients with minor depression, paroxetine was not more efficacious but was more cognitively toxic than placebo. One trial included patients with dementia.
Sertraline	10[f] (N = 1,817)	50–200	Sertraline was more efficacious than placebo and as efficacious as amitriptyline, fluoxetine, fluvoxamine, imipramine, nortriptyline, and venlafaxine. Sertraline was better tolerated than imipramine and venlafaxine. Greater cognitive improvement occurred with sertraline than with nortriptyline or fluoxetine. Trials included long-term-care patients and patients with dementia of the Alzheimer's type.

[a] Allard et al. 2004; Andersen et al. 1994; Kyle et al. 1998; Navarro et al. 2001; Nyth and Gottfries 1990; Nyth et al. 1992; Roose et al. 2004b. [b] Kasper et al. 2005. [c] Altamura et al. 1989; Devanand et al. 2005; Doraiswamy et al. 2001; Evans et al. 1997; Feighner and Cohn 1985; Finkel et al. 1999; Kasper et al. 2005; Petracca et al. 2001; Schone and Ludwig 1993; Taragano et al. 1997; Tollefson et al. 1995; Wehmeier et al. 2005. [d] Phanjoo et al. 1991; Rahman et al. 1991; Rossini et al. 2005; Wakelin 1986. [e] Burrows et al. 2002; Dunner et al. 1992; Geretsegger et al. 1995; Guillibert et al. 1989; Katona et al. 1998; Mulsant et al. 1999, 2001b; Rapaport et al. 2003; Schatzberg et al. 2002; Schone and Ludwig 1993. [f] Bondareff et al. 2000; Cohn et al. 1990; Doraiswamy et al. 2003; Finkel et al. 1999; Forlenza et al. 2001; Lyketsos et al. 2003; Newhouse et al. 2000; Oslin et al. 2000, 2003; Rossini et al. 2005; Schneider et al. 2003; Sheikh et al. 2004a.

trast, some published studies—including one randomized, placebo-controlled trial—suggest that SSRIs may be efficacious in the treatment of behavioral disturbances associated with dementia, including not only agitation and disinhibition but also delusions and hallucinations (Nyth and Gottfries 1990; Nyth et al. 1992; Pollock et al. 1997, 2002).

In older patients, SSRI starting dosages are typically half the minimal efficacious dosage (see Table 16–3), and the dosage is usually doubled after 1 week. All the SSRIs can be administered in a single daily dose except for fluvoxamine, which should be given in two divided doses. Although even the most frail older patients typically tolerate these drugs relatively well (Oslin et al. 2000), some patients experience some gastrointestinal distress (e.g., nausea) during the first few days of treatment. The syndrome of inappropriate secretion of antidiuretic hormone (SIADH) with significant hyponatremia is a rare but potentially dangerous adverse effect that is observed almost exclusively in the elderly (Fabian et al. 2004).

Recent data have demonstrated that the use of SSRIs is associated with a small but significant increase in the risk of gastrointestinal or postsurgical bleeding (Dalton et al. 2006; Movig et al. 2003). Since SSRIs may act synergistically with other medications that increase the risk of gastrointestinal bleeding, such as nonsteroidal anti-inflammatory drugs (NSAIDs) or low-dose aspirin, SSRIs should be used cautiously in older patients treated with these medications (Dalton et al. 2006).

SSRIs can also be associated with bradycardia and should be started with great caution in patients with low heart rates (e.g., patients taking β-blockers). Even though they can occur, extrapyramidal symptoms are rare in older patients (Mamo et al. 2000), and SSRIs are well tolerated by most

patients with Parkinson's disease (Richard and Kurlan 1997).

Other Newer Antidepressants

Only limited controlled data support the efficacy and safety of bupropion, duloxetine, mirtazapine, nefazodone, or venlafaxine in older patients (Table 16–5). Nevertheless, due to their usually favorable side-effect profiles in younger patients and their various mechanisms of action, these drugs are the preferred alternatives in older patients who do not respond to or who cannot tolerate SSRIs (Alexopoulos et al. 2001). Still, recent controlled data suggest that venlafaxine may be less safe than sertraline in a frail elderly population, without evidence for an increase in efficacy (Oslin et al. 2003). Thus, in the absence of systematic research in older patients, newer agents should be used cautiously (Oslin et al. 2003; Rabins and Lyketsos 2005).

Bupropion

Published data supporting the safety and efficacy of bupropion in geriatric depression are limited to two small controlled trials (see Table 16–5) and one small open study (Steffens et al. 2001). Expert consensus favors the use of bupropion—alone or as an augmentation agent—in older depressed patients who have not responded to SSRIs or who cannot tolerate them (Alexopoulos et al. 2001). In particular, bupropion can be helpful for patients who complain of nausea, diarrhea, unbearable fatigue or sexual dysfunction when treated with SSRIs (Nieuwstraten and Dolovich 2001; Thase et al. 2005b). Although augmentation with bupropion has been reported to be helpful in younger and older patients who were partial responders to SSRIs or venlafaxine (Bodkin et al. 1997; Spier 1998), the safety of this combination has not been established (see below).

TABLE 16–3. Pharmacokinetic properties of selective serotonin reuptake inhibitors

	Half-life (days), including active metabolite(s)	Proportionality of dosage to plasma concentration	Risk of uncomfortable withdrawal symptoms	Age-related pharmacokinetic changes?	Efficacious dosage range in elderly (mg/day)[a]
Citalopram	1–3	Linear across therapeutic range	Low	Yes	20–40
Escitalopram	1–3	Linear across therapeutic range	Low	Yes	10–20
Fluoxetine	7–10	Nonlinear at higher dosages	Very low	Yes	20–40
Fluvoxamine	0.5–1	Nonlinear at higher dosages	Moderate	Yes	50–300
Paroxetine	1	Nonlinear at higher dosages	Moderate	Yes	20–40
Sertraline	1–3	Linear across therapeutic range	Low	No	50–200

[a]Starting dosage is typically half of the lower efficacious dosage; all the selective serotonin reuptake inhibitors can be administered in single daily doses except for fluvoxamine, which should be given in two divided doses.

TABLE 16–4. Newer antidepressants' inhibition of cytochrome P450 and potential for clinically significant drug-drug interaction

	Cytochrome P450				Potential for clinically significant drug-drug interaction
	1A2	2C9/2C19	2D6	3A4	
Bupropion	0	0	+ +	0	Moderate
Citalopram	+	0	+	0	Low
Duloxetine	0	0	+	+	Low
Escitalopram	+	0	+	0	Low
Fluoxetine	+	+ +	+ + +	+ +	High
Fluvoxamine	+ + +	+ + +	+	+ +	High
Mirtazapine	0	0	0	+	Low
Nefazodone	0	+	0	+ + +	High
Paroxetine	+	+	+ + +	+	Moderate
Sertraline	+	+	+	+	Low
Venlafaxine	0	0	0	0	Low

Note. 0 = minimal or no inhibition; + = mild inhibition; + + = moderate inhibition; + + + = strong inhibition.

Source. Belpaire et al. 1998; Brosen et al. 1993; Crewe et al. 1992; Ereshefsky and Dugan 2000; Gram et al. 1993; Greenblatt et al. 1998, 1999; Greene and Barbhaiya 1997; Hua et al. 2004; Iribarne et al. 1998; Jeppesen et al. 1996; Kashuba et al. 1998; Kobayashi et al. 1995; Kotlyar et al. 2005; Pollock 1999; Preskorn and Magnus 1994; Preskorn et al. 1997; Rasmussen et al. 1998; Rickels et al. 1998; Solai et al. 1997, 2002; Spina et al. 2002; von Moltke et al. 1995, 2001; Weigmann et al. 2001.

TABLE 16–5. Summary of published randomized controlled trials of bupropion, duloxetine, mirtazapine, nefazodone, and venlafaxine for acute treatment of geriatric depression

	Number of published trials (cumulative number of older participants)	Dosages studied (mg/day)	Comments
Bupropion	2[a] (N=163)	100–450	Bupropion was as efficacious as imipramine and paroxetine.
Duloxetine	0	NA	NA
Mirtazapine	2[b] (N=370)	15–45	Mirtazapine was as efficacious as low-dose (total daily dose 30–90 mg) amitriptyline and marginally superior to paroxetine.
Nefazodone	0	NA	NA
Venlafaxine	6[c] (N=621)	50–150	Venlafaxine was as efficacious as citalopram, clomipramine, dothiepin, nortriptyline, and sertraline, and was more efficacious than trazodone. It was less well tolerated than sertraline, as well tolerated as citalopram and dothiepin, and better tolerated than clomipramine, nortriptyline, and trazodone.

[a]Branconnier et al. 1983; Doraiswamy et al. 2001; Weihs et al. 2000.
[b]Hoyberg et al. 1996; Schatzberg et al. 2002.
[c]Allard et al. 2004; Gasto et al. 2003; Mahapatra and Hackett 1997; Oslin et al. 2003; Smeraldi et al. 1998; Trick et al. 2004.

In addition to the three small geriatric trials supporting its safety, controlled data on the use of bupropion in patients with heart disease (Kiev et al. 1994; Roose et al. 1991), in smokers (Tashkin et al. 2001), and in patients with neuropathic pain (Semenchuk et al. 2001) confirm clinical experience that bupropion is relatively well tolerated by medically ill patients. Bupropion is contraindicated in patients with seizure disorders or who are at risk for seizure disorders (e.g., poststroke patients). However, the sustained-release preparation of bupropion appears to be associated with a very low incidence of seizure, comparable to other antidepressants (Dunner et al. 1998). Bupropion has also been associated with the onset of psychosis in case reports (Howard and Warnock 1999), and it is prudent to avoid this medication in psychotic patients or in patients at risk for the development of psychotic symptoms. The propensity of bupropion to induce psychosis in patients at risk has been attributed to its action on dopaminergic neurotransmission (Howard and Warnock 1999). The same mechanism has been hypothesized to underlie the association of bupropion with gait disturbance and falls in some patients (Joo et al. 2002; Szuba and Leuchter 1992). Bupropion is a moderate inhibitor of cytochrome P450 2D6 (Kotlyar et al. 2005). It appears to be metabolized by the cytochrome P450 isoform 2B6 (Hesse et al. 2000, 2004), and adverse effects of bupropion such as seizures or gait disturbance may be more likely in patients who take drugs that can inhibit cytochrome P450 2B6, such as fluoxetine or paroxetine (Joo et al. 2002).

Duloxetine

Duloxetine is the newest antidepressant approved in the United States. Like venlafaxine, duloxetine is a dual serotonin-norepinephrine reuptake inhibitor (SNRI) (Chalon et al. 2003). Randomized con-trolled trials in younger patients support its efficacy and tolerability in the treatment of major depression (Hudson et al. 2005; Kirwin and Goren 2005). It is also approved for the treatment of pain associated with diabetic neuropathy (Goldstein et al. 2005), and some data support its efficacy in the treatment of stress urinary incontinence (Mariappan et al. 2005). Published data on duloxetine in the elderly are limited to two publications. In a pooled analysis of patients age 55 and older ($N=$ 299) who participated in eight placebo-controlled trials, duloxetine was found to be efficacious in the treatment of depression and to alleviate associated pain symptoms (Nelson et al. 2005). A small pharmacokinetic study in 12 older and 12 younger healthy volunteers suggests that age has a minimal effect on duloxetine pharmacokinetics and that specific dose recommendations for the elderly are not warranted (Skinner at al. 2004). Similarly, on the basis of currently available data, duloxetine appears to have a low likelihood to be involved in clinically significant drug-drug interactions (Hua et al. 2004) (Table 16–4).

The effect of duloxetine on the reuptake of norepinephrine raises some concerns on its use in older patients with heart disease (Davidson et al. 2005; Johnson et al., in press; Oslin et al. 2003). In younger healthy patients, duloxetine has only a modest effect on heart rate and blood pressure and no clinically meaningful effect on electrocardiographic parameters (Thase et al. 2005c). However, it often takes many years before specific drug toxicity is recognized in older patients (see related discussion elsewhere in this chapter on SSRIs; venlafaxine, another SNRI; and atypical antipsychotics). Thus, in the absence of evidence suggesting any clear advantage over other antidepressants (Hansen et al. 2005; Vis et al. 2005), it is prudent not to use duloxetine as a first-line agent until its safety has been established in a large number of older patients with a variety of physical illnesses (Oslin et al. 2003; Rabins and Lyketsos 2005).

Mirtazapine

The antidepressant activity of mirtazapine has been attributed to its blockade of α_2 autoreceptors, resulting in a direct enhancement of noradrenergic neurotransmission and an increase in synaptic levels of serotonin (5-hydroxytryptamine [5-HT]), indirectly enhancing neurotransmission mediated by serotonin type 1A (5-HT$_{1A}$) receptors. In addition, like the antinausea drugs granisetron and ondansetron, mirtazapine inhibits the 5-HT$_2$ and 5-HT$_3$ serotonin receptors. Thus, mirtazapine could be particularly helpful for patients who do not tolerate SSRIs due to sexual dysfunction (Gelenberg et al. 2000; Montejo et al. 2001), tremor (Pact and Giduz 1999), or severe nausea (Pedersen and Klysner 1997). In one case series, mirtazapine was successfully used to treat depression in 19 mixed-age oncology patients who were receiving chemotherapy (Thompson 2000). In some cases it has been combined with SSRIs (Pedersen and Klysner 1997). However, such a combination should be used very cautiously because its safety has not been established and it has been associated with a serotonin syndrome in an older patient (Benazzi 1998).

There are no published placebo-controlled trials and only two comparator-controlled trials of mirtazapine in geriatric depression (Hoyberg et al. 1996; Schatzberg et al. 2002) (Table 16–5). Consistent with this paucity of controlled data, experts favor the use of mirtazapine as a third-line drug in older depressed patients who have failed to respond or to tolerate SSRIs or venlafaxine (Alexopoulos et al. 2001). While mirtazapine has also been used to treat depression in frail nursing home patients (Roose et al. 2003) and in older patients with dementia (Raji and Brady 2001), there are concerns about its impact on cognition. It has been shown to significantly impair driving performance in two placebo- and active comparator–controlled trials in healthy volunteers (Ridout et al. 2003; Wingen et al. 2005) and to cause delirium in older patients with organic brain syndromes (Bailer et al. 2000). This deleterious impact on cognition is possibly due to mirtazapine's antihistaminergic and sedative effect. Other adverse effects of mirtazapine include weight gain with lipid increase (Nicholas et al. 2003), and neutropenia or even agranulocytosis (Hutchison 2001; Stimmel et al. 1997). While these hematological adverse effects are very rare, they may occur more frequently in patients with compromised immune function (Stimmel et al. 1997).

Nefazodone

Given the absence of any controlled trial in geriatric depression, mediocre outcomes in an open study (Saiz-Ruiz et al. 2002), and reports that the incidence of hepatic toxicity or even liver failure is 10- to 30-fold higher with nefazodone than with other antidepressants (Carvajal et al. 2002; Lucena et al. 1999), nefazodone is very rarely used in older patients. When it is prescribed, one needs to be mindful of potentially problematic drug-drug interactions due to its strong inhibition of the cytochrome P450 3A4, an isozyme responsible for the metabolism of the majority of drugs, including alprazolam, triazolam, carbamazepine, or cyclosporin (Rickels et al. 1998; Spina et al. 2002) (Table 16–4). Also, since older persons metabolize nefazodone more slowly than younger patients, geriatric doses should be about 50% of the doses used in younger adults (Barbhaiya et al. 1996). Finally, a cognitive study in a small group of healthy volunteers found that a higher dosage of nefazodone (i.e.,

200 mg twice daily) was associated with impairment of cognitive and memory functions (van Laar et al. 1995).

Venlafaxine

Like duloxetine, venlafaxine is a SNRI: it inhibits the reuptake of both serotonin and norepinephrine (Harvey et al. 2000). Published geriatric data are from six randomized controlled trials (see Table 16–5) and several case series or open trials (Amore et al. 1997; Dahmen et al. 1999; Dierick 1996; Khan et al. 1995), including in older patients with atypical depression (Roose et al. 2004a), dysthymic disorder (Devanand et al. 2004), and poststroke depression (Dahmen et al. 1999).

In younger depressed patients, several meta-analyses suggest that venlafaxine produces a similar rate of response but a higher rate of remission than SSRIs (Shelton et al. 2005; Smith et al. 2002; Stahl et al. 2002; Thase et al. 2001). This difference in remission rates seems to be most marked in women age 50 and older (Thase et al. 2005a). Also, some open data support the use of venlafaxine in geriatric patients whose symptoms have failed to respond to SSRIs (Whyte et al. 2004). However, venlafaxine exhibits a clear dose-response relationship (Kelsey 1996), and younger patients require higher dosages (i.e., 225 mg/day or more) to obtain the benefits of its dual-action (Harvey et al. 2000). Since venlafaxine pharmacokinetics is similar in younger and older patients (Klamerus et al. 1996), geriatric patients may similarly require high dosages, which are associated with some safety concerns (see below). Venlafaxine can also be useful in the treatment of older patients with generalized anxiety disorder (Katz et al. 2002) or chronic pain syndromes (Grothe et al. 2004). For the treatment of pain syndromes, higher dosages (i.e., 225 mg/day or more) are usually needed, since venlafaxine's antinociceptive effect seems to be mediated through its adrenergic action (Harvey et al. 2000; Schreiber et al. 1999).

Venlafaxine does not inhibit any of the major cytochrome P450 isoenzymes, and thus it is unlikely to cause clinically significant drug-drug interactions (Table 16–4). However, venlafaxine is metabolized by CYP 2D6, and its concentration can increase markedly in genetically poor metabolizers or in patients who are treated with drugs that inhibit this isozyme (Whyte et al. 2006). Even at low doses, venlafaxine inhibits the reuptake of serotonin. Thus, it shares the side-effect profile of SSRIs, including not only nausea, diarrhea, headaches, and excessive sweating but also syndrome of inappropriate antidiuretic hormone and hyponatremia (Kirby et al. 2002), sexual dysfunction (Montejo et al. 2001), serotonin syndrome (McCue et al. 2001; Perry 2000), and discontinuation symptoms (even with the extended-release preparation of venlafaxine) (Fava et al. 1997). In fact, venlafaxine has been associated with the most severe and protracted antidepressant discontinuation syndromes we have observed.

Venlafaxine is also associated with adverse effects that can be linked to its action on the adrenergic system. Adverse effects usually seen with tricyclic antidepressants (TCAs) have been described, including dry mouth, constipation, urinary retention, increased ocular pressure, cardiovascular problems, and transient agitation (Aragona et al. 1998; Benazzi 1997). Most are usually benign, but cardiovascular adverse effects are of concern in the elderly. Most clinicians are aware that venlafaxine can cause hypertension, generally in a dose-dependent fashion (Thase 1998; Zimmer et al. 1997). It has also been associated with clinically significant hypotension, electrocardiographic changes, arrhythmia, and acute ischemia (Davidson et al. 2005; Johnson et al., in press; Lessard et al. 1999; Reznik et al. 1999). In

Great Britain, the National Institute for Clinical Excellence has recommended that venlafaxine should not be prescribed to patients with preexisting heart disease, that an electrocardiogram should be obtained at baseline, and that blood pressure and cardiac functions should be monitored in those patients taking higher doses (National Collaborating Centre for Mental Health 2004). In a randomized trial conducted under double-blind conditions in older nursing home residents, venlafaxine was found to be less well tolerated and less safe than sertraline without evidence for an increase in efficacy (Oslin et al. 2003). Therefore, at present, it seems prudent not to use venlafaxine as a first-line agent in older patients but to reserve it for those who do not respond to SSRIs (Alexopoulos et al. 2001; Mulsant et al. 2001a; Whyte et al. 2004).

Tricyclic Antidepressants and Monoamine Oxidase Inhibitors

TCAs and monoamine oxidase inhibitors (MAOIs) have become third- and fourth-line drugs in the treatment of late-life depression because of their adverse effects and the special precautions their use in older patients entails (Mottram et al. 2006; Mulsant et al. 2001a; Wilson and Mottram 2004). The tertiary-amine TCAs—amitriptyline, clomipramine, doxepin, and imipramine—can cause significant orthostatic hypotension and anticholinergic effects, including cognitive impairment, and they should be avoided in the elderly (Beers 1997). MAOIs, now rarely used in older depressed patients, are discussed later in this section.

When one needs to use a TCA in an older patient, the secondary amines desipramine and nortriptyline are preferred because of their lower propensity to cause orthostasis and falls, their linear pharmacokinetics, and their more modest anti-

cholinergic effects. Typically, the entire dose of desipramine or nortriptyline can be given at bedtime. The relatively narrow therapeutic index (i.e., the plasma level range separating efficacy and toxicity) of the secondary amines necessitates monitoring of plasma levels and electrocardiograms in older patients. After initiation of desipramine at 50 mg and nortriptyline at 25 mg, plasma levels can be obtained after 5–7 days and dosages adjusted linearly, targeting plasma levels of 200–400 ng/mL for desipramine and 50–150 ng/mL for nortriptyline. These narrow ranges may ensure efficacy while decreasing risks of cognitive toxicity and other side effects. Similar to the tertiary TCAs, desipramine and nortriptyline are type 1 antiarrhythmics: they have quinidine-like effects on cardiac conduction and should not be used in patients who have or are at risk for conduction defects (Roose et al. 1991).

Most anticholinergic side effects of desipramine or nortriptyline (e.g., dry mouth, constipation) resolve with time or else can usually be mitigated with symptomatic treatment (Mulsant et al. 1999; Rosen et al. 1993). However, TCAs have been associated with cognitive worsening (Reifler et al. 1989) and with less cognitive improvement than sertraline (Bondareff et al. 2000; Doraiswamy et al. 2003) or other SSRIs.

Even though they have been found to be efficacious in older depressed patients (Georgotas et al. 1986), MAOIs are now rarely used due to the significant hypotension that can be associated with their use and the risk of life-threatening hypertensive or serotonergic crises associated with dietary noncompliance or drug interactions. When MAOIs are used, phenelzine may be preferred to tranylcypromine because it has been more extensively studied in older patients (Georgotas et al. 1983, 1986). A typical starting dosage would be

15 mg/day with a target dosage of 45–90 mg/day in three divided doses. Patients need to be advised about dietary restrictions and should be instructed to inform any health providers (including pharmacists) that they are taking an MAOI.

Psychostimulants

Small double-blind trials suggest that methylphenidate is generally well tolerated and modestly efficacious for medically burdened depressed elders (Satel and Nelson 1989; Wallace et al. 1995). Methylphenidate may also have specific utility in treating the apathy and anergia accompanying late-life depression or dementia. Nonetheless, caution is advised regarding the possible exacerbation of anxiety, psychosis, anorexia, and hypertension that may be associated with methylphenidate as well as its potential interactions with warfarin. Recently, interest has been renewed in using methylphenidate to augment antidepressant response to SSRIs (Lavretsky et al. 2006). Given that SSRIs may inhibit dopamine release, contributing to apathy in this population with diminished dopaminergic function, further exploration of methylphenidate as an augmenting agent is warranted.

Experience with other dopaminergic medications—such as pemoline, piribedil, pramipexole, and ropinirole—in cognitively impaired elders has been more limited than experience with methylphenidate, but there have been encouraging reports (Eisdorfer et al. 1968; Nagaraja and Jayashree 2001; Ostow 2002). It should also be noted that paradoxically, sleepiness has been reported as a side effect in Parkinson's disease patients taking pramipexole and ropinirole (Etminan et al. 2001). The wakefulness-promoting agent modafinil, which appears to induce a calm alertness through nondopaminergic mechanisms, may also have utility in treating residual apathy and fatigue, but systematic geriatric data are currently nonexistent.

Antipsychotic Medications

As in other age groups, atypical antipsychotics are being prescribed as first-line drugs for the treatment of psychotic symptoms of any etiology in late life (Rapoport et al. 2005). An increasing number of studies support the efficacy of these agents in the treatment of older patients with schizophrenia, behavioral and psychological symptoms of dementia, or delirium. At the same time, a series of reports are raising questions regarding their tolerability and safety in older patients (discussed later in this subsection). In the face of the rapidly changing knowledge base, this section summarizes the data relevant to the use of antipsychotics in older patients.

Comparisons of Conventional and Atypical Antipsychotics

As in other age groups, atypical antipsychotics have become first-line drugs for the treatment of psychotic symptoms of any etiology in late life (Rapoport et al. 2005). Despite this major shift in prescribing practice, only seven published randomized controlled trials have compared atypical and conventional antipsychotics in older patients: 1) olanzapine, risperidone, and promazine were compared in patients with behavioral and psychological symptoms of dementia (Gareri et al. 2004); 2) olanzapine and haloperidol were compared in two trials involving older patients with schizophrenia (Barak et al. 2002; Kennedy et al. 2003) and one trial involving patients with behavioral and psychological symptoms of dementia (Verhey et al. 2006); and 3) risperidone and haloperidol were compared in three trials in patients with behavioral and psychological symptoms of dementia (Chan et al. 2001;

De Deyn et al. 1999; Suh et al. 2004). In addition, two randomized controlled trials of relevance to geriatric patients compared oral haloperidol with olanzapine or risperidone (Han et al. 2004; Skrobik et al. 2004). Overall, in these nine trials, olanzapine and risperidone have shown similar or superior efficacy and tolerability to promazine or haloperidol. In particular, they were associated with fewer and less severe extrapyramidal symptoms. In addition to these controlled data, several large case series (e.g., Curran et al. 2005; Frenchman et al. 1997) and expert opinion (Alexopoulos et al. 2004) also support that a shift away from conventional antipsychotics may benefit the elderly who are particularly prone to develop extrapyramidal symptoms or tardive dyskinesia (Caligiuri et al. 2000; del Miller et al. 2005; Dolder and Jeste 2003; Jeste 2004; Jeste et al. 1995; Pollock and Mulsant 1995).

A highly publicized meta-analysis and an FDA warning have noted a nearly twofold increase in the rate of death in older patients with behavioral and psychological symptoms of dementia treated with atypical antipsychotics when compared with patients randomly assigned to receive placebo (Kuehn 2005; Schneider et al. 2005). Other reports have questioned whether atypical antipsychotics cause fewer falls (Hien et al. 2005; Landi et al. 2005) or even extrapyramidal symptoms (Lee et al. 2004; Rochon et al. 2005; van Iersel et al. 2005) than conventional antipsychotics, particularly when doses are increased. Studies suggest that conventional antipsychotics have a lower risk of cerebrovascular events (Percudani et al. 2005), venous thromboembolism (Liperoti et al. 2005b), and pancreatitis (Koller et al. 2003). By contrast, a series of meta-analyses and large pharmacoepidemiologic studies have found that conventional antipsychotics have comparable (or even higher) risks for diabetes mellitus (Feldman et al. 2004), cerebro-

vascular events (Finkel et al. 2005; Liperoti et al. 2005a; Moretti et al. 2005), stroke (Gill et al. 2005; Herrmann et al. 2004), or death (Ray et al. 2001; Wang et al. 2005). Given the current uncertainty regarding the safety of both conventional and atypical antipsychotics—and the absence of consistent evidence supporting the efficacy or safety of drugs from alternative classes (Sink et al. 2005)—clinicians need to consider their risk-benefit ratio for each individual patient (Rabins and Lyketsos 2005). Similarly, in the absence of data supporting differential efficacy (Schneider et al. 2001; Sink et al. 2005), the selection of a specific drug to treat a specific patient should be guided by the strength of the available evidence relevant to the disorder being treated and, in the absence of such evidence, on the differing side-effect profiles of the drugs currently available.

Risperidone

Of the six atypical antipsychotics currently available in the United States, risperidone has the most published geriatric data for a variety of conditions (Alexopoulos et al. 2004; Schneider et al. 2005; Sink et al. 2005). Its efficacy and safety in the treatment of behavioral and psychological symptoms of dementia have been demonstrated in several randomized, placebo-controlled trials (Brodaty et al. 2003; De Deyn et al. 1999, 2005b; Katz et al. 1999; Sink et al. 2005), and randomized comparisons with haloperidol (Chan et al. 2001; De Deyn et al. 1999; Suh et al. 2004), promazine and olanzapine (Gareri et al. 2004), or olanzapine (Fontaine et al. 2003; Mulsant et al. 2004), and uncontrolled studies or large case series (e.g., Irizarry et al. 1999; Herrmann et al. 1998; Lane et al. 2002; Lavretsky and Sultzer 1998; Rainer et al. 2001; Zarate et al. 1997).

The efficacy and safety of risperidone in the treatment of late-life schizophrenia are supported by one randomized comparison with olanzapine (Harvey et al. 2003; Jeste et al. 2003a) and one randomized open-label study of cross-over from conventional antipsychotics to risperidone or olanzapine (Ritchie et al. 2003, 2006). The parallel study showed similar efficacy between olanzapine and risperidone but more weight gain and less cognitive improvement with olanzapine. In the cross-over study, patients switched to olanzapine were more likely to complete the switching process and to show an improvement in psychological quality of life. The results from these two controlled trials are supported by a large body of uncontrolled data in older patients with schizophrenia and other psychotic disorders (e.g., Davidson et al. 2000; Madhusoodanan et al. 1999a, 1999b; Sajatovic et al. 1996; Zarate et al. 1997). In addition, an analysis of the patients with schizophrenia age 65 and older ($N=57$) who participated in randomized studies of the long-acting injectable ("depot" or Consta) risperidone found it was well tolerated and produced significant symptomatic improvements (Lasser et al. 2004).

One randomized comparison with haloperidol (Han andKim 2004) and some uncontrolled data (e.g., Horikawa et al. 2003; Liu et al. 2004; Mittal et al. 2004; Parellada et al. 2004) support the efficacy and tolerability of risperidone in the treatment of delirium. However, there have been several case reports of delirium induced by risperidone (e.g., Kato et al. 2005; Ravona-Springer et al. 1998; Tavcar et al. 1998). One small randomized comparison with clozapine ($N=10$; Ellis et al. 2000) and several open trials of low-dose risperidone in the treatment of patients with Parkinson's disease and drug-induced psychosis or with Lewy body dementia have

had inconsistent results, with clear worsening of parkinsonian symptoms in some studies (e.g., Leopold 2000; Meco et al. 1997; Mohr et al. 2000; Rich et al. 1995; Workman et al. 1997). Thus, risperidone should be used with great caution in the treatment of these disorders (Parkinson Study Group 1999).

As other atypical antipsychotics, the efficacy and safety of risperidone in younger patients with bipolar disorder (and possibly other mood disorders) (Andreescu et al. 2006) are well established. However, there are no efficacy data in older patients with bipolar disorder that would favor the selection of a specific atypical antipsychotic for these patients. As a result, experts favor the use of mood stabilizers except in the presence of severe mania or mania with psychosis, in which case they favor combining risperidone, olanzapine, or quetiapine with a mood stabilizer (Alexopoulos et al. 2004; Sajatovic et al. 2005b; Young et al. 2004).

Commonly reported side effects of risperidone include orthostatic hypotension (on initiation of treatment) and extrapyramidal symptoms that are dose-dependent (Katz et al. 1999). At a given dosage, concentrations of risperidone (and possibly of its active metabolites paliperidone or 9-hydoxyrisperidone) seem to increase with age (Aichhorn et al. 2005; Maxwell et al. 2002). Therefore, typical dosages should be between 0.5 and 2 mg/day for older dementia patients and below 4 mg/day for older nondementia patients. Of all the atypical antipsychotics, risperidone appears to be the most likely to be associated with hyperprolactinemia (Kinon et al. 2003). Risperidone causes only moderate EEG abnormalities (Centorrino et al. 2002), and it is rarely associated with cognitive impairment, probably because of its low affinity for muscarinic receptors (Harvey et al. 2003; Mulsant et al. 2004).

Like other antipsychotics, risperidone can cause weight gain, diabetes, or dyslipidemia. It is more likely to do so than aripiprazole and ziprasidone but less likely than clozapine or olanzapine (Alexopoulos et al. 2004; American Diabetes Association et al. 2004; Feldman et al. 2004).

Olanzapine

After risperidone, olanzapine has the most published geriatric data. Its efficacy and safety in the treatment of behavioral and psychological symptoms of dementia have been demonstrated in several randomized placebo-controlled trials (Clark et al. 2001; De Deyn et al. 2004; Street et al. 2000) and in randomized comparisons with haloperidol (Verhey et al. 2006), promazine and risperidone (Gareri et al. 2004), and risperidone (Fontaine et al. 2003; Mulsant et al. 2004). Of note, the study by Street and colleagues (2000) found an inverted dose-response relationship (i.e., patients receiving 15 mg/day had worse outcomes than patients receiving 5 mg/day), suggesting that higher doses may be toxic in these patients (see discussion later in this subsection). As discussed above, the efficacy and safety of olanzapine in the treatment of late-life schizophrenia have been demonstrated in two randomized comparisons with haloperidol (Barak et al. 2002; Kennedy et al. 2003) and two randomized comparisons with risperidone (Harvey et al. 2003; Jeste et al. 2003a; Ritchie et al. 2003, 2006).

In one of only three published randomized controlled trials of the pharmacotherapy of delirium, and the largest to date, olanzapine and haloperidol were found to be comparable in efficacy (Skrobik et al. 2004). However, caution is needed when using olanzapine in patients with delirium since some controlled trials have reported some cognitive worsening in dementia patients treated with olanzapine (Kennedy et al. 2005; Mulsant et al. 2004), and several case reports of delirium induced by olanzapine have been published (Lim et al. 2006; Morita et al. 2004; Samuels and Fang 2004). Similarly, two controlled trials suggest that olanzapine may not be a drug of choice in treating drug-induced psychosis in patients with Parkinson's disease. In one placebo-controlled study, olanzapine was not significantly different from placebo in terms of psychotic symptoms and was significantly worse in terms of parkinsonian symptoms and activities of daily living (Breier et al. 2002). In another small randomized study ($N=15$), olanzapine was not as efficacious as clozapine and was more toxic (Goetz et al. 2000). The need for caution when olanzapine is used to treat psychosis in patients with Parkinson's disease or Lewy body dementia is reinforced by several open trials or case series: although a few have shown positive results (e.g., Cummings et al. 2002; Sa et al. 2001), most have reported a significant worsening of motor symptoms in these patients (e.g., Marsh et al. 2001; Molho and Factor 1999; Onofrj et al. 2000; Parkinson Study Group 1999; Z. Walker et al. 1999; Wolters et al. 1996).

The evidence supporting the efficacy and safety of olanzapine in younger patients with bipolar disorder and other mood disorders (Andreescu et al. 2006; Shelton et al. 2001; Thase 2002) is particularly strong. However, as discussed earlier, there are no relevant data in older patients with mood disorders (Alexopoulos et al. 2004; Sajatovic et al. 2005a, 2005b; Young et al. 2004). Similarly, there are no relevant geriatric data on the rapidly dissolving or the intramuscular preparations of olanzapine (Belgamwar and Fenton 2005).

On review of all evidence available in 2004, a consensus conference concluded

TABLE 16–6. Receptor blockade of atypical antipsychotics

	D_2	5-HT$_2$	M_1	α_2
Aripiprazole	*	++	0	+
Clozapine	+	++	+++	+
Olanzapine	++	++	+++	+
Quetiapine	+	++	+	++
Risperidone	+++	+++	0	++
Ziprasidone	++	++	0	+

Note. * = high affinity partial agonist; α_2 = alpha-adrenergic type 2; D_2 = dopamine type 2; 5-HT$_2$ = 5-hydroxytryptamine (serotonin) type 2; M_1 = muscarinic type 1; 0 = none; + = minimal; ++ = intermediate; +++ = high.

that among the six atypical antipsychotics, clozapine and olanzapine are associated with the highest risk for diabetes and cause the greatest weight gain and dyslipidemia (American Diabetes Association et al. 2004). However, this consensus was based on data in younger patients with psychotic and mood disorders. Olanzapine has been associated with significant increases in concentrations of glucose and lipids (Melkersson and Hulting 2001), which can occur even in the absence of weight gain but appear to be reversible on discontinuation of the drug (Lindenmayer et al. 2001). There are only very limited relevant geriatric data, and it is possible that the risks for metabolic problems are different in older patients, in particular those with dementia (Etminan et al. 2003; Feldman et al. 2004; Hwang et al. 2003; Micca et al. 2006). Other common side effects include sedation and gait distrubance. Extrapyramidal symptoms appear to be dose-dependent and are rare at the lower dosages typically used in treating older patients (5–10 mg/day). Olanzapine has also been associated with electroencephalographic abnormalities (Centorrino et al. 2002), and its strong blocking of the muscarinic receptor (Chew et al. 2005; Mulsant et al. 2003) (Table 16–6) may explain why it has been associated with constipation in a large se-

ries of long-term-care patients (Martin et al. 2003); decreased efficacy at higher doses in a randomized trial in older agitated or psychotic patients with dementia (Street et al. 2000); a differential cognitive effect from risperidone in randomized trials involving older patients with schizophrenia (Harvey et al. 2003) or dementia (Mulsant et al. 2004); worsening of cognition in a large placebo-controlled trial in older nonagitated, nonpsychotic patients with Alzheimer's disease (Kennedy et al. 2005); and frank delirium in some clinical cases (Lim et al. 2006; Morita et al. 2004; Samuels and Fang 2004). Patients who are older, females, nonsmokers, or on a drug that inhibits the cytochrome P450 1A2 (e.g., fluvoxamine or ciprofloxacin) have higher concentrations of olanzapine and may be at higher risk for adverse effects (Gex-Fabry et al. 2003). Because of its adverse-effect profile, experts do not recommend olanzapine as a first-line antipsychotic in older patients with cognitive impairment, constipation, diabetes, diabetic neuropathy, dyslipidemia, obesity, xerophthalmia, or xerostomia (Alexopoulos et al. 2004).

Quetiapine

Results of randomized controlled trials in older patients with behavioral and psychological symptoms of dementia—still un-published but presented at conferences (Schneider et al. 2005)—and published but uncontrolled or unblinded data in older patients with primary psychotic disorders, dementia, or delirium suggest that quetiapine is effective for these disorders (Kim et al. 2003; Madhusoodanan et al. 2000; McManus et al. 1999; Mintzer et al. 2004; Pae et al. 2004; Sasaki et al. 2003; Tariot et al. 2000; Yang et al. 2005). To date, the strongest published geriatric data on the use of quetiapine in late life are in patients with Parkinson's disease and drug-induced psychosis (Fernandez et al. 1999, 2002; Menza et al. 1999; Targum and Abbott 2000). The overall efficacy and good tolerability of quetiapine in patients at high risk for extrapyramidal symptoms make quetiapine the first-line antipsychotic for older patients with Parkinson's disease, dementia with Lewy body, or tardive dyskinesia (Alexopoulos et al. 2004; Poewe 2005). Quetiapine can cause somnolence or dizziness (Jaskiw et al. 2004; Yang et al. 2005), but the incidence of these adverse effects can be minimized by a slower dose titration. The risk for weight gain, diabetes, or dyslipidemia associated with the use of quetiapine appears similar to the risk of risperidone but lower than the risk of clozapine or olanzapine (American Diabetes Association et al. 2004; Feldman et al. 2004).

Clozapine

Clozapine is still considered the drug of choice for younger patients with treatment-refractory schizophrenia (Meltzer 1998), and one small case series suggests that it can be similarly helpful for the treatment of older patients with primary psychotic disorders that are refractory to other treatments (Sajatovic et al. 1997). A randomized, controlled trial comparing clozapine and chlorpromazine in older patients with

schizophrenia (Howanitz et al. 1999) and one large case series (Barak et al. 1999) also support the use of clozapine in moderate dosages (i.e., around 50–200 mg/day) in older patients with primary psychotic disorders. The strongest published geriatric studies of clozapine are focused on the treatment of drug-induced psychosis in patients with Parkinson's disease (Ellis et al. 2000; Goetz et al. 2000; Parkinson Study Group 1999). The results of these studies suggest that clozapine at low dosages (12.5–50 mg/day) is the preferred treatment for this condition (Parkinson Study Group 1999). However, the use of clozapine in older patients is severely limited due to its significant hematologic, neurologic and cognitive, metabolic, and cardiac adverse effects (Alvir et al. 1993; Centorrino et al. 2002, 2003; Koller et al. 2001; Melkersson and Hulting 2001; Modai et al. 2000; Sernyak et al. 2002).

Aripiprazole and Ziprasidone

Aripiprazole and ziprasidone are the latest atypical antipsychotics to become available in the United States. On the basis of their lower impact on glucose, lipids, and weight (American Diabetes Association et al. 2004), and their lack of affinity for the muscarinic receptor (see Table 16–6) and thus their low potential to cause cognitive impairment, aripiprazole and ziprasidone are attractive medications for older patients with psychosis. However, their use in older patients has been limited to a second-line treatment so far due to the almost total absence of geriatric data (Alexopoulos et al. 2004).

One randomized controlled trial of aripiprazole in older patients with behavioral and psychological symptoms of dementia has been published (De Deyn et al. 2005a). Other geriatric data are limited to two publications (Jeste et al. 2003b;

Madhusoodanan et al. 2004). There is only one published case series (Berkowitz 2003) and one pharmacokinetic study (Wilner et al. 2000) on oral ziprasidone in the elderly. In addition, there are two published reports on the use of intramuscular ziprasidone, with no adverse cardiovascular or electrocardiographic changes observed in a total of 38 older patients (Greco et al. 2005; Kohen et al. 2005). However, in the absence of systematic study, there is lingering concern regarding the potential effects of ziprasidone on cardiac conduction, and ziprasidone should not be used in older patients with QTc prolongation or congestive heart failure (Alexopoulos et al. 2004).

Mood Stabilizers

As a class, mood stabilizers are high-risk medications for elderly patients. There is a paucity of controlled studies and an abundance of concern regarding their potential toxicity, problematic side effects, and drug interactions. Lithium continues to be used for older patients with bipolar disorder and, less commonly, for antidepressant augmentation. Beyond their approved indications, anticonvulsants are often deployed in the management of agitation accompanying dementia. Despite its age-associated risks, lithium is still used commonly in elders with bipolar disorder (Umapathy et al. 2000). Currently, there is no consensus as to whether it is still appropriate to prescribe lithium as a first-line mood stabilizer for elders, nor is there agreement on the management of secondary mania (Sajatovic et al. 2005b; Young et al. 2004).

Lithium

Open and naturalistic trials suggest that lithium is efficacious in the acute treatment and prophylaxis of mania in older patients (Eastham et al. 1998; Wylie et al.

1999). However, reductions in renal clearance and decreased total body water significantly affect the pharmacokinetics of lithium in older patients, increasing the risk of toxicity. Moreover, specific medical comorbidities common in late life—such as renal dysfunction, hyponatremia, dehydration, and heart failure—also exacerbate the risk of toxicity. Thiazide diuretics, angiotensin-converting enzyme inhibitors, and nonsteroidal anti-inflammatory drugs may precipitate toxicity by further diminishing the renal clearance of lithium. For all these reasons, older patients require lower dosages than younger patients to produce similar serum lithium levels.

Elders are more sensitive to neurological side effects at lower lithium levels. This sensitivity may be a consequence of increased permeability of the blood-brain barrier and subtle changes in sodium-lithium countertransport. Neurotoxicity may manifest as coarse tremor, slurred speech, ataxia, hyperreflexia, and muscle fasciculations. Cognitive impairment has been observed with levels well below 1 mEq/L, and frank delirium has been reported with serum levels as low as 1.5 mEq/L (Sproule et al. 2000). Consequently, older patients are typically treated with target levels of lithium as low as 0.4–0.8 mEq/L.

In addition to lithium levels, electrolytes and the electrocardiogram should be checked regularly. Older patients are at higher risk for lithium-induced hypothyroidism and should have their thyroid-stimulating hormone concentration monitored at 6-month intervals. Lithium toxicity can be fatal or can produce persistent central nervous system impairment. Thus, it is a medical emergency that requires careful correction of fluid and electrolyte imbalances and that may require administration of aminophylline and mannitol (or even hemodialysis) to increase lithium excretion.

Anticonvulsants

Anticonvulsants are used as alternatives to lithium in the treatment of bipolar disorder and as alternatives to antipsychotics for the symptomatic management of agitation accompanying dementia. In general, side effects are more tolerable and less severe than those of lithium. Furthermore, there may be a subgroup of bipolar patients with dysphoria or rapid cycling who respond poorly to lithium but do well with anticonvulsants (Post et al. 1998). Similarly, given its putative etiology, mania associated with dementia and other neurological illness ("secondary mania") may respond preferentially to anticonvulsants (Shulman 1997).

Valproate

Valproate is a broad-spectrum anticonvulsant that has been approved in the United States for the treatment of mania. Small case series have suggested that valproic acid is relatively well tolerated by older bipolar patients (Kando et al. 1996; Noaghiul et al. 1998) and those with agitation in the context of dementia (Kunik et al. 1998). Nonetheless, there have been four negative placebo-controlled trials in which valproate was not better than placebo in treating agitation of dementia (Sink et al. 2005; Tariot et al. 2005).

Sedation, nausea, weight gain, and hand tremors are common dose-related side effects. Mild stomach upset may be decreased by use of the enteric-coated divalproex salt. Thrombocytopenia is possible in more than half of elderly patients treated with valproate and may ensue at lower total drug levels than in younger patients (Conley et al. 2001). Also dose-related are reversible elevations in liver enzymes and transient elevations in blood ammonia levels (Davis et al. 1994). Liver failure and pancreatitis are rare. Valproate has other metabolic effects of concern to aging patients, such as increases in bone turnover and reductions of serum folate, with concomitant elevations in plasma homocysteine concentrations (Sato et al. 2001; Schwaninger et al. 1999).

The pharmacokinetics of valproate vary according to formulation, and valproic acid, divalproex sodium, and its extended-release preparation are not interchangeable. Valproate is principally metabolized by mitochondrial β-oxidation and secondarily by the cytochrome P450 system; typical half-lives are in the range of 5–16 hours and are not affected by aging alone. Concomitant administration of valproate will increase concentrations of phenobarbital, primidone, carbamazepine, diazepam, and lamotrigine. Conversely, concurrent administration of carbamazepine, lamotrigine, topiramate, and phenytoin may decrease levels of valproate. Fluoxetine and erythromycin may potentiate the effects of valproate. Changes in protein binding due to drug interactions are no longer considered clinically important beyond causing the misinterpretation of total (i.e., free and bound) drug levels (Benet and Hoener 2002). Valproate binding to plasma proteins is generally reduced in the elderly, suggesting that use of free drug levels may be preferable (Kodama et al. 2001).

Carbamazepine

Carbamazepine is effective for the acute treatment and prophylaxis of mania in younger patients (Post et al. 1998). In a placebo-controlled trial in 51 nursing home patients, carbamazepine was also found to be efficacious in treating agitation and aggression associated with dementia (Tariot et al. 1998).

Carbamazepine is primarily eliminated by cytochrome P450 3A4, and its clearance is reduced with aging (Bernus et al. 1997). Its interactions with other drugs are protean and complex. Carbamazepine concentrations are increased to potential toxicity by cytochrome P450 3A4 inhibitors such as macrolide antibiotics, antifungals, and some antidepressants (see Table 16–3). Cytochrome P450 3A4 inducers—such as phenobarbital, phenytoin, and carbamazepine itself—will lower its concentration and the concentrations of many drugs metabolized by this isoenzyme (Spina et al. 1996). Side effects of carbamazepine include nausea, dizziness, ataxia, and neutropenia. Older patients are at higher risk for drug-induced leukopenia and agranulocytosis, ataxia, and, of course, drug interactions (Cates and Powers 1998). Oxcarbamazepine, the 10-keto analog of carbamazepine, is a less potent cytochrome P450 3A4 inducer, and although studied in some small trials in bipolar patients, it has not been studied in dementia (Lima 2000).

Gabapentin and Pregabalin

Although gabapentin is used in bipolar disorder, trials have not borne out its effectiveness and there are only anecdotal reports of its use in dementia (Pande et al. 2000). Nonetheless, it has a generally favorable side-effect profile and modest anxiolytic and analgesic effects, particularly for neuropathic pain. Gabapentin does not bind to plasma proteins and is not metabolized, being eliminated by renal excretion. In patients with renal impairment, neurological adverse effects such as ataxia, involuntary movements, disorganized thinking, excitation, and extreme sedation have been noted. Even in the absence of renal dysfunction, elderly patients may be prone to excessive sedation. Therefore, in the elderly, initial doses of 100 mg twice a day are more prudent than the 900 mg/day recommended as a starting dosage for younger patients with epilepsy.

Pregabalin is a structural congener of gabapentin. It has an improved pharmacokinetic profile and may be helpful for neuropathic pain in the elderly. Nonetheless, it is a controlled substance, and there are no data in the geriatric population (Guay 2005).

Lamotrigine

Lamotrigine is approved in the United States for the maintenance treatment of bipolar disorder to prevent mood episodes (depressive, manic, or mixed episodes). Data from a randomized controlled trial support that lamotrigine is more effective than placebo in treating bipolar disorder in older patients (Sajatovic et al. 2005a).

Somnolence, rashes, and headaches have been observed in a significant number of older patients. In contrast with many other mood stabilizers and antidepressants, lamotrigine does not seem to be associated with weight gain (Morell et al. 2003).

In geriatric patients, rashes were the most common reason for study withdrawal, but they were less frequent with lamotrigine (3%) than with carbamazepine (19%) (Brodie et al. 1999). Severe rashes including Stevens-Johnson syndrome or toxic epidermal necrolysis have been observed in about 0.3% of adult patients (Messenheimer 1998). At the first sign of rash or other evidence of hypersensitivity (e.g., fever, lymphadenopathy), unless the signs are clearly not drug-related, lamotrigine should be discontinued and the patient should be evaluated. The incidence of rashes can be reduced by using a slower dose titration. Also, because valproate increases lamotrigine plasma concentration, the titration of lamotrigine needs to be slowed down and its target dosage needs to be halved in patients who are receiving valproate.

Anxiolytics

Social isolation, financial concerns, and declining intellectual and physical function may predispose elders to anxiety. New-onset anxiety is a frequent accompaniment of physical illness, depression, or medication side effects. The SSRIs and venlafaxine have displaced the long-acting benzodiazepines (e.g., diazepam) and medications with very short half-lives (e.g., alprazolam) as initial treatments for anxiety in late life, whereas the intermediate half-life benzodiazepine lorazepam and the nonbenzodiazepines (e.g., zaleplon, zolpidem) have become the most commonly used hypnotics.

Benzodiazepines and Nonbenzodiazepine Hypnotics

Detrimental effects of the benzodiazepines in elders frequently outweigh any short-term symptomatic relief that they may provide. Continuous benzodiazepine use increases the risk of falls, hip fractures, and cognitive impairment in elderly patients (Sorock and Shimkin 1988). The popular nonbenzodiazepine zolpidem was found in a very large case-control study to double the risk of hip fracture, after controlling for age, gender, and medical conditions (Wang et al. 2001). Single small doses of diazepam, nitrazepam, and temazepam have caused significant impairment in memory and psychomotor performance in elderly subjects (Nikaido et al. 1990; Pomara et al. 1989).

Nevertheless, treatment with benzodiazepines may be indicated for a few weeks in the acute treatment of depression-related sleep disturbance when the primary pharmacotherapy is an antidepressant. Relative contraindications include heavy snoring (because it suggests sleep apnea), dementia (because such patients are at increased risk for daytime confusion, im-

pairment in activities of daily living, and daytime sleepiness), and the use of other sedating medications or alcohol.

In the elderly, compounds with long half-lives (clonazepam, diazepam, and flurazepam) should be avoided. Also, several drugs with shorter half-lives (i.e., alprazolam, triazolam, midazolam, and the nonbenzodiazepines zaleplon and zolpidem) undergo phase 1 hepatic metabolism by cytochrome P450 3A4 that is subject to specific interactions and apparently age-associated decline (Freudenreich and Menza 2000; Greenblatt et al. 1991). Sedatives with very short half-lives may also increase the likelihood that confused elders will awake in the middle of the night to stagger off to the bathroom. Oxazepam and lorazepam have acceptable half-lives that do not increase with age, are not subject to drug interactions, and have no active metabolites. Lorazepam is preferred for inducing sleep because oxazepam has a relatively slow and erratic absorption. Lorazepam is available in appropriately small doses (0.5-mg pills) and is well absorbed intramuscularly.

Buspirone

The anxiolytic buspirone, a partial 5-HT$_{1A}$ agonist, may be beneficial for some anxious patients and appears to be well tolerated by the elderly without the sedation or addiction liability of the benzodiazepines (Steinberg 1994). Thus, it may be helpful for elders with generalized anxiety disorder who are prone to falls, confusion, or chronic lung disease. Nonetheless, buspirone may take several weeks to exert an anxiolytic effect; has no cross-tolerance with benzodiazepines; and may have side effects such as dizziness, headache, and nervousness (Strand et al. 1990). Unlike the SSRIs, buspirone is of limited use for panic or obsessive-compulsive disorders. The pharmacokinetics of buspirone are not

TABLE 16–7. Cholinesterase inhibitors

Drug	Clearance	Dosing	Significant side effects	Pharmacodynamics
Donepezil	Half-life, 70–80 hr Cytochrome P450 3A4, 2D6	5–10 mg/day Start at 5 mg qhs	Mild nausea, diarrhea, agitation	Reversible acetylcholinesterase inhibition
Galantamine	Half-life, 7 hr Cytochrome P450 2D6, 3A4	8–24 mg/day divided bid Start at 4 mg bid	Moderate nausea, vomiting, diarrhea, anorexia, tremor, insomnia	Reversible acetylcholinesterase inhibition; nicotinic modulation may increase acetylcholine release
Rivastigmine	Half-life, 1.25 hr Renal	6–12 mg/day divided bid Start at 1.5 mg bid, retitrate if drug stopped	Severe nausea, vomiting, anorexia, weight loss, sweating, dizziness	Pseudoirreversible acetylcholinesterase inhibition, also butylcholinesterase inhibition

affected by age or gender, but coadministration with verapamil, diltiazem, erythromycin, or itraconazole will substantially increase buspirone concentrations, and overenthusiastic combinations with serotonergic medications may result in the serotonin syndrome (Mahmood and Sahajwalla 1999). Buspirone should be started at 5 mg three times a day and gradually increased by 5-mg increments every week to a maximum dosage of 60 mg/day.

Cognitive Enhancers

Cholinesterase Inhibitors

Four of the five currently approved drugs for Alzheimer's disease in the United States (tacrine, donepezil, rivastigmine, and galantamine) are cholinesterase inhibitors (Table 16–7). The use of tacrine is no longer recommended because of its potential hepatotoxic effects. The principal side effects of these medications are concentration dependent and result from their peripheral cholinergic actions. With these side effects

in mind, clinicians should be aware of the drugs' specific pathways of elimination and potential pharmacokinetic drug interactions with cytochrome P450 2D6/3A4 inhibitors and cytochrome P450 3A4 inducers when prescribing donepezil and galantamine (Carrier 1999; Crismon 1998). Rivastigmine will be affected by renal function, and FDA warnings have emphasized the need for careful dose titration (and retitration if restarting) to prevent severe vomiting. Drugs with potent anticholinergic effects directly antagonize cholinesterase inhibitors (Chew et al. 2005; Mulsant et al. 2003).

The currently available cognitive enhancers have been demonstrated in controlled trials to result in modest improvements in cognition and function (Cummings 2000). A rapid symptomatic deterioration may occur when these drugs are discontinued, and no evidence suggests that they alter the underlying neuropathology of Alzheimer's disease or its eventual progression. Before initiating anticholinesterase therapy, it is imperative that unnecessary anticholinergic medications be discontinued. In patients with diminished cognitive reserve, even small anticholinergic effects can substantially impair cognition (Chew et al. 2005; Mulsant et al. 2003; Nebes et al. 2005). Cholinesterase inhibitors may have a role to play in the prevention and treatment of behavioral and psychological symptoms of dementia (Sink et al. 2005), but more research is needed in this area.

NMDA Receptor Antagonist

Memantine, the first drug of this class, has been approved by the FDA for the treatment of moderate to severe Alzheimer's disease. Glutaminergic overstimulation may cause excitotoxic neuronal damage. As an uncompetitive antagonist with moderate affinity for NMDA receptors, memantine may attenuate neurotoxicity without interfering with glutamate's normal physiological actions. In patients with moderate to severe Alzheimer's disease, a daily dosage of 20 mg of memantine was well tolerated and significantly slowed the rate of deterioration compared with placebo in a 28-week U.S. multicenter trial (Reisberg et al. 2003). A 6-month, placebo-controlled study in 401 donepezil-treated patients showed benefits of the combination therapy on cognition and activities of daily living relative to baseline (Tariot et al. 2004). In both studies, memantine was well tolerated, although it may cause confusion in some patients. It does not appear to be implicated in drug-drug interactions, but it is excreted by the kidneys and its dosage may need to be reduced in patients with significant impairment in renal function.

References

Aichhorn W, Weiss U, Marksteiner J, et al: Influence of age and gender on risperidone plasma concentrations. J Psychopharmacol. 19(4):395–401, 2005

Alexopoulos GS, Katz IR, Reynolds CF 3rd, et al: Pharmacotherapy of depression in older patients: a summary of the expert consensus guidelines. J Psychiatr Pract 7:361–376, 2001

Alexopoulos GS, Streim J, Carpenter D, Docherty JP, Expert Consensus Panel for Using Antipsychotic Drugs in Older Patients: Using antipsychotic agents in older patients. J Clin Psychiatry 65 (suppl 2):5–104, 2004

Allard P, Gram L, Timdahl K, et al: Efficacy and tolerability of venlafaxine in geriatric outpatients with major depression: a double-blind, randomised 6-month comparative study. Int J Geriatr Psychiatry 19:1123–1130, 2004

Altamura AC, De Novellis F, Guercetti G, et al: Fluoxetine compared with amitriptyline in elderly depression: a controlled clinical trial. Int J Clin Pharmacol Res 9:391–396, 1989

Alvir JJ, Lieberman JA, Safferman AZ, et al: Clozapine-induced agranulocytosis: incidence and risk factors in the United States. N Engl J Med 329:162–167, 1993

American Diabetes Association, American Psychiatric Association, American Association of Clinical Endocrinologists, et al: Consensus development conference on antipsychotic drugs and obesity and diabetes. Diabetes Care 27(2):596–601, 2004

Amore M, Ricci M, Zanardi R, et al: Long-term treatment of geropsychiatric depressed patients with venlafaxine. J Affect Disord 46:293–296, 1997

Andersen G, Vestergaard K, Lauritzen L: Effective treatment of poststroke depression with the selective serotonin reuptake inhibitor citalopram. Stroke 25:1099–1104, 1994

Andreescu C, Mulsant BH, Rothschild AJ, et al: Pharmacotherapy of major depression with psychotic features: what is the evidence? Psychiatric Annals 35(1):31–38, 2006

Aragona M, Inghilleri M: Increased ocular pressure in two patients with narrow angle glaucoma treated with venlafaxine. Clin Neuropharmacol 21:130–131, 1998

Arranz FJ, Ros S: Effects of comorbidity and polypharmacy on the clinical usefulness of sertraline in elderly depressed patients: an open multicentre study. J Affect Disord 46:285–291, 1997

Bailer U, Fischer P, Kufferle B, et al: Occurrence of mirtazapine-induced delirium in organic brain disorder. Int Clin Psychopharmacol 15:239–243, 2000

Barak Y, Wittenberg N, Naor S, et al: Clozapine in elderly psychiatric patients: tolerability, safety, and efficacy. Compr Psychiatry 40:320–325, 1999

Barak Y, Shamir E, Zemishlani H, et al: Olanzapine vs haloperidol in the treatment of elderly chronic schizophrenia patients. Progr Neuropsychopharmacol Biol Psychiatry 26(6):1199–1202, 2002

Barbhaiya RH, Buch AB, Greene DS: A study of the effect of age and gender on the pharmacokinetics of nefazodone after single and multiple doses. J Clin Psychopharmacol 16:19–25, 1996

Beers MH: Explicit criteria for determining potentially inappropriate medication use by the elderly. Arch Intern Med 157:1531–1536, 1997

Belgamwar RB, Fenton M: Olanzapine IM or velotab for acutely disturbed/agitated people with suspected serious mental illnesses. Cochrane Database of Systematic Reviews, Issue 2, Art No CD003729; DOI: 10.1002/14651858.CD003729, 2005

Belpaire FM, Wijnant P, Temmerman A, et al: The oxidative metabolism of metoprolol in human liver microsomes: inhibition by the selective serotonin reuptake inhibitors. Eur J Clin Pharmacol 54:261–264, 1998

Benazzi F: Urinary retention with venlafaxine-haloperidol combination. Pharmacopsychiatry 30:27, 1997

Benazzi F: Serotonin syndrome with mirtazapine-fluoxetine combination. Int J Geriatr Psychiatry 13:495–496, 1998

Benet LZ, Hoener B: Changes in plasma protein binding have little clinical relevance. Clin Pharmacol Ther 71:115–121, 2002

Berkowitz A: Ziprasidone for dementia in elderly patients: case review. J Psychiatr Pract 9(6):469–473, 2003

Bernus I, Dickinson RG, Hooper WD: Anticonvulsant therapy in aged patients. Clinical pharmacokinetic considerations. Drugs Aging 10:278–289, 1997

Bodkin JA, Lasser RA, Wines JD Jr, et al: Combining serotonin reuptake inhibitors and bupropion in partial responders to antidepressant monotherapy. J Clin Psychiatry 58:137–145, 1997

Bondareff W, Alpert M, Friedhoff AJ, et al: Comparison of sertraline and nortriptyline in the treatment of major depressive disorder in late life. Am J Psychiatry 157:729–736, 2000

Branconnier RJ, Cole JO, Ghazvinian S, et al: Clinical pharmacology of bupropion and imipramine in elderly depressives. J Clin Psychiatry 44(5 pt 2):130–133, 1983

Breier A, Sutton VK, Feldman PD, et al: Olanzapine in the treatment of dopamimetic-induced psychosis in patients with Parkinson's disease. Biol Psychiatry 52(5):438–445, 2002

Brodaty H, Ames D, Snowdon J, et al: A randomized placebo-controlled trial of risperidone for the treatment of aggression, agitation, and psychosis of dementia. J Clin Psychiatry 64(2):134–143, 2003

Brodie MJ, Overstall PW, Giorgi L: Multicentre, double-blind, randomised comparison between lamotrigine and carbamazepine in elderly patients with newly diagnosed epilepsy. The UK Lamotrigine Elderly Study Group. Epilepsy Res 37:81–87, 1999

Brosen K, Skjelbo E, Rasmussen BB, et al: Fluvoxamine is a potent inhibitor of cytochrome P4501A2. Biochem Pharmacol 45:1211–1214, 1993

Burrows AB, Salzman C, Satlin A, et al: A randomized, placebo-controlled trial of paroxetine in nursing home residents with non-major depression. Depress Anxiety 15(3):102–110, 2002

Caligiuri MR, Jeste DV, Lacro JP: Antipsychotic-induced movement disorders in the elderly: epidemiology and treatment recommendations. Drugs Aging 17:363–384, 2000

Carrier L: Donepezil and paroxetine: possible drug interaction. J Am Geriatr Soc 47:1037, 1999

Carvajal GP, Garcia D, Sanchez SA, et al: Hepatotoxicity associated with the new antidepressants. J Clin Psychiatry 63:135–137, 2002

Cates M, Powers R: Concomitant rash and blood dyscrasias in geriatric psychiatry patients treated with carbamazepine. Ann Pharmacother 32:884–887, 1998

Centorrino F, Price BH, Tuttle M, et al: EEG abnormalities during treatment with typical and atypical antipsychotics. Am J Psychiatry 159:109–115, 2002

Centorrino F, Albert MJ, Drago-Ferrante G, et al: Delirium during clozapine treatment: incidence and associated risk factors. Pharmacopsychiatry 36(4):156–160, 2003

Chalon SA, Granier LA, Vandenhende FR, et al: Duloxetine increases serotonin and norepinephrine availability in healthy subjects: a double-blind, controlled study. Neuropsychopharmacology 28(9):1685–1693, 2003

Chan WC, Lam LC, Choy CN, et al: A double-blind randomised comparison of risperidone and haloperidol in the treatment of behavioural and psychological symptoms in Chinese dementia patients. Int J Geriatr Psychiatry 16:1156–1162, 2001

Chew ML, Mulsant BH, Rosen J, et al: Serum anticholinergic activity and cognition in patients with moderate to severe dementia. Am J Geriatr Psychiatry 13:535–538, 2005

Clark WS, Street JS, Feldman PD, et al: The effects of olanzapine in reducing the emergence of psychosis among nursing home patients with Alzheimer's disease. J Clin Psychiatry 62:34–40, 2001

Cohn CK, Shrivastava R, Mendels J, et al: Double-blind, multicenter comparison of sertraline and amitriptyline in elderly depressed patients. J Clin Psychiatry 51 (suppl B):28–33, 1990

Conley EL, Coley KC, Pollock BG, et al: Prevalence and risk of thrombocytopenia with valproic acid: experience at a psychiatric teaching hospital. Pharmacotherapy 21:1325–1330, 2001

Crewe HK, Lennard MS, Tucker GT, et al: The effect of selective serotonin re-uptake inhibitors on cytochrome P4502D6 (CYP 2D6) activity in human liver microsomes. Br J Clin Pharmacol 34:262–265, 1992

Crismon ML: Pharmacokinetics and drug interactions of cholinesterase inhibitors administered in Alzheimer's disease. Pharmacotherapy 18:47–54, 1998

Cummings JL: Cholinesterase inhibitors: a new class of psychotropic compounds. Am J Psychiatry 157:4–15, 2000

Cummings JL, Street J, Masterman D, et al: Efficacy of olanzapine in the treatment of psychosis in dementia with Lewy bodies. Dement Geriatr Cogn Disord 13(2):67–73, 2002

Curran S, Turner D, Musa S, et al: Psychotropic drug use in older people with mental illness with particular reference to antipsychotics: a systematic study of tolerability and use in different diagnostic groups. Int J Geriatr Psychiatry 20(9):842–847, 2005

Dahmen N, Marx J, Hopf HC, et al: Therapy of early poststroke depression with venlafaxine: safety, tolerability, and efficacy as determined in an open, uncontrolled clinical trial. Stroke 30:691–692, 1999

Dalton SO, Sorensen HT, Johansen C: SSRIs and upper gastrointestinal bleeding: what is known and how should it influence prescribing? CNS Drugs 20(2):143–151, 2006

Davidson J, Watkins L, Owens M, et al: Effects of paroxetine and venlafaxine XR on heart rate variability in depression. J Clin Psychopharmacol 25(5):480–484, 2005

Davidson M, Harvey PD, Vervarcke J, et al: A long-term, multicenter, open-label study of risperidone in elderly patients with psychosis. On behalf of the Risperidone Working Group. Int J Geriatr Psychiatry 15:506–514, 2000

Davis R, Peters DH, McTavish D: Valproic acid. A reappraisal of its pharmacological properties and clinical efficacy in epilepsy. Drugs 47:332–372, 1994

De Deyn PP, Rabheru K, Rasmussen A, et al: A randomized trial of risperidone, placebo, and haloperidol for behavioral symptoms of dementia. Neurology 53:946–955, 1999

De Deyn PP, Carrasco MM, Deberdt W, et al: Olanzapine versus placebo in the treatment of psychosis with or without associated behavioral disturbances in patients with Alzheimer's disease. Int J Geriatr Psychiatry 19(2):115–126, 2004

De Deyn PP, Jeste DV, Swanik R, et al: Aripiprazole for the treatment of psychosis in patients with Alzheimer's disease: a randomized placebo-controlled study. J Clin Psychopharmacol 25(5):463–467, 2005a

De Deyn PP, Katz IR, Brodaty H, et al: Management of agitation, aggression, and psychosis associated with dementia: a pooled analysis including three randomized, placebo-controlled double-blind trials in nursing home residents treated with risperidone. Clin Neurol Neurosurg 107(6):497–508, 2005b

Devanand DP, Pelton GH, Marston K, et al: Sertraline treatment of elderly patients with depression and cognitive impairment. Int J Geriatr Psychiatry 18(2):123–130, 2003

Devanand DP, Juszczak N, Nobler MS, et al: An open treatment trial of venlafaxine for elderly patients with dysthymic disorder. J Geriatr Psychiatry Neurol 17(4):219–224, 2004

Devanand DP, Nobler MS, Cheng J, et al: Randomized, double-blind, placebo-controlled trial of fluoxetine treatment for elderly patients with dysthymic disorder. Am J Geriatr Psychiatry 13(1):59–68, 2005

Dierick M: An open-label evaluation of the long-term safety of oral venlafaxine in depressed elderly patients. Ann Clin Psychiatry 8:169–178, 1996

Dolder CR, Jeste DV: Incidence of tardive dyskinesia with typical versus atypical antipsychotics in very high risk patients. Biol Psychiatry 53(12):1142–1145, 2003

Doraiswamy PM, Khan ZM, Donahue RM, et al: Quality of life in geriatric depression: a comparison of remitters, partial responders, and nonresponders. Am J Geriatr Psychiatry 9:423–428, 2001

Doraiswamy PM, Krishnan KR, Oxman T, et al: Does antidepressant therapy improve cognition in elderly depressed patients? J Gerontol A Biol Sci Med Sci 58(12):M1137–M1144, 2003

Dunner DL, Cohn JB, Walshe TD, et al: Two combined, multicenter double-blind studies of paroxetine and doxepin in geriatric patients with major depression. J Clin Psychiatry 53 (suppl):57–60, 1992

Dunner DL, Zisook S, Billow AA, et al: A prospective safety surveillance study for bupropion sustained-release in the treatment of depression. J Clin Psychiatry 59:366–373, 1998

Eastham JH, Jeste DV, Young RC: Assessment and treatment of bipolar disorder in the elderly. Drugs Aging 12:205–224, 1998

Eisdorfer C, Conner JF, Wilkie FL: The effect of magnesium pemoline on cognition and behavior. J Gerontol 23:283–288, 1968

Ellis T, Cudkowicz ME, Sexton PM, et al: Clozapine and risperidone treatment of psychosis in Parkinson's disease. J Neuropsychiatry Clin Neurosci 12:364–369, 2000

Ereshefsky L, Dugan D: Review of the pharmacokinetics, pharmacogenetics, and drug interaction potential of antidepressants: focus on venlafaxine. Depress Anxiety 12 (suppl 1):30–44, 2000

Etminan M, Samii A, Takkouche B, et al: Increased risk of somnolence with the new dopamine agonists in patients with Parkinson's disease: a meta-analysis of randomised controlled trials. Drug Saf 24:863–868, 2001

Etminan M, Streiner DL, Rochon PA: Exploring the association between atypical neuroleptic agents and diabetes mellitus in older adults. Pharmacotherapy 23(11):1411–1415, 2003

Evans M, Hammond M, Wilson K, et al: Treatment of depression in the elderly: effect of physical illness on response. Int J Geriatr Psychiatry 12:1189–1194, 1997

Fabian TJ, Amico JA, Kroboth PD, et al: Paroxetine-induced hyponatremia in older adults: a 12-week prospective study. Arch Intern Med 164(3):327–332, 2004

Fava M, Mulroy R, Alpert J, et al: Emergence of adverse events following discontinuation of treatment with extended-release venlafaxine. Am J Psychiatry 154:1760–1762, 1997

Feighner JP, Cohn J: Double-blind comparative trials of fluoxetine and doxepin in geriatric patients with major depressive disorder. J Clin Psychiatry 46(3 pt 2):20–25, 1985

Feldman PD, Hay LK, Deberdt W, et al: Retrospective cohort study of diabetes mellitus and antipsychotic treatment in a geriatric population in the United States. J Am Med Dir Assoc 5(1):38–46, 2004

Fernandez HH, Friedman JH, Jacques C, et al: Quetiapine for the treatment of drug-induced psychosis in Parkinson's disease. Mov Disord 14:484–487, 1999

Fernandez HH, Trieschmann ME, Burke MA, et al: Quetiapine for psychosis in Parkinson's disease versus dementia with Lewy bodies. J Clin Psychiatry 63(6):513–515, 2002

Finkel SI, Richter EM, Clary CM, et al: Comparative efficacy of sertraline vs. fluoxetine in patients age 70 or over with major depression. Am J Geriatr Psychiatry 7:221–227, 1999

Finkel S, Kozma C, Long S, et al: Risperidone treatment in elderly patients with dementia: relative risk of cerebrovascular events versus other antipsychotics. Int Psychogeriatrics 17(4):617–629, 2005

Flint AJ: Generalised anxiety disorder in elderly patients: epidemiology, diagnosis and treatment options. Drugs Aging 22(2):101–114, 2005

Fontaine CS, Hynan LS, Koch K, et al: A double-blind comparison of olanzapine versus risperidone in the acute treatment of dementia-related behavioral disturbances in extended care facilities. J Clin Psychiatry 64(6):726–730, 2003

Forlenza OV, Almeida OP, Stoppe A Jr, et al: Antidepressant efficacy and safety of low-dose sertraline and standard-dose imipramine for the treatment of depression in older adults: results from a double-blind, randomized, controlled clinical trial. Int Psychogeriatrics 13(1):75–84, 2001

Frenchman IB, Prince T: Clinical experience with risperidone, haloperidol, and thioridazine for dementia-associated behavioral disturbances. Int Psychogeriatr 9:431–435, 1997

Freudenreich O, Menza M: Zolpidem-related delirium: a case report. J Clin Psychiatry 61:449–450, 2000

Furlan PM, Kallan MJ, Ten Have T, et al: Cognitive and psychomotor effects of paroxetine and sertraline on healthy elderly volunteers. Am J Geriatr Psychiatry 9:429–438, 2001

Gareri P, Cotroneo A, Lacava R, et al: Comparison of the efficacy of new and conventional antipsychotic drugs in the treatment of behavioral and psychological symptoms of dementia (BPSD). Arch Gerontol Geriatrics Suppl 9:207–215, 2004

Gasto C, Navarro V, Marcos T, et al: Single-blind comparison of venlafaxine and nortriptyline in elderly major depression. J Clin Psychopharmacol 23(1):21–26, 2003

Gelenberg AJ, Laukes C, McGahuey C, et al: Mirtazapine substitution in SSRI-induced sexual dysfunction. J Clin Psychiatry 61:356–360, 2000

Georgotas A, Friedman E, McCarthy M, et al: Resistant geriatric depressions and therapeutic response to monoamine oxidase inhibitors. Biol Psychiatry 18:195–205, 1983

Georgotas A, McCue RE, Hapworth W, et al: Comparative efficacy and safety of MAOIs versus TCAs in treating depression in the elderly. Biol Psychiatry 21:1155–1166, 1986

Geretsegger C, Stuppaeck CH, Mair M, et al: Multicenter double blind study of paroxetine and amitriptyline in elderly depressed inpatients. Psychopharmacology (Berl) 119:277–281, 1995

Gex-Fabry M, Balant-Gorgia AE, Balant LP: Therapeutic drug monitoring of olanzapine: the combined effect of age, gender, smoking, and comedication. Ther Drug Monit 25(1):46–53, 2003

Gill SS, Rochon PA, Herrmann N, et al: Atypical antipsychotic drugs and risk of ischaemic stroke: population based retrospective cohort study. BMJ 330(7489): 445, 2005

Glassman AH, O'Connor CM, Califf RM, et al; Sertraline Antidepressant Heart Attack Randomized Trial (SADHEART) Group: Sertraline treatment of major depression in patients with acute MI or unstable angina. JAMA 288(6):701–709, 2002

Goetz CG, Blasucci LM, Leurgans S, et al: Olanzapine and clozapine: comparative effects on motor function in hallucinating PD patients. Neurology 55:789–794, 2000

Goldstein DJ, Lu Y, Detke MJ, et al: Duloxetine vs placebo in patients with painful diabetic neuropathy. Pain 116(1–2):109–118, 2005

Goodnick PJ, Hernandez M: Treatment of depression in comorbid medical illness. Expert Opin Pharmacother 1:1367–1384, 2000

Gram LF, Hansen MG, Sindrup SH, et al: Citalopram: interaction studies with levomepromazine, imipramine, and lithium. Ther Drug Monit 15:18–24, 1993

Greco KE, Tune LE, Brown FW, et al: A retrospective study of the safety of intramuscular ziprasidone in agitated elderly patients. J Clin Psychiatry 66(7):928–929, 2005

Greenblatt DJ, Harmatz JS, Shapiro L, et al: Sensitivity to triazolam in the elderly. N Engl J Med 324:1691–1698, 1991

Greenblatt DJ, von Moltke LL, Harmatz JS, et al: Drug interactions with newer antidepressants: role of human cytochromes P450. J Clin Psychiatry 59 (suppl 15):19–27, 1998

Greenblatt DJ, von Moltke LL, Harmatz JS, et al: Human cytochromes and some newer antidepressants: kinetics, metabolism, and drug interactions. J Clin Psychiatry 19 (suppl 1):23S–35S, 1999

Greene DS, Barbhaiya RH: Clinical pharmacokinetics of nefazodone. Clin Pharmacokinet 33:260–275, 1997

Grothe DR, Scheckner B, Albano D: Treatment of pain syndromes with venlafaxine. Pharmacotherapy 24(5):621–629, 2004

Guay DR: Pregabalin in neuropathic pain: a more "pharmaceutically elegant" gabapentin? Am J Geriatr Pharmacother 3:274–287, 2005

Guillibert E, Pelicier Y, Archambault JC, et al: A double-blind, multicentre study of paroxetine versus clomipramine in depressed elderly patients. Acta Psychiatr Scand Suppl 350:132–134, 1989

Han CS, Kim YK: A double-blind trial of risperidone and haloperidol for the treatment of delirium. Psychosomatics 45(4):297–301, 2004

Hansen RA, Gartlehner G, Lohr KN, et al: Efficacy and safety of second-generation antidepressants in the treatment of major depressive disorder. Ann Intern Med 143(6):415–426, 2005

Harvey AT, Rudolph RL, Preskorn SH: Evidence of the dual mechanisms of action of venlafaxine. Arch Gen Psychiatry 57:503–509, 2000

Harvey PD, Napolitano JA, Mao L, et al: Comparative effects of risperidone and olanzapine on cognition in elderly patients with schizophrenia or schizoaffective disorder. Int J Geriatr Psychiatry 18:820–829, 2003

Herrmann N, Rivard MF, Flynn M, et al: Risperidone for the treatment of behavioral disturbances in dementia: a case series. J Neuropsychiatry Clin Neurosci 10:220–223, 1998

Herrmann N, Mamdani M, Lanctot KL: Atypical antipsychotics and risk of cerebrovascular accidents. Am J Psychiatry 161(6): 1113–1115, 2004

Hesse LM, Venkatakrishnan K, Court MH, et al: CYP2B6 mediates the in vitro hydroxylation of bupropion: potential drug interactions with other antidepressants. Drug Metab Dispos 28:1176–1183, 2000

Hesse LM, He P, Krishnaswamy S, et al: Pharmacogenetic determinants of interindividual variability in bupropion hydroxylation by cytochrome P450 2B6 in human liver microsomes. Pharmacogenetics 14(4):225–238, 2004

Hien le TT, Cumming RG, Cameron ID, et al: Atypical antipsychotic medications and risk of falls in residents of aged care facilities. J Am Geriatr Soc 53(8):1290–1295, 2005

Horikawa N, Yamazaki T, Miyamoto K, et al: Treatment for delirium with risperidone: results of a prospective open trial with 10 patients. Gen Hosp Psychiatry 25:289–292, 2003

Howanitz E, Pardo M, Smelson DA, et al: The efficacy and safety of clozapine versus chlorpromazine in geriatric schizophrenia. J Clin Psychiatry 60:41–44, 1999

Howard WT, Warnock JK: Bupropion-induced psychosis. Am J Psychiatry 156:2017–2018, 1999

Hoyberg OJ, Maragakis B, Mullin J, et al: A double-blind multicentre comparison of mirtazapine and amitriptyline in elderly depressed patients. Acta Psychiatr Scand 93:184–190, 1996

Hua TC, Pan A, Chan C, et al: Effect of duloxetine on tolterodine pharmacokinetics in healthy volunteers. Br J Clin Pharmacol 57(5):652–656, 2004

Hudson JI, Wohlreich MM, Kajdasz DK, et al: Safety and tolerability of duloxetine in the treatment of major depressive disorder: analysis of pooled data from eight placebo-controlled clinical trials. Hum Psychopharmacol 20(5):327–341, 2005

Hutchison LC: Mirtazapine and bone marrow suppression: a case report. J Am Geriatr Soc 49:1129–1130, 2001

Hwang JP, Yang CH, Lee TW, et al: The efficacy and safety of olanzapine for the treatment of geriatric psychosis. J Clin Psychopharmacol 23(2):113–118, 2003

Iribarne C, Picart D, Dreano Y, et al: In vitro interactions between fluoxetine or fluvoxamine and methadone or buprenorphine. Fundam Clin Pharmacol 12(2):194–199, 1998

Irizarry MC, Ghaemi SN, Lee-Cherry ER, et al: Risperidone treatment of behavioral disturbances in outpatients with dementia. J Neuropsychiatry Clin Neurosci 11:336–342, 1999

Jaskiw GE, Thyrum PT, Fuller MA, et al: Pharmacokinetics of quetiapine in elderly patients with selected psychotic disorders. Clin Pharmacokinet 43(14):1025–1035, 2004

Jeppesen U, Gram L, Vistisen K: Dose-dependent inhibition of CYP1A2, CYP2C19, and CYP2D6 by citalopram, fluoxetine, fluvoxamine, and paroxetine. Eur J Clin Pharmacol 51:73–78, 1996

Jeste DV: Tardive dyskinesia rates with atypical antipsychotics in older adults. J Clin Psychiatry 65 (suppl 9):21–24, 2004

Jeste DV, Caligiuri MP, Paulsen JS, et al: Risk of tardive dyskinesia in older patients: a prospective longitudinal study of 266 outpatients. Arch Gen Psychiatry 52:756–765, 1995

Jeste DV, Barak Y, Madhusoodanan S, et al: International multisite double-blind trial of the atypical antipsychotics risperidone and olanzapine in 175 elderly patients with chronic schizophrenia. Am J Geriatr Psychiatry 11(6):638–647, 2003a

Jeste DV, De Deyn P, Carson W, et al: Aripiprazole in dementia of the Alzheimer's type. J Am Geriatr Soc 51(suppl):543, 2003b

Johnson EM, Whyte E, Mulsant BH, et al: Cardiovascular changes associated with venlafaxine in the treatment of late life depression. Am J Geriatr Psychiatry (in press)

Joo JH, Lenze EJ, Mulsant BH, et al: Risk factors for falls during treatment of late-life depression. J Clin Psychiatry 63:936–941, 2002

Kando JC, Tohen M, Castillo J, et al: The use of valproate in an elderly population with affective symptoms. J Clin Psychiatry 57:238–240, 1996

Karp JF, Weiner D, Seligman K, et al: Body pain and treatment response in late-life depression. Am J Geriatr Psychiatry 13:188–194, 2005

Kasckow JW, Mohamed S, Thallasinos A, et al: Citalopram augmentation of antipsychotic treatment in older schizophrenia patients. Int J Geriatr Psychiatry 16(12):1163–1167, 2001

Kashuba AD, Nafziger AN, Kearns GL, et al: Effect of fluvoxamine therapy on the activities of CYP1A2, CYP2D6, and CYP3A as determined by phenotyping. Clin Pharmacol Ther 64:257–268, 1998

Kasper S, de Swart H, Andersen HF: Escitalopram in the treatment of depressed elderly patients. Am J Geriatr Psychiatry 13(10): 884–891, 2005

Kato D, Kawanishi C, Kishida I, et al: Delirium resolving upon switching from risperidone to quetiapine: implication of CYP2D6 genotype. Psychosomatics 46(4):374–375, 2005

Katona CLE, Hunter BN, Bray J: A double-blind comparison of the efficacy and safety of paroxetine and imipramine in the treatment of depression with dementia. Int J Geriatr Psychiatry 13:100–108, 1998

Katz IR, Jeste DV, Mintzer JE, et al: Comparison of risperidone and placebo for psychosis and behavioral disturbances associated with dementia: a randomized, double-blind trial. Risperidone Study Group. J Clin Psychiatry 60:107–115, 1999

Katz IR, Reynolds CF 3rd, Alexopoulos GS, et al: Venlafaxine ER as a treatment for generalized anxiety disorder in older adults: pooled analysis of five randomized placebo-controlled clinical trials. J Am Geriatr Soc 50(1):18–25, 2002

Kelsey JE: Dose-response relationship with venlafaxine. J Clin Psychopharmacol 16 (3 suppl 2):21S–26S; discussion 26S–28S, 1996

Kennedy JS, Jeste D, Kaiser CJ, et al: Olanzapine vs haloperidol in geriatric schizophrenia: analysis of data from a double-blind controlled trial. Int J Geriatr Psychiatry 18(11):1013–1020, 2003

Kennedy J, Deberdt W, Siegal A, et al: Olanzapine does not enhance cognition in non-agitated and non-psychotic patients with mild to moderate Alzheimer's dementia. Int J Geriatr Psychiatry 20(11):1020–1027, 2005

Khan A, Rudolph R, Baumel B, et al: Venlafaxine in depressed geriatric outpatients: an open-label clinical study. Psychopharmacol Bull 31:753–758, 1995

Kiev A, Masco HL, Wenger TL, et al: The cardiovascular effects of bupropion and nortriptyline in depressed outpatients. Ann Clin Psychiatry 6:107–115, 1994

Kim KY, Bader GM, Kotlyar V, et al: Treatment of delirium in older adults with quetiapine. J Geriatr Psychiatry Neurol 16(1):29–31, 2003

Kinon BJ, Stauffer VL, McGuire HC, et al: The effects of antipsychotic drug treatment on prolactin concentrations in elderly patients. J Am Med Dir Assoc 4(4): 189–194, 2003

Kirby D, Harrigan S, Ames D: Hyponatraemia in elderly psychiatric patients treated with selective serotonin reuptake inhibitors and venlafaxine: a retrospective controlled study in an inpatient unit. Int J Geriatr Psychiatry 17(3):231–237, 2002

Kirwin JL, Goren JL: Duloxetine: a dual serotonin-norepinephrine reuptake inhibitor for treatment of major depressive disorder. Pharmacotherapy 25(3):396–410, 2005

Klamerus KJ, Parker VD, Rudolph RL, et al: Effects of age and gender on venlafaxine and O-desmethylvenlafaxine pharmacokinetics. Pharmacotherapy 16:915–923, 1996

Kobayashi K, Yamamoto T, Chiba K, et al: The effects of selective serotonin reuptake inhibitors and their metabolites on S-mephenytoin 4'-hydroxylase activity in human liver microsomes. Br J Clin Pharmacol 40:481–485, 1995

Kodama Y, Kodama H, Kuranari M, et al: Gender- or age-related binding characteristics of valproic acid to serum proteins in adult patients with epilepsy. Eur J Pharm Biopharm 52:57–63, 2001

Kohen I, Preval H, Southard R, et al: Naturalistic study of intramuscular ziprasidone versus conventional agents in agitated elderly patients: retrospective findings from a psychiatric emergency service. Am J Geriatr Pharmacother 3(4):240–245, 2005

Koller E, Schneider B, Bennett K, et al: Clozapine-associated diabetes. Am J Med 111: 716–723, 2001

Koller EA, Cross JT, Doraiswamy PM, et al: Pancreatitis associated with atypical antipsychotics: from the Food and Drug Administration's MedWatch surveillance system and published reports. Pharmacotherapy 23(9):1123–1130, 2003

Kotlyar M, Brauer LH, Tracy TS, et al: Inhibition of CYP2D6 activity by bupropion. J Clin Psychopharmacol 25(3):226–229, 2005

Kroenke K, West SL, Swindle R, et al: Similar effectiveness of paroxetine, fluoxetine, and sertraline in primary care: a randomized trial. JAMA 286:2947–2955, 2001

Kuehn BM: FDA warns antipsychotic drugs may be risky for elderly. JAMA 293(20):2462, 2005

Kunik ME, Puryear L, Orengo CA, et al: The efficacy and tolerability of divalproex sodium in elderly demented patients with behavioral disturbances. Int J Geriatric Psychiatry 13:29–34, 1998

Kyle CJ, Petersen HE, Overo KF: Comparison of the tolerability and efficacy of citalopram and amitriptyline in elderly depressed patients treated in general practice. Depress Anxiety 8:147–153, 1998

Landi F, Onder G, Cesari M, et al; Silver Network Home Care Study Group: Psychotropic medications and risk for falls among community-dwelling frail older people: an observational study. J Gerontol A Biol Sci Med Sci 60(5):622–626, 2005

Lane HY, Chang YC, Su MH, et al: Shifting from haloperidol to risperidone for behavioral disturbances in dementia: safety, response predictors, and mood effects. J Clin Psychopharmacol 22:4–10, 2002

Lasser RA, Bossie CA, Zhu Y, et al: Efficacy and safety of long-acting risperidone in elderly patients with schizophrenia and schizoaffective disorder. Int J Geriatr Psychiatry 19(9):898–905, 2004

Lavretsky H, Sultzer D: A structured trial of risperidone for the treatment of agitation in dementia. Am J Geriatr Psychiatry 6:127–135, 1998

Lavretsky H, Park S, Siddarth P, et al: Methylphenidate-enhanced antidepressant response to citalopram in the elderly: a double-blind, placebo-controlled pilot trial. Am J Geriatr Psychiatry 142:181–185, 2006

Lee PE, Gill SS, Freedman M, et al: Atypical antipsychotic drugs in the treatment of behavioural and psychological symptoms of dementia: systematic review. BMJ 329(7457):75, 2004

Lenze EJ, Mulsant BH, Shear MK, et al: Anxiety symptoms in elderly patients with depression: what is the best approach to treatment? Drugs Aging 19:753–760, 2002

Lenze EJ, Mulsant BH, Shear MK, et al: Efficacy and tolerability of citalopram in the treatment of late-life anxiety disorders: results from an 8-week randomized, placebo-controlled trial. Am J Psychiatry 162:146–150, 2005

Leopold NA: Risperidone treatment of drug-related psychosis in patients with parkinsonism. Mov Disord 15:301–304, 2000

Lessard E, Yessine MA, Hamelin BA, et al: Influence of CYP2D6 activity on the disposition and cardiovascular toxicity of the antidepressant agent venlafaxine in humans. Pharmacogenetics 9:435–443, 1999

Lim CJ, Trevino C, Tampi RR: Can olanzapine cause delirium in the elderly? Ann Pharmacother 40(1):135–138, 2006

Lima JM: The new drugs and the strategies to manage epilepsy. Curr Pharm Des 6:873–878, 2000

Lindenmayer JP, Nathan AM, Smith RC: Hyperglycemia associated with the use of atypical antipsychotics. J Clin Psychiatry 62 (suppl 23):30–38, 2001

Liperoti R, Gambassi G, Lapane KL, et al: Cerebrovascular events among elderly nursing home patients treated with conventional or atypical antipsychotics. J Clin Psychiatry 66(9):1090–1096, 2005a

Liperoti R, Pedone C, Lapane KL, et al: Venous thromboembolism among elderly patients treated with atypical and conventional antipsychotic agents. Arch Intern Med 165(22):2677–2682, 2005b

Liu CY, Juang YY, Liang HY, et al: Efficacy of risperidone in treating the hyperactive symptoms of delirium. Int Clin Psychopharmacol 19(3):165–168, 2004

Lucena MI, Andrade RJ, Gomez-Outes A, et al: Acute liver failure after treatment with nefazodone. Dig Dis Sci 44:2577–2579, 1999

Lyketsos CG, DelCampo L, Steinberg M, et al: Treating depression in Alzheimer disease: efficacy and safety of sertraline therapy, and the benefits of depression reduction: the DIADS. Arch Gen Psychiatry 60(7): 737–746, 2003

Madhusoodanan S, Brecher M, Brenner R, et al: Risperidone in the treatment of elderly patients with psychotic disorders. Am J Geriatr Psychiatry 7:132–138, 1999a

Madhusoodanan S, Suresh P, Brenner R, et al: Experience with the atypical antipsychotics—risperidone and olanzapine in the elderly. Ann Clin Psychiatry 11:113–118, 1999b

Madhusoodanan S, Brenner R, Alcantra A: Clinical experience with quetiapine in elderly patients with psychotic disorders. J Geriatr Psychiatry Neurol 13:28–32, 2000

Madhusoodanan S, Brenner R, Gupta S, et al: Clinical experience with aripiprazole treatment in ten elderly patients with schizophrenia or schizoaffective disorder: retrospective case studies. CNS Spectr 9(11):862–867, 2004

Mahapatra SN, Hackett D: A randomised, double-blind, parallel-group comparison of venlafaxine and dothiepin in geriatric patients with major depression. Int J Clin Pract 51:209–213, 1997

Mahmood I, Sahajwalla C: Clinical pharmacokinetics and pharmacodynamics of buspirone, an anxiolytic drug. Clin Pharmacokinet 36:277–287, 1999

Mamo DC, Sweet RA, Mulsant BH, et al : The effect of nortriptyline and paroxetine on extrapyramidal signs and symptoms: a prospective double-blind study in depressed elderly patients. Am J Geriatr Psychiatry 8:226–231, 2000

Mariappan P, Ballantyne Z, N'Dow JMO, et al: Serotonin and noradrenaline reuptake inhibitors (SNRI) for stress urinary incontinence in adults. Cochrane Database of Systematic Reviews, Issue 3, Art No CD004742; DOI:10.1002/14651858. CD004742, 2005

Marsh L, Lyketsos C, Reich SG: Olanzapine for the treatment of psychosis in patients with Parkinson's disease and dementia. Psychosomatics 42:477–481, 2001

Martin H, Slyk MP, Deymann S, et al: Safety profile assessment of risperidone and olanzapine in long-term care patients with dementia. J Am Med Dir Assoc 4(4):183–188, 2003

Maxwell RA, Sweet RA, Mulsant BH, et al: Risperidone and 9-hydroxyrisperidone concentrations are not dependent on age or creatinine clearance among elderly subjects. J Geriatr Psychiatry Neurol 15(2):77–81, 2002

McCue RE, Joseph M: Venlafaxine- and trazodone-induced serotonin syndrome. Am J Psychiatry 158:2088–2089, 2001

McManus DQ, Arvanitis LA, Kowalcyk BB: Quetiapine, a novel antipsychotic: experience in elderly patients with psychotic disorders. Seroquel Trial 48 Study Group. J Clin Psychiatry 60:292–298, 1999

Meco G, Alessandri A, Giustini P, et al: Risperidone in levodopa-induced psychosis in advanced Parkinson's disease: an open-label, long-term study. Mov Disord 12: 610–612, 1997

Melkersson KI, Hulting AL: Insulin and leptin levels in patients with schizophrenia or related psychoses—a comparison between different antipsychotic agents. Psychopharmacology 154:205–212, 2001

Meltzer HY: Suicide in schizophrenia: risk factors and clozapine treatment. J Clin Psychiatry 59 (suppl 3):15–20, 1998

Menza MM, Palermo B, Mark M: Quetiapine as an alternative to clozapine in the treatment of dopamimetic psychosis in patients with Parkinson's disease. Ann Clin Psychiatry 11:141–144, 1999

Messenheimer JA: Rash in adult and pediatric patients treated with lamotrigine. Can J Neurol Sci 25:S14–S18, 1998

Micca JL, Hoffmann VP, Lipkovich I, et al: Retrospective analysis of diabetes risk in elderly patients with dementia in olanzapine clinical trials. Am J Geriatr Psychiatry 14(1):62–70, 2006

Miller del D, McEvoy JP, Davis SM, et al: Clinical correlates of tardive dyskinesia in schizophrenia: baseline data from the CATIE schizophrenia trial. Schizophr Res 80(1):33–43, 2005

Mintzer JE, Mullen JA, Sweitzer DE: A comparison of extrapyramidal symptoms in older outpatients treated with quetiapine or risperidone. Curr Med Res Opin 20(9):1483–1491, 2004

Mittal D, Jimerson NA, Neely EP, et al: Risperidone in the treatment of delirium: results from a prospective open-label trial. J Clin Psychiatry 65(5):662–667, 2004

Modai I, Hirschmann S, Rava A, et al: Sudden death in patients receiving clozapine treatment: a preliminary investigation. J Clin Psychopharmacol 20:325–327, 2000

Mohr E, Mendis T, Hildebrand K, et al: Risperidone in the treatment of dopamine-induced psychosis in Parkinson's disease: an open pilot trial. Mov Disord 15:1230–1237, 2000

Molho ES, Factor SA: Worsening of motor features of parkinsonism with olanzapine. Mov Disord 14:1014–1016, 1999

Montejo AL, Llorca G, Izquierdo JA, et al: Incidence of sexual dysfunction associated with antidepressant agents: a prospective multicenter study of 1022 outpatients. Spanish Working Group for the Study of Psychotropic-Related Sexual Dysfunction. J Clin Psychiatry 62 (suppl 3):10–21, 2001

Moretti R, Torre P, Antonello RM, et al: Olanzapine as a possible treatment of behavioral symptoms in vascular dementia: risks of cerebrovascular events. A controlled, open-label study. J Neurol 252(10):1186–1193, 2005

Morita T, Tei Y, Shishido H, et al: Olanzapine-induced delirium in a terminally ill cancer patient. J Pain Symptom Manage 28(2):102–103, 2004

Morrell MJ, Isojarvi J, Taylor AE, et al: Higher androgens and weight gain with valproate compared with lamotrigine for epilepsy. Epilepsy Res 54:189–199, 2003

Mottram P, Wilson K, Strobl J: Antidepressants for depressed elderly. Cochrane Database of Systematic Reviews, Issue 1, Art No CD003491; DOI: 10.1002/14651858:CD003491, 2006

Movig KL, Janssen MW, de Waal MJ, et al: Relationship of serotonergic antidepressants and need for blood transfusion in orthopedic surgical patients. Arch Intern Med 163(19):2354–2358, 2003

Mulsant BH, Pollock BG, Nebes RD, et al: A double-blind randomized comparison of nortriptyline and paroxetine in the treatment of late-life depression: 6-week outcome. J Clin Psychiatry 60 (suppl 20):16–20, 1999

Mulsant BH, Alexopoulos GS, Reynolds CF 3rd, et al: The PROSPECT Study Group. Pharmacological treatment of depression in older primary care patients: the PROSPECT algorithm. Int J Geriatr Psychiatry 16:585–592, 2001a

Mulsant BH, Pollock BG, Nebes R, et al: A twelve-week, double-blind, randomized comparison of nortriptyline and paroxetine in older depressed inpatients and outpatients. Am J Geriatr Psychiatry 9:406–414, 2001b

Mulsant BH, Pollock BG, Kirshner M, et al: Serum anticholinergic activity in a community-based sample of older adults: relationship with cognitive performance. Arch Gen Psychiatry 60:198–203, 2003

Mulsant BH, Gharabawi GM, Bossie CA, et al: Correlates of anticholinergic activity in patients with dementia and psychosis treated with risperidone or olanzapine. J Clin Psychiatry 65(12):1708–1714, 2004

Murray V, von Arbin M, Bartfai A, et al: Double-blind comparison of sertraline and placebo in stroke patients with minor depression and less severe major depression. J Clin Psychiatry 66(6):708–716, 2005

Nagaraja D, Jayashree S: Randomized study of the dopamine receptor agonist piribedil in treatment of mild cognitive impairment. Am J Psychiatry 158:1517–1519, 2001

National Collaborating Centre for Mental Health: Management of Depression in Primary and Secondary Care. Clinical Guideline 23. London, National Institute for Clinical Excellence, 2004

Navarro V, Gasto C, Torres X, et al: Citalopram versus nortriptyline in late-life depression: a 12-week randomized single-blind study. Acta Psychiatr Scand 103: 435–440, 2001

Nebes RD, Pollock BG, Meltzer CC, et al: Cognitive effects of serum anticholinergic activity and white matter hyperintensities. Neurology 65:1487–1489, 2005

Nelson JC, Wohlreich MM, Mallinckrodt CH, et al: Duloxetine for the treatment of major depressive disorder in older patients. Am J Geriatr Psychiatry 13(3):227–235, 2005

Nemeroff CB: Comorbidity of mood and anxiety disorders: the rule, not the exception? Am J Psychiatry 159:3–4, 2002

Newhouse PA, Krishnan KR, Doraiswamy P, et al: A double-blind comparison of sertraline and fluoxetine in depressed elderly outpatients. J Clin Psychiatry 61:559–568, 2000

Nicholas LM, Ford AL, Esposito SM, et al: The effects of mirtazapine on plasma lipid profiles in healthy subjects. J Clin Psychiatry 64(8):883–889, 2003

Nieuwstraten CE, Dolovich LR: Bupropion versus selective serotonin-reuptake inhibitors for treatment of depression. Ann Pharmacother 35(12):1608–1613, 2001

Nikaido AM, Ellinwood EH Jr, Heatherly DG, et al: Age-related increase in CNS sensitivity to benzodiazepines as assessed by task difficulty. Psychopharmacology (Berl) 100:90–97, 1990

Noaghiul S, Narayan M, Nelson JC: Divalproex treatment of mania in elderly patients. Am J Geriatr Psychiatry 6:257–262, 1998

Nyth AL, Gottfries CG: The clinical efficacy of citalopram in treatment of emotional disturbances in dementia disorders. A Nordic multicentre study. Br J Psychiatry 157:894–901, 1990

Nyth AL, Gottfries CG, Lyby K, et al: A controlled multicenter clinical study of citalopram and placebo in elderly depressed patients with and without concomitant dementia. Acta Psychiatr Scand 86:138–145, 1992

Olafsson K, Jorgensen S, Jensen HV, et al: Fluvoxamine in the treatment of demented elderly patients: a double-blind, placebo-controlled study. Acta Psychiatr Scand 85:453–456, 1992

Onofrj M, Thomas A, Bonanni L, et al: Leucopenia induced by low dose clozapine in Parkinson's disease recedes shortly after drug withdrawal. Clinical case descriptions with commentary on switch-over to olanzapine. Neurol Sci 21:209–215, 2000

Oslin DW, Streim JE, Katz IR, et al: Heuristic comparison of sertraline with nortriptyline for the treatment of depression in frail elderly patients. Am J Geriatr Psychiatry 8:141–149, 2000

Oslin DW, Ten Have TR, Streim JE, et al: Probing the safety of medications in the frail elderly: evidence from a randomized clinical trial of sertraline and venlafaxine in depressed nursing home residents. J Clin Psychiatry 64(8):875–882, 2003

Ostow M: Pramipexole for depression. Am J Psychiatry 159:320–321, 2002

Pact V, Giduz T: Mirtazapine treats resting tremor, essential tremor, and levodopa-induced dyskinesias. Neurology 53:1154, 1999

Pae CU, Lee SJ, Lee CU, et al: A pilot trial of quetiapine for the treatment of patients with delirium. Hum Psychopharmacol 19(2):125–127, 2004

Pande AC, Crockatt JG, Janney C, et al: Gabapentin in bipolar disorder: a placebo-controlled trial of adjunctive therapy. Bipolar Disord 2 (3 pt 2):249–255, 2000

Parellada E, Baeza I, de Pablo J, et al: Risperidone in the treatment of patients with delirium. J Clin Psychiatry 65(3):348–353, 2004

Parkinson Study Group: Low-dose clozapine for the treatment of drug-induced psychosis in Parkinson's disease. N Engl J Med 340:757–763, 1999

Pedersen L, Klysner R: Antagonism of selective serotonin reuptake inhibitor-induced nausea by mirtazapine. Int Clin Psychopharmacol 12:59–60, 1997

Percudani M, Barbui C, Fortino I, et al: Second-generation antipsychotics and risk of cerebrovascular accidents in the elderly. J Clin Psychopharmacol 25(5):468–470, 2005

Perry NK: Venlafaxine-induced serotonin syndrome with relapse following amitriptyline. Postgrad Med J 76:254–256, 2000

Petracca GM, Chemerinski E, Starkstein SE: A double-blind, placebo-controlled study of fluoxetine in depressed patients with Alzheimer's disease. Int Psychogeriatrics 13: 233–240, 2001

Phanjoo AL, Wonnacott S, Hodgson A: Double-blind comparative multicentre study of fluvoxamine and mianserin in the treatment of major depressive episode in elderly people. Acta Psychiatr Scand 83:476–479, 1991

Poewe W: Treatment of dementia with Lewy bodies and Parkinson's disease dementia. Movement Disord 20 (suppl 12):S77–S82, 2005

Pollock BG: Adverse reactions of antidepressants in elderly patients. J Clin Psychiatry 60 (suppl 20):4–8, 1999

Pollock BG, Mulsant BH: Antipsychotics in older patients: a safety perspective. Drugs Aging 6:312–323, 1995

Pollock BG, Mulsant BH, Sweet R, et al: An open pilot study of citalopram for behavioral disturbances of dementia. Am J Geriatr Psychiatry 5:70–78, 1997

Pollock BG, Rosen J, Mulsant BH: Antipsychotics and selective serotonin reuptake inhibitors for the treatment of behavioral disturbances in dementia of the Alzheimer type: a review of clinical data. Consultant Pharmacist 11:1251–1258, 1999

Pollock BG, Mulsant BH, Rosen J, et al: Comparison of citalopram, perphenazine, and placebo for the acute treatment of psychosis and behavioral disturbances in hospitalized, demented patients. Am J Psychiatry 159:460–465, 2002

Pomara N, Deptula D, Medel M, et al: Effects of diazepam on recall memory: relationship to aging, dose, and duration of treatment. Psychopharmacol Bull 25:144–148, 1989

Post RM, Frye MA, Denicoff KD, et al: Beyond lithium in the treatment of bipolar illness. Neuropsychopharmacology 19:206–219, 1998

Preskorn SH, Magnus RD: Inhibition of hepatic P-450 isoenzymes by serotonin selective reuptake inhibitors: in vitro and in vivo findings and their implications for patient care. Psychopharmacol Bull 30:251–259, 1994

Preskorn SH, Alderman J, Greenblatt DJ, et al: Sertraline does not inhibit cytochrome P450 3A-mediated drug metabolism in vivo. Psychopharmacol Bull 33:659–665, 1997

Rabins PS, Lyketsos CG: Antipsychotic drugs in dementia: what should be made of the risks? JAMA 294:1963–1965, 2005

Rahman MK, Akhtar MJ, Savla NC, et al: A double-blind, randomised comparison of fluvoxamine with dothiepin in the treatment of depression in elderly patients. Br J Clin Pract 45:255–258, 1991

Rainer MK, Masching AJ, Ertl MG, et al: Effect of risperidone on behavioral and psychological symptoms and cognitive function in dementia. J Clin Psychiatry 62:894–900, 2001

Raji MA, Brady SR: Mirtazapine for treatment of depression and comorbidities in Alzheimer disease. Ann Pharmacother 35:1024–1027, 2001

Rampello L, Chiechio S, Nicoletti G, et al: Prediction of the response to citalopram and reboxetine in post-stroke depressed patients. Psychopharmacology (Berl) 173 (1–2):73–78, 2004

Rapaport MH, Schneider LS, Dunner DL, et al: Efficacy of controlled-release paroxetine in the treatment of late-life depression. J Clin Psychiatry 64(9):1065–1074, 2003

Rapoport M, Mamdani M, Shulman KI, et al: Antipsychotic use in the elderly: shifting trends and increasing costs. Int J Geriatr Psychiatry 20(8):749–753, 2005

Rasmussen A, Lunde M, Poulsen DL, et al: A double-blind, placebo-controlled study of sertraline in the prevention of depression in stroke patients. Psychosomatics 44(3): 216–221, 2003

Rasmussen BB, Nielsen TL, Brosen K: Fluvoxamine is a potent inhibitor of the metabolism of caffeine in vitro. Pharmacol Toxicol 83:240–245, 1998

Ravona-Springer R, Dolberg OT, Hirschmann S, et al: Delirium in elderly patients treated with risperidone: a report of three cases. J Clin Psychopharmacol 18(2):171–172, 1998

Ray WA, Meredith S, Thapa PB, et al: Antipsychotics and the risk of sudden cardiac death. Arch Gen Psychiatry 58:1161–1167, 2001

Reifler BV, Teri L, Raskind M: Double-blind trial of imipramine in Alzheimer's disease in patients with and without depression. Am J Psychiatry 146:45–49, 1989

Reisberg B, Doody R, Stoffler A, et al; Memantine Study Group: Memantine in moderate-to-severe Alzheimer's disease. N Engl J Med 348:1333–1341, 2003

Reznik I, Rosen Y, Rosen B: An acute ischaemic event associated with the use of venlafaxine: a case report and proposed pathophysiological mechanisms. J Psychopharmacol 13:193–195, 1999

Rich SS, Friedman JH, Ott BR: Risperidone versus clozapine in the treatment of psychosis in six patients with Parkinson's disease and other akinetic-rigid syndromes. J Clin Psychiatry 56:556–559, 1995

Richard IH, Kurlan R: A survey of antidepressant drug use in Parkinson's disease. Parkinson Study Group. Neurology 49:1168–1170, 1997

Rickels K, Schweizer E, Case WG, et al: Nefazodone in major depression: adjunctive benzodiazepine therapy and tolerability. J Clin Psychopharmacol 18:145–153, 1998

Ridout F, Meadows R, Johnsen S, et al: A placebo controlled investigation into the effects of paroxetine and mirtazapine on measures related to car driving performance. Hum Psychopharmacol 18(4): 261–269, 2003

Ritchie CW, Chiu E, Harrigan S, et al: The impact upon extrapyramidal side effects, clinical symptoms and quality of life of a switch from conventional to atypical antipsychotics (risperidone or olanzapine) in elderly patients with schizophrenia. Int J Geriatr Psychiatry 18(5):432–440, 2003

Ritchie CW, Chiu E, Harrigan S, et al: A comparison of the efficacy and safety of olanzapine and risperidone in the treatment of elderly patients with schizophrenia: an open study of six months duration. Int J Geriatr Psychiatry 21(2):171–179, 2006

Robinson R, Schultz S, Castillo C, et al: Nortriptyline versus fluoxetine in the treatment of depression and in short-term recovery after stroke: a placebo-controlled, double-blind study. Am J Psychiatry 157: 351–359, 2000

Rocca P, Calvarese P, Faggiano F, et al: Citalopram versus sertraline in late-life nonmajor clinically significant depression: a 1-year follow-up clinical trial. J Clin Psychiatry 66(3):360–369, 2005

Rochon PA, Stukel TA, Sykora K, et al: Atypical antipsychotics and parkinsonism. Arch Intern Med 165(16):1882–1888, 2005

Roose SP, Dalack GW, Glassman AH, et al: Cardiovascular effects of bupropion in depressed patients with heart disease. Am J Psychiatry 148:512–516, 1991

Roose SP, Nelson JC, Salzman C, et al: Mirtazapine in the Nursing Home Study Group: Open-label study of mirtazapine orally disintegrating tablets in depressed patients in the nursing home. Curr Med Res Opin 19(8):737–746, 2003

Roose SP, Miyazaki M, Devanand D, et al: An open trial of venlafaxine for the treatment of late-life atypical depression. Int J Geriatr Psychiatry 19(10):989–994, 2004a

Roose SP, Sackeim HA, Krishnan KR, et al; Old-Old Depression Study Group: Antidepressant pharmacotherapy in the treatment of depression in the very old: a randomized, placebo-controlled trial. Am J Psychiatry 161(11):2050–2059, 2004b

Rosen J, Sweet R, Pollock BG, et al: Nortriptyline in the hospitalized elderly: tolerance and side effect reduction. Psychopharmacol Bull 29:327–331, 1993

Rossini D, Serretti A, Franchini L, et al: Sertraline versus fluvoxamine in the treatment of elderly patients with major depression: a double-blind, randomized trial. J Clin Psychopharmacol 25(5):471–475, 2005

Sa DS, Lang AE: Olanzapine and clozapine: comparative effects on motor function in hallucinating PD patients. Neurology 57: 747, 2001

Saiz-Ruiz J, Ibanez A, Diaz-Marsa M, et al: Nefazodone in the treatment of elderly patients with depressive disorders: a prospective, observational study. CNS Drugs 16(9):635–643, 2002

Sajatovic M, Ramirez LF, Vernon L, et al: Outcome of risperidone therapy in elderly patients with chronic psychosis. Int J Psychiatry Med 26:309–317, 1996

Sajatovic M, Jaskiw G, Konicki PE, et al: Outcome of clozapine therapy for elderly patients with refractory primary psychosis. Int J Geriatr Psychiatry 12:553–558, 1997

Sajatovic M, Gyulai L, Calabrese JR, et al: Maintenance treatment outcomes in older patients with bipolar I disorder. Am J Geriatr Psychiatry 13:305–311, 2005a

Sajatovic M, Madhusoodanan S, Coconcea N: Managing bipolar disorder in the elderly: defining the role of the newer agents. Drugs Aging 22(1):39–54, 2005b

Samuels S, Fang M: Olanzapine may cause delirium in geriatric patients. J Clin Psychiatry 65(4):582–583, 2004

Sasaki Y, Matsuyama T, Inoue S, et al: A prospective, open-label, flexible-dose study of quetiapine in the treatment of delirium. J Clin Psychiatry 64(11):1316–1321, 2003

Satel SL, Nelson JC: Stimulants in the treatment of depression: a critical overview. J Clin Psychiatry 50:241–249, 1989

Sato Y, Kondo I, Ishida S, et al: Decreased bone mass and increased bone turnover with valproate therapy in adults with epilepsy. Neurology 57:445–449, 2001

Schatzberg AF, Kremer C, Rodrigues HE, et al; Mirtazapine vs Paroxetine Study Group: Double-blind, randomized comparison of mirtazapine and paroxetine in elderly depressed patients. Am J Geriatr Psychiatry 10(5):541–550, 2002

Schneider LS, Olin JT: Efficacy of acute treatment for geriatric depression. Int Psychogeriatr 7 (suppl):7–25, 1995

Schneider LS, Tariot PN, Lyketsos CG, et al: National Institute of Mental Health Clinical Antipsychotic Trials of Intervention Effectiveness (CATIE): Alzheimer disease trial methodology. Am J Geriatr Psychiatry 9:346–360, 2001

Schneider LS, Nelson JC, Clary CM, et al; Sertraline Elderly Depression Study Group: An 8-week multicenter, parallel-group, double-blind, placebo-controlled study of sertraline in elderly outpatients with major depression. Am J Psychiatry 160(7): 1277–1285, 2003

Schneider LS, Dagerman KS, Insel P: Risk of death with atypical antipsychotic drug treatment for dementia: meta-analysis of randomized placebo-controlled trials. JAMA 294(15):1934–1943, 2005

Schone W, Ludwig M: A double-blind study of paroxetine compared with fluoxetine in geriatric patients with major depression. J Clin Psychopharmacol 13 (6 suppl 2): 34S–39S, 1993

Schreiber S, Backer MM, Pick CG: The antinociceptive effect of venlafaxine in mice is mediated through opioid and adrenergic mechanisms. Neurosci Lett 273:85–88, 1999

Schwaninger M, Ringleb P, Winter R, et al: Elevated plasma concentrations of homocysteine in antiepileptic drug treatment. Epilepsia 40:345–350, 1999

Semenchuk MR, Sherman S, Davis B: Double-blind, randomized trial of bupropion SR for the treatment of neuropathic pain. Neurology 57:1583–1588, 2001

Serebruany VL, Glassman AH, Malinin AI, et al; Sertraline AntiDepressant Heart Attack Randomized Trial Study Group: Platelet/endothelial biomarkers in depressed patients treated with the selective serotonin reuptake inhibitor sertraline after acute coronary events: the Sertraline AntiDepressant Heart Attack Randomized Trial (SADHART) Platelet Substudy. Circulation 108(8):939–944, 2003

Sernyak MJ, Leslie DL, Alarcon RD, et al: Association of diabetes mellitus with use of atypical neuroleptics in the treatment of schizophrenia. Am J Psychiatry 159:561–566, 2002

Sheikh JI, Cassidy EL, Doraiswamy PM, et al: Efficacy, safety, and tolerability of sertraline in patients with late-life depression and comorbid medical illness. J Am Geriatr Soc 52(1):86–92, 2004a

Sheikh JI, Lauderdale SA, Cassidy EL: Efficacy of sertraline for panic disorder in older adults: a preliminary open-label trial. Am J Geriatr Psychiatry 12(2):230, 2004b

Shelton RC, Tollefson GD, Tohen M, et al: A novel augmentation strategy for treating resistant major depression. Am J Psychiatry 158:131–134, 2001

Shelton C, Entsuah R, Padmanabhan SK, et al: Venlafaxine XR demonstrates higher rates of sustained remission compared to fluoxetine, paroxetine or placebo. Int Clin Psychopharmacol 20(4):233–238, 2005

Shulman KI: Disinhibition syndromes, secondary mania and bipolar disorder in old age. J Affect Disord 46:175–182, 1997

Sink KM, Holden KF, Yaffe K: Pharmacological treatment of neuropsychiatric symptoms of dementia: a review of the evidence. JAMA 293(5):596–608, 2005

Skinner MH, Kuan HY, Skerjanec A, et al: Effect of age on the pharmacokinetics of duloxetine in women. Br J Clin Pharmacol 57(1):54–61, 2004

Skrobik YK, Bergeron N, Dumont M, et al: Olanzapine vs haloperidol: treating delirium in a critical care setting. Intens Care Med 30(3):444–449, 2004

Smeraldi E, Rizzo F, Crespi G: Double-blind, randomized study of venlafaxine, clomipramine and trazodone in geriatric patients with major depression. Primary Care Psychiatry 4:189–195, 1998

Smith D, Dempster C, Glanville J, et al: Efficacy and tolerability of venlafaxine compared with selective serotonin reuptake inhibitors and other antidepressants: a meta-analysis. Br J Psychiatry 180:396–404, 2002

Solai LK, Mulsant BH, Pollock BG, et al: Effect of sertraline on plasma nortriptyline levels in depressed elderly. J Clin Psychiatry 58:440–443, 1997

Solai LK, Mulsant BH, Pollock BG: Selective serotonin reuptake inhibitors for late-life depression: a comparative review. Drugs Aging 18:355–368, 2001

Solai LK, Pollock BG, Mulsant BH, et al: Effect of nortriptyline and paroxetine on CYP2D6 activity in depressed elderly patients. J Clin Psychopharmacol 22:481–486, 2002

Sorock GS, Shimkin EE: Benzodiazepine sedatives and the risk of falling in a community-dwelling elderly cohort. Arch Intern Med 148:2441–2444, 1988

Spier SA: Use of bupropion with SRIs and venlafaxine. Depress Anxiety 7:73–75, 1998

Spina E, Pisani F, Perucca E: Clinically significant pharmacokinetic drug interactions with carbamazepine. An update. Clin Pharmacokinet 31:198–214, 1996

Spina E, Scordo MG: Clinically significant drug interactions with antidepressants in the elderly. Drugs Aging 19(4):299–320, 2002

Sproule BA, Hardy BG, Shulman KI: Differential pharmacokinetics of lithium in elderly patients. Drugs Aging 16:165–177, 2000

Stahl SM, Entsuah R, Rudolph RL: Comparative efficacy between venlafaxine and SSRIs: a pooled analysis of patients with depression. Biol Psychiatry 52(12):1166–1174, 2002

Steffens DC, Doraiswamy PM, McQuoid DR: Bupropion SR in the naturalistic treatment of elderly patients with major depression. Int J Geriatr Psychiatry 16:862–865, 2001

Steinberg JR: Anxiety in elderly patients. A comparison of azapirones and benzodiazepines. Drugs Aging 5:335–345, 1994

Stimmel GL, Dopheide JA, Stahl SM: Mirtazapine: an antidepressant with noradrenergic and specific serotonergic effects. Pharmacotherapy 17:10–21, 1997

Strand M, Hetta J, Rosen A, et al: A double-blind controlled trial in primary care patients with generalized anxiety: a comparison between buspirone and oxazepam. J Clin Psychiatry 51(suppl):40–45, 1990

Street JS, Clark WS, Gannon KS, et al: Olanzapine treatment of psychotic and behavioral symptoms in patients with Alzheimer disease in nursing care facilities: a double-blind, randomized, placebo-controlled trial. The HGEU Study Group. Arch Gen Psychiatry 57:968–976, 2000

Street JS, Clark WS, Kadam DL, et al: Long-term efficacy of olanzapine in the control of psychotic and behavioral symptoms in nursing home patients with Alzheimer's dementia. Int J Geriatr Psychiatry 16 (suppl 1):S62–S70, 2001

Suh GH, Son HG, Ju YS, et al: A randomized, double-blind, crossover comparison of risperidone and haloperidol in Korean dementia patients with behavioral disturbances. Am J Geriatr Psychiatry 12(5):509–516, 2004

Szuba MP, Leuchter AF: Falling backward in two elderly patients taking bupropion. J Clin Psychiatry 53:157–159, 1992

Taragano FE, Lyketsos CG, Mangone CA, et al: A double-blind, randomized, fixed-dose trial of fluoxetine vs. amitriptyline in the treatment of major depression complicating Alzheimer's disease. Psychosomatics 38:246–252, 1997

Targum SD, Abbott JL: Efficacy of quetiapine in Parkinson's patients with psychosis. J Clin Psychopharmacol 20:54–60, 2000

Tariot PN, Erb R, Podgorski CA, et al: Efficacy and tolerability of carbamazepine for agitation and aggression in dementia. Am J Psychiatry 155:54–61, 1998

Tariot PN, Salzman C, Yeung PP, et al: Long-term use of quetiapine in elderly patients with psychotic disorders. Clin Ther 22:1068–1084, 2000

Tariot PN, Farlow MR, Grossberg GT, et al; Memantine Study Group: Memantine treatment in patients with moderate to severe Alzheimer disease already receiving donepezil: a randomized controlled trial. JAMA 291(3):317–324, 2004

Tariot PN, Raman R, Jakimovich L, et al; Alzheimer's Disease Cooperative Study, Valproate Nursing Home Study Group: Divalproex sodium in nursing home residents with possible or probable Alzheimer disease complicated by agitation: a randomized, controlled trial. Am J Geriatr Psychiatry 13:942–949, 2005

Tashkin D, Kanner R, Bailey W, et al: Smoking cessation in patients with chronic obstructive pulmonary disease: a double-blind, placebo-controlled, randomised trial. Lancet 357:1571–1575, 2001

Tavcar R, Dernovsek MZ: Risperidone-induced delirium. Can J Psychiatry 43(2):194, 1998

Thase ME: Effects of venlafaxine on blood pressure: a meta-analysis of original data from 3744 depressed patients. J Clin Psychiatry 59:502–508, 1998

Thase ME: What role do atypical antipsychotic drugs have in treatment-resistant depression? J Clin Psychiatry 63:95–103, 2002

Thase ME, Entsuah AR, Rudolph RL: Remission rates during treatment with venlafaxine or selective serotonin reuptake inhibitors. Br J Psychiatry 178:234–241, 2001

Thase ME, Entsuah R, Cantillon M, et al: Relative antidepressant efficacy of venlafaxine and SSRIs: sex-age interactions. J Womens Health 14(7):609–616, 2005a

Thase ME, Haight BR, Richard N, et al: Remission rates following antidepressant therapy with bupropion or selective serotonin reuptake inhibitors: a meta-analysis of original data from 7 randomized controlled trials. J Clin Psychiatry 66(8):974–981, 2005b

Thase ME, Tran PV, Wiltse C, et al: Cardiovascular profile of duloxetine, a dual reuptake inhibitor of serotonin and norepinephrine. J Clin Psychopharmacol 25(2): 132–140, 2005c

Thompson DS: Mirtazapine for the treatment of depression and nausea in breast and gynecological oncology. Psychosomatics 41:356–359, 2000

Tollefson GD, Bosomworth JC, Heiligenstein JH, et al: A double-blind, placebo-controlled clinical trial of fluoxetine in geriatric patients with major depression. The Fluoxetine Collaborative Study Group. Int Psychogeriatr 7:89–104, 1995

Trappler B, Cohen CI: Use of SSRIs in "very old" depressed nursing home residents. Am J Geriatr Psychiatry 6:83–89, 1998

Trick L, Stanley N, Rigney U, et al: A double-blind, randomized, 26-week study comparing the cognitive and psychomotor effects and efficacy of 75 mg (37.5 mg b.i.d.) venlafaxine and 75 mg (25 mg mane, 50 mg nocte) dothiepin in elderly patients with moderate major depression being treated in general practice. J Psychopharmacol 18:205–214, 2004

Umapathy C, Mulsant BH, Pollock BG: Bipolar disorder in the elderly. Psychiatr Ann 30:473–480, 2000

van Iersel MB, Zuidema SU, Koopmans RT, et al: Antipsychotics for behavioral and psychological problems in elderly people with dementia: a systematic review of adverse events. Drugs Aging 22(10):845–858, 2005

van Laar MW, van Willigenburg AP, Volkerts ER: Acute and subchronic effects of nefazodone and imipramine on highway driving, cognitive functions, and daytime sleepiness in healthy adult and elderly subjects. J Clin Psychopharmacol 15:30–40, 1995

Verhey FR, Verkaaik M, Lousberg R, Olanzapine-Haloperidol in Dementia Study Group: Olanzapine versus haloperidol in the treatment of agitation in elderly patients with dementia: results of a randomized controlled double-blind trial. Dement Geriatr Cogn Disord 21(1):1–8, 2006

Vis PM, van Baardewijk M, Einarson TR: Duloxetine and venlafaxine-XR in the treatment of major depressive disorder: a meta-analysis of randomized clinical trials. Ann Pharmacother 39(11):1798–1807, 2005

von Moltke LL, Greenblatt DJ, Court MH, et al: Inhibition of alprazolam and desipramine hydroxylation in vitro by paroxetine and fluvoxamine: comparison with other selective serotonin reuptake inhibitor antidepressants. J Clin Psychopharmacol 15: 125–131, 1995

von Moltke LL, Greenblatt DJ, Giancarlo GM, et al: Escitalopram (S-citalopram) and its metabolites in vitro: cytochromes mediating biotransformation, inhibitory effects, and comparison to R-citalopram. Drug Metab Dispos 29:1102–1109, 2001

Wakelin JS: Fluvoxamine in the treatment of the older depressed patient; double-blind, placebo-controlled data. Int Clin Psychopharmacol 1:221–230, 1986

Walker Z, Grace J, Overshot R, et al: Olanzapine in dementia with Lewy bodies: a clinical study. Int J Geriatr Psychiatry 14:459–466, 1999

Wallace AE, Kofoed LL, West AN: Double-blind placebo-controlled trial of methylphenidate in older, depressed, medically ill patients. Am J Psychiatry 152:929–931, 1995

Wang PS, Bohn RL, Glynn RJ, et al: Zolpidem use and hip fractures in older people. J Am Geriatr Soc 49:1685–1690, 2001

Wang PS, Schneeweiss S, Avorn J, et al: Risk of death in elderly users of conventional vs atypical antipsychotic medications. N Engl J Med 353(22):2335–2341, 2005

Wehmeier PM, Kluge M, Maras A, et al: Fluoxetine versus trimipramine in the treatment of depression in geriatric patients. Pharmacopsychiatry 38(1):13–16, 2005

Weigmann H, Gerek S, Zeisig A, et al: Fluvoxamine but not sertraline inhibits the metabolism of olanzapine: evidence from a therapeutic drug monitoring service. Ther Drug Monit 23:410–413, 2001

Weihs KL, Settle EC Jr, Batey SR, et al: Bupropion sustained release versus paroxetine for the treatment of depression in the elderly. J Clin Psychiatry 61:196–202, 2000

Whyte EM, Mulsant BH: Post-stroke depression: epidemiology, pathophysiology, and biological treatment. Biol Psychiatry 52: 253–264, 2002

Whyte EM, Basinski J, Farhi P, et al: Geriatric depression treatment in nonresponders to selective serotonin reuptake inhibitors. J Clin Psychiatry 65(12):1634–1641, 2004

Whyte E, Romkes M, Mulsant BH, et al: CYP2D6 genotype and venlafaxine-XR concentrations in depressed elderly. Int J Geriatr Psychiatry 21:1–8, 2006

Wilner KD, Tensfeldt TG, Baris B, et al: Single- and multiple-dose pharmacokinetics of ziprasidone in healthy young and elderly volunteers. Br J Clin Pharmacol 49 (suppl 1):15S–20S, 2000

Wilson K, Mottram P: A comparison of side effects of selective serotonin reuptake inhibitors and tricyclic antidepressants in older depressed patients: a meta-analysis. Int J Geriatr Psychiatry 19(8):754–762, 2004

Wingen M, Bothmer J, Langer S, et al: Actual driving performance and psychomotor function in healthy subjects after acute and subchronic treatment with escitalopram, mirtazapine, and placebo: a crossover trial. J Clin Psychiatry 66:436–443, 2005

Wolters EC, Jansen EN, Tuynman-Qua HG, et al: Olanzapine in the treatment of dopaminomimetic psychosis in patients with Parkinson's disease. Neurology 47:1085–1087, 1996

Workman RH Jr, Orengo CA, Bakey AA, et al: The use of risperidone for psychosis and agitation in demented patients with Parkinson's disease. J Neuropsychiatry Clin Neurosci 9:594–597, 1997

Wylie ME, Mulsant BH, Pollock BG, et al: Age of onset in geriatric bipolar disorder: effects on clinical presentation and treatment outcomes in an inpatient sample. Am J Geriatr Psychiatry 7:77–83, 1999

Wylie ME, Miller MD, Shear MK, et al: Fluvoxamine pharmacotherapy of anxiety disorders in late life: preliminary open-trial data. J Geriatr Psychiatry Neurol 13: 43–48, 2000

Yang CH, Tsai SJ, Hwang JP: The efficacy and safety of quetiapine for treatment of geriatric psychosis. J Psychopharmacol 19: 661–666, 2005

Young RC, Gyulai L, Mulsant BH, et al: Pharmacotherapy of bipolar disorder in old age: review and recommendations. Am J Geriatr Psychiatry 12(4):342–357, 2004

Zarate CA Jr, Baldessarini RJ, Siegel AJ, et al: Risperidone in the elderly: a pharmacoepidemiologic study. J Clin Psychiatry 58: 311–317, 1997

Zimmer B, Kant R, Zeiler D, et al: Antidepressant efficacy and cardiovascular safety of venlafaxine in young vs old patients with comorbid medical disorders. Int J Psychiatry Med 27:353–364, 1997

Study Questions

Select the single best response for each question.

1. Psychopharmacological treatment of late-life psychiatric illness has significantly improved clinical function and quality of life for patients. However, systemic side effects from psychotropic medications are a vexing problem in this population. Many side effects are due to anticholinergic, antihistaminic, and antiadrenergic effects. All of the following clinical problems are referable to anticholinergic effects *except*

    A. Constipation.
    B. Urinary retention.
    C. Sedation.
    D. Delirium.
    E. Cognitive dysfunction.

2. The selective serotonin reuptake inhibitors (SSRIs) have become the first-line agents in the treatment of mood disorders in older adults. Which of the following is true regarding the use of SSRIs in older patients?

    A. Due to their pharmacokinetic profiles and low risk for drug-drug interactions, sertraline and fluoxetine are the preferred SSRIs.
    B. Several controlled trials have demonstrated the effectiveness of SSRIs in anxiety disorders in elderly patients.
    C. Despite not being technically "antipsychotic," SSRIs have been shown to be efficacious in treating delusions and hallucinations in dementia.
    D. SSRIs may cause the syndrome of inappropriate secretion of antidiuretic hormone (SIADH) with hypernatremia, which may lead to delirium.
    E. SSRIs are poorly tolerated in Parkinson's disease.

3. Other contemporary antidepressants may be clinically indicated in the older patient for various psychiatric symptoms. Which of the following is true?

    A. Bupropion is contraindicated in seizure disorder patients, but it is recommended for poststroke depression.
    B. Because it may energize a fatigued depressed patient, bupropion is the antidepressant of choice in psychotic depression.
    C. Venlafaxine has different pharmacokinetic properties depending on the patient's age; thus, lower doses are typically effective for older patients.
    D. Venlafaxine significantly reduces the risk for a withdrawal syndrome when treatment is interrupted or discontinued.
    E. Mirtazapine inhibits $5\text{-}HT_2$ and $5\text{-}HT_3$ receptors, making it an attractive choice for elderly depressed patients with severe nausea.

4. Newer agents have largely supplanted the tricyclic antidepressants (TCAs). However, some TCAs may be useful for certain patients. The secondary, rather than tertiary, amine structures are associated with less side-effect burden. Which of the following TCAs is a secondary amine and thus likely to be more tolerable by older patients?

   A. Amitriptyline.
   B. Desipramine.
   C. Imipramine.
   D. Doxepin.
   E. Clomipramine.

5. The atypical antipsychotic agents have been quickly integrated into geriatric psychiatric practice, as they are in general more tolerable than the older typical agents. Which of the following is true regarding this group of antipsychotic agents?

   A. When used for drug-induced psychosis in Parkinson's disease, clozapine should be used at dosages between 100 and 200 mg/day.
   B. Olanzapine has been associated with elevated glucose and lipids, but only when there is simultaneous weight gain.
   C. Because of risk of extrapyramidal symptoms in elderly patients, the dosage of risperidone should be limited to less than 1 mg/day.
   D. Quetiapine does not show affinity for muscarinic receptors and is a viable alternative to clozapine for drug-induced psychosis in Parkinson's disease.
   E. Ziprasidone's use in elderly patients is limited by its high degree of muscarinic receptor affinity and resultant risk of cognitive impairment.

6. Mood stabilizers may be useful in elderly patients, both for patients with long-established bipolar disorders and for behavioral acting-out in dementing illness. Which of the following is true?

   A. Because of their greater safety profile in older patients, anticonvulsants are now prescribed much more commonly than lithium for elderly bipolar patients.
   B. Older patients are subject to lithium toxicity at lower serum lithium levels than younger adults, with cognitive impairment reported at levels even lower than 1 mEq/L.
   C. Thrombocytopenia is a rare complication of valproate use in elderly patients.
   D. Aging alone typically increases the half-life of valproate metabolism by a factor of 2 to 3.
   E. Carbamazepine is a cytochrome P450 inhibitor and thus can inhibit its own metabolism, increasing serum levels.

7. Which of these cholinesterase inhibitors is notably affected by renal function and carries an FDA warning about dose titration?

   A. Tacrine.
   B. Donepezil.
   C. Rivastigmine.
   D. Galantamine.
   E. Physostigmine.

Individual and Group Psychotherapy

Ann K. Aspnes, M.A.

Thomas R. Lynch, Ph.D.

Psychotherapy has been shown to be an effective treatment for a number of mental disorders seen in older adults. As a treatment modality it can be particularly useful for older adult psychiatric patients who cannot or will not tolerate medication or who are dealing with stressful conditions, interpersonal difficulties, limited levels of social support, or recurrent episodes of the disorder. However, it has been estimated that only 10% of older adults in need of psychiatric services actually receive professional care, and there has been minimal utilization of mental health services in this age group (Abrahams and Patterson 1978; Friedhoff 1994; Weissman et al. 1981).

Many practitioners assume that older adults have negative attitudes toward psychotherapy. Although research on attitudes toward treatment in elderly samples is not conclusive, contrary to clinical lore, growing descriptive research suggests that older adults may prefer counseling over medication treatment. In a community sample of 462 nondepressed older adults, 68% agreed with a statement that professional counseling or therapy helps most depressed people feel better. Interestingly, 56% of the same sample reported that they believed antidepressant medications to be addictive, and only 4% disagreed (Vitt et al. 1999). Older adults have also been shown to report a greater number of positive attitudes toward mental health professionals and to be less concerned than younger adults with stigmas attached to seeking treatment for depression (Rokke and Scogin 1995). Regardless, attitudinal barriers to treatment occur in samples of both younger and older adults (Allen et al. 1998), and patient preferences or biases toward treatment should be considered before referral for psychotherapy.

In this chapter we review the theoretical and empirical evidence for psychotherapy in older adults. The material is organized by type of disorder and, for each disorder, type of therapy. We begin by reviewing what is known about common factors that influence outcome across modalities. When possible, we evaluate the evidence with respect to quality of data, generalizability, and long-term effects of treatment.

Common Factors

Simply stated, the goals of psychotherapy are to enhance human coping and to reduce human suffering.

Most therapies consist of some type of therapeutic feedback to enhance patient awareness or to change patient behavior (Goldfried et al. 1997, 1998). Therapist feedback may help patients by influencing cognitive and attentional biases for problematic stimuli (Beck et al. 1979; Hayes et al. 1996; Klerman et al. 1984; Strupp and Binder 1984). Thus, therapists can be seen to work toward helping patients refocus attention toward aspects of themselves that have previously been avoided or overattended so that they can gain new perspectives about themselves or improve their ability to solve problems (Goldfried et al. 1997). Therapeutic feedback may function optimally when corrective information regarding ineffective behavior is balanced by validation of behavior that is effective (Linehan 1993).

Therapy also typically occurs within the context of some type of interpersonal relationship. Some have argued that relationship factors account for as much as 80% of the variance in treatment outcomes (Andrews 1998). However, research has not confirmed this assertion. Contrary to the belief that the therapeutic relationship is the salient curative feature, relationship variables have been shown to produce only 10% of the variance in outcomes, essentially equivalent to the variance attributed to specific therapeutic approaches (Horvath and Symonds 1991; Luborsky et al. 2002; Martin et al. 2000).

In general, older adults will respond to many of the therapeutic interventions used with younger populations. The pace of therapy should be slower, and fonts for written material should be larger. In addition, providing memory aids can be very help-

ful. For example, in our work we audiotape each session and ask the patient to review the session during the week before the next meeting. Additional areas to consider are listed below.

- Medical illness or problematic medicines can exacerbate symptoms of a mental disorder. During assessment it is important to obtain a medical history and a medication list.
- Social desirability factors should be considered when obtaining self reports. A nonjudgmental stance on the part of the clinician will likely help disclosure.
- The clinician should actively work against stereotypes of elderly persons as being withdrawn, rigid, lonely, dependent, or unable to learn.
- Older adults may have difficulty remembering troublesome events. The clinician should consider consulting family members or longtime friends.
- Some patients may avoid feedback about their problems as a way to reduce anxiety. Patients should be advised that change will likely involve some discomfort as they learn to cope differently (e.g., being assertive if normally avoidant).
- Cognitive deficits can impede learning speed and memory. Therapists may need to slow the pace when teaching skills and may need to ask patients to summarize issues covered.

Depression

Cognitive-Behavioral Therapy

Cognitive-behavioral therapy (CBT) interventions have been the most frequently studied therapies and have repeatedly been found useful in treating depression in older adults (Koder et al. 1996; Scogin and McElreath 1994; Thompson and Gallagher 1984; Thompson et al. 1987). CBT techniques currently in use generally combine earlier work that used either solely cognitive or solely behavioral therapies and now encompass a wide variety of treatment protocols. Cognitive therapies focus on problematic thoughts that may perpetuate depression. The goal is to change and adapt cognitive patterns away from negative thoughts that have become automatic. By changing the thoughts, therapists hope to change underlying dysfunctional attitudes that are hypothesized to result in relapse (Floyd and Scogin 1998).

More purely behavioral interventions are derived from classic learning theory in which problem behaviors are viewed as the result of specific antecedent stimuli and consequential events that reinforce, punish, or maintain behavioral responses (e.g., Dougher and Hackbert 1994). Genetics and biology are considered to play important roles in the development of psychopathology; however, theorists believe that biological predispositions can be mediated by skill acquisition and learning that occurs throughout the lifespan. This therapeutic approach views depression as a state in which there is a relative shift toward an increase in dysphoric or hopeless affective reactions and a concomitant reduction in the frequency of reinforcing overt activities. Problem behaviors are analyzed functionally. For example, dysphoric responses (e.g., sad facial expressions, self-denigration) may function to reduce hostility or increase sympathy by caregivers, yet over time the lack of recovery or recurrent depression may be seen as aversive to caregivers (Biglan 1991; Coyne 1976; Dougher and Hackbert 1994). Behavioral techniques include monitoring behavior and affect patterns, assigning pleasant events, stimulus control, limiting worry and depressive ruminations with time limits, behavioral exposure, and skills training (relaxation, problem-solving, interpersonal skills).

In a study comparing cognitive, behavioral, and brief psychodynamic therapy to waiting-list control subjects, Thompson and colleagues (1987) found that all of the treatment modalities led to comparable and clinically significant reductions of depression. All three treatment regimens included individual treatment twice weekly for 4 weeks and weekly thereafter, totaling 16–20 sessions. Overall, 52% of the sample attained complete remission after treatment, and 18% showed significant improvement with some enduring depressive symptoms. These rates are comparable to treatment outcomes in younger adult populations and response to pharmacotherapy (O'Rourke and Hadjistavropoulos 1997; Thompson et al. 1987). Follow-up research indicated that at 12 months after treatment, 58% of the sample was depression free and that at 24 months, 70% of the sample was not depressed. Like in acute treatment, no differences were found between treatment modalities at follow-up (Gallagher-Thompson et al. 1990), although in previous research with a smaller sample size depressed geriatric patients in cognitive and behavioral therapies maintained the gains longer than those treated with brief psychodynamic therapy (Gallagher and Thompson 1982).

In the first known randomized trial examining CBT as a medication augmentation strategy, Thompson et al. (2001) assessed 102 depressed older adults. Patients were assigned to one of three treatment conditions: 1) CBT alone, 2) medication alone, or 3) combined CBT and medication. Although all three groups showed improvements in depressive symptoms over 16–20 weeks of treatment, the combined-therapy group had the greatest improvements. A significant difference was found between the combined-therapy and the medication-only groups. The CBT-alone group showed similar improvements as the combined-therapy group, but the superiority of CBT alone over medication alone did not reach a significant level. This study supports conclusions by Reynolds et al. (1999) that a combined medication plus psychotherapy approach may be optimal for the treatment of depression in older adults.

A related therapy for elderly depression that utilizes elements associated with both cognitive and behavioral interventions described above examines problems associated with social problem solving. Social problem-solving therapy (PST) is based on a model in which ineffective coping under stress is hypothesized to lead to a breakdown of problem-solving abilities and subsequent depression (Nezu 1987; Thompson and Gallagher 1984). Patients are taught a structured format for solving problems that considers problem details, present goals, multiple solutions, specific solution advantages, and assessing the final solution in context. PST ideally refines and augments patients' present strategies to improve their ability to handle day-to-day problems. Like interpersonal psychotherapy, PST bolsters an area of weakness in individuals with depression. PST attempts to increase coping and buffer factors that maintain and aggravate depression (Hegel et al. 2002a). One of the attractions of PST is that it can be delivered in a limited space of time. A positive trend in the research examines adaptations of PST to be used in primary care facilities. Because many older adults do not seek treatment for depression beyond their primary care health providers, this is an ideal place to deliver psychotherapies for depression in older adults.

Arean et al. (1993) examined the efficacy of PST in a randomized, controlled trial of 74 clinically depressed older adults (age 55 or older). Patients were assigned to one of three treatment conditions: PST, reminiscence therapy, or a waiting-list control condition. After 12 weekly sessions, both therapies showed significant reductions in depressive symptoms at posttreatment and at a 3-month follow-up relative to control subjects. However, a significantly greater number of patients in the PST group than in the reminiscence therapy group were classified as improved or in remission after treatment.

Several studies have evaluated the adaptation of problem-solving treatment in primary care (PST-PC) (Hegel et al. 2002a; Mynors-Wallis 2001; Unutzer et al. 2001; Williams et al. 2000). In one study, primary care treatment options were compared in a population of older adults with depression or dysthymia (Williams et al. 2000). Subjects were randomly assigned to treatment with an antidepressant, treatment with a placebo, or PST-PC. Subjects who received PST-PC did not show significant improvements over subjects who received placebos. The antidepressant treatment group did show significant improvements over placebo. However, Unutzer et al. (2002) found that patients who received PST-PC as part of a comprehensive treatment, including antidepressant medication, psychoeducation, and case management, had significantly less depressive symptomatology than usual-care patients immediately after treatment. Patients in the intervention experienced increasing symptom reduction up to a 12-month follow-up. These findings suggest that the ideal use of PST-PC for older adults might include augmentation with medication and other treatment strategies.

PST-PC has advantages because it requires only brief training and has been shown to be almost equally effective whether delivered by a nurse practitioner or a medical doctor (Mynors-Wallis 2001). However, in a recent study, previous training of therapists in cognitive-behavioral interventions proved to be a significant predictor of treatment improvement (Hegel et al. 2002b). This difficulty may be mitigated in primary care multidisciplinary teams by placing a point person trained in cognitive-behavioral interventions within each team.

Interpersonal Psychotherapy

Interpersonal psychotherapy (IPT) is a manualized treatment that focuses on four components that are hypothesized to lead to or maintain depression. Whatever its etiology, depression is seen to persist in a social context. The four components of treatment focus are 1) grief (e.g., death of spouse); 2) interpersonal disputes (e.g., conflict with adult children); 3 role transitions (e.g., retirement); and 4) interpersonal deficits (e.g., lack of assertiveness skills). Techniques utilized in treatment include role-playing, communication analysis, clarification of the patient's wants and needs, and links between affect and environmental events (Hinrichsen 1997). Frank and colleagues (1993) developed separate treatment manuals for interpersonal therapy in late life and interpersonal maintenance therapy for older patients. These manuals include adaptations specific for use in elderly patients, including flexibility in length of sessions, long-standing role disputes, and the need to help the patient with practical problems.

Controlled trials in populations of depressed adults have demonstrated the efficacy of IPT for the treatment of acute depression (Frank and Spanier 1995; Hinrichsen 1997). Interpersonal therapy has also been found to be as effective in the acute treatment of major depressive disorder in elderly patients as nortriptyline (Sloane et al. 1985). Of additional importance are findings that elderly patients in IPT treatment were less likely to drop out of treatment than were those taking nortriptyline because of the medication's side effects.

IPT in combination with nortriptyline has been shown to be an effective treatment for depression in geriatric samples (Reynolds et al. 1992, 1994). In an attempt to understand more about the treatment of elderly patients with recurrent depression, Reynolds et al. (1992) selected patients only if they reported at least one prior episode of depression. Seventy-eight percent (116 of 148) remitted during the acute phase of treatment (8–14 weeks). During the continuation phase, 15% (18 of 116) experienced relapse of major depression; therefore, a total of 66% of patients recovered fully (Reynolds et al. 1992, 1994). The authors concluded that older patients with recurrent major depression can be successfully treated with a combination of antidepressant medication and IPT and that older patients respond as well, albeit more slowly, as middle-aged patients (Reynolds et al. 1997).

Psychodynamic Psychotherapy

Psychodynamic psychotherapy is based on psychoanalytical theory, which views current interpersonal and emotional experience as having been influenced by early childhood experience (Bibring 1952). Revised conceptualizations have emphasized how relationships are internalized and transformed into a sense of self (e.g., Kernberg 1976; M. Klein 1952; Kohut and Wolf 1978; Mahler 1952). Psychopathology is theorized as being related to arrestments in the development of the self, and depression is viewed as a symptom state resulting from unresolved intrapsychic conflict that may be activated by life events such as loss. During therapy patients are encouraged to develop insight into their past experience and how this experience influences their current relationships.

Although short-term psychodynamic therapy has been less studied than other treatments for older adults (e.g., CBT, IPT), there have been several indications that short-term psychodynamic therapy, particularly as conducted by Thompson, Gallagher-Thompson, and colleagues, is an effective means to treat depression in samples of older adults. In studies with random assignment to a waiting-list control condition, short-term psychodynamic therapy, or cognitive-behavioral therapy, no significant differences were found between the types of psychotherapy at the end of treatment nor at 12- and 24-month follow-ups (Gallagher-Thompson et al. 1990; Thompson et al. 1987). Additional research on depressed caregivers demonstrated an interaction between the mode of therapy and length of caregiving, such that those who had been providing care for less than 44 months appeared to achieve greater improvement with dynamic therapy, whereas longer-term caregivers seemed to obtain greater benefit from CBT (Gallagher-Thompson and Steffen 1994). The authors suggested that the long-term caregivers needed the skills learned in CBT to care for family members with more pronounced deficits and requiring more complicated care. These interesting results call for additional controlled trials comparing different treatment modalities, continued component analysis research, and continued research that examines which type of treatment works best with which type of patient.

Group Psychotherapy

Our review of the literature found nine published reports on controlled studies of group treatments for noncognitively impaired elderly persons with depression. Perrotta and Meacham (1982) reported that group reminiscence therapy was no more effective than a waiting-list control condition. In contrast, self-management therapy and education groups were both equally effective and were superior to a waiting-list control condition (Rokke et al.

1999). In comparisons with medications, one nonrandomized controlled study found that cognitive-behavioral and psychodynamic group therapies were both more effective than placebo pill but less effective than tricyclics (Jarvik et al. 1982) and that although the cognitive-behavioral and psychodynamic groups were equivalent on most measures of depression and anxiety, the CBT group had lower posttreatment scores on one depression measure (Steuer 1984). A randomized, controlled study found that cognitive therapy with or without alprazolam (an anxiolytic) was more effective than alprazolam alone (Beutler et al. 1987). Also, the addition of behavioral group therapy to standard hospital care (which presumably included medication) led to higher remission rates among inpatients than standard care alone (Brand and Clingempeel 1992). In a recent study, antidepressant medication plus clinical management alone was compared with the same therapy with the addition of dialectical behavior therapy (DBT) skills training and scheduled telephone coaching sessions (Lynch et al. 2003). At 6-month follow-up, 73% of medication plus DBT patients were in remission, compared with only 38% of medication-only patients, a significant difference. Only patients receiving DBT showed significant improvements from pretreatment to posttreatment on scores of dependency and adaptive coping, which are theorized to create vulnerability to depression (Lynch et al. 2003). This treatment modality has also been adapted to older adults with comorbid depression and personality disorders and shows some promising results as detailed in the "Axis II Disorders" section (Lynch et al., in press). Another recent study compared CBT group therapy with case management and a combination of the two in a sample of low-income older adults (Arean et al. 2005). Patients receiving case management showed greater improvement than the CBT group at a 12-month follow-up, though the difference was not significant. Patients receiving the combined treatment showed significantly less depression than either case management or CBT group at 12-month follow-up.

In summary, certain group therapy interventions, particularly cognitive-behavioral groups, appear promising for use with depressed older adults. Group therapy may also offer advantages for many elders; it is generally less expensive than individual treatment, and the social network provided by group therapy may provide significant therapeutic benefits to elders experiencing a loss of interpersonal relationships through the death of friends and spouses.

Anxiety Disorders

Anxiety Symptoms

According to epidemiological sampling, anxiety disorders are the most prevalent mental disorders diagnosed among community-dwelling older adults (Regier et al. 1988). The prevalence of anxiety disorders among younger adults was estimated at 7.3% of the population; a slightly lower rate of 5.5% was reported among older adults (Regier et al. 1988). Review of these reports, however, suggests that the rate of anxiety disorders in older adults may be underestimated due to older adults' reluctance to report symptoms, confusion of anxiety symptoms with symptoms of physical illness, and a lack of measurement instruments validated for geriatric populations. A review of eight community surveys revealed that prevalence rates for anxiety disorders in older adults ranged from 0.7% to 18.6% (Flint 1994). Another possible explanation for the range in reported prevalence rates is that the symptomatic makeup of anxiety disorders in older adults differs

from that seen in younger adults. Indeed, older adults tend to report anxiety symptoms that do not necessarily fit a specific disorder. A naturalistic survey of primary care patients found that in older adults diagnosed with anxiety disorders, the most prevalent diagnosis was anxiety disorder not otherwise specified (Stanley et al. 2001). A portion of the empirical work on the psychotherapeutic treatment of anxiety in older adults focuses on symptoms rather than specific diagnostic categories.

The most frequently used and the most well-substantiated treatments for anxiety in older adults are based on behavioral therapies. Specifically, a variety of relaxation training techniques have been pilot tested as a treatment strategy for older adults. Preliminary work by DeBerry (1982a, 1982b) showed that progressive muscle relaxation and meditation relaxation techniques reduced anxiety symptoms more effectively than treatment control conditions in older adults. Scogin and associates (1992) assessed the use of progressive muscle relaxation and imaginal relaxation, with mixed results. Both relaxation training groups showed improvements in state anxiety and anxiety symptoms after training, but there was no significant improvement in trait anxiety.

In a 1-year follow-up assessment (Rickard et al. 1984) of older adults who had responded to relaxation training with a significant decrease in anxiety symptoms, the improvements from the pretraining assessment to the 1-year follow-up in state anxiety, trait anxiety, psychological symptoms, and relaxation level were all significant. Study participants also showed a nonsignificant trend of continuing treatment gains from posttreatment to 1-year follow-up. Given the small sample size of 26 study participants, these results indicate the potential promise of using relaxation strategies to treat distinct anxiety symptoms.

Relaxation training does have some advantages for treating mild anxiety in older adults. The strategies can be taught in brief individual or group sessions. Theoretically, the strategies can be delivered during a regular visit to a primary care physician. Like many behavioral strategies, relaxation training has the advantage of masquerading as skills training for patients who might avoid traditional psychotherapy. Also, patients with cognitive deficits, who may have difficulty with more cognitive strategies, may benefit from purely behavioral strategies.

CBT is a potentially useful treatment for anxiety symptoms. Unfortunately, the bulk of literature assessing CBT for anxiety in older adults describes case reports or suffers from problematic methodology. An exception is a randomized trial conducted by Barrowclough and colleagues (2001) comparing CBT and supportive counseling delivered in patients' homes for the treatment of anxiety symptoms in older adults (over age 55) who met criteria for a range of anxiety disorders. Despite a strong effort in the recruitment phase of this study, which originally identified 179 potentially eligible older adults, only 55 individuals qualified. Further attrition due to dropouts or changes in health status among study participants reduced the final sample to 33. Participants who received CBT showed significantly greater decreases in self-reported anxiety symptoms after treatment than did participants who received supportive counseling. Although the CBT participants also showed a stronger decreasing trend from posttreatment to 12-month follow-up in clinician-rated anxiety symptoms, the differences between the two treatment groups on this measure did not reach statistical significance ($P < 0.08$). At the 12-month follow-up, the number of participants in the CBT group who attained criteria for treatment response was significantly higher than in the supportive counseling group. Despite some of the weaknesses of this study, the results did support the efficacy of CBT for anxiety in older adults and did so in comparison to supportive counseling rather than a weaker treatment comparison, such as standard care. Certainly, more empirical support is needed to establish the efficacy of CBT as a treatment for anxiety symptoms in older adults. Barrowclough and colleagues have shown at the very least that the use of CBT in an older population deserves further investigation.

Generalized Anxiety Disorder

Among older adults, generalized anxiety disorder (GAD) is the most commonly diagnosed anxiety disorder. Based on Epidemiological Catchment Area surveys, it is estimated that up to 1.9% of older adults currently experience GAD (Blazer et al. 1991). Although researchers tend to agree that rates of GAD are lower in older adults than in younger populations, several researchers have suggested that GAD is still underdiagnosed in this population (Fuentes and Cox 1997; Palmer et al. 1997; Stanley and Novy 2000). Diagnostic criteria for GAD in younger adults may fail to take into account different ways that older adults experience anxiety. Older adults may focus on different targets of worry and on somatic symptoms that can be confused with medical illness. Evidence also suggests that GAD often appears in conjunction with depressive symptoms, which confuse both diagnostic criteria and the focal point for treatment strategies. One study reported that 91% of individuals with GAD diagnoses also met criteria for depression (Lindesay et al. 1989). In a sample of older adults, 60% of those who met criteria for GAD also endorsed comorbid depressive episodes. The problems of variant symptom presentations, overemphasis on somatic symptoms, and depressive comorbidity create confusion in both diagnoses and treatment choices.

Given the issue of comorbidity with depression, the previously reported success of CBT in the treatment of depression in older adults makes it a logical area of treatment research for GAD in older adults. Because of the nature of CBT, this treatment will also theoretically expose a variety of cognitive patterns of worry regardless of content and the cognitive and behavioral antecedents that link anxiety to somatic symptoms. CBT appears to be the best-equipped form of psychotherapy to manage the diagnostic and treatment issues that exist in older populations with GAD. Treatment research on GAD in late life is limited. Not surprisingly, though, the bulk of this literature focuses on the efficacy of CBT in this population (Mohlman and Gorman 2005; Stanley and Novy 2000; Stanley et al. 1996, 2004; Wetherell et al. 2003).

In a randomized trial, Stanley et al. (2003) compared the efficacy of CBT to that of a minimal contact condition. The researchers' treatment protocol included education training, relaxation training, cognitive restructuring, and exposure to anxiety-provoking stimuli. Compared with the minimal contact condition, participation in CBT was associated with significantly greater improvements over time in GAD severity, anxiety, and depression. These marked improvements in depression and anxiety symptoms were demonstrated in both self-report measures and clinician ratings. CBT participants reported a significant within-group improvement in the severity of GAD symptoms from the point of their assessment immediately after the completion of the treatment protocol to an assessment 12 months after treatment completion. These findings suggest that CBT may not only provide effective immediate therapy but may also promote long-term gains in the management of GAD.

Because of the tendency for older adults to seek treatment for mental disorders in primary care facilities, current research is exploring an adaptation of CBT protocols that can be delivered in primary care. In a pilot study, Stanley and associates (2004) presented a shortened CBT protocol for use in a primary care setting. This therapy was administered in eight sessions, either within the medical clinic or in the patients' homes. The treatment focused on six issues: education, relaxation training, cognitive therapy, problem-solving strategies, gradual exposure treatment, and sleep management. Further details may be found in the treatment manual (Stanley et al. 2004). Compared with a usual-care control condition, CBT was associated with significant decreases in GAD severity, anxiety symptoms, and depression symptoms. Although the sample size was very small ($N = 12$), the positive results provide preliminary utility for the use of CBT in primary care settings. Although CBT has strong promise for treating GAD in older adults, further empirical research must be conducted to verify its efficacy in this population.

Substance Use Disorders

Limited research is available on the prevalence of substance use disorders in older people, much less on the treatment of substance use disorders. With the exception of alcohol use, most substance use in late life is thought to be an extension of substance use from earlier periods of life (Oslin et al. 2000). Although medical comorbidity becomes an increasing factor in older adults, most substance use in late life is presumed to differ from younger populations' use more because of cohort differences than developmental differences. Treatment research on substance use in this population is nearly absent but is greatly needed.

The only substance whose use has been studied comprehensively in older adults is alcohol. Alcohol dependence is estimated to be lower in older adults than in younger cohorts. According to Epidemiological Catchment Area surveys, current alcohol dependence and abuse prevalence rates ranged from 1.4% in North Carolina to 3.7% in Maryland in adults over age 65 in comparison to a prevalence rate of 8.6% in all adult Americans (Adams et al. 1993). Regular alcohol use that falls below diagnostic criteria can still be problematic in older adults. Given the possibility of interactions with prescription medications and increased risk of physical illness, lower levels of alcohol can be potentially dangerous for older adults (Fingerhood 2000; Moore et al. 1999).

Research on effective therapy for alcohol-related disorders in older adults is sparse. In the review literature, standard treatment for older adults is to "mainstream" them into therapeutic groups for adults of any age, such as Alcoholics Anonymous. This treatment choice appears to be only moderately effective in older adults (Satre et al. 2004). In fact some researchers suggest that older adults will demonstrate better treatment gains in peer support groups and age-specific treatment protocols (Dupree et al. 1984; Schonfeld et al. 2000).

Schonfeld and colleagues (2000) compared the success of veterans age 60 and above who completed a cognitive-behavioral treatment for substance abuse with veterans who dropped out of the treatment program. Although the dropouts do not constitute an unbiased treatment control comparison group, the dropouts do allow some level of comparison between those who received full treatment and those who did not. Of the 110 veterans who enrolled in the program, 61 dropped out. The treatment program consisted of 22 weekly group sessions, including components of health education, cognitive-behavioral treatment, and self-management strategies. The cognitive-behavioral and self-management strategies focused especially on identifying and managing situations that were risky for substance abuse, coping with depression and anxiety without substance abuse, and reestablishing goals after a relapse. Analysis found that the veterans who completed treatment were significantly more likely to have remained abstinent even after a brief relapse than were those who had dropped out of treatment. This study has several limitations, including a lack of division between alcohol abuse and other substance abuse and a biased control comparison group. However, given the positive preliminary findings, especially in a difficult-to-treat population in which 34.2% were homeless, this study shows a clear incentive to investigate the use of age-specific cognitive-behavioral treatments for substance abuse in older adults.

As in other Axis I disorders such as depression and generalized anxiety disorder, brief interventions in primary care have received increasing attention for the treatment of alcohol use in older adults. Because primary care physicians are most likely to identify overuse of alcohol in their patients, this is a natural area in which to develop treatment protocols. In one study, adults age 65 and older either received a brief cognitive-behavioral intervention from their physician or just a general health booklet (Fleming et al. 1999). The intervention consisted of two 10- to 15-minute counseling sessions in which the physician discussed consequences of alcohol consumption and personal cues for alcohol consumption. The physician also instructed the patient to keep a diary card of his or her drinking behavior and made a drinking agreement with each patient to control his or her alcohol consumption. The researchers found that at 3-month and 12-month follow-ups, the patients who had received the intervention drank significantly less than those who received only a health booklet. Patients who participated in the intervention also had significantly less binge drinking and excessive drinking than those who did not receive the intervention.

The empirical studies described above provide groundwork for further research in this area. Age-specific cognitive-behavioral treatment techniques show promise for the treatment of alcohol abuse in older adults. One avenue of research might examine group interventions to take advantage of peer support, whereas a second avenue of research might investigate primary care interventions to take advantage of older adults' relationships with their physicians.

Axis II Disorders

According to the DSM-IV and DSM-IV-TR (American Psychiatric Association 1994, 2000), a personality disorder is an enduring pattern of inner experience (e.g., cognition, affect, impulse control) and behavior (e.g., interpersonal difficulties) that has an onset in adolescence or early adulthood, is stable over time, deviates considerably from normal cultural expectations, and causes distress or impairment in functioning. Although a recent meta-analysis concludes that rates of personality disorders among older adults are essentially equivalent to rates observed in younger age groups (Abrams and Horowitz 1999), others contend that rates of personality disorders decline over age (Solomon 1981; Tyrer 1988).

Growing empirical evidence suggests that elderly depressed patients with comorbid personality disorder are generally less responsive to treatment, including antidepressant medications and psychotherapy (Abrams 1996; Abrams et al. 1994; Pilkonis and Frank 1988; Thompson et al.

1988; Vine and Steingart 1994; also see Gradman et al. 1999 for a review). However, with the exception of case studies, no published outcome study has specifically focused on treating late-life personality disorders.

Gradman et al. (1999) reviewed seven treatment studies of older adults in which personality disorder was examined. However, only one of these studies included a randomized control. In their randomized, controlled trial, Thompson et al. (1988) examined 75 elderly outpatients who met diagnostic criteria for major depression. The researchers then compared the outcomes of short-term cognitive (Beck et al. 1979), behavioral (Lewinsohn et al. 1973), and psychodynamic therapy (Horowitz et al. 1980). Therapy sessions were held twice a week for the first 4 weeks and once a week for the remaining 16–20 sessions. Although it was not the specific focus of the study, the authors examined the effect of personality disorder on outcome using the Structured Interview for DSM-III Personality Disorders (Stangl et al. 1985). Results indicated that the likelihood of treatment failure was approximately four times greater for patients diagnosed with personality disorders (37%) than for those without (9.5%). In addition, the authors reported that individuals with passive-aggressive or compulsive personality disorders were more likely to experience treatment failure, whereas those with dependent or avoidant personality disorders were more likely to have their treatment succeed. A 2-year follow-up of this study concluded that patients with avoidant and mixed personality disorders were at a higher risk of relapse (Rose et al. 1991).

Methodological differences across studies also limit the ability to make strong conclusions. Treatments were often not clearly defined, standardized instruments varied across studies or were not used at all, and measures of treatment adherence were not obtained. Gradman et al. (1999) concluded that disorders such as dependent and avoidant personality disorder may respond better to treatment because patients with these disorders are more likely to comply with suggestions by the therapist and to work in a collaborative way. However, as Morse and Lynch (2000) point out, rates of Cluster A disorders may be higher than previously thought among older adults, and consequently treatments that specifically target noncompliance may prove more relevant (e.g., DBT).

As mentioned above (see "Group Psychotherapy"), DBT has been successfully modified to treat depression in older adults using a group skills training format (Lynch et al. 2003). Extending this work, Lynch and colleagues (in press) at Duke University have examined DBT as an augmentation to medication in depressed older adults with personality disorders. There was a nonsignificant trend toward patients in the DBT condition having higher rates of remission and lower depressive symptoms than patients in the medication only condition immediately following treatment and at 6-month follow-up. Patients in the DBT group showed significantly lower levels of interpersonal sensitivity and interpersonal aggression at posttreatment and follow-up assessments compared with individuals in the control condition group.

Treatments for Dementia

The development of psychosocial interventions for dementia is a complicated area of research. Unlike some of the other disorders discussed in this chapter, dementia is unlikely to remit as a result of psychotherapy. Researchers in this area have struggled to find distinct goals and outcomes to focus on. Because the dementia as a whole is not expected to abate, researchers have chosen specific variables to focus on in older adults with dementia, such as global quality of life, affective states, disruptive behavioral symptoms, functional impairment, and prevention of self-harm.

Because of the cognitive deterioration experienced, most empirical research on interventions for dementia is based on behavioral strategies. These therapies generally train those who care for the individuals with dementia—whether in the community or in inpatient facilities—to manage patient behavior using principles of operant conditioning. In a treatment efficacy study with Alzheimer's disease patients and their spouses (Bourgeois et al. 2002), 63 spousal caregivers were assigned to one of three test conditions: patient change, self-change, or control. Subjects in the patient-change group assessed individual problem behaviors in their spouses and then individually developed behavioral management strategies, such as distracting the patient or using physical prompts. The self-change intervention focused on teaching the caregivers specific strategies to manage personal stress, including increasing pleasant activities, enhancing problem-solving strategies, and practicing relaxation techniques. Patients whose spouses participated in the patient-change group showed a significant decrease in the frequency of problem behaviors from a pretreatment baseline to evaluations after treatment, at 3 months, and at 6 months. Both intervention groups showed significant decreases in aggressive behavior at 3 months and 6 months, as well as significant improvements in the caregivers' moods after treatment and at 6 months. These findings suggest that interventions for caregivers that combine self-care and behavioral management strategies might prove most effective.

Cognitive symptoms such as disorientation and confusion can cause distress and injury in patients and increased stress in caregivers. One proposed psychotherapeutic technique to cope with the cognitive symptoms of dementia is reality orientation therapy. The purpose of this therapy is to continuously reorient patients' attention to the present situation and surroundings by repeating who they are and where they are. Reality orientation is often augmented by group classes that provide reorienting information. In a randomized treatment-control study, inpatients with Alzheimer's disease completed either a series of reality orientation therapy cycles or standard care (Zanetti et al. 1995). Patients who completed reality orientation therapy showed significantly better cognitive outcomes than those in the control condition at an 8-month checkpoint. However, participants in reality orientation therapy did not differ in terms of affect measures or decline in their ability to complete normal activities of daily living. One concern in the use of this therapy is that reality orientation may itself be distressing to confused patients. One patient in the treatment group did become emotionally distressed and was subsequently removed from the treatment protocol. In some patients, though, reality orientation may be a positive component to include in a wider behavioral treatment protocol to target cognitive decline in patients with dementia.

Because individuals with dementia are often at risk for anxiety, depression, or other negative affective states, certain behavioral therapies have directly targeted depressive symptoms in patients. One such therapy was evaluated in a study by Teri and colleagues (1997). Two therapy protocols were assessed: behavior therapy with pleasant events and behavior therapy with problem solving. In both therapies, the therapists helped the caregiver develop behavioral strategies in response to the patient's behavior. Participants in the pleasant-events group were also encouraged to increase pleasant activities. Participants in the problem-solving group were taught systematic problem-solving strategies along with the behavior therapy. Immediately after treatment, there were no significant improvements. However, at 6 months, both therapy groups showed significant improvements over baseline measures in patients' depressive symptoms and patients' cognitive status scores. Both problem solving around problem behaviors and introducing more pleasant events into patients' experience may function as successful behavioral management strategies for depressive moods in patients with dementia.

Although different behavioral interventions have shown success in either promoting positive outcomes or decreasing negative outcomes, each intervention appears to target a limited number of symptoms experienced by patients with dementia. Further research should examine more comprehensive treatment interventions that take advantage of behavioral management through controlling the environment, delivering direct interventions to patients, and educating caregivers on how to use behavioral strategies to manage patient behavior. Comprehensive treatments may also contain different behavioral components that target different symptoms of dementia. For example, one intervention might include increasing pleasant events to reduce depression, reality orientation to increase cognitive function, and caregiver training to promote effective care for patients.

Conclusion

It is becoming increasingly evident that psychotherapy offers significant promise for the treatment of psychopathology in elderly persons and at times may be the treatment of choice in terms of both efficacy and patient preference. We encourage practitioners to select treatments that have been tested using randomized clinical trials not based on theoretical preference or ease of application. Use of treatments without this type of empirical support can slow or reduce recovery.

Future research should continue to examine the beneficial effects of strategies combining medication and psychotherapy. In addition, research examining the mechanisms of change and issues associated with treatment response by disorder and type of therapy remain to be more fully developed. Finally, continued research needs to focus on populations with treatment-resistant illness (e.g., personality disorders and comorbid disorders).

References

Abrahams RB, Patterson RD: Psychological distress among the community elderly: prevalence, characteristics and implications for service. Int J Aging Hum Dev 9:1–18, 1978

Abrams RC: Personality disorders in the elderly. Int J Geriatr Psychiatry 11:759–763, 1996

Abrams RC, Horowitz SV: Personality disorders after age 50: a meta-analytic review of the literature, in Personality Disorders in Older Adults: Emerging Issues in Diagnosis and Treatment. Edited by Rosowsky E, Abrams RC. Mahwah, NJ, Erlbaum, 1999, pp 55–68

Abrams RC, Rosendahl E, Card C, et al: Personality disorder correlates of late and early onset depression. J Am Geriatr Soc 42:727–731, 1994

Adams WL, Yuan Z, Barboriak JJ, et al: Alcohol-related hospitalizations of elderly people: prevalence and geographic variation in the United States. JAMA 270:1222–1225, 1993

Allen R, Walker Z, Shergill P, et al: Attitudes to depression in hospital inpatients: a comparison between older and younger subjects. Aging Ment Health 2:36–39, 1998

American Psychiatric Association: Diagnostic and Statistical Manual of Mental Disorders, 4th Edition. Washington, DC, American Psychiatric Association, 1994

American Psychiatric Association: Diagnostic and Statistical Manual of Mental Disorders, 4th Edition, Text Revision. Washington, DC, American Psychiatric Association, 2000

Andrews HB: The myth of the scientist-practitioner: a reply. Aust Psychol 35:60–63, 1998

Arean PA, Perri MG, Nezu AM, et al: Comparative effectiveness of social problem-solving therapy and reminiscence therapy as treatments for depression in older adults. J Consult Clin Psychol 61:1003–1010, 1993

Arean PA, Gum A, McCulloch CE, et al: Treatment of depression in low-income older adults. Psychol Aging 20:601–609, 2005

Barrowclough C, King P, Colville J, et al: A randomized trial of the effectiveness of cognitive-behavioral therapy and supportive counseling for anxiety symptoms in older adults. J Consult Clin Psychol 69:756–762, 2001

Beck AT, Rush AJ, Shaw BF, et al: Cognitive Therapy of Depression. New York, Guilford, 1979

Beutler LE, Scogin F, Kirkish P, et al: Group cognitive therapy and alprazolam in the treatment of depression in older adults. J Consult Clin Psychol 55:550–556, 1987

Bibring E: The problem of depression. Psyche 6:81–101, 1952

Biglan A: Distressed behavior and its context. Behav Anal 14:157–169, 1991

Blazer D, George LK, Hughes D: The epidemiology of anxiety disorders: an age comparison, in Anxiety in the Elderly: Treatment and Research. Edited by Salzman C, Lebowitz BD. New York, Springer, 1991, pp 17–30

Bourgeois MS, Schulz R, Burgio LD, et al: Skills training for spouses of patients with Alzheimer's disease: outcomes of an intervention study. Journal of Clinical Geropsychology 8:53–73, 2002

Brand E, Clingempeel WG: Group behavioral therapy with depressed geriatric inpatients: an assessment of incremental efficacy. Behav Ther 23:475–482, 1992

Coyne JC: Depression and the response of others. J Abnorm Psychol 85:186–193, 1976

DeBerry S: The effects of meditation-relaxation on anxiety and depression in a geriatric population. Psychotherapy: Theory, Research and Practice 19:512–521, 1982a

DeBerry S: An evaluation of progressive muscle relaxation on stress related symptoms in a geriatric population. Int J Aging Hum Dev 14:255–269, 1982b

Dougher MJ, Hackbert L: A behavior-analytic account of depression and a case report using acceptance-based procedures. Behav Anal 17:321–334, 1994

Dupree LW, Broskowski H, Schonfeld LI: The Gerontology Alcohol Project: a behavioral treatment program for elderly alcohol abusers. Gerontologist 24:510–516, 1984

Fingerhood M: Substance abuse in older people. J Am Geriatr Soc 48:985–995, 2000

Fleming MFM, Manwell LB, Barry KLP, et al: Brief physician advice for alcohol problems in older adults: a randomized community-based trial. J Fam Pract 48:378–384, 1999

Flint AJ: Epidemiology and comorbidity of anxiety disorders in the elderly. Am J Psychiatry 15:640–649, 1994

Floyd M, Scogin F: Cognitive-behavior therapy for older adults: how does it work? Psychotherapy 35:459–463, 1998

Frank E, Spanier C: Interpersonal psychotherapy for depression: overview, clinical efficacy, and future directions. Clinical Psychology Science and Practice 2:349–369, 1995

Frank E, Frank N, Cornes C, et al: Interpersonal psychotherapy in the treatment of late-life depression, in New Applications of Interpersonal Psychotherapy. Edited by Klerman GL, Weissman MM. Washington, DC, American Psychiatric Press, 1993, pp 167–198

Friedhoff AJ: Consensus Development Conference statement: diagnosis and treatment of depression in late life, in Diagnosis and Treatment of Depression in Late Life: Results of the NIH Consensus Development Conference. Edited by Schneider LSM, Reynolds CF III, Lebowitz BD, et al. Washington, DC, American Psychiatric Press, 1994, pp 491–511

Fuentes K, Cox BJ: Prevalence of anxiety disorders in elderly adults: a critical analysis. J Behav Ther Exp Psychiatry 28:269–279, 1997

Gallagher DE, Thompson LW: Treatment of major depressive disorder in older adult outpatients with brief psychotherapies. Psychotherapy: Theory, Research and Practice 19:482–490, 1982

Gallagher-Thompson D, Steffen AM: Comparative effects of cognitive-behavioral and brief psychodynamic psychotherapies for depressed family caregivers. J Consult Clin Psychol 62:543–549, 1994

Gallagher-Thompson D, Hanley-Peterson P, Thompson LW: Maintenance of gains versus relapse following brief psychotherapy for depression. J Consult Clin Psychol 58:371–374, 1990

Goldfried MR, Castonguay LG, Hayes AM, et al: A comparative analysis of the therapeutic focus in cognitive-behavioral and psychodynamic-interpersonal sessions. J Consult Clin Psychol 65:740–748, 1997

Goldfried MR, Raue PJ, Castonguay LG: The therapeutic focus in significant sessions of master therapists: a comparison of cognitive-behavioral and psychodynamic-interpersonal interventions. J Consult Clin Psychol 66:803–810, 1998

Gradman TJ, Thompson LW, Gallagher-Thompson D: Personality disorders and treatment outcome, in Personality Disorders in Older Adults: Emerging Issues in Diagnosis and Treatment. Edited by Rosowsky E, Abrams RC. Mahwah, NJ, Erlbaum, 1999, pp 69–94

Hayes AM, Castonguay LG, Goldfried MR: Effectiveness of targeting the vulnerability factors of depression in cognitive therapy. J Consult Clin Psychol 64:623–627, 1996

Hegel MTP, Barrett JE, Cornell JE, et al: Predictors of response to problem solving treatment of depression in primary care. Behav Ther 33:511–527, 2002a

Hegel MT, Imming J, Cyr-Provost M, et al: Role of allied behavioral health professionals in a collaborative stepped care treatment model for depression in primary care: Project IMPACT. Families, Systems and Health 20:265–277, 2002b

Hinrichsen GA: Interpersonal psychotherapy for depressed older adults. J Geriatr Psychiatry 30:239–257, 1997

Horowitz MJ, Wilner N, Kaltreider N, et al: Signs and symptoms of posttraumatic stress disorder. Arch Gen Psychiatry 37:85–92, 1980

Horvath AO, Symonds BD: Relation between working alliance and outcome in psychotherapy: a meta-analysis. J Couns Psychol 38:139–149, 1991

Jarvik LF, Mintz J, Steuer JL, et al: Treating geriatric depression: a 26-week interim analysis. J Am Geriatr Soc 30:713–717, 1982

Kernberg OF: Technical considerations in the treatment of borderline personality organization. J Am Psychoanal Assoc 24:795–829, 1976

Klein M: The origins of transference. Int J Psychoanal 33:433–438, 1952

Klerman GL, Weissman MM, Rounsaville BJ, et al: Interpersonal Psychotherapy of Depression. New York, Basic Books, 1984

Koder DA, Brodaty H, Anstey KJ: Cognitive therapy for depression in the elderly. Int J Geriatr Psychiatry 11:97–107, 1996

Kohut H, Wolf ES: The disorders of the self and their treatment: an outline. Int J Psychoanal 59:413–425, 1978

Lewinsohn PM, Lobitz WC, Wilson S: "Sensitivity" of depressed individuals to aversive stimuli. J Abnorm Psychol 81:259–263, 1973

Lindesay J, Briggs K, Murphy E: The Guy's/Age Concern Survey: prevalence rates of cognitive impairment, depression and anxiety in an urban elderly community. Br J Psychiatry 155:317–329, 1989

Linehan MM: Cognitive-behavioral treatment of borderline personality disorder. New York, Guilford, 1993

Luborsky L, Rosenthal R, Diguer L, et al: The dodo bird verdict is alive and well—mostly. Clinical Psychology Science and Practice 9:2–12, 2002

Lynch TR, Morse JQ, Mendelson T, et al: Dialectical behavior therapy for depressed older adults: a randomized pilot study. Am J Geriatr Psychiatry 11:33–45, 2003

Lynch TR, Cheavens JS, Cukrowicz KC, et al: Treatment of older adults with comorbid personality disorder and depression: a dialectical behavior therapy approach. Int J Geriatr Psychiatry (in press)

Mahler MS: On child psychosis and schizophrenia: autistic and symbiotic infantile psychoses. Psychoanal Study Child 7:286–305, 1952

Martin DJ, Garske JP, Davis MK: Relation of the therapeutic alliance with outcome and other variables: a meta-analytic review. J Consult Clin Psychol 68:438–450, 2000

Mohlman J, Gorman JM: The role of executive functioning in CBT: a pilot study with anxious older adults. Behav Res Ther 43:447–465, 2005

Moore AA, Morton SC, Beck JC, et al: A new paradigm for alcohol use in older persons. Med Care 37:165–179, 1999

Morse JQ, Lynch TR: Personality disorders in late-life. Curr Psychiatry Rep 2:24–31, 2000

Mynors-Wallis LM: Pharmacotherapy is more effective than psychotherapy for elderly people with minor depression or dysthymia. Evidence-Based Healthcare 5:61, 2001

Nezu AM: A problem-solving formulation of depression: a literature review and proposal of a pluralistic model. Clin Psychol Rev 7:121–144, 1987

O'Rourke N, Hadjistavropoulos T: The relative efficacy of psychotherapy in the treatment of geriatric depression. Aging Ment Health 1:305–310, 1997

Oslin DW, Katz IR, Edell WS, et al: Effects of alcohol consumption on the treatment of depression among elderly patients. Am J Geriatr Psychiatry 8:215–220, 2000

Palmer BW, Jeste DV, Sheikh JI: Anxiety disorders in the elderly: DSM-IV and other barriers to diagnosis and treatment. J Affect Disord 46:183–190, 1997

Perrotta P, Meacham JA: Can a reminiscing intervention alter depression and self-esteem? Int J Aging Hum Dev 14:23–30, 1982

Pilkonis PA, Frank E: Personality pathology in recurrent depression: Nature, prevalence, and relationship to treatment response. Am J Psychiatry 145:435–441, 1988

Regier DA, Boyd JH, Burke JD, et al: One-month prevalence of mental disorders in the United States: based on five epidemiologic catchment area sites. Arch Gen Psychiatry 45:977–986, 1988

Reynolds CF 3rd, Frank E, Perel JM, et al: Combined pharmacotherapy and psychotherapy in the acute and continuation treatment of elderly patients with recurrent major depression: a preliminary report. Am J Psychiatry 149:1687–1692, 1992

Reynolds CF 3rd, Frank E, Perel JM, et al: Treatment of consecutive episodes of major depression in the elderly. Am J Psychiatry 151:1740–1743, 1994

Reynolds CF 3rd, Frank E, Houck PR, et al: Which elderly patients with remitted depression remain well with continued interpersonal psychotherapy after discontinuation of antidepressant medication? Am J Psychiatry 154:958–962, 1997

Reynolds CF 3rd, Frank E, Perel JM, et al: Nortriptyline and interpersonal psychotherapy as maintenance therapies for recurrent major depression: a randomized controlled trial in patients older than 59 years. JAMA 281:39–45, 1999

Rickard HC, Scogin F, Keith S: A one-year follow-up of relaxation training for elders with subjective anxiety. Gerontologist 34:121–122, 1984

Rokke PD, Scogin F: Depression treatment preferences in younger and older adults. Journal of Clinical Geropsychology 1:243–257, 1995

Rokke PD, Tomhave JA, Jocic Z: The role of client choice and target selection in self-management therapy for depression in older adults. Psychol Aging 14:155–169, 1999

Rose J, Schwarz M, Steffen AM, et al: Personality disorder and outcome in the treatment of depressed elders: two year follow-up. Poster presented at the 44th Annual Conference of the Gerontological Society of America, San Francisco, CA, November 22–26, 1991

Satre DD, Mertens JR, Weisner C: Gender differences in treatment outcomes for alcohol dependence among older adults. J Stud Alcohol 65:638–642, 2004

Schonfeld L, Dupree LW, Dickson-Fuhrmann E, et al: Cognitive-behavioral treatment of older veterans with substance abuse problems. J Geriatr Psychiatry Neurol 13:124–129, 2000

Scogin F, McElreath L: Efficacy of psychosocial treatments for geriatric depression: a quantitative review. J Consult Clin Psychol 62:69–73, 1994

Scogin F, Rickard HC, Keith S, et al: Progressive and imaginal relaxation training for elderly persons with subjective anxiety. Psychol Aging 7:419–424, 1992

Sloane RB, Staples FR, Schneider LSM: Interpersonal therapy versus nortriptyline for depression in the elderly: case reports and discussion, in Clinical and Pharmacological Studies of Psychiatric Disorders. Edited by Burrows G, Norman TR, Dennerstein L. London, John Libbey, 1985, pp 344–346

Solomon K: Personality disorders and the elderly, in Personality Disorders: Diagnosis and Management. Edited by Lion JR. Baltimore, MD, Williams & Wilkins, 1981, pp 310–338

Stangl D, Pfohl B, Zimmerman M, et al: A structured interview for the DSM-III personality disorders—a preliminary report. Arch Gen Psychiatry 42:591–596, 1985

Stanley MA, Novy DM: Cognitive-behavior therapy for generalized anxiety in late life: an evaluative overview. J Anxiety Disord 14:191–207, 2000

Stanley MA, Beck JG, Glassco JD: Treatment of generalized anxiety in older adults: a preliminary comparison of cognitive-behavioral and supportive approaches. Behav Ther 27:565–581, 1996

Stanley MA, Roberts RE, Bourland SL, et al: Anxiety disorders among older primary care patients. Journal of Clinical Geropsychology 7:105–116, 2001

Stanley MA, Beck JG, Novy DM, et al: Cognitive behavioral treatment of late-life generalized anxiety disorder. J Consult Clin Psychol 71:309–319, 2003

Stanley MA, Diefenbach GJ, Hopko DR: Cognitive behavioral treatment for older adults with generalized anxiety disorder: a therapist manual for primary care settings. Behav Modif 28:73–117, 2004

Steuer JL: Cognitive-behavioral and psychodynamic group psychotherapy in treatment of geriatric depression. J Consult Clin Psychol 52:180–189, 1984

Strupp HH, Binder J: Psychotherapy in a New Key. New York, Basic Books, 1984

Teri L, Logsdon RG, Uomoto J, et al: Behavioral treatment of depression in dementia patients: a controlled clinical trial. J Gerontol B Psychol Sci Soc Sci 52:P159–P166, 1997

Thompson LW, Gallagher D: Efficacy of psychotherapy in the treatment of late-life depression. Advances in Behaviour Research and Therapy 6:127–139, 1984

Thompson LW, Gallagher D, Breckenridge JS: Comparative effectiveness of psychotherapies for depressed elders. J Consult Clin Psychol 55:385–390, 1987

Thompson LW, Gallagher D, Czirr R: Personality disorder and outcome in the treatment of late-life depression. J Geriatr Psychiatry 21:133–146, 1988

Thompson LW, Coon DW, Gallagher-Thompson D, et al: Comparison of desipramine and cognitive/behavioral therapy in the treatment of elderly outpatients with mild-to-moderate depression. Am J Geriatr Psychiatry 9:225–240, 2001

Tyrer P: Personality Disorders: Diagnosis, Management and Course. Kent, England, Wright/Butterworth Scientific, 1988

Unutzer JM, Katon WM, Williams JWJ, et al: Improving primary care for depression in late life: the design of a multicenter randomized trial. Med Care 39:785–799, 2001

Unutzer J, Katon W, Callahan CM, et al: Collaborative care management of late-life depression in the primary care setting. JAMA 288:2836–2845, 2002

Vine RG, Steingart AB: Personality disorder in the elderly depressed. Can J Psychiatry 39:392–398, 1994

Vitt CM, Idler EL, Leventhal H, et al: Attitudes toward treatment and help-seeking preferences in an elderly sample. Poster presented at the 52nd Annual Meeting of the Gerontological Society of America, San Francisco, CA, November 19–23, 1999

Weissman MM, Myers JK, Thompson WD: Depression and its treatment in a U.S. urban community—1975–1976. Arch Gen Psychiatry 38:417–421, 1981

Wetherell JL, Gatz M, Craske MG: Treatment of generalized anxiety disorder in older adults. J Consult Clin Psychol 71:31–40, 2003

Williams JW Jr, Barrett J, Oxman T, et al: Treatment of dysthymia and minor depression in primary care: a randomized controlled trial in older adults. JAMA 284:1519–1526, 2000

Zanetti O, Frisoni GB, De Leo D, et al: Reality orientation therapy in Alzheimer disease: useful or not? a controlled study. Alzheimer Dis Assoc Disord 9:132–138, 1995

Study Questions

Select the single best response for each question.

1. Psychotherapy may be a preferred model for certain geropsychiatric conditions. Which of the following is true regarding the general issue of psychotherapy for older patients?

    A. Because of the availability of Medicare, over 50% of older patients with psychiatric illnesses receive professional mental health care, unlike younger patients for whom insurance coverage is often problematic.

    B. Descriptive research regularly shows that older patients prefer psychopharmacological treatment to psychotherapy.

    C. Part of older patients' preference for psychopharmacological therapy is because few elders are concerned about "addiction" to antidepressants.

    D. Objective research confirms that "relationship factors" account for 80% of the variance in treatment outcomes with psychotherapy.

    E. None of the above.

2. In conducting psychotherapy with older patients, several factors specific to this age group should be taken into close account. All of the following are true *except*

    A. Older adults rarely respond to therapeutic interventions used with younger patients.

    B. Medical illnesses or medications may exacerbate psychiatric symptoms.

    C. The clinician must work against stereotypes about elderly patients.

    D. Older adults may not easily remember troubling earlier life events.

    E. Cognitive deficits may affect the progress of psychotherapy.

3. Cognitive-behavioral psychotherapy models may be considered for older patients. Which of the following is true?

    A. The Thompson et al. study (1987) showed cognitive and behavioral therapy to be superior to brief psychodynamic therapy in reducing depression symptoms.

    B. The studies by Thompson et al. (2001) and Reynolds et al. (1999) both concluded that combined medication and psychotherapy were optimal in the treatment of depression in older adults.

    C. A logistical limitation of social problem-solving therapy is that it is not adaptable to the primary care clinic.

    D. All of the above.

    E. None of the above.

4. Another useful model of psychotherapy for depressed older adults is interpersonal psychotherapy (IPT). This model is based on four components of interpersonal relationships that lead to and maintain depressive states. These four components include all of the following *except*

    A. Grief.

    B. Interpersonal disputes.

    C. Role transitions.

    D. Interpersonal deficits.

    E. Intrapsychic or psychodynamic conflict.

5. Various psychotherapy models can be utilized for the management of anxiety disorders in older patients. Which of the following is true?

   A. The most frequently used and well-substantiated psychotherapy model for geriatric anxiety symptoms is cognitive-behavioral therapy (CBT).

   B. Behavioral therapy such as progressive muscle relaxation training is contraindicated for patients with cognitive impairment.

   C. CBT appears to be the best-equipped psychotherapy model for generalized anxiety disorder (GAD) in older patients.

   D. A major limitation of CBT for geriatric anxiety states is that it cannot be conducted in the primary care clinic.

   E. Elderly patients with GAD infrequently exhibit simultaneous depressive symptoms.

CHAPTER 18

Working With the Family of the Older Adult

Lisa P. Gwyther, M.S.W.

Given heterogeneity and the need for individualized family assessment and treatment, no single model exists for working with families of older adults. Despite the need for family-specific treatment, there are patterns of family issues based on consistent trajectories of psychiatric illness. Perhaps the most specific guidance in the literature comes from clinical research on families of older adults with progressive degenerative dementias (Sorensen et al. 2002).

Over the course of an older adult's degenerative dementia, families will confront depression, delusions, agitation, behavioral changes, and other psychiatric symptoms in their cognitively impaired relatives (Lyketsos et al. 2000; Olin et al. 2002; Tractenberg et al. 2002). The burden on the family can be great, information can be insufficient, and doubt can be overwhelming (Gwyther

2000). Families caring for older members with dementia need reminders from psychiatrists to focus on maintaining family quality of life as well as quality of care within the constraints imposed by psychiatric, functional, and behavioral changes (Hughes et al. 1999).

This chapter takes a chronological approach to working with families over the course of the dementia of an older adult. Dementias are the focus because of ample evidence that dementia is more disruptive of family life, more likely to result in negative mental health outcomes for family caregivers (especially females) (Pinquart and Sorensen 2006). Compared with family caregivers of older adults with normal cognition, family caregivers of older adults with Alzheimer's disease spend more hours per week providing care, with measurable negative impacts on caregivers' mental

I gratefully acknowledge support for preparing this manuscript from grant 5P50 AG0 5128 from the National Institute on Aging to the Joseph and Kathleen Bryan Alzheimer's Disease Research Center at Duke University Medical Center and from grant 5R01 AG19605, "Stress, Serotonin Genes and Health Disparities," from the National Institute on Aging to the Duke University Behavioral Medicine Research Center.

health, personal and family time (Langa et al. 2001), and family relationships. Psychiatrists working with families of persons with dementia should expect to treat vulnerable primary family caregivers as well as families in conflict.

Family Care for Older Adults With Dementia

Half of family caregivers live with the older adult over a disease course of 3–20 years. Despite the high rates of shared residence, increasing evidence suggests that 20% of older adults with moderate to severe dementia live alone, often with extensive supervision and assistance from local and long-distance family caregivers.

Certain trends emerge from studies of family care in dementia. A shift is occurring away from the direct provision of care by families toward more long-distance care or family care coordination. Dementia care may precipitate moves by retired adult children or a move by the older person to be closer to adult children. More female family caregivers are employed full- or part-time, and employment appears to have unanticipated benefits as well as commonly assumed burdens associated with role overload. Dementia care frequently precipitates the family's first experience seeking help from public or private agencies and even from other family members. Finally, increasing evidence shows that the lack of an affordable, available long-term-care system is pushing the limits of family capacity and solidarity.

Family care is universally preferred, based in strong family values that cross cultural and ethnic lines. Yet exclusive reliance on family care has well-documented personal and social costs. Family caregivers may become overwhelmed, exhausted, depressed, or anxious. Many family caregivers report loss of pleasure, motivation,

friends, activities, privacy, intimacy, or identity. Gradual and sometimes sudden loss of the person as he or she once was can precipitate significant grief in family members.

Research even documents that premature death is associated with spousal caregiver strain in the care of persons with Alzheimer's disease, suggesting an urgent public health preventive or protective focus for work with spouses of older adults with dementia (Schulz and Beach 1999).

Despite this apparent investment of families in care for older adults, some families never comprehend minimal safety risks associated with dementia care. Elder mistreatment—whether abuse or passive or active neglect—may be associated with exceeding these family limits (Fulmer et al. 2005). Families may feel powerless and overwhelmed when they cannot predictably control the symptoms and course of dementia. The role of the psychiatrist with the family becomes one of assessment of tolerance limits, education, treatment of psychiatric consequences of caregiver burden, and management of family expectations of the disease course and of themselves.

Despite a research focus on primary family caregivers, often a change in primary caregiver occurs when a spouse dies or when siblings pass a cognitively impaired parent among themselves in a futile attempt to equalize responsibility.

Increasing dependency, loss, and grief are realities of family care in Alzheimer's disease, but not all family outcomes are negative or burdensome. Although depression is the most frequently reported psychiatric symptom among caregivers of Alzheimer's disease patients, some families express pride in their care as a legacy of commitment to family values.

The following clinical reminders about family care may prove useful in working with families of older adults:

1. Family care is an adaptive challenge: the family is not necessarily the problem, nor is the family necessarily the obstacle to effective care. Few incentives (financial, religious, or counseling) will make an unwilling family assume care. The reverse is equally true. Few disincentives will keep a determined spouse or child from honoring his or her commitment.

2. The family is rarely one voice. Different perceptions and expectations of close and distant family members frequently precipitate family conflict. There is no perfectly fair and equal division of family care responsibility. Families can expect a permanent imbalance in the normal give and take of family relationships while working toward a more equitable sharing of responsibility.

3. Few families have the luxury of one person needing care at a time. There is much less manipulation by dependent elders than there are real unmet dependency needs. There is more underreporting of burden and underutilization of services than the reverse.

4. There is no one right or ideal way or place to offer family care. Many families are forced to choose between equally unacceptable options. Successful family caregivers gather information, take direct action when possible, and often reframe things they cannot change in more positive terms. ("It could be worse—at least she is still with me.")

5. Successful family caregivers are flexible in adjusting expectations of themselves, of the older adult, and of other family members to fit the needs and capacities of all. Coping with family care is facilitated by a sense of humor; a strong faith, belief, or value system; creativity; practical problem-solving skills; and emotional support from other family members or friends.

6. Families caring for older adults with dementia must define and negotiate complex situations, perform physically intimate tasks, manage emotions and communication, modify expectations, and capitalize on the older adult's preserved capacities.

7. A family caregiver's knowledge of an available service, need for the service, and access to the service do not necessarily lead to appropriate and timely use of that service.

8. There is no perfect control in a family care situation. Families are better off if they work on their reactions to stress or lack of control.

9. Denial is a common defense of family caregivers. Some people need to deny the inevitable outcome (loss of a beloved spouse or eventual placement of a parent in a nursing home) to provide hopeful, consistent daily care.

10. A primary caregiver at home is efficient and preferred. Primary caregivers need breaks and backup people and services to supplement their personalized care. Even in ideal situations, contingency plans are necessary.

Goals in Working With Families of Older Adults

Clinical goals with families of older adults will vary with presenting problems and family resources. Common goals in working with families of older adults with dementia are to normalize variability, to address safety and security issues, to mobilize secondary family support, to facilitate appropriate decision making at care transitions, and to help family members accept help or let go of direct care as necessary. In essence, the family is forced to adapt to a new normal in family life, often with active resistance from the member with dementia. Well-timed psychiatric help in interpreting the family's and the elder's reluctance to accept new realities can promote appropriate decision making.

Other goals in working with family caregivers include treatment of affective, substance abuse, and anxiety disorders of the caregiver and individual or family treatment around issues of grief, loss, or conflict in family relationships that limit the effectiveness of care. In general, family work should enhance the effectiveness of family care and coping, enhance the self-efficacy of caregivers (Fortinsky 2002a), and enhance the family's satisfaction with their preferred levels of involvement.

Psychiatrists working with family caregivers over time will monitor the quality of family care; the mental health, capacity, and vulnerability of caregivers; and the impact of the demands of care on family relationships (Yates et al. 1999). Psychiatrists should be especially alert to escalating anxiety, self-neglect, suicidal ideation, depression, or anger in caregivers and abuse or neglect of the patient. These indications should prompt immediate recommendations for treatment, respite, or relinquishment of primary care responsibility. Negative caregiver outcomes on which to focus therapeutic efforts include decrements in mental health, social participation, and personal or family time and loss of privacy.

Interdisciplinary Partnerships

Focused work with families of older adults holds great potential for positive outcomes, particularly in the context of an interdisciplinary partnership or team (Fortinsky et al. 2002b). Research suggests that social workers' individual and family counseling with family caregivers can mobilize and sustain community and secondary family support, reduce primary caregiver depression, and even delay nursing home placement (Mittelman et al. 1996).

Psychiatrists may work collaboratively with social workers or nurses. These mental health professionals can provide sustained or timely assistance at care transitions. The psychiatrist's role is to assess and treat a family caregiver's psychiatric illness and to treat the cognitively impaired patient's psychiatric symptoms. The social worker or nurse may provide case management, monitoring family capacity and tolerance while educating the family about common symptoms and care transitions over time.

Some families will resist referrals to social workers. These families may respond to descriptions of the social worker as an expert consumer guide or family consultant. A family consultant can offer assessment and intervention as well as information. Families can learn from family consultants how to be their own case managers with minimal professional support at key care transitions. The family consultant at any one time may be a teacher, coach, advocate, counselor, cheerleader, peer, or support person who can provide energy and a fresh perspective to promote family resilience.

Referrals to well-developed and validated psychoeducational group treatment programs have demonstrated equally positive results (Ostwald et al. 1999). Participation in peer counseling or support groups can have positive outcomes for active caregiver participants (Pillemer and Suitor 1996).

Another way to monitor goals in the psychiatric treatment of families of older adults is to base treatment on known precipitants of the breakdown of family care. Major precipitants of placement include both patient and caregiver factors (Yaffe et al. 2002). One of the patient factors that strongly predicts placement is disruptive psychiatric and behavioral symptoms. Changes in behavior and personality are also major causes of caregiver burden and depression. To the extent that psychiatric consultation is available to the older adult for treatment of psychiatric symptoms and to the extent the family can be taught non-pharmacological approaches (see Chapter 15, "Agitation and Suspiciousness"), the health of the family and caregivers and effective home care for the older adult can be preserved.

Other predictors of family care breakdown are affective, substance abuse, or anxiety disorders of the primary caregiver and unresolved family conflict. Treating depression in a family caregiver generally has a positive impact on the mood, function, and behavior of the cognitively impaired older adult (Brodaty and Luscombe 1998), and the reverse is equally true.

The Family as Information Seeker

Families are more likely than older adults with dementia to initiate and seek psychiatric care throughout the course of the illness. The stigma of psychiatric illness often delays psychiatric diagnosis, and ethnic and cultural beliefs that equate cognitive decline with normal aging can produce the same result. Psychiatrists must remind families that a specific diagnosis suggests treatment options. Stigma is best addressed by correcting misconceptions or lack of information. An unconvinced family can be told that Alzheimer's disease is a brain disorder that can and does happen to anyone. The brain becomes the vulnerable organ in dementia, and psychiatric symptoms are brain symptoms just as angina is a symptom of a heart disorder. When damaged, both organs require special diagnosis and care.

Many family caregivers do not seek a diagnosis until the patient's psychiatric symptoms (such as suspiciousness) or the patient's personality changes (such as uncharacteristic irritability) disrupt family life. Unfortunately, the patient is most likely to resist an evaluation once psychiatric and behavioral symptoms are present, and psychiatrists are understandably reluctant to talk to family members without the consent of the patient. An evaluation can be facilitated if the psychiatrist agrees to see the older adult about a less threatening symptom such as headaches, loss of interest, or low energy.

Diagnostic Office Visits

Although the older adult is entitled to initial time alone with the psychiatrist, later time alone with family informants will be invaluable to the psychiatrist in assessing the impact of functional loss and other family stressors. Most family caregivers prefer to talk privately with the psychiatrist to avoid confronting the older adult with his or her symptoms or decline. It may be helpful to have two family members accompany the patient for an evaluation. One family member can distract or sit with the older adult while another family member has a private conversation with the psychiatrist.

Initial Communication With Older Adults and Their Families

Initial communication with older adults diagnosed with dementia and their families will be in response to common emotional reactions to a degenerative diagnosis. Elders and family members may express doubts about the diagnosis. Rather than confront the doubt and denial, it is often more helpful to suggest that the family behave as if the diagnosis of Alzheimer's disease had been confirmed while awaiting confirmation based on progression. Asking directly about common early changes such as difficulty handling money or increased irritability may highlight expectable changes and offer a preview of psychiatric expertise. Sometimes, explanations of apathy and loss of executive function help families understand why efforts to get the elder to try harder to function effectively may prove frustrating and futile.

Initial family sessions often elicit fear from family caregivers for their interdependent future or genetic risk.

Frustration is another common theme that emerges in early family treatment. Family caregivers frequently express frustration with the elder's obsessive need for repetition and reassurance. Clearing up misconceptions about the presumed intentionality of the elder's resistance or the elder's confabulations to fill in gaps in memory helps families cope with these changes. Encouraging the family to get angry at the disease rather than at professionals, services, or each other can be extremely helpful. Families should be reminded that conflict among their members will only limit needed help. It is important for the family to understand that the elder's realistic dependency does not imply weakness of character or will.

Fatigue and exhaustion are common themes in work with families of older adults. Encouraging rest, exercise, and energy economies can be helpful for family members. Guilt is another common theme in family work. Family members express guilt at losing patience, and they appreciate reminders from psychiatrists that everyone experiences regret based on unique but certain limits.

Key themes, tailored to the family's capacity to understand them, should be highlighted and repeated in writing to distant or absent family members after a psychiatric evaluation. Older couples in first marriages are generally more comfortable facing threatening health information together. Spouses of older adults with Alzheimer's disease are often put off by attempts to separate them from their impaired spouse. Providing the same information at the same time helps older couples preserve their couple identity and accept the psychiatric recommendations as a mutual adaptive challenge.

Family Expectations of Psychiatrists

Vulnerable family caregivers may seek a private place and time, undivided professional attention, and the comfort of familiar initial polite small talk. Families want psychiatrists to listen without a rush to implied understanding or suggestions. Families of older adults expect to be asked what they have tried in coping with their relative's impairment. Even more, these families appreciate the psychiatrist asking about what else is going on within the family.

Older spouse caregivers may expect advice from an authoritative expert and immediate cures for the dementia patient's most disruptive symptoms. These older spouse caregivers expect explanations about why antipsychotic medications do not "treat" wandering as well as environmental and activity strategies do. They need specific referrals to the Alzheimer's Association's Safe Return identification system as well as help in coping with the toll created by the prolonged hypervigilance needed to protect a wandering spouse.

Families of older adults want psychiatrists to tailor information and education relevant to their immediate, pressing concerns. For example, a family concerned about the increasingly combative behavior of an older adult male may be helped by a psychiatrist who responds, "First, let's get the guns out of the house" (Spangenberg et al. 1999).

When depleted primary caregivers are confronting the range of behavioral symptoms of older adults with Alzheimer's disease, they may look to the psychiatrist to lend energy, a proactive attitude, and perspective. Later, families want acknowledgement of their contributions to the older adult's quality of life, or absolution or forgiveness for what they were unable to achieve despite their best intentions. The psychiatrist must be careful with well-intentioned efforts to commend families for doing "a great job." Some family caregivers are quick to point out, "I am not her caregiver—I am her husband and I promised to take care of her in sickness and in health."

Families also appreciate preventive self-care reminders from psychiatrists, but vague suggestions that caregivers need to take care of themselves often frustrate overwhelmed families that have few resources (Burton et al. 1997). Family members need help translating principles of respite in ways that are congruent with their personal values and cultural expectations. Specific examples may help. For example, some husbands respond to statements such as "family care without respite is like expecting your car to run on empty. It doesn't." Respite options can be presented as opportunities to "recharge your battery."

Also, increasing evidence shows that encouraging physical activity (King and Brassington 1997) and actively assessing and treating sleep disorders in older adults and their family caregivers are associated with positive care and family outcomes (McCurry et al. 2005).

Families also look to psychiatrists for decisional support or help in mobilizing other family members. Psychiatric expertise in family systems and family communication is extremely relevant at these points.

Family caregivers expect psychiatrists to let them express and learn how to manage unacceptable feelings, such as anger toward the older adult, toward other family members or service providers, or toward God. These families appreciate psychiatrists who create new choices by reframing the problem or situation. The primary family caregiver may seek permission from the psychiatrist to be less than perfect or a good-enough-for-now family caregiver. At such times, a psychiatrist's use of humor and compassion can produce dramatic results.

Assessing the Family of an Older Adult

A targeted assessment of the family of an older adult may result in referrals to Alzheimer's Association services, private or public geriatric care management, family or peer counseling, home help, day programs, assisted living, or nursing home care. Cultural values, expectations, and health beliefs will influence how and when families decide to pursue referrals, as well as their receptivity to family treatment by psychiatrists.

One of the most useful ways to elicit a picture of family functioning is to ask the family to describe a typical day. Clues about how much time the patient is left alone and about potential safety risks come from such open-ended questions. The psychiatrist should probe further if the caregiver hints about increased use of alcohol or psychoactive medications in response to stress. Older husband caregivers are particularly at risk of increased alcohol use in response to care demands.

The psychiatrist should be alert for positive activities such as regular exercise, social stimulation, and secondary family support. A husband caring for his wife may be frustrated by her loss of interest in cooking. A suggestion to try regular restaurant meals at a familiar diner may conserve his energy and better meet the couple's nutritional and social needs.

Questions about a typical day often elicit family anger at the patient's apathy and withdrawal or a family's lack of awareness of safety issues. The family may complain that the cognitively impaired older adult is becoming more irritable and jealous of grandchildren. Probing may reveal that the impaired grandparent is still providing child care despite significant declines in judgment or function.

It is wise to assess the home and neighborhood environment. People with dementia are easy targets for exploitation by telephone and mail fraud and people who come to the door. High-crime neighborhoods pose additional risks. An older adult who spends his time at the corner store buying alcohol and cigarettes may be especially vulnerable.

The psychiatrist should ask specifically about the primary caregiver's health. The psychiatrist should be alert to offhand comments such as "I'm fine as long as he can drive me to chemotherapy." The caregiver should be asked about his or her sleep and how it is affected by the older adult's sleep pattern. Many family caregivers will report being frustrated, overwhelmed, edgy, or exhausted but will deny having depression, anxiety, or psychiatric symptoms. Although psychiatrists are well advised to respond promptly to poorly controlled rage or suicidal or violent threats, skillful probing may be required to elicit frank symptoms.

A brief review of family relationships may further elicit new or resurfacing family conflict that can complicate care. A distant, estranged sister may insist that her local sister is exaggerating their mother's dependency needs in an attempt to take control. The psychiatrist's written explanation of the mother's need for constant supervision may mobilize support from the distant daughter or at least may reassure the local daughter that her supervision is in fact what her mother needs. The psychiatrist must be alert to reports by family caregivers of exacerbated somatic symptoms or chronic illnesses that may not be attributed to caregiver burden.

Another key to effective family assessment is to ask about other family commitments. A daughter backing up her mother's care of her father may be distracted by anxiety about her husband's failing business or a child's drug addiction. Cultural expectations must be carefully assessed along with each family member's subjective perceptions of financial resources. When paid or formal services are needed, family decision making is often related to subjective perceptions of future financial adequacy rather than the objective cost or affordability of services. Some family members may be saving for a rainy day, whereas others may value preserving their inheritance above meeting the elder's current care needs.

It is wise to assess family styles, strengths, and goals. Some families cope well with end-of-life care for an immobile or incontinent older adult but are unable to tolerate the disruptive behaviors or sleep patterns of persons with moderate dementia. Families who have coped with chronic mental illness or substance abuse in other members may have well-developed coping strategies or support systems such as Alcoholics Anonymous that help them adapt to care for an impaired elder.

Finally, assessment should include some review of the family's experience with previous and current help, both family help and help from paid services. Previous family conflict over elder care will limit the family's willingness to ask for help. If the last home care worker stole from them or never showed up, the family is unlikely to accept another home health referral. Key questions about previous and current help are about adequacy, quality, and dependability. If a family believes the help they give each other is adequate, dependable, or sufficient, they are often unwilling to consider formal services.

Selecting Interventions for Families of Older Adults

Families of persons with dementia need a continuing source of reliable information. Referrals to the Alzheimer's Association (800-272-3900; http://www.alz.org) and the Alzheimer's Disease Education and Referral Center of the National Institute on Aging (800-438-4380; http://www.nia.nih.gov/alzheimers) meet this need.

Combined interventions have been shown to enhance positive caregiver outcomes. Combining individual and family counseling, family education, support group participation, and sustained availability of a care manager are associated with decreased caregiver burden and depression; decreases in the elder's disruptive symptoms; and increased caregiver satisfaction, subjective well-being, and self-efficacy (Sorensen et al. 2002). Psychoeducational and psychotherapeutic interventions produce the most consistent short-term effects on all outcome measures. Although interventions with dementia caregivers appear effective in meta-analyses, effects are small and domain-specific rather than global. For example, a reasonable multimodal approach to treating an elder's disruptive agitation could include treatment of depression in the elder or in the family caregiver with pharmacological and nonpharmacological strategies, participation by the family caregiver in psychoeducational, skills training, or caregiver support groups, and participation by the elder and the family caregiver in structured exercise programs.

Nonpharmacological approaches to the treatment of depression in elder-care family dyads could be based on increasing the frequency of individually selected pleasant events (Teri et al. 1997). Once the elder and caregiver have identified which activities are the most enjoyable, the goal becomes one of increasing the frequency and duration of these activities relative to less enjoyable daily activities.

Referrals to support groups should be balanced and not oversold. Research on participation in support groups documents specific benefits from experiential similarity, consumer information, coping and survivor models, expressive or advocacy outlets, and (for some participants) the creation of substitute family or social outlets. Indeed, early studies of support group participation showed that participants knew more about Alzheimer's disease and services (although participants did not necessarily use that information) and that participants felt less isolated and misunderstood than nonparticipants. There are, however, realistic limits to the benefits of support group participation.

One support group does not fit all. African Americans frequently do not understand the need to talk about family business among strangers. In an open mutual help group with revolving membership, not all participants will be dealing with the same care issues. The exclusive focus on Alzheimer's disease as just one aspect of family life may not meet family needs. Some families cannot get to meetings regularly, and some groups are not consistently available. These factors limit the benefits of such a minimalist intervention. The benefits of participation can be enhanced by encouraging families to shop around for a group that best meets their needs and by reminding them that they may be able to obtain comparable social support from groups to which they already belong, such as a church or retiree organization, or even from online sources such as discussion boards and online discussion groups dedicated to Alzheimer's disease.

Educational Strategies With Families of Older Adults

Many families are too overwhelmed at a first psychiatric consultation to absorb information or instructions. Teachable moments with families come at crisis points with specific psychiatric symptoms such as accusations of family theft or spousal infidelity or when the older adult asks his or her spouse to find his "real" wife or husband.

A medicine metaphor is appropriate. The timing and "dosing" of information may enhance effective use of that information in adapting care over time. Some families have read or heard inaccurate or partially correct information about symptoms that can be easily corrected, such as myths about all older men with dementia becoming sexual predators. Just like medication management in geriatrics, the maxim "start low and go slow" applies equally well to family education about dementia. Overwhelming families with too many treatment suggestions or referrals is just as likely to lead to poor compliance as is changing multiple medication regimens all at once. Finally, information should be presented in hopeful terms, such as "treating your depression should have positive effects on your husband's mood as well" or "many families surprise themselves with their resilience."

The presentation of information in a timed and dosed manner also offers opportunities for repetition of key themes. The key messages for family caregivers listed in Table 18–1 can be presented at intervals and in "doses" that are based on the frequency of contact with the family, the family's need to know, and the family's capacity to understand.

Responding to Families Over the Course of Progressive Impairment

Over the course of a dementia, family caregivers become not only information seekers but also care managers, consumer advocates, surrogate decision makers, and health care providers. It is difficult enough to negotiate these complex roles, and it is even more difficult if the family caregiver is burdened by role overload. Assessing caregiver vulnerability can be facilitated by asking family members to self-assess their pressure points, or signs of increasing caregiver overload (Kaufer et al. 1998).

Clinical red flags may signal imminent danger resulting from the caregiver's precarious health. Unsubtle hints may be comments such as "after my last stroke," "before he totaled the car," or "sometimes I feel like just letting him wander away." Pursuing these threads with standard clinical protocols is certainly warranted.

Other issues surface when working with families of moderately impaired older adults. Isolation of the caregiver and elder is common as friends drop off in response to disruptive behavioral symptoms or the need for constant supervision of the older adult. Families need to be reminded that being vulnerable does not make older people grateful or lovable and that cabin fever among co-residing elders and family caregivers is a real threat to mental health and safety. Families are especially sensitive to elders who confuse or mistake family identities or suggest that family members are impostors. Making suggestions that family caregivers say something like "I'll try to do it like your mother would" may help them to understand.

TABLE 18–1. Key messages for family caregivers

1. Be willing to listen to the older adult, but understand that you cannot fix or do everything he or she may want or need. Know that it will not necessarily get easier, but things will change, and the experience will change you forever.

2. You are living with a situation you did not create, and your choices are limited by circumstances beyond your control. Seek options that are good enough for now.

3. You can only do what seems best at the time. Identify what you can and will tolerate, then set limits and call in reinforcements. Doubts are inevitable.

4. Find someone with whom you can be brutally honest, express those feelings, and move on.

5. Solving problems is much easier than living with the solutions. It is tempting for distant relatives to second-guess or criticize. Hope for the best but plan for the worst.

6. It is not always possible to compare how one person handles things to how another relative would handle it if the positions were reversed.

7. The older adult is not unhappy or upset because of what you have done. He or she is living with unwanted dependency. Sick people often take out their frustration on close family members.

8. Considering what is best for your family involves compromise among competing needs, loyalties, and commitments. Everyone may get some of what he or she needs. Think twice before giving up that job, club, or church group. Make realistic commitments, and avoid making promises that include the words *always*, *never*, or *forever*.

9. Find ways to let your older relative give to or help you. He or she needs to feel purposeful, appreciated, and loved.

10. Take time to celebrate small victories when things go well.

Family members need to be warned not to give up cherished activities—social engagement has positive mental health effects at any age, and maintenance of a strong religious faith or community has been shown to have positive effects on elders and family caregivers. Expressive outlets such as sports, the arts, or advocacy can help families cope with frustration and anger. Prayer, meditation, exercise, massage, and yoga in combination with active treatment of depression or anxiety are all worthy treatment recommendations. An elder's participation at an adult day center can be presented to the family as a source of social stimulation for the elder and a stress-reduction strategy for the family caregiver (Zarit et al. 1998).

Helping Families Assess Capacity of Older Adults

Many families turn to psychiatrists to assess the judgment and decision-making capacity of older adults, whether it is related to handling money, health decisions, living alone, or driving.

Handling money and health care decisions should be addressed soon after diagnosis to ensure time for patients to select a surrogate. Often families seek psychiatric consultation when family conflict surfaces over the patient's selection of a surrogate or the surrogate's handling of the older adult's funds. Questions about whether the patient had sufficient capacity at the time he or she wrote a will or assigned power of attorney can become adversarial and unrelated to family treatment.

Effective work with families regarding capacity is done early with a preventive focus. It is wise for one family member to make sure bills are paid. This can be done with different levels of involvement of the patient, from decision making about which bills to pay to signing checks.

Assessment and Limitations on Driving

Families can be encouraged to assess driving capacity based on observations of current driving, with reminders that dementia affects judgment, reaction time, and problem solving. Psychiatric assessment of the patient along with current observations from the family will provide direction on when driving should be limited. Unfortunately, by the time there is evidence of a decline in driving abilities, many patients cannot adequately report or judge their safety on the road. Anonymous reports to the department of motor vehicles may lead to required testing or removal of the patient's license, but the absence of a license rarely stops a determined older adult with dementia.

Driving is one area in which the family must be encouraged and prepared to assess capacity over time. The signs listed in Table 18–2 may guide family observations and reports to the psychiatrist.

Psychiatrists may suggest a range of successful ways to limit driving, such as the following:

- A prescription reminder to stop driving can be tempered with a qualifier such as "until the end of your treatment." The patient's forgetfulness can be put to work for the psychiatrist. However, patients have been known to keep driving, making comments such as "That doctor doesn't know anything."
- Shaving the patient's keys, substituting another key, removing a distributor cap,

TABLE 18–2. Signs of decline in driving skills

Incorrect signaling

Trouble navigating turns

Moving into the wrong lane

Confusion on exits

Parking in inappropriate places

Driving at inappropriate speed

Delayed responses to unexpected situations

Failure to anticipate dangerous situations

Scrapes or dents on car, garage, or mailbox

Becoming lost in familiar places

Arriving unusually late for a short-distance drive

Receiving moving violations or warnings about near misses

Confusing the brake and accelerator

Stopping in traffic for no apparent reason

or otherwise disabling a car can sometimes reduce the need to confront the patient with lost skills. However, patients have been known to fix the car, replace the keys, or even buy a new car while the old one was "in the shop."
- The car could be sold, moved to an undisclosed location, or put up on blocks. One family of a taxi driver put the taxi on blocks in the backyard to help the patient remember that it was broken.
- The family can also work on solutions that limit the need for driving—delivery services, senior vans, or offers of regular rides to church or for visits. Some families find that a taxi charge account works best.

Addressing Questions of Capacity to Live Alone

Families may go to extremes to keep an older adult with dementia in a familiar environment, allowing values of autonomy and choice to temporarily trump safety. In addition to psychiatric assessment of the patient's cognition, judgment, functional impairment, and decision-making capacity, the psychiatrist can suggest that the family consider the following questions:

- Can he or she use the telephone to call for help from a family member or to call 911? Will he or she respond inappropriately to telemarketers? Have mysterious packages or bills for unusual items begun appearing? Does he or she make repetitive calls every few minutes to the police or the same family member at work or at home?
- Can he or she get to the store or to regular activities? Does he or she overbuy or underbuy certain items?
- Can he or she handle money and pay bills, or is he or she willing to let others do this for him or her?
- Can he or she take medicine appropriately, on time, and in correct doses? Does he or she self-medicate or risk overdoses of unnecessary medications?
- Is he or she bathing, changing clothes, and dressing appropriately for the weather?
- Is he or she leaving the house after dark or traveling in dangerous areas alone? Does he or she let strangers in or buy from or contribute to questionable causes based on visits to his or her home?
- Is he having problems positioning his body to use a toilet, or is he urinating in wastebaskets or outdoors?
- Is he or she falling or getting lost by wandering outside a safe area?
- Are there significant changes in his or her appetite, weight, sleep, appearance, or eating habits?
- Is discreet surveillance by neighbors, friends, or family readily available?

The question of discreet surveillance is paramount. Persons with moderate dementia may live alone successfully if they have regular contact with, surveillance by, or checking from neighbors or family members. Environmental demand varies considerably and must be assessed along with patient variables.

Families and Institutionalization of the Older Adult

Not only does family stress not stop at the door of the nursing home, but ample evidence shows that families experience the greatest burden, disruption, and conflict in the time immediately before and after nursing home placement. Family members may seek psychiatric services to deal with guilt, grief, and often anger toward the nursing facility, reimbursement system, and each other. Many families are disappointed by the lack of medical or psychiatric treatment available to residents of nursing homes. Families should be encouraged to work with the facility and the nursing home ombudsman while dealing with their affective, anxiety, and grief symptoms.

Conclusion

Work with families of older adults is about adaptation to change and loss. Much of psychiatric treatment of families helps them modify expectations for new dependency while learning to forgive themselves and others for inevitable doubts and mistakes. Interdisciplinary partnerships and teamwork with the Alzheimer's Association or with nurses or social workers offer the most effective and efficient models for psychiatric services to families of older adults. There is often as much need for "timed and dosed" patient and family education as there is need for treatment of specific psychiatric symptoms or syndromes of the elder or family members. Families will expect psychiatrists to provide active treatment and monitoring of psychiatric symptoms, reassurance, interpretation of information, and referrals. In addition, it is always helpful to acknowledge losses and contributions to care by individual family members, to encourage caregiver self-care, to offer authoritative absolution for inevitable mistakes, and to offer decisional support, especially with transitions in care or with end-of-life care.

References

Brodaty H, Luscombe G: Psychological morbidity in caregivers is associated with depression in patients with dementia. Alzheimer Dis Assoc Disord 1:62–70, 1998

Burton LC, Newsom JT, Schulz R, et al: Preventive health behaviors among spousal caregivers. Prev Med 26:162–169, 1997

Fortinsky RH, Kercher K, Burant CJ: Measurement and correlates of family caregiver self-efficacy for managing dementia. Aging Ment Health 6:153–160, 2002a

Fortinsky RH, Unson CG, Garcia RI: Helping family caregivers by linking primary care physicians with community-based dementia care services. Dementia 1(2):227–240, 2002b

Fulmer T, Paveza G, Van de Weerd C, et al: Dyadic vulnerability and risk profiling for elder neglect. Gerontologist 45(4):525–534, 2005

Gwyther LP: Family issues in dementia: finding a new normal. Neurol Clin 18:993–1010, 2000

Hughes SL, Giobie-Hurder A, Weaver FM, et al: Relationships between caregiver burden and health-related quality of life. Gerontologist 39:534–545, 1999

Kaufer DI, Cummings JL, Christine D, et al: Assessing the impact of neuropsychiatric symptoms in Alzheimer's disease: the Neuropsychiatric Inventory Caregiver Distress Scale. J Am Geriatr Soc 46:210–215, 1998

King AC, Brassington G: Enhancing physical and psychological functioning in older family caregivers: the role of regular physical activity. Ann Behav Med 19:91–100, 1997

Langa KM, Chernew ME, Kabeto MU, et al: National estimates of the quantity and cost of informal caregiving for the elderly with dementia. J Gen Intern Med 16:770–776, 2001

Lyketsos CG, Steinberg M, Tschanz JT: Mental and behavioral disturbances in dementia: findings from the Cache County Study on Memory in Aging. Am J Psychiatry 157:708–714, 2000

McCurry SM, Gibbons LE, Logsdon RG, et al: Nighttime insomnia treatment and education for Alzheimer's disease: a randomized controlled trial. J Am Geriatr Soc 53(5):793–802, 2005

Mittelman MS, Ferris SH, Shulman E, et al: A family intervention to delay nursing home placement of patients with Alzheimer disease: a randomized controlled trial. JAMA 276:1725–1731, 1996

Olin JT, Schneider LS, Katz IR, et al: Provisional diagnostic criteria for depression of Alzheimer's disease. Am J Geriatr Psychiatry 10:125–128, 2002

Ostwald SK, Hepburn KW, Caron W, et al: Reducing caregiver burden: a randomized psychoeducational intervention for caregivers of persons with dementia. Gerontologist 39:299–309, 1999

Pillemer K, Suitor JJ: "It takes one to help one": effects of similar others on the well-being of caregivers. J Gerontol B Psychol Sci Soc Sci 51:S250–S257, 1996

Pinquart M, Sorensen S: Gender differences in caregiver stressors, social resources, and health: an updated meta-analysis. J Gerontol B Psychol Sci Soc Sci 61(1):P33–P45, 2006

Schulz R, Beach SR: Caregiving as a risk factor for mortality: the Caregiver Health Effects Study. JAMA 282:2215–2219, 1999

Sorensen S, Pinquart M, Duberstein P, et al: How effective are interventions with caregivers? An updated meta-analysis. Gerontologist 42:356–372, 2002

Spangenberg KB, Wagner MT, Hendrix S, et al: Firearm presence in households of patients with Alzheimer's disease and other dementias. J Am Geriatr Soc 47:1183–1186, 1999

Teri L, Logsdon RG, Uomoto J, et al: Behavioral treatment of depression in dementia patients: a controlled clinical trial. J Gerontol B Psychol Sci Soc Sci 52:P159–P166, 1997

Tractenberg RE, Weiner MF, Thal LJ: Estimating the prevalence of agitation in community-dwelling persons with Alzheimer's disease. J Neuropsychiatry Clin Neurosci 14: 11–18, 2002

Yaffe K, Fox P, Newcomer R, et al: Patient and caregiver characteristics and nursing home placement in patients with dementia. JAMA 287:2090–2097, 2002

Yates ME, Tennstedt S, Chang BH: Contributors to and mediators of psychological well-being for informal caregivers. J Gerontol B Psychol Sci Soc Sci 54:P12–P22, 1999

Zarit SH, Stephens MA, Townsend A, et al: Stress reduction for family caregivers: effects of adult day care use. J Gerontol B Psychol Sci Soc Sci 53:S267–S277, 1998

Study Questions

Select the single best response for each question.

1. Which of the following is true regarding care of elderly patients with dementia in the community?

    A. Fifty percent of older patients with moderate or severe dementia live alone with some level of supervision.

    B. Spousal caregiver strain from care for patients with dementia is associated with increased risk of premature death.

    C. Anxiety symptoms are the most commonly reported psychiatric symptoms in caregivers of patients with dementia.

    D. Dependent elders are much more likely to engage in manipulative behavior than to have legitimate unmet dependency needs.

    E. Defensive denial of inevitable bad outcomes in dementia must be discouraged and avoided for caregivers to give appropriate dementia care.

2. In working with dementia patients and their families, psychiatrists are advised to attend to many parallel issues in both patients and family members. All of the following are true *except*

    A. Psychiatrists should monitor the mental health, capacity, and vulnerability of caregivers as well as patients.

    B. Caregivers' self-neglect and patient neglect by caregivers are both important areas for surveillance.

    C. A common goal in working with families of older adults with dementia is to address safety and security issues.

    D. Affective, anxiety, and substance abuse disorders of primary caregivers do not predict breakdown of family care.

    E. Major precipitants of patient placement include both patient and caregiver factors.

3. The conduct of office visits with dementia patients and family caregivers calls for the psychiatrist to make certain commonsense changes to clinical routine. Which of the following is true?

    A. The psychiatrist should rigorously preserve patient confidentiality and not speak to family members unless the patient is present.

    B. The patient should not be accompanied to the physician's office by more than one family member as this confuses the patient and leads to excessive boundary management challenges.

    C. Older couples with long relationships often prefer to face medical challenges together rather than singly.

    D. Psychiatrists should not encourage family members to remove weapons from the home of patients with dementia, as this is an invasion of privacy.

    E. The psychiatrist should not encourage physical activity for the patient with dementia as the patient needs to preserve energy for cognitive tasks.

4. The psychiatrist caring for patients with dementia also needs to assess the family members of the patient. Which of the following is *not* true?

    A. Older husbands who are caregivers are at increased risk of alcohol abuse.
    B. Caregivers should be encouraged to pursue regular exercise.
    C. The caregiver has a need for social stimulation while caring for a dependent elder.
    D. Secondary family support should be assessed.
    E. The psychiatrist should not directly address the caregiver's own health, as this is a matter for that person's own physician.

5. Driving is often a contentious issue in dementia. Which of the following is *not* true regarding driving by cognitively impaired patients?

    A. Dementia leads to decreased judgment.
    B. Increased reaction time is common in dementia.
    C. Patients with dementia will respect the loss of their driver's license and cease to try to drive.
    D. Mechanically disabling the car reduces the need to confront the patient with his or her lost skills.
    E. Families should proactively arrange for alternative transportation to decrease the incentive for the patient to try to drive.

Clinical Psychiatry in the Nursing Home

Joel E. Streim, M.D.

Ira R. Katz, M.D., Ph.D.

Nursing homes provide long-term care for elderly patients with chronic illness and disability as well as rehabilitation and convalescent care for those recovering from acute illness. As documented in other reviews (Katz et al. 2000; Streim et al. 1996), clinical studies have consistently provided evidence that the diagnosis, management, and treatment of mental disorders is an important component of nursing home care. At present, the delivery of mental health services is being shaped by several factors, including growing scientific knowledge, availability of new treatments, evolving federal regulations, public dissemination of survey data, and changes in the medical marketplace. In this chapter we review current information on the psychiatric problems that are common in the nursing home, discuss current trends affecting clinical care, and present a conceptual model for the organization of mental health services.

Prevalence of Psychiatric Disorders

Epidemiological studies conducted over the past 15 years have uniformly reported high prevalence rates for psychiatric disorders among nursing home residents. Rovner and colleagues (1990a) reported the prevalence of psychiatric disorders among persons newly admitted to a proprietary chain of nursing homes to be 80.2%. Parmelee and associates (1989) found psychiatric disorders diagnosed according to DSM-III-R (American Psychiatric Association 1987) criteria in 91% of the residents of a large urban geriatric center. On the basis of psychiatric interviews of subjects in randomly selected samples, other investigators found prevalence rates of DSM-III (American Psychiatric Association 1980) or DSM-III-R disorders to be as high as 94% (Chandler and Chandler 1988; Rovner et al. 1986; Tariot et al. 1993).

Although some studies reported lower rates, those investigations used less rigorous methods for sampling or diagnosis (Burns et al. 1988; Custer et al. 1984; German et al. 1986; National Center for Health Statistics 1987; Teeter et al. 1976). In one study, Rovner and colleagues (1990a) found that 67.4% of residents had dementia, 10.4% had depressive disorders, and 2.4% had schizophrenia or other psychotic disorders. Subsequent data from the Medical Expenditures Panel Survey (MEPS) revealed that 70%–80% of residents have cognitive impairment and 20% have a diagnosis of a depressive disorder (Krauss and Altman 1998). Although the MEPS data were not derived from clinical interviews, they indicate prevalence rates of dementia and depression that are greater than the prevalence rates found in nursing home studies a decade earlier.

These prevalence data also suggest that nursing homes are de facto neuropsychiatric institutions, although they were not originally intended for this purpose. The challenge of providing long-term-care services in nursing homes is therefore complicated by the extensive psychiatric comorbidity found in this setting.

Cognitive Disorders and Behavioral Disturbances

In all studies, the most common psychiatric disorder was dementia, with prevalence rates of 50%–75% (Chandler and Chandler 1988; Katz et al. 1989; Parmelee et al. 1989; Rovner et al. 1986, 1990a; Tariot et al. 1993; Teeter et al. 1976). Alzheimer's disease (DSM-III-R primary degenerative dementia) accounted for about 50%–60% of cases of dementia, and vascular dementia accounted for about 25%–30% (Barnes and Raskind 1980; Rovner et al. 1986, 1990a). Other causes of dementia were reported with lower prevalence and greater variability between sites. The prevalence of Lewy body dementia has not been ascertained in nursing home populations.

Delirium is common in nursing homes and occurs primarily in patients made more vulnerable by a dementing illness. Available studies indicated that approximately 6%–7% of residents were delirious at the time of evaluation (Barnes and Raskind 1980; Rovner et al. 1986, 1990a). However, this figure probably underestimates

the number of patients who have reversible toxic or metabolic components of their cognitive impairment. In one study, investigators found that nearly 25% of impaired residents had potentially reversible conditions (Sabin et al. 1982); in another study it was found that 6%–12% of residential care patients with dementia actually improved in cognitive performance over the course of 1 year (Katz et al. 1991). In the nursing home, as in other settings, the most common reversible cause of cognitive impairment may be cognitive toxicity from drugs used to treat medical or psychiatric disorders.

The clinical features of dementing disorders include treatable psychiatric symptoms—such as hallucinations, delusions, and depression—that can contribute to disability. Psychotic symptoms have been reported in approximately 25%–50% of residents with a primary dementing illness (Berrios and Brook 1985; Chandler and Chandler 1988; Rovner et al. 1986, 1990a; Teeter et al. 1976). Clinically significant depression is seen in approximately 25% of patients with dementia; one-third of such patients exhibit symptoms of secondary major depression (Parmelee et al. 1989; Rovner et al. 1986, 1990a).

MEPS data revealed that 30% of residents exhibit behavioral problems, including 11.8% with verbal abuse, 9.1% with physical abuse, 14.5% with socially inappropriate behavior, 12.5% with resistance to care, and 9.4% with wandering (Krauss and Altman 1998). In earlier studies, behavioral disturbances were found in up to 75% of residents, and multiple behavior problems were found in at least half (Chandler and Chandler 1988; Cohen-Mansfield 1986; National Center for Health Statistics 1979; Rovner et al. 1986, 1990a; Tariot et al. 1993; Zimmer et al. 1984). It is likely that the lower rates reported in the MEPS reflect a different method of case ascertainment, rather than improvement in behavioral management leading to a decrease in prevalence.

In addition to impaired ability to perform activities of daily living (ADLs), disturbances of behavior have been identified as the most common reasons that patients with dementia are admitted to nursing homes (Steele et al. 1990), and disruptive behaviors frequently complicate care after admission (Cohen-Mansfield et al. 1989; Teeter et al. 1976; Zimmer et al. 1984).

The majority of psychiatric consultations in long-term-care settings are for the evaluation and treatment of behavioral disturbances (Loebel et al. 1991) such as pacing and wandering, verbal abusiveness, disruptive shouting, physical aggression, and resistance to necessary care. Behavioral disturbances most frequently occur in patients with dementia, often in those with psychotic symptoms—an association that remains even after controlling for level of cognitive impairment (Rovner et al. 1990b). Agitation and hyperactivity can also be caused by agitated depression, delirium, sensory deprivation or overload, occult physical illness, pain, constipation, urinary retention, and adverse drug effects (including akathisia due to neuroleptics) (Cohen-Mansfield and Billig 1986).

In addition to agitation, symptoms such as apathy, inactivity, and withdrawal occur among nursing home residents. Although these symptoms are less disturbing to staff and less frequently lead to psychiatric consultation, they can be disabling and may be associated with decreases in socialization and self-care.

Depression

Depressive disorders represent the second most common psychiatric diagnosis in nursing home residents. Most studies in United States nursing homes show depression prevalence rates of 15%–50%, depending on the population studied and the instruments used, whether major depression or depressive symptoms are being reported, and whether primary depression and depression occurring secondary to dementia are considered together or separately (Baker and Miller 1991; Chandler and Chandler 1988; Hyer and Blazer 1982; Katz et al. 1989; Lesher 1986; Parmelee et al. 1989; Rovner et al. 1986, 1990a, 1991; Tariot et al. 1993; Teeter et al. 1976). Studies from other countries have shown similar rates (Ames 1990, 1991; Ames et al. 1988; Harrison et al. 1990; Horiguchi and Inami 1991; Mann et al. 1984; Snowdon 1986; Snowdon and Donnelly 1986; Spagnoli et al. 1986; Trichard et al. 1982).

Approximately 6%–10% of all nursing home residents, and 20%–25% of those who are cognitively intact, meet DSM-III or DSM-III-R criteria for major depression; the latter figure is an order of magnitude greater than rates among community-dwelling elderly persons (Blazer and Williams 1980; Kramer et al. 1985).

The prevalence of less severe but clinically significant (e.g., minor or subsyndromal) depression is even higher. In one study, Parmelee and associates (1992a) reported that the 1-year incidence of major depression was 9.4% and that patients with preexisting minor depression were at increased risk; the incidence of minor depression among those who were euthymic at baseline was 7.4%. Other smaller-scale studies have shown comparable rates (Foster et al. 1991; Katz et al. 1989). These data show that minor depression in nursing home residents appears to be a risk factor for major depression and might represent an opportunity for preventive treatment in this population.

Depression among nursing home residents tends to be persistent. Although there may be moderate decreases in self-rated depression in the initial 2 weeks after nursing home admission (Engle and Graney 1993), Ames et al. (1988) found that only

17% of patients with diagnosable depressive disorders had recovered after an average 3.6 years of follow-up. Evidence for morbidity associated with depression comes from studies that showed an increase in pain complaints among residents with depression (Parmelee et al. 1991) and an association between depression and biochemical markers of subnutrition (Katz et al. 1993). In addition to its association with morbidity, depression has been found to be associated with an increase in mortality rate, with effect sizes ranging from 1.6 to 3 (Ashby et al. 1991; Katz et al. 1989; Parmelee et al. 1992b; Rovner et al. 1991). There is, however, controversy about the mechanism involved. Whereas Rovner and colleagues (1991) reported that the increased mortality rate remained apparent after controlling for the patients' medical diagnoses and level of disability, Parmelee and associates (1992a) found that the effect could be attributed to the interrelationships among depression, disability, and physical illness. Resolution of this issue will require further study.

The literature on depression as it presents in patients with significant medical illness is marked by recurring questions about the extent to which diagnostic criteria developed in younger and healthier adults remain valid among patients with significant psychiatric-medical comorbidity. It might seem logical to expect that the somatic and vegetative symptoms that characterize major depression in other populations lose their diagnostic value among long-term-care residents and that long-term-care patients who have symptoms consistent with a diagnosis of major depressive disorder may instead be experiencing a combination of medical symptoms and an existential reaction to disease, disability, and residential care placement. However, it has been demonstrated that DSM diagnostic criteria remain valid as predictors of treatment response and that

the symptoms of major depression in frail elderly patients residing in nursing homes characterize a disease similar to that which occurs among younger adult psychiatric patients residing in the community (Katz et al. 1990), even though most nursing home patients have concurrent medical illnesses and disabilities that complicate diagnosis and treatment.

In addition to the high level of complexity that characterizes major depression among nursing home residents, there is evidence for heterogeneity in these patients that may reflect the existence of clinically relevant subtypes of depression. The treatment study by Katz and colleagues (1990) demonstrated that measures of self-care deficits and serum levels of albumin were highly intercorrelated and that both predicted a lack of response to treatment with nortriptyline. Therefore, although this study demonstrated that major depression is a specific, treatable disorder—even in long-term-care patients with medical comorbidity—there is also evidence in this setting for a treatment-relevant subtype of depression characterized by high levels of disability and low levels of serum albumin. This latter condition may be related to failure to thrive in infants, as discussed by Braun and colleagues (1988) and by Katz et al. (1993).

Progress in Treatment of Psychiatric Disorders in the Nursing Home

An appreciation of the unique characteristics of nursing home populations—particularly the extremes of old age and the high prevalences of cognitive impairment, psychiatric-medical comorbidity, and disability, all in the context of residential long-term-care institutions—has led to increased recognition that results of efficacy studies conducted in general adult outpatient populations may not be readily generalizable to nursing home residents. Although the number of randomized controlled studies is limited, there is a growing body of literature on treatment outcomes in the nursing home.

Nonpharmacological Management of Behavioral Disturbances

Since 1990, more than 60 studies have been published describing nonpharmacological interventions for behavioral disturbances associated with dementia in the nursing home setting. Few are randomized controlled trials. The reader is referred to comprehensive reviews of these studies by Cohen-Mansfield (2001) and Snowden et al. (2003).

Several nonpharmacological interventions have been shown to be effective. One promising approach combined enhanced activities, guidelines for the use of psychotropic medication, and educational rounds for nursing home staff (Rovner et al. 1996). In a randomized clinical trial, this approach was shown to reduce the prevalence of problem behaviors and the use of antipsychotic drugs and physical restraints. Individualized consultation for staff nurses about the management of patients with dementia was also shown to diminish the use of physical restraints (L.K. Evans et al. 1997). Reductions in agitation were also observed in a study of a daytime physical activity intervention combined with a nighttime program to decrease noise and sleep-disruptive nursing care practices (Alessi 1999). Other programs decrease behavioral difficulties through modifications in the physical environment. Research on individualized behavioral interventions for patients with behavioral disturbances of dementia has been limited to case series and small-scale controlled trials that are often difficult to replicate, although some of the results are promising (Allen-Burge et al. 1999).

Psychotherapy

The growing evidence for the efficacy of psychotherapy in other settings suggests that it may be of value for treating mental disorders of aging in patients whose cognitive abilities allow them to participate. However, a search of the MEDLINE and PsycINFO databases for the terms *psychotherapy* and *nursing homes* from 1987 to the time of writing this chapter identified only a small number of controlled studies of the effectiveness of specific psychotherapeutic modalities, individual or group, for nursing home residents.

Controlled research on psychotherapeutic interventions has included studies of task-oriented versus insight-oriented therapy (Moran and Gatz 1987); reality orientation (Baines et al. 1987); reminiscence groups (Baines et al. 1987; Goldwasser et al. 1987; McMurdo and Rennie 1993; Orten et al. 1989; Rattenbury and Stones 1989; Youssef 1990); exercise, activity, and progressive relaxation groups (Bensink et al. 1992; McMurdo and Rennie 1993); supportive group psychotherapy (Goldwasser et al. 1987; Williams-Barnard and Lindell 1992); validation therapy (Toseland et al. 1997); cognitive or cognitive-behavioral group therapies (Abraham et al. 1992; Zerhusen et al. 1991); focused visual imagery therapy (Abraham et al. 1997); and a psychosocial activity intervention (Beck et al. 2002). With the exception of the investigations by Abraham and colleagues, patients in most of these studies were not selected on the basis of specific psychiatric symptoms or syndromes, but rather on the basis of age, cognitive status, or mobility.

Some of these studies reported improvements on measures of communication, behavior, cognitive performance, mood, social withdrawal, physical function, somatic preoccupation, self-esteem, perceived locus of control, and life satisfaction. Case reports and demonstration projects by experienced clinicians also documented the value of psychotherapy for treating depressed nursing home residents (Leszcz et al. 1985; Sadavoy 1991). Overall, there is a paucity of research on the outcomes of well-described psychotherapies among nursing home residents who have well-characterized psychiatric disorders. Nevertheless, the available evidence from nursing home research, considered together with outcomes of psychotherapy for older adults in other clinical settings, suggests that psychotherapy should be regarded as an important component of mental health treatment for the more cognitively intact nursing home residents with depression.

Pharmacotherapy

Pharmacological treatments are commonly used in nursing homes for dementia and its psychiatric and behavioral complications and for depression. For a more comprehensive review of the evidence for pharmacological treatment of neuropsychiatric symptoms of dementia, the reader is referred to the article by Sink and colleagues (2005).

Some earlier studies provided evidence for the efficacy of conventional antipsychotic drugs in managing agitation and related symptoms in nursing home residents with dementia, but the effect sizes were often modest, and high placebo response rates were common (Barnes et al. 1982; Schneider et al. 1990). Subsequently, three multicenter, randomized, double-blind, placebo-controlled clinical trials have demonstrated the efficacy of risperidone, an atypical antipsychotic agent, for the treatment of psychotic symptoms and agitated behavior in nursing home residents with dementia (Brodaty et al. 2003; DeDeyn et al. 1999; Katz et al. 1999). The results showed that risperidone had antipsychotic

effects and also had independent effects on aggression or agitation. The study by DeDeyn and colleagues included a comparison group treated with haloperidol. Follow-up studies suggested that risperidone may cause less tardive dyskinesia than do typical antipsychotic agents (Jeste et al. 2000). A randomized clinical trial of olanzapine versus placebo in nursing home residents showed efficacy similar to that of risperidone (Street et al. 2000). Randomized controlled trials of aripiprazole and quetiapine in nursing home patients with dementia complicated by psychosis or agitation were completed but not yet published at the time this chapter was written.

These controlled clinical trials examined only the acute effects of treatment, typically for 6–12 weeks of treatment, and little is known about the effectiveness of treatment for longer periods. However, there is evidence to suggest that the need for and benefit from antipsychotic drug treatment changes over the course of months in nursing home patients with dementia. Two double-blind, placebo-controlled studies of antipsychotic drug discontinuation demonstrated that the majority of patients who had been receiving longer-term treatment could be withdrawn from these agents without reemergence of psychosis or agitated behaviors (Bridges-Parlet et al. 1997; Cohen-Mansfield et al. 1999). This finding is consistent with results from previous discontinuation studies, in which only 16%–22% of patients who had been receiving medications on a chronic basis exhibited increased agitation when the drugs were withdrawn (Barton and Hurst 1966; Risse et al. 1987; Semla et al. 1994). Therefore, it is important to reevaluate on a regular basis the need for continuing antipsychotic drug treatment.

Since 2003, analyses of safety data from randomized controlled studies of atypical antipsychotic drugs in elderly patients with dementia, including the aforementioned nursing home studies, have revealed significantly increased risks of cerebrovascular adverse events and mortality in this population. Although elevated risks were not found in every study, pooled analyses showed that the rate of cerebrovascular adverse events (including stroke and transient ischemic attacks) is greater than the rate found with placebo by 2.3% in elderly patients treated with risperidone, 0.9% in those treated with olanzapine, and 0.7% in those treated with aripiprazole. Most of the affected individuals had known cerebrovascular risk factors prior to starting drug treatment. These findings led to regulatory warnings in the United States, Canada, and the United Kingdom regarding the safety of these drugs in elderly patients with dementia.

The U.S. Food and Drug Administration (FDA) also warned that elderly patients with dementia-related psychosis who are treated with atypical antipsychotics have a risk of death between 1.6 and 1.7 times greater than those treated with placebo (4.5% vs. 2.6%); with a reminder that atypical antipsychotics are not FDA-approved for the treatment of patients with dementia-related psychosis. Consistent with this FDA warning, a meta-analysis by Schneider and colleagues (2005), examining results of 15 randomized controlled trials, many of which were conducted in nursing home patients, found that the risk of mortality was 3.5% in elderly patients treated with atypical antipsychotics versus 2.3% of patients receiving placebo. Although no placebo-controlled trials of ziprasidone or clozapine are known to have been conducted in elderly patients with dementia, it is reasonable to view the increased mortality as a class effect. Although the FDA mortality warning applies to all atypical antipsychotics but not to conventional antipsychotic drugs, a study by Wang and colleagues (2005) found a significantly higher adjusted risk of death in elderly patients taking conventional antipsychotics compared with those taking atypical antipsychotic medications, whether or not the patients had dementia or resided in a nursing home. The authors suggested that conventional antipsychotic medications are at least as likely as atypical agents to increase the risk of death in older adults, and that conventional drugs should not be used to replace atypical agents discontinued in response to the FDA warning.

In light of the concerns about risks of antipsychotic drugs in elderly nursing home residents with dementia, experts in the field have suggested that nonpharmacological approaches should be considered first when treating noncognitive behavioral symptoms. However, for those nursing home patients whose behavioral symptoms do not respond to nonpharmacological interventions, the decision to use an atypical antipsychotic should be based on a careful assessment of individual risk-benefit profile.

Three randomized clinical trials evaluated the efficacy of mood-stabilizing anticonvulsant drugs for the treatment of agitation and aggression in nursing home residents. The first was a study of carbamazepine that showed it to be effective for agitation and aggression but not for psychotic symptoms such as delusions and hallucinations (Tariot et al. 1998). In this study, nursing reports indicated that less staff time was required for patient care in the group treated with carbamazepine. Another placebo-controlled study evaluated divalproex and found evidence for its efficacy in reducing agitated behavior (Porsteinsson et al. 2001), although sedation and diminished oral intake may be problems in elderly nursing home residents with dementia. However, the most recent controlled trial of divalproex, in 153 nursing home residents with Alzheimer's dementia complicated by agitation, showed no treatment benefit (Tariot et al. 2005).

Acetylcholinesterase inhibitors have been shown to delay the decline in cognitive function in patients with mild to moderate Alzheimer's disease. However, little is known about the effects of these agents in more advanced dementia, which is commonly found in nursing home populations. One randomized clinical trial of donepezil in nursing home residents showed effects on cognitive performance that were comparable to those observed in less impaired outpatients (Tariot et al. 2001). A few studies have examined the effects of acetylcholinesterase inhibitors on behavioral disturbances, usually as a secondary outcome measure in outpatients, and some findings suggested that these agents may be useful for treating such disturbances in nursing home residents (Cummings et al. 2005; Kaufer et al. 1998; J.C. Morris et al. 1998). Prospective trials are needed to evaluate effects on behavioral disturbances in nursing home populations.

There have been only four randomized clinical trials evaluating the effects of antidepressants in nursing home residents. The first study, which was placebo controlled, showed a positive response to nortriptyline for treatment of major depression in a long-term-care population with high levels of medical comorbidity (Katz et al. 1990). In the second study, patients were randomly assigned to receive regular or low-dosage nortriptyline, and significant plasma level–response relationships were demonstrated in cognitively intact patients (Streim et al. 2000). These findings again confirmed the validity of the diagnosis of depression in nursing home residents in the context of significant medical comorbidity and disability. However, in patients with dementia, the plasma level–response relationship was significantly different, suggesting that the depression occurring in dementia might be a treatment-relevant subtype of depression or a distinct disorder.

A controlled antidepressant trial in nursing home residents with late-stage Alzheimer's disease showed no significant benefits of sertraline over placebo (Magai et al. 2000). Available open-label studies of the efficacy of serotonin reuptake inhibitors (SRIs) in nursing home residents with depression have had mixed results, some consistent with the findings of Magai and coworkers, suggesting that SRIs may be less effective for depression in patients with dementia than in those who are cognitively intact (see Oslin et al. 2000; Rosen et al. 2000; Trappler and Cohen 1996, 1998).

Although the SRIs might be expected to be well tolerated by frail elderly nursing home patients because of their side-effect profile, there is evidence that these drugs can cause serious adverse events in this population. Thapa et al. (1998) demonstrated that the use of SRIs was associated with a nearly twofold increase in the risk of falls in nursing home residents, comparable to the risk found with tricyclic antidepressant drugs. Investigators in the United Kingdom reported that antidepressant use was associated with better physical functioning but also with greater frequency of falls in residential care patients (Arthur et al. 2002). A recently completed randomized trial found that venlafaxine was less well tolerated compared with sertraline in frail nursing home patients without conferring more treatment benefits, as might be expected from an agent with mixed serotonergic and noradrenergic effects (Oslin et al. 2003).

Deficient Mental Health Care as an Impetus for Nursing Home Reform

Although psychiatric disorders are extraordinarily common among nursing home residents, and efficacious treatments exist, psychiatric services are often not adequate. Historically, nursing home design, staffing, programs, services, and funding have not evolved to meet the needs of patients with mental disorders (Streim and Katz 1994). This mismatch of psychiatric needs and available treatment led not only to neglect but also to inappropriate treatment, in which psychiatric problems were often mismanaged by using physical or chemical restraints.

Physical Restraints

A 1977 survey of American nursing home residents showed that 25% of 1.3 million people were restrained by geriatric chairs, cuffs, belts, or similar devices, primarily in an attempt to control behavioral symptoms (National Center for Health Statistics 1979). Other early surveys demonstrated rates of restraint as high as 85%. Potential adverse effects of restraints include an increased risk of falls and other injuries (Capezuti et al. 1996), as well as functional decline, skin breakdown, physiological effects of immobilization stress, disorganized behavior, and demoralization.

Although mechanical restraints have frequently been used in attempts to control agitation, they do not, in fact, decrease behavioral disturbances (Werner et al. 1989), and cross-national studies indicated that it is possible to manage nursing home residents without such measures (Cape 1983; Evans and Strumpf 1989; Innes and Turman 1983).

Misuse of Psychotropic Drugs

Concerns about inadequate and inappropriate care have also focused on the overuse of psychotropic drugs in nursing home residents, especially the misuse of these drugs as "chemical restraints" to control patient behaviors. Studies in the 1970s and 1980s reported that approximately 50% of residents had orders for psychotropic medications, with 20%–40% taking antipsychotic drugs and 10%–40% taking anxiolytics or hypnotics (Avorn et al. 1989; Beers et al. 1988; Buck 1988; Burns et al. 1988; Cohen-Mansfield 1986; Custer et al. 1984; DeLeo et al. 1989; Ray et al. 1980; Teeter et al. 1976; Zimmer et al. 1984). Psychotropic drugs were frequently prescribed without adequate regard for the residents' psychiatric diagnosis or medical status (Avorn et al. 1989; Zimmer et al. 1984).

Despite evidence for the efficacy of antipsychotic drugs in managing psychosis and agitation in nursing home residents with dementia, patients with nonpsychotic behavioral problems may be appropriately managed with other medications, behavioral treatments, interpersonal approaches, or environmental interventions. Moreover, it is important to note that, whereas all the evidence for the efficacy of antipsychotic medications comes from short-term studies, these medications are frequently prescribed for long-term treatment. In this context, concerns about overuse of antipsychotic drugs were supported by findings from drug discontinuation studies (cited above).

Inadequate Treatment of Depression

Although the focus of public concern and regulatory scrutiny in the 1970s and 1980s was on overprescription of antipsychotic medications in patients with dementia, undertreatment of other psychiatric conditions in the nursing home has also been a serious problem. The Institute of Medicine (1986) report "Improving the Quality of Care in Nursing Homes," which did much to stimulate nursing home reform, highlighted problems both in the overuse of antipsychotic drugs and in the underuse of antidepressants for treatment of affective disorders. Similarly, in reviewing epidemiological studies on the use of psychotropics in nursing homes, Murphy (1989) noted that antidepressants were the one class of drugs that appeared to be underused and that as a result, major depression in this setting often remained untreated.

Federal Regulations and Psychiatric Care in the Nursing Home

The misuse of physical and chemical restraints was a rallying point for advocacy groups that urged the federal government to institute a process of nursing home reform. Apparently in response to this and other concerns, Congress enacted the Nursing Home Reform Act as part of the Omnibus Budget Reconciliation Act of 1987 (OBRA-87) (Public Law 100-203). This legislation provided for government regulation of the operation of nursing facilities and of the care that they provide (Elon and Pawlson 1992). The legislation also directed the Health Care Financing Administration (HCFA; now renamed) to issue guidelines that assist federal and state surveyors in interpreting the regulations (Health Care Financing Administration 1992a). Mental health screening, assessment, care planning, and treatment are addressed under sections of the regulations that pertain to resident assessment, resident rights and facility practices, and quality of care.

Regulations requiring comprehensive assessment for all residents (Health Care Financing Administration 1991) led to development of a uniform Resident Assessment Instrument, which includes the Minimum Data Set (MDS) (J.N. Morris et al. 1990). This instrument must be adminis-

tered on a regular basis by members of an interdisciplinary health care team; usually a nurse is responsible for its completion (Health Care Financing Administration 1992c). Areas of assessment relevant to mental illness and behavior include mood, cognition, communication, functional status, medications, and other treatments.

Responses on the MDS suggesting that there may be a need to reevaluate a patient's clinical status and treatment plan serve as triggers for completing Resident Assessment Protocols (RAPs). These protocols 1) define medical conditions, psychiatric disorders, adverse treatment effects, functional impairments, and disabilities that are common among nursing home residents, 2) note differential diagnoses and potential causal and aggravating factors, 3) outline procedures for evaluation, and 4) list key elements of management or treatment (Health Care Financing Administration 1992c). The MDS and RAPs together are designed as a two-stage assessment system, with a screening survey followed by a focused clinical evaluation. RAP problem areas related to mental disorders and behavior include delirium, cognitive loss and dementia, psychosocial well-being, mood state, behavior problems, psychotropic drug use, and physical restraints. The individual RAPs are designed to 1) help nursing home staff recognize common signs and symptom clusters that are indicators of clinically significant problems, 2) conduct evaluations that use standardized algorithms, and 3) determine whether it is necessary to alter the treatment plan. The regulations hold facilities responsible for ensuring that RAPs are followed appropriately. Although physicians have no mandated role in this process, physician involvement is clearly necessary for proper diagnosis and treatment of conditions covered by the RAPs (Elon and Pawlson 1992). Psychiatric consultation may be needed when RAPs indicate a need for the evaluation of problems related to mental health.

Regulations related to resident rights and facility practices restrict the use of physical restraints and antipsychotic drugs when they are "administered for purposes of discipline or convenience and not required to treat the resident's medical symptoms" (Health Care Financing Administration 1991, p. 48,875 [tag F204]). Regulations related to quality of care further require that residents not receive "unnecessary drugs" and specify that antipsychotic drugs may not be given "unless these are necessary to treat a specific condition as diagnosed and documented in the clinical record" (p. 48,910 [tag F307]). An unnecessary drug is defined as any drug used 1) in excessive dose (including duplicate therapy), 2) for excessive duration, 3) without adequate monitoring, 4) without adequate indications for its use, 5) in the presence of adverse consequences that indicate that it should be reduced or discontinued, or 6) for any combination of the first five reasons (Health Care Financing Administration 1991). The guidelines based on these regulations further limit the use of antipsychotic drugs, antianxiety agents, sedative-hypnotics, and related drugs (Health Care Financing Administration 1992a). For each of these classes, the guidelines specify a list of acceptable indications, upper limits for daily doses, requirements for monitoring treatment and adverse effects, and time frames for attempting dose reductions and discontinuation. These guidelines were updated in 2000 to reflect new clinical knowledge and the availability of new drugs approved by the FDA (Health Care Financing Administration 2000). In addition to addressing the use of psychotropic drugs, the interpretive guidelines also outline conditions for the use of physical restraints.

To minimize concerns about federal interference with medical practice, the current guidelines include qualifying statements that recognize cases in which strict adherence to prescribing limits is "clinically contraindicated." Thus, the physician's options for treating nursing home residents need not be restricted by the regulations if the clinical rationale—explaining that the benefits of treatment (in terms of symptom relief, improved health status, or improved functioning) outweigh the risks—is clearly documented in the medical record. Although the facility, not the physician, is accountable for compliance with the regulations, the physician's clinical reasoning and judgment play a critical role in the process of ensuring quality care.

Although much of the emphasis of the federal regulations is on eliminating inappropriate treatment, there are also requirements for the provision of necessary and appropriate care for residents with mental health problems. Under the provisions designed to ensure quality of care, federal regulations define a need for geriatric psychiatry services in nursing homes, requiring that "the facility must ensure that a resident who displays mental or psychosocial adjustment difficulties receives appropriate services to correct the assessed problem" (Health Care Financing Administration 1991, p. 48,896 [tag F272]).

More recently, within the scope of its responsibility as a payer, HCFA developed a system for assessing the quality of care provided in United States nursing homes. To enable surveyors to compare individual facilities within the same state, HCFA introduced quality indicators (QIs) derived from MDS data (Clark 1999). There are 24 QIs in 11 different domains, including behavior and emotional problems, cognitive patterns, and psychotropic drug use. Whenever a review in any of these areas results in a citation of deficiency, a plan of correction must be developed and submitted for approval. This system is a first step in monitoring quality of care, although the face validity of some of the QIs has been questioned and the results of quality surveys may be difficult to interpret. Nevertheless, the results from every nursing home surveyed are available for public inspection on the Centers for Medicare and Medicaid Services Web site, and consumers of nursing home services (and their families) are beginning to pay attention to the QI reports.

Changing Patterns of Psychiatric Care

Since the implementation of the Nursing Home Reform Act in 1990, there have been significant changes in nursing home care, including mental health care. Some of these changes may be attributed to the process of conducting surveys and enforcing federal regulations; however, several other factors appear to have contributed, including the dissemination of information about regulatory requirements, availability and marketing of new medications, advances in scientific knowledge from nursing home research, and cumulative effects of professional education regarding good clinical practice. Increasing consumer awareness is also likely to have played a role.

Shifts in Antipsychotic Drug Use

Studies of the effect of federal regulations in the early years after implementation showed a substantial decline in the use of antipsychotic drugs (Shorr et al. 1994) and physical restraints (Hawes et al. 1997) and increases in antidepressant use (Lantz et al. 1996). One study reported that greater reductions in antipsychotic use during this period were found in nursing facilities with an emphasis on psychosocial care, a less severe case mix, and a higher nurse-to-resident ratio (Svarstad et al. 2001). Soon after the regulations were introduced, several investigators developed educational programs for physicians, nurses,

and aides, teaching practice principles consistent with federal guidelines. Studies evaluating these educational interventions demonstrated reductions of 23%–72% in the use of antipsychotic drugs (Avorn et al. 1992; Meador et al. 1997; Ray et al. 1993; Rovner et al. 1992; Schnelle et al. 1992). Studies of the appropriateness of antipsychotic use examining documentation of OBRA-approved diagnostic indications and appropriate target symptoms, and dosing within the recommended limits in the HCFA guidelines, suggest relatively high rates of compliance with the OBRA regulations (Llorente et al. 1998; Siegler et al. 1997). Although the changes found by the studies were generally interpreted as an indication of improvement in care, the studies did not examine health care outcomes or the effect on residents' quality of life (Snowden and Roy-Byrne 1998) and did not address concerns that reductions in medication use might have an adverse effect on patients who required antipsychotic treatment.

In contrast to the declining rates of antipsychotic use in the early 1990s, Online Survey Certification and Reporting (OSCAR) data showed a reversal in this trend from 1995 to 1999, with the national rate for antipsychotic drug use in nursing homes increasing from 16% to 19.4% during that period (American Society of Consultant Pharmacists 2000). Despite this increase, a survey conducted by the Office of the Inspector General of the Department of Health and Human Services, based on data from the year 2000, found that psychotropic drugs were appropriately prescribed in 85% of 485 cases reviewed (Office of Inspector General 2001c).

However, the Office of the Inspector General findings are contradicted by a large retrospective analysis of Medicare databases merged to minimum data set assessments from the same time period (Briesacher et al. 2005). In this analysis, 27.6% of all

Medicare beneficiaries in nursing homes received antipsychotic drugs during 2000–2001, and of the treated patients, only 41.8% received antipsychotic therapy within federal prescribing guidelines. There are still no prospective studies that have examined the effect of compliance with the federal guidelines or of the changing rates of psychotropic drug use on resident outcomes such as symptom control, functional status, and quality of life.

The increased rates of antipsychotic drug use, coupled with the safety concerns related to the risk of cardiovascular adverse events and mortality, have prompted a closer look at alternatives to antipsychotic drug treatment of behavioral disturbances in nursing home residents with dementia. A study by Fossey and colleagues (2006), conducted in the wake of the safety findings described earlier in this chapter, examined 12-month outcomes of an intervention providing training and support to nursing home staff for psychosocial approaches to managing agitated behavior associated with dementia. The rate of antipsychotic drug use was 19.1% lower in the intervention homes, with no significant differences in the level of agitated or disruptive behavior between intervention and control facilities. Thus, it appears that a significant proportion of residents may be managed with less risk without a concomitant increase in behavioral problems. Nevertheless, changes in the prevalence of antipsychotic drug use specifically in response to safety concerns have not yet been documented in nursing home populations.

Increase in Antidepressant Drug Use

Despite the decline in use of antipsychotic drugs in the early 1990s, there was an increase in the use of antidepressants from 12.6% to 24.9% (a 97.6% increase) between 1991 and 1997 (Health Care Financing Administration 1998). Since the mid-1990s, there has been emerging evidence of further increases in the prevalence of antidepressant use. According to OSCAR data (American Society of Consultant Pharmacists 2000), 35.5% of United States nursing home patients had prescriptions for antidepressant medication in 2001, ranging from 27.9% in Hawaii to 62.7% in Utah. A study of five Pennsylvania nursing homes similarly found that 47.6% of residents were taking antidepressants (Datto et al. 2002). Before 1990, fewer than 15% of residents with a known diagnosis of depression were receiving antidepressant medication (Heston et al. 1992).

Considered together, these data represent an extraordinary change in the pattern of drug use in a population that has traditionally received inadequate pharmacotherapy for depression. The dramatic increase in antidepressant prescriptions is probably due in part to the wide availability of newer antidepressants that are thought to be well tolerated by elderly nursing home residents with medical-psychiatric comorbidity. Aggressive marketing to primary care physicians may also play a role. With current antidepressant drug use rates that appear comparable to or greater than the estimated prevalence of depression in nursing homes, it is possible that a significant proportion of antidepressant prescriptions are intended for indications other than depression, such as sleep, pain, or agitation. Research is needed to determine whether the reported changes in prescribing have had a positive effect on the mental health of nursing home residents with depression.

Decline in Physical Restraint Use

Although questions remain about the interpretation of trends in psychotropic drug use (Lantz et al. 1996), the effect of the federal regulations on restraints appears to be positive, with several studies showing significant reductions in the use of physical restraints (Castle et al. 1997). One study found restraint use rates of 37.4% in 1990 (before OBRA-87 implementation in October 1990) and 28.1% in 1993 (after introduction of the standardized Resident Assessment Instrument required by OBRA-87) (Hawes et al. 1997). Siegler et al. (1997) found that restraint use could be significantly reduced without a resultant increase in antipsychotic or benzodiazepine use. There are no published studies showing an increase in fall-related injuries associated with lower rates of physical restraint use.

Special Care Units

Encouraged by consumer demand to better meet the needs of nursing home residents with dementia, 10% of United States nursing homes had established special care units (SCUs) by 1991. A decade later, it was estimated that 22% of nursing homes had designated SCUs for patients with dementia. Research on the effectiveness of SCUs is difficult to interpret and generalize because of the heterogeneity of these facilities (Office of Technology Assessment 1992; Ohta and Ohta 1988). Of note, more than 90% of residents in SCUs have behavior problems (Wagner et al. 1995).

Some studies indicate that the facilities, services, and programs offered by SCUs may not be significantly better than those available on conventional nursing home units. A case-control study of 625 patients in 31 SCUs and 32 traditional units found that residence in an SCU was associated with reduced use of physical restraints but not with less use of "pharmacological restraints" (Sloane et al. 1991). A subsequent study that included data on more than 1,100 residents in 48 SCUs reported that the use of physical restraints was not different, and the likelihood of psychotropic

medication use was actually greater, for patients on SCUs than for their counterparts on traditional units (Phillips et al. 2000). These authors suggested that residents of SCUs might even receive a poorer quality of care than that provided to similar residents in traditional units. Although evidence suggests that mobility may be maintained for longer among residents of SCUs (Saxton et al. 1998), others have found that the rate of decline in ADL function is not significantly slower for SCU residents (Phillips et al. 1997).

Studies showing benefits of SCUs for behavioral disturbances are limited, and randomized clinical trials reporting positive outcomes of SCU residency have been limited to reduced frequency of catastrophic reactions (Swanson et al. 1993)—sudden agitated behavior in response to overwhelming external stimuli. Some studies have demonstrated psychological benefits not only for patients (Lawton et al. 1998) but also for caregivers (Kutner et al. 1999; Wells and Jorm 1987), with evidence of increased family involvement (Hansen et al. 1988; Sloane et al. 1998).

Despite the efforts of these investigators, there is still insufficient knowledge about the essential elements of treatment in SCUs, and evidence for the effectiveness of these units has not been adequately demonstrated.

Subacute Care in Nursing Homes

Over the past 20 years, many patients have been discharged to nursing homes that serve as step-down facilities, providing subacute medical treatment, convalescent care, and rehabilitation services.

In general, short-stay residents—patients who, after relatively brief stays in nursing homes, are discharged to the community or die—differ from long-term-care patients in that they are younger; more likely to be admitted directly from an acute-care hospital; less likely to have irreversible cognitive impairment, incontinence, or ambulatory dysfunction; and more likely to have a primary diagnosis of hip fracture, stroke, or cancer. The objectives of mental health care for short-stay patients are related not so much to managing behavior problems associated with dementia as to helping patients cope with disease and disability, to searching for reversible causes of cognitive impairment, and to treating disorders such as depression and anxiety that can be impediments to rehabilitation and recovery.

In short, the objectives of mental health care for these patients are similar to the goals of traditional consultation-liaison psychiatry in the general hospital. As the opportunities for psychiatric intervention follow these patients from the acute-care hospital into the nursing homes, the services required may need to be more frequent or intensive than those usually available to long-term-care residents. Enhanced mental health services will increase opportunities for tradeoffs in which an increased investment in psychiatric care can lead to more independent functioning and more rapid discharge to the community. It is hoped that the benefits of mental health care, in terms of both cost offsets and improved quality of life, will provide a strong incentive for insurers, public and private, to establish reimbursement policies that facilitate such treatment.

Adequacy of Care

The high prevalence of psychiatric problems and the federal mandate to ensure quality of care define a need for geriatric mental health services in nursing homes (Smith et al. 1990). Although the OBRA regulations are having the intended impact (Snowden and Roy-Byrne 1998) and have resulted in measurable improvements in patient care, it has not been shown that the federal requirements for assessment and treatment of mental disorders have led to improved case identification, access to mental health care, receipt of appropriate care, or improved health care outcomes. Medicare claims data in 1992, 2 years after implementation of the Nursing Home Reform Act of 1987, indicated that only 36% of residents with a mental illness received psychiatric services (Smyer et al. 1994), and evidence shows continued low levels of mental health treatment in nursing homes (Shea et al. 2000).

There are also concerns that required assessments using the MDS *after* admission do not provide adequate detection of depression (Brown et al. 2002; Office of Inspector General 2001b; Schnelle et al. 2001). In examining the data from 1,492 nursing homes across five states, Brown and coworkers (2002) found that 11% of residents were identified on the MDS as depressed, half the rate that was expected on the basis of epidemiological studies that used direct clinical assessments. Of the 11% detected, only 55% received antidepressant therapy. Thus, even when mental disorders are identified, detection does not routinely result in treatment.

Limited access to care appears to be at least part of the problem. In a survey of nursing homes across six states, conducted by Reichman et al. (1998), 47.6% of 899 respondents indicated that the frequency of on-site psychiatric consultation was inadequate. Directors of nursing judged 38% of nursing home residents as needing a psychiatric evaluation, but more than one-fourth of rural facilities and more than one-fifth of small facilities reported that no psychiatric consultant was available to them. Meeting the demand for mental

health treatment may also be more difficult for nursing facilities that are part of a
chain or contain Medicaid beds (Castle
and Shea 1997). Thus, there is evidence
that the federal requirement that patients
receive services to "attain or maintain the
highest practicable physical, mental, and
psychosocial well-being" has not remedied
the problem of access to mental health
services in United States nursing homes
(Colenda et al. 1999).

Even among patients whose mental disorders are recognized and for whom treatment is initiated, there is evidence that
treatment is often inadequate. A report by
Brown et al. (2002) indicated that, of nursing home residents known to be depressed
and receiving antidepressants, 32% were
taking doses less than the manufacturers'
recommended minimum effective dose
for treating depression. In a survey of five
nursing homes, Datto and colleagues (2002)
found 47% of patients were taking antidepressants, but nearly half of these patients were still depressed. Although a small
proportion of these residents may have
been in the early stages of treatment, before a treatment response could reasonably be expected, it appears likely that
many residents did not receive proper follow-up care with required dose adjustments or changes in therapy for those who
were not responsive to initial treatment.
This finding points to a need for nursing
home providers to improve adherence to
practice guidelines for the follow-up care
of depression.

A recently introduced federal QI focuses on persistence of depression. Prescription of an antidepressant suggests that
depression has been recognized and diagnosed and that the first step has been taken
to manage it. However, persistence of depression in a patient who is receiving an
antidepressant drug suggests that the treatment may not be adequate. Thus, if the

proportion of depressed patients receiving
antidepressants is high, it may indicate
that the facility is doing a good job of recognizing depression and initiating treatment, but it may also suggest it is not doing an adequate job of monitoring patients'
response to treatment and modifying treatments as needed to produce optimal outcomes.

Mental Health Care in Nursing Homes: A Model for Service Delivery

The high prevalence of psychiatric disorders in nursing homes argues for the importance of establishing systems that incorporate mental health into the basic
services provided (Borson et al. 1987). In
addition, several factors argue for the importance of the professional components
of care: 1) the complex nature of the psychiatric disorders exhibited by nursing
home residents, 2) the need to evaluate
medical as well as social and environmental factors as causes of mental health problems, 3) the potential benefits of specific
treatments, and 4) the need for careful
monitoring to assess treatment responses
and prevent serious adverse effects of medications. Thus, clinical needs demand that
mental health services in nursing homes
have two distinct but interacting systems:
one that is intrinsic to the facility and con-
textual, another that is professional and
concerned primarily with the delivery of
specific treatments.

It has been suggested that mental health
training should be provided to facility
staff to develop basic skills in assessment
and clinical management that can help staff
handle problems that occur when specific
professional services are lacking. However,
it is important to recognize that the intrinsic and the professional systems cannot

readily replace each other and that adequate care requires both. Although there is a real need for staff training, a realistic goal is to develop staff skills that complement rather than replace the activities of mental health professionals. This two-system model has obvious implications with respect to the financing of mental health services in nursing homes: it demonstrates the need to fund mental health care both as a necessary part of the per diem costs of nursing home care and as a reimbursable professional service.

Although the intrinsic and the professional systems for mental health services are distinct, they must interact: Geriatric psychiatrists and psychologists and geropsychiatric nurse-practitioners can play important intrinsic roles as administrative and staff consultants, in-service educators, moderators of case conferences, participants in interdisciplinary team meetings, and contributors in other activities familiar to the consultation-liaison psychiatrist. Facility staff must be effective in recognizing problems, facilitating referral, supporting treatment, and monitoring outcome to enable the professional system to function optimally.

Intrinsic System

The intrinsic system of mental health care in nursing homes can be conceptualized as including a wide range of components: design of the environment; implementation of psychosocial programs; formulation of institutional policies and procedures for assessment, care delivery, monitoring, and quality improvement; and optimization of the ways in which staff and residents interact. The importance of the intrinsic system is recognized in nursing home regulations that require training of nursing aides; in the nursing staff assessments required for completion of the MDS and RAPs; and in OBRA requirements that nursing homes provide assessments, treatment planning,

and services to attain or maintain the highest practicable level of mental and physical well-being for each resident. Because psychiatric disorders are common in nursing homes, nurses and aides should be knowledgeable about the nature of the cognitive and functional deficits associated with dementia and the manifestations of delirium and depression. Staff members should understand how to modify their approach to working with residents when cognitive impairment or communication deficits interfere with care. Staff should also know how to apply basic principles of behavioral psychology to identify the causes of agitation and related behavioral symptoms in patients with dementia, as well as how to plan environmental and behavioral interventions.

Professional System

The intrinsic system for mental health services as described above is necessary but not sufficient to meet the needs of nursing home residents. In addition, the services of mental health professionals are important in evaluating the interactions between medical and mental health problems, in establishing psychiatric diagnoses, and in planning and administering specific treatments for mental disorders. This component of the professional system must encompass medically oriented psychiatric care, including psychopharmacological treatment. The complexity of psychopharmacological treatment in frail nursing home residents with medical comorbidity requires that the skills of psychiatrists knowledgeable in geriatrics be an integral part of the professional system.

The professional system should include care with a psychosocial focus as well as a biomedical focus. For example, psychiatrists, psychologists, and psychiatric nurse-practitioners with specific expertise in behavioral treatment may be successful in evaluating the antecedents and causes of agitation and related symptoms among patients with dementia and in developing environmental and behavioral interventions, even when efforts by the facility's nursing staff have proven ineffective.

Integration of the professional and intrinsic components of mental health care in the nursing home is required because of the inherent interdependence of these systems. To conduct valid assessments and make diagnoses, mental health professionals must rely on nursing home staff to report their shift-by-shift observations of residents' behavior and other clinical signs. Mental health professionals must also depend on nursing home staff to implement and monitor the treatments they prescribe. Conversely, to succeed in providing appropriate mental health care to nursing home residents, staff members in the intrinsic system must have access to ongoing consultation from, and must receive direct support from, mental health professionals who are knowledgeable in geriatrics.

References

Abraham IL, Neundorfer MM, Currie LJ: Effects of group interventions on cognition and depression in nursing home residents. Nurs Res 41:196–202, 1992

Abraham IL, Onega LL, Reel SJ, et al: Effects of cognitive group interventions on depressed frail nursing home residents, in Depression in Long Term and Residential Care: Advances in Research and Treatment. Edited by Rubinstein RL, Lawton MP. New York, Springer, 1997, pp 154–168

Alessi CA: A randomized trial of a combined physical activity and environmental intervention in nursing home residents: do sleep and agitation improve? J Am Geriatr Soc 47:784–791, 1999

Allen-Burge R, Stevens AB, Burgio LD: Effective behavioral interventions for decreasing dementia-related challenging behavior in nursing homes. Int J Geriatr Psychiatry 14:213–228, 1999

American Association for Geriatric Psychiatry, American Geriatrics Society, American Psychiatric Association: Psychotherapeutic medications in the nursing home. J Am Geriatr Soc 40:946–949, 1992

American Psychiatric Association: Diagnostic and Statistical Manual of Mental Disorders, 3rd Edition. Washington, DC, American Psychiatric Association, 1980

American Psychiatric Association: Diagnostic and Statistical Manual of Mental Disorders, 3rd Edition, Revised. Washington, DC, American Psychiatric Association, 1987

American Society of Consultant Pharmacists: Fact Sheet. Alexandria, VA, American Society of Consultant Pharmacists, September, 2000

Ames D: Depression among elderly residents of local-authority residential homes: its nature and the efficacy of intervention. Br J Psychiatry 156:667–675, 1990

Ames D: Epidemiological studies of depression among the elderly in residential and nursing homes. Int J Geriatr Psychiatry 6:347–354, 1991

Ames D, Ashby D, Mann AH, et al: Psychiatric illness in elderly residents of part III homes in one London borough: prognosis and review. Age Ageing 17:249–256, 1988

Arthur A, Matthews R, Jagger C, et al: Factors associated with antidepressant treatment in residential care: changes between 1990 and 1997. Int J Geriatr Psychiatry 17:54–60, 2002

Ashby D, Ames D, West CR, et al: Psychiatric morbidity as prediction of mortality for residents of local authority homes for the elderly. Int J Geriatr Psychiatry 6:567–575, 1991

Avorn J, Langer E: Induced disability in nursing home patients: a controlled trial. J Am Geriatr Soc 30:397–400, 1982

Avorn J, Dreyer P, Connelly K, et al: Use of psychoactive medication and the quality of care in rest homes: findings and policy implications of a statewide study. N Engl J Med 320:227–232, 1989

Avorn J, Soumerai SD, Everitt DE, et al: A randomized trial of a program to reduce the use of psychoactive drugs in nursing homes. N Engl J Med 327:168–173, 1992

Baines S, Saxby P, Ehlert K: Reality orientation and reminiscence therapy. Br J Psychiatry 151:222–231, 1987

Baker FM, Miller CL: Screening a skilled nursing home population for depression. J Geriatr Psychiatry Neurol 4:218–221, 1991

Banziger G, Roush S: Nursing homes for the birds: a control-relevant intervention with bird feeders. Gerontologist 23:527–531, 1983

Barnes RD, Raskind MA: DSM-III criteria and the clinical diagnosis of dementia: a nursing home study. J Gerontol 36:20–27, 1980

Barnes R, Veith R, Okimoto J, et al: Efficacy of antipsychotic medications in behaviorally disturbed dementia patients. Am J Psychiatry 139:1170–1174, 1982

Barton R, Hurst L: Unnecessary use of tranquilizers in elderly patients. Br J Psychiatry 112:989–990, 1966

Beck CK, Vogelpohl TS, Rasin JH, et al: Effects of behavioral interventions on disruptive behavior and affect in demented nursing home residents. Nurs Res 51:219–228, 2002

Beers M, Avon J, Soumerai SB, et al: Psychoactive medication use in intermediate-care facility residents. JAMA 260:3016–3020, 1988

Bensink GW, Godbey KL, Marshall MJ, et al: Institutionalized elderly: relaxation, locus of control, self-esteem. J Gerontol Nurs 18:30–36, 1992

Berrios GE, Brook P: Delusions and psychopathology of the elderly with dementia. Acta Psychiatr Scand 75:296–301, 1985

Blazer DG, Williams CD: Epidemiology of dysphoria and depression in an elderly population. Am J Psychiatry 137:439–444, 1980

Borson S, Liptzin B, Nininger J, et al: Psychiatry and the nursing home. Am J Psychiatry 144:1412–1418, 1987

Borson S, Loebel JP, Kitchell M, et al: Psychiatric assessments of nursing home residents under OBRA-87: should PASARR be reformed? Pre-Admission Screening and Annual Review. J Am Geriatr Soc 45:1173–1181, 1997

Braun JV, Wykle MH, Cowling WR: Failure to thrive in older persons: a concept derived. Gerontologist 28:809–812, 1988

Bridges-Parlet S, Knopman D, Steffes S: Withdrawal of neuroleptic medications from institutionalized dementia patients: results of a double-blind, baseline-treatment-controlled pilot study. J Geriatr Psychiatry Neurol 10:119–126, 1997

Briesacher BA, Limcangco R, Simoni-Wastila L, et al: The quality of antipsychotic drug prescribing in nursing homes. Arch Intern Med 165:1280–1285, 2005

Brodaty H, Ames D, Snowdon J, et al: A randomized placebo-controlled trial of risperidone for the treatment of aggression, agitation, and psychosis of dementia. J Clin Psychiatry 64:134–143, 2003

Brown MN, Lapane KL, Luisi AF: Management of depression in older nursing home residents. J Am Geriatr Soc 50:69–76, 2002

Buck JA: Psychotropic drug practice in nursing homes. J Am Geriatr Soc 36:409–418, 1988

Burns BJ, Taube CA: Mental health services in general medical care and in nursing homes, in Mental Health Policy for Older Americans: Protecting Minds at Risk. Edited by Fogel BS, Furino A, Gottlieb GL. Washington, DC, American Psychiatric Press, 1990, pp 63–84

Burns BJ, Larson DB, Goldstrom ID, et al: Mental disorder among nursing home patients: preliminary findings from the National Nursing Home Survey Pretest. Int J Geriatr Psychiatry 3:27–35, 1988

Cape RD: Freedom from restraint. Gerontologist 23:217, 1983

Capezuti E, Evans L, Strumpf N, et al: Physical restraint use and falls in nursing home residents. J Am Geriatrics Soc 44:627–633, 1996

Castle NG, Shea D: Institutional factors of nursing homes that predict the provision of mental health services. J Ment Health Adm 24:44–54, 1997

Castle NG, Fogel B, Mor V: Risk factors for physical restraint use in nursing homes: pre- and post-implementation of Nursing Home Reform Act. Gerontologist 37:737–747, 1997

Chandler JD, Chandler JE: The prevalence of neuropsychiatric disorders in a nursing home population. J Geriatr Psychiatry Neurol 1:71–76, 1988

Clark TR (ed): Nursing Home Survey Procedures and Interpretive Guidelines. A Resource for the Consultant Pharmacist. Alexandria, VA, American Society of Consultant Pharmacists, 1999, pp 1–8

Cohen-Mansfield J: Agitated behaviors in the elderly: preliminary results in the cognitively deteriorated. J Am Geriatr Soc 34: 722–727, 1986

Cohen-Mansfield J: Nonpharmacologic interventions for inappropriate behaviors in dementia: a review, summary, and critique. Am J Geriatr Psychiatry 9:361–381, 2001

Cohen-Mansfield J, Billig N: Agitated behaviors in the elderly: a conceptual review. J Am Geriatr Soc 34:711–721, 1986

Cohen-Mansfield J, Marx MS, Rosenthal AS: A description of agitation in a nursing home. J Gerontol 44:M77–M84, 1989

Cohen-Mansfield J, Lipson S, Werner P, et al: Withdrawal of haloperidol, thioridazine, and lorazepam in the nursing home: a controlled, double-blind study. Arch Intern Med 159:1733–1740, 1999

Colenda CC, Streim JE, Greene JA, et al: The impact of the Omnibus Budget Reconciliation Act of 1987 (OBRA '87) on psychiatric services in nursing homes. Am J Geriatr Psychiatry 7:12–17, 1999

Cummings JL, Koumaras B, Chen M, et al: Effects of rivastigmine treatment on the neuropsychiatric and behavioral disturbances of nursing home residents with moderate and severe probable Alzheimer's disease: a 26-week, multicenter, open-label study. Am J Geriatr Pharmacother 3:137–148, 2005

Custer RL, Davis JE, Gee SC: Psychiatric drug usage in VA nursing home care units. Psychiatr Ann 14:285–292, 1984

Datto C, Oslin D, Streim J, et al: Pharmacological treatment of depression in nursing home residents: a mental health services perspective. J Geriatr Psychiatry Neurol 15:141–146, 2002

DeDeyn PP, Rabheru K, Rasmussen A, et al: A randomized trial of risperidone, placebo, and haloperidol for behavioral symptoms of dementia. Neurology 53:946–955, 1999

DeLeo D, Stella AG, Spagnoli A: Prescription of psychotropic drugs in geriatric institutions. Int J Geriatr Psychiatry 4:11–16, 1989

Elon R, Pawlson LG: The impact of OBRA on medical practice within nursing facilities. J Am Geriatr Soc 40:958–963, 1992

Engle VF, Graney MJ: Stability and improvement of health after nursing home admission. J Gerontol 48:S17–S23, 1993

Evans LK, Strumpf NE: Tying down the elderly: a review of the literature on physical restraint. J Am Geriatr Soc 37:65–74, 1989

Evans JM, Chutka DS, Fleming KC, et al: Medical care of nursing home residents. Mayo Clin Proc 70:694–702, 1995

Evans LK, Strumpf NE, Allen-Taylor SL, et al: A clinical trial to reduce restraints in nursing homes. J Am Geriatr Soc 45:675–681, 1997

Fossey J, Ballard C, Juszczak E, et al: Effect of enhanced psychosocial care on antipsychotic use in nursing home residents with severe dementia: cluster randomized trial. Br Med J 332:756–761, 2006

Foster JR, Cataldo JK, Boksay IJE: Incidence of depression in a medical long-term care facility: findings from a restricted sample of new admissions. Int J Geriatr Psychiatry 6:13–20, 1991

Gabrel C, Jones A: The National Nursing Home Survey: 1995 Summary. Vital Health Stat 13(146):1–83, 2000

German PS, Shapiro S, Kramer M: Nursing home study of eastern Baltimore epidemiologic catchment area, in Mental Illness in Nursing Homes: Agenda for Research. Edited by Harper MS, Lebowitz BD. Rockville, MD, National Institute of Mental Health, 1986, pp 21–40

Goldwasser AN, Auerbach SM, Harkins SW: Cognitive, affective, and behavioral effects of reminiscence group therapy of demented elderly. Int J Aging Hum Dev 25: 209–222, 1987

Grant LA, Kane RA, Stark AJ: Beyond labels: nursing home care for Alzheimer's disease in and out of special care units. J Am Geriatr Soc 43:569–576, 1995

Hansen SS, Patterson MA, Wilson RW: Family involvement on a dementia unit: the Resident Enrichment and Activity Program. Gerontologist 28:508–510, 1988

Harrison R, Savla N, Kafetz K: Dementia, depression, and physical disability in a London borough: a survey of elderly people in and out of residential care and implications for future developments. Age Ageing 19:97–103, 1990

Hawes C, Mor V, Phillips CD, et al: The OBRA-87 nursing home regulations and implementation of the Resident Assessment Instrument: effects on process quality. J Am Geriatr Soc 45:977–985, 1997

Health Care Financing Administration: Medicare and Medicaid: Requirements for Long Term Care Facilities, Final Regulations. Fed Regist 56:48865–48921, 1991

Health Care Financing Administration: Medicare and Medicaid Programs: Preadmission Screening and Annual Resident Review. Fed Regist 57:56450–56504, 1992a

Health Care Financing Administration: Medicare and Medicaid: Resident Assessment in Long Term Care Facilities. Fed Regist 57:61614–61733, 1992b

Health Care Financing Administration: State Operations Manual: Provider Certification (Transmittal No 250). Washington, DC, Health Care Financing Administration, 1992c

Health Care Financing Administration: Report to Congress: Study of Private Accreditation (Deeming) of Nursing Homes, Regulatory Incentives and Non-Regulatory Incentives, and Effectiveness of the Survey and Certification System. Washington, DC, 1998. Available at http://cms.hhs.gov/medicaid/reports/default.asp. Accessed July 17, 2003.

Health Care Financing Administration: Appendix PP: Guidance to Survivors—Long Term Care Facilities, in Medicare State Operations Manual: Provider Certification (Transmittal No 15). Washington, DC, Health Care Financing Administration, April 2000, pp 121–164. Available at http://cms.hhs.gov/manuals/pm_trans/R15SOM.pdf. Accessed October 19, 2003.

Heston LL, Garrard J, Makris L, et al: Inadequate treatment of depressed nursing home elderly. J Am Geriatr Soc 40:1117–1122, 1992

Holmes D, Teresi J, Weiner A, et al: Impact associated with special care units in long-term care facilities. Gerontologist 30:178–181, 1990

Horiguchi J, Inami Y: A survey of the living conditions and psychological states of elderly people admitted to nursing homes in Japan. Acta Psychiatr Scand 83:338–341, 1991

Hyer L, Blazer DG: Depressive symptoms: impact and problems in long term care facilities. International Journal of Behavioral Gerontology 1:33–44, 1982

Innes EM, Turman WG: Evolution of patient falls. Q Rev Biol 9:30–35, 1983

Institute of Medicine, Committee on Nursing Home Regulation: Improving the Quality of Care in Nursing Homes. Washington, DC, National Academy Press, 1986

Jeste DV, Okamoto A, Napolitano J, et al: Low incidence of persistent tardive dyskinesia in elderly patients with dementia treated with risperidone. Am J Psychiatry 157:1150–1155, 2000

Katz IR, Lesher E, Kleban M, et al: Clinical features of depression in the nursing home. Int Psychogeriatr 1:5–15, 1989

Katz IR, Simpson GM, Curlik SM, et al: Pharmacological treatment of major depression for elderly patients in residential care settings. J Clin Psychiatry 51 (suppl):41–48, 1990

Katz IR, Parmelee P, Brubaker K: Toxic and metabolic encephalopathies in long-term care patients. Int Psychogeriatr 3:337–347, 1991

Katz IR, Beaston-Wimmer P, Parmelee PA, et al: Failure to thrive in the elderly: exploration of the concept and delineation of psychiatric components. J Geriatr Psychiatry Neurol 6:161–169, 1993

Katz IR, Jeste DV, Mintzer JE, et al: Comparison of risperidone and placebo for psychosis and behavioral disturbances associated with dementia: a randomized, double-blind trial. J Clin Psychiatry 60:107–115, 1999

Katz IR, Streim JE, Smith BD: Psychiatric aspects of long-term care, in Kaplan and Sadock's Comprehensive Textbook of Psychiatry, 7th Edition, Vol 2. Edited by Sadock BJ, Sadock VA. Philadelphia, PA, Lippincott Williams & Wilkins, 2000, pp 3145–3150

Kaufer D, Cummings JL, Christine D: Differential neuropsychiatric symptom responses to tacrine in Alzheimer's disease: relationship to dementia severity. J Neuropsychiatry Clin Neurosci 10:55–63, 1998

Kramer M, German PS, Anthony JC, et al: Patterns of mental disorders among the elderly residents of eastern Baltimore. J Am Geriatr Soc 33:236–245, 1985

Krantz DS, Schulz PR: Personal control and health: some applications to crises of middle and old age. Advances in Environmental Psychology 2:23–57, 1980

Krauss NA, Altman BM: Characteristics of Nursing Home Residents—1996. MEPS Research Findings No 5 (AHCPR Publ No 99-0006). Rockville, MD, Agency for Health Care Policy and Research, 1998

Kutner N, Mistretta E, Barnhart H, et al: Family members' perceptions of quality of life change in dementia SCU residents. J Appl Gerontol 18:423–439, 1999

Langer E, Rodin J: The effects of choice and enhanced personal responsibility for the aged: a field experiment in an institutional setting. J Pers Soc Psychol 34:191–198, 1976

Lantz MS, Giambanco V, Buchalter EN: A ten-year review of the effect of OBRA-87 on psychotropic prescribing practices in an academic nursing home. Psychiatr Serv 47:951–955, 1996

Lasser RA, Sunderland T: Newer psychotropic medication use in nursing home residents. J Am Geriatr Soc 46:202–207, 1998

Lawton MP, Van Haitsma K, Klapper J, et al: A stimulation-retreat special care unit for elders with dementing illness. Int Psychogeriatr 10:379–395, 1998

Lesher E: Validation of the Geriatric Depression Scale among nursing home residents. Clinics in Gerontology 4:21–28, 1986

Leszcz M, Sadavoy J, Feigenbaum E, et al: A men's group psychotherapy of elderly men. Int J Group Psychother 33:177–196, 1985

Llorente MD, Olsen EJ, Leyva O, et al: Use of antipsychotic drugs in nursing homes: current compliance with OBRA regulations. J Am Geriatr Soc 46:198–201, 1998

Loebel JP, Borson S, Hyde T, et al: Relationships between requests for psychiatric consultations and psychiatric diagnoses in long-term care facilities. Am J Psychiatry 148:898–903, 1991

Magai C, Kennedy G, Cohen CI, et al: A controlled clinical trial of sertraline in the treatment of depression in nursing home patients with late-stage Alzheimer's disease. Am J Geriatr Psychiatry 8:66–74, 2000

Mann AH, Graham N, Ashby D: Psychiatric illness in residential homes for the elderly: a survey in one London borough. Age Ageing 13:257–265, 1984

McMurdo MET, Rennie L: A controlled trial of exercise by residents of old people's homes. Age Ageing 22:11–15, 1993

Meador KG, Taylor JA, Thapa PB, et al: Predictors of antipsychotic withdrawal or dose reduction in a randomized controlled trial of provider education. J Am Geriatr Soc 45:207–210, 1997

Montgomery SA, Åsberg M: A new depression scale designed to be sensitive to change. Br J Psychiatry 134:381–382, 1979

Moran JA, Gatz M: Group therapies for nursing home adults: an evaluation of two treatment approaches. Gerontologist 27:588–591, 1987

Morris JC, Cyrus PS, Orazem J, et al: Metrifonate benefits cognitive, behavioral, and global function in patients with Alzheimer's disease. Neurology 50:1222–1230, 1998

Morris JN, Hawes C, Fries BE, et al: Designing the national resident assessment instrument for nursing homes. Gerontologist 30:293–307, 1990

Murphy E: The use of psychotropic drugs in long-term care (editorial). Int J Geriatr Psychiatry 4:1–2, 1989

National Center for Health Statistics: The National Nursing Home Survey (DHEW Publ No PHS-79-1794). Hyattsville, MD, National Center for Health Statistics, 1979

National Center for Health Statistics: Use of nursing homes by the elderly: preliminary data from the 1985 National Nursing Home Survey (DHHS Publ No PHS-87-1250). Hyattsville, MD, National Center for Health Statistics, 1987

Nyth AL, Gottfries CG: The clinical efficacy of citalopram in treatment of emotional disturbances in dementia disorders. A Nordic multicentre study. Br J Psychiatry 157:894–901, 1990

Office of Inspector General: Medicare Payments for Psychiatric Services in Nursing Homes: A Follow-Up (Publ No OEI-02-99-00140). Washington, DC, U.S. Department of Health and Human Services, 2001a. Available at http://oig.hhs.gov/oei/reports/oei-02-99-00140.pdf. Accessed July 17, 2003.

Office of Inspector General: Nursing Home Resident Assessment, Quality of Care (Publ No OEI-02-99-00040). Washington, DC, U.S. Department of Health and Human Services, 2001b. Available at http://oig.hhs.gov/oei/reports/oei-02-99-00040.pdf. Accessed July 17, 2003.

Office of Inspector General: Psychotropic Drug Use in Nursing Homes (Publ No OEI-02-00-00490). Washington, DC, U.S. Department of Health and Human Services, 2001c. Available at http://oig.hhs.gov/oei/reports/oei-02-00-00490.pdf. Accessed July 17, 2003.

Office of Technology Assessment: Special Care Units for People With Alzheimer's and Other Dementias: Consumer Education, Research, Regulatory, and Reimbursement Issues (OTA-H-543). Washington, DC, U.S. Government Printing Office, August 1992

Ohta RJ, Ohta BM: Special units for Alzheimer's disease patients: a critical look. Gerontologist 28:803–808, 1988

Omnibus Budget Reconciliation Act of 1987, Pub. L. No. 100-203. Subtitle C: Nursing home reform. Washington, DC

Orten JD, Allen M, Cook J: Reminiscence groups with confused nursing center residents: an experimental study. Soc Work Health Care 14:73–86, 1989

Oslin DW, Streim JE, Katz IR, et al: Heuristic comparison of sertraline with nortriptyline for the treatment of depression in frail elderly patients. Am J Geriatr Psychiatry 8:141–149, 2000

Oslin DW, Ten Have TR, Streim JE, et al: Probing the safety of medications in the frail elderly: evidence from a randomized clinical trial of sertraline and venlafaxine in depressed nursing home residents. J Clin Psychiatry 64:875–882, 2003

Parmelee PA, Katz IR, Lawton MP: Depression among institutionalized aged: assessment and prevalence estimation. J Gerontol 44:M22–M29, 1989

Parmelee PA, Katz IR, Lawton MP: The relation of pain to depression among institutionalized aged. J Gerontol 46:P15–P21, 1991

Parmelee PA, Katz IR, Lawton MP: Depression and mortality among institutionalized aged. J Gerontol 47:P3–P10, 1992a

Parmelee PA, Katz IR, Lawton MP: Incidence of depression in long-term care settings. J Gerontol 47:M189–M196, 1992b

Phillips CD, Sloane PD, Hawes C, et al: Effects of residence in Alzheimer's disease special care units on functional outcomes. JAMA 278:1340–1344, 1997

Phillips CD, Spry KM, Sloane PD, et al: Use of physical restraints and psychotropic medications in Alzheimer special care units in nursing homes. Am J Public Health 90:92–96, 2000

Porsteinsson AP, Tariot PN, Erb R, et al: Placebo-controlled study of divalproex sodium for agitation in dementia. Am J Geriatr Psychiatry 9:58–66, 2001

Rattenbury C, Stones MJ: A controlled evaluation of reminiscence and current topics discussion groups in a nursing home context. Gerontologist 29:768–771, 1989

Ray WA, Federspiel CF, Schaffner W: A study of antipsychotic drug use in nursing homes: epidemiologic evidence suggesting misuse. Am J Public Health 70:485–491, 1980

Ray WA, Taylor JA, Meador KG, et al: Reducing antipsychotic drug use in nursing homes. A controlled trial of provider education. Arch Intern Med 153:713–721, 1993

Reichman WE, Coyne AC, Borson S, et al: Psychiatric consultation in the nursing home. A survey of six states. Am J Geriatr Psychiatry 6:320–327, 1998

Rhoades J, Krauss N: Nursing Home Trends, 1987 and 1996. MEPS Chartbook No 3 (AHCPR Publ No 99-0032). Rockville, MD, Agency for Health Care Policy and Research, 1999

Risse SC, Cubberley L, Lampe TH, et al: Acute effects of neuroleptic withdrawal in elderly dementia patients. Journal of Geriatric Drug Therapy 2:65–77, 1987

Rosen J, Mulsant BH, Pollock BG: Sertraline in the treatment of minor depression in nursing home residents: a pilot study. Int J Geriatr Psychiatry 15:177–180, 2000

Rovner BW, Kafonek S, Filipp L, et al: Prevalence of mental illness in a community nursing home. Am J Psychiatry 143:1446–1449, 1986

Rovner BW, German PS, Broadhead J, et al: The prevalence and management of dementia and other psychiatric disorders in nursing homes. Int Psychogeriatr 2:13–24, 1990a

Rovner BW, Lucas-Blaustein J, Folstein MF, et al: Stability over one year in patients admitted to a nursing home dementia unit. Int J Geriatr Psychiatry 5:77–82, 1990b

Rovner BW, German PS, Brant LJ, et al: Depression and mortality in nursing homes. JAMA 265:993–996, 1991

Rovner BW, Edelman BA, Cox MP, et al: The impact of antipsychotic drug regulations (OBRA 1987) on psychotropic prescribing practices in nursing homes. Am J Psychiatry 149:1390–1392, 1992

Rovner BW, Steele CD, Shmuely Y, et al: A randomized trial of dementia care in nursing homes. J Am Geriatr Soc 44:7–13, 1996

Sabin TD, Vitug AJ, Mark VH: Are nursing home diagnosis and treatment inadequate? JAMA 248:321–322, 1982

Sadavoy J: Psychotherapy for the institutionalized elderly, in Practical Psychiatry in the Nursing Home: A Handbook for Staff. Edited by Conn DK, Herrman N, Kaye A, et al. Toronto, ON, Canada, Hogrefe & Huber, 1991, pp 217–236

Saxton J, Silverman M, Ricci E, et al: Maintenance of mobility in residents of an Alzheimer's special care facility. Int Psychogeriatr 10:213–224, 1998

Schneider LS, Pollack VE, Lyness SA: A meta-analysis of controlled trials of neuroleptic treatment in dementia. J Am Geriatr Soc 38:553–563, 1990

Schneider LS, Dagerman KS, Insel P: Risk of death with atypical antipsychotic drug treatment for dementia: meta-analysis of randomized placebo-controlled trials. JAMA 294:1934–1943, 2005

Schnelle JF, Newman DR, White M, et al: Reducing and managing restraints in long-term-care facilities. J Am Geriatr Soc 40: 381–385, 1992

Schnelle JF, Wood S, Schnelle ER, et al: Measurement sensitivity and the Minimum Data Set depression quality indicator. Gerontologist 41:401–405, 2001

Schulz PR: Effect of control and predictability on the psychological well-being of the institutionalized aged. J Pers Soc Psychol 33:563–573, 1976

Semla TP, Palla K, Poddig B, et al: Effect of the Omnibus Reconciliation Act 1987 on antipsychotic prescribing in nursing home residents. J Am Geriatr Soc 42:648–652, 1994

Shea DG, Russo PA, Smyer MA: Use of mental health services by persons with a mental illness in nursing facilities: initial impacts of OBRA 87. J Aging Health 12:560–578, 2000

Shorr RI, Fought RL, Ray WA: Changes in antipsychotic drug use in nursing homes during implementation of the OBRA-87 regulations. JAMA 271:358–362, 1994

Siegler EL, Capezuti E, Maislin G, et al: Effects of a restraint reduction intervention and OBRA '87 regulations on psychoactive drug use in nursing homes. J Am Geriatr Soc 45:791–796, 1997

Sink KM, Holden KF, Yaffe K: Pharmacological treatment of neuropsychiatric symptoms of dementia: a review of the evidence. JAMA 293:596–608, 2005

Sloane PD, Mathew LS, Scarborough M, et al: Physical and pharmacologic restraint of nursing home patients with dementia: impact of specialized units. JAMA 265:1278–1282, 1991

Sloane PD, Mitchell CM, Preisser JS, et al: Environmental correlates of resident agitation in Alzheimer's disease special care units. J Am Geriatr Soc 46:862–869, 1998

Smith M, Buckwalter KC, Albanese M: Geropsychiatric education programs. Providing skills and understanding. J Psychosoc Nurs Ment Health Serv 28:8–12, 1990

Smyer M, Brannon D, Cohn M: Improving nursing home care through training and job redesign. Gerontologist 32:327–333, 1992

Smyer MA, Shea DG, Streit A: The provision and use of mental health services in nursing homes: results from the National Medical Expenditure Survey. Am J Public Health 84:284–287, 1994

Snowden M, Roy-Byrne P: Mental illness and nursing home reform: OBRA-87 ten years later. Omnibus Budget Reconciliation Act. Psychiatr Serv 49:229–233, 1998

Snowden M, Sato K, Roy-Byrne P: Assessment and treatment of nursing home residents with depression or behavioral symptoms associated with dementia. J Am Geriatr Soc 51:1305–1317, 2003

Snowdon J: Dementia, depression, and life satisfaction in nursing homes. Int J Geriatr Psychiatry 1:85–91, 1986

Snowdon J, Donnelly N: A study of depression in nursing homes. J Psychiatr Res 20:327–333, 1986

Spagnoli A, Forester G, MacDonald A, et al: Dementia and depression in Italian geriatric institutions. Int J Geriatr Psychiatry 1:15–23, 1986

Steele C, Rovner BW, Chase GA, et al: Psychiatric symptoms and nursing home placement in Alzheimer's disease. Am J Psychiatry 147:1049–1051, 1990

Street JS, Clark WS, Gannon KS, et al: Olanzapine treatment of psychotic and behavioral symptoms in patients with Alzheimer disease in nursing care facilities: a double-blind, randomized, placebo-controlled trial. Arch Gen Psychiatry 57:968–976, 2000

Streim JE, Katz IR: Federal regulations and the care of patients with dementia in the nursing home. Med Clin North Am 78:895–909, 1994

Streim JE, Rovner BW, Katz IR: Psychiatric aspects of nursing home care, in Comprehensive Review of Geriatric Psychiatry–II, 2nd Edition. Edited by Sadavoy J, Lazarus LW, Jarvik LF, et al. Washington, DC, American Psychiatric Press, 1996, pp 907–936

Streim JE, Oslin DW, Katz IR, et al: Drug treatment of depression in frail elderly nursing home residents. Am J Geriatr Psychiatry 8:150–159, 2000

Svarstad BL, Mount JK, Bigelow W: Variations in the treatment culture of nursing homes and responses to regulations to reduce drug use. Psychiatr Serv 52:666–672, 2001

Swanson E, Maas M, Buckwalter K: Catastrophic reactions and other behaviors of Alzheimer's residents: special unit compared with traditional units. Arch Psychiatr Nurs 7:292–299, 1993

Tariot PN, Podgorski CA, Blazina L, et al: Mental disorders in the nursing home: another perspective. Am J Psychiatry 150:1063–1069, 1993

Tariot PN, Erb R, Podgorski CA, et al: Efficacy and tolerability of carbamazepine for agitation and aggression in dementia. Am J Psychiatry 155:54–61, 1998

Tariot PN, Cummings JL, Katz IR, et al: A randomized, double-blind, placebo-controlled study of the efficacy and safety of donepezil in patients with Alzheimer's disease in the nursing home setting. J Am Geriatr Soc 49:1590–1599, 2001

Tariot PN, Raman R, Jakimovich L, et al: Divalproex sodium in nursing home residents with possible or probable Alzheimer's disease complicated by agitation: a randomized, controlled trial. Am J Geriatr Psychiatry 13:942–949, 2005

Teeter RB, Garetz FK, Miller WR, et al: Psychiatric disturbances of aged patients in skilled nursing homes. Am J Psychiatry 133:1430–1434, 1976

Thapa PB, Gideon P, Cost CW, et al: Antidepressants and the risk of falls among nursing home residents. N Engl J Med 339:875–882, 1998

Toseland RW, Diehl M, Freeman K, et al: The impact of validation group therapy on nursing home residents with dementia. J Appl Gerontol 61:31–50, 1997

Trappler B, Cohen CI: Using fluoxetine in "very old" depressed nursing home residents. Am J Geriatr Psychiatry 4:258–262, 1996

Trappler B, Cohen CI: Use of SSRIs in "very old" depressed nursing home residents. Am J Geriatr Psychiatry 6:83–89, 1998

Trichard L, Zabow A, Gillis LS: Elderly persons in old age homes: a medical, psychiatric and social investigation. S Afr Med J 61:624–627, 1982

Wagner AW, Teri L, Orr-Rainey N: Behavior problems of residents with dementia in special care units. Alzheimer Dis Assoc Disord 9:121–127, 1995

Wang PS, Schneeweiss S, Avorn J, et al: Risk of death in elderly users of conventional vs atypical antipsychotic medications. N Engl J Med 353:2335–2341, 2005

Wells Y, Jorm FA: Evaluation of a special nursing home unit for dementia sufferers: a randomized controlled comparison with community care. Aust N Z J Psychiatry 21:524–531, 1987

Werner P, Cohen-Mansfield J, Braun J, et al: Physical restraint and agitation in nursing home residents. J Am Geriatr Soc 37:1122–1126, 1989

Williams-Barnard CL, Lindell AR: Therapeutic use of "prizing" and its effect on self-concept of elderly clients in nursing homes and group homes. Issues Ment Health Nurs 13:1–17, 1992

Youssef FA: The impact of group reminiscence counseling on a depressed elderly population. Nurse Pract 15:32–38, 1990

Zerhusen JD, Boyle K, Wilson W: Out of the darkness: group cognitive therapy for depressed elderly. J Psychosoc Nurs Ment Health Serv 29:16–21, 1991

Zimmer JG, Watson N, Treat A: Behavioral problems among patients in skilled nursing facilities. Am J Public Health 74:1118–1121, 1984

Study Questions

Select the single best response for each question.

1. The prevalence of psychiatric disorders in nursing home residents has been the subject of several studies. Which of the following is *not* true?

    A. Interview-based studies have found prevalence rates of psychiatric illness in nursing home residents as high as 94%.

    B. The Rovner et al. study (1990) found that two-thirds of nursing home residents had dementia.

    C. The Medical Expenditures Panel Survey (MEPS) found a rate of depressive disorders in nursing home residents of 20%.

    D. The MEPS study was based on clinical interviews.

    E. Rovner et al. (1990) found a prevalence of psychiatric illness of 80% in new nursing home admissions.

2. Among psychiatric illnesses in nursing home residents, disorders of cognitive impairment are of great importance. Which of the following is true?

    A. Among dementia subtypes, Alzheimer's disease accounts for 75% of cases, with Lewy body dementia the second most common dementia.

    B. Delirium has been found in 20% of nursing home residents, primarily due to underlying dementia.

    C. Psychotic symptoms are seen in 25%–50% of dementia patients in nursing homes.

    D. Most psychiatric consultations in nursing homes are for psychotic episodes.

    E. Behavioral disturbance in dementia is solely due to cognitive impairment.

3. In addition to cognitive disorders, mood disorders are common psychiatric illnesses in nursing home residents. Which of the following is true?

    A. Depressive disorders are the second most common psychiatric illness in nursing home residents.

    B. The rate of mood disorders in nursing home residents in the United States is substantially higher than in other industrialized nations.

    C. Depression in nursing home residents increases morbidity, but not mortality, rates.

    D. Because of concurrent chronic medical illnesses, the DSM-IV-TR diagnostic criteria for mood disorders are not clinically valid in nursing home residents.

    E. There is a subtype of depression in nursing home residents featuring low serum albumin, high levels of psychosocial disability, and prompt response to treatment with nortriptyline.

4. Intervention for psychiatric illnesses in nursing home residents is a major clinical focus of the geropsychiatrist. Which of the following is true?

   A. A program of daytime physical activity and nursing interventions to promote nighttime sleep may decrease depression, but not agitation.
   B. Outcome studies on psychotherapy models in nursing home residents are derived from illness-specific interventions.
   C. Risperidone has been shown to have a beneficial effect on psychotic symptoms but not independent effects on agitation or aggression.
   D. Risperidone has been repeatedly demonstrated to have beneficial long-term effects on psychosis in nursing home residents.
   E. The majority of nursing home residents who are withdrawn from antipsychotic agents do not experience a reemergence of psychosis.

5. Several concerns noted in the 1970s and 1980s in the United States led to various legal and regulatory initiatives to improve the psychiatric care in nursing homes. Which of the following is true?

   A. A 1977 survey in the United States revealed that 10% of nursing home residents were physically restrained.
   B. Mechanical restraints independently decrease physical agitation.
   C. Nursing home patients with nonpsychotic causes of agitation nonetheless require antipsychotic medications.
   D. The 1986 Institute of Medicine report found that antipsychotic drugs were being overused in nursing homes.
   E. The 1986 Institute of Medicine report found that antidepressant drugs were being overused in nursing homes.

6. Concern had been raised about the use of "unnecessary drugs" in psychiatrically ill nursing home patients. All of the following constitute an "unnecessary drug" use *except*

   A. Drug used at an excessive dose.
   B. Drug used for excessive duration.
   C. Drug used with inadequate monitoring.
   D. Drug used despite adverse consequences.
   E. Drug used for other than FDA-approved indications ("off-label").

Answer Guide

Chapter 1:
Demography and Epidemiology of
Psychiatric Disorders in Late Life

Select the single best response for each question.

1. The "old-old" populace (older than age 85) is projected to reach what number of persons by the year 2050?

    A. 10 million.
    B. 12 million.
    C. 20 million.
    D. 25 million.
    E. 27 million.

    The correct response is option **C**.

    The oldest old among us are projected to reach 20 million by the year 2050 and to make up 5% of the United States population at that time (Blazer 2000). **(p. 3)**

2. The geriatric population is expected to increase to how many by the year 2030?

    A. 30 million.
    B. 40 million.
    C. 50 million.
    D. 60 million.
    E. 70 million.

    The correct response is option **E**.

    The size of the elderly population in the United States is expected to dramatically increase in the next decades, reaching 70 million by the year 2030 (Federal Interagency Forum on Aging Related Statistics 2000). **(p. 4)**

3. Case identification in geriatrics is particularly germane because

    A. Distinction between a case and a noncase is easily established.
    B. Epidemiologists cannot assist the clinician in identifying meaningful clusters of symptoms.
    C. Many of the symptoms and signs of a psychiatric disorder in late life may be ubiquitous with the aging process.

D. Clinicians particularly favor case identification based on severity of functional impediment.

E. Most older adults ideally fit the psychiatric diagnosis they receive.

The correct response is option **C**.

Many of the symptoms and signs of a psychiatric disorder in late life may be ubiquitous with the aging process, thus blurring the distinction between cases and noncases.

The absolute distinction between a case and a noncase—that is, persons requiring psychiatric attention versus those who do not require such care—is not easily established. Epidemiologists can assist the clinician in identifying meaningful clusters of symptoms and significant degrees of symptom severity. Some authors define a case on the basis of severity of physical, psychological, and social impairment secondary to the symptoms. This approach to case identification is less popular among clinicians, who are more inclined to "treat a disease" than to "improve function." Most older adults do not ideally fit the psychiatric diagnosis that they receive. **(pp. 4–5)**

4. The NIMH ECA program (1984) established the two most prevalent disorders of the elderly as

A. Depressive and anxiety disorders.
B. Depressive and cognitive disorders.
C. Depressive and psychotic disorders.
D. Anxiety and cognitive disorders.
E. Anxiety and psychotic disorders.

The correct response is option **D**.

According to the NIMH ECA program (Regier et al. 1984), the two most prevalent disorders in people age 65 or older were an anxiety disorder (5.5%) and severe cognitive impairment (4.9%) (Regier et al. 1988). **(p. 6)**

5. The most frequently reported psychiatric symptom(s) of the elderly is (are)

A. Depression.
B. Fatigue.
C. Problems with sleep.
D. Anxiety related.
E. C and D.

The correct response is option **E**.

The most frequently reported symptoms are problems with sleep and symptoms of anxiety. **(p. 7)**

6. Suicide in the elderly

A. Is highest in the 65–74 sector.
B. Is highest in the 78–84 sector.
C. Is inversely correlated with age.
D. Is most pronounced in white men older than 70.
E. Has demonstrated a cohort effect of an increased rate with more modern manufacture of domestic gas.

The correct response is option **D**.

The highest suicide rates are found in white males older than 70. Suicide rates have been positively correlated with age.

The rate of gas poisoning has dramatically decreased with the conversion of domestic gas to methane. **(p. 15)**

7. Major depression has *not* been associated with

   A. Having functional limitation.
   B. External locus of control.
   C. Poorer self-perceived health.
   D. Perceived loneliness.
   E. Being unmarried.

The correct response is option **B**.

In the Longitudinal Aging Study Amsterdam (LASA; Beekman et al. 1995), major depression was associated with being unmarried; having functional limitation, perceived loneliness, internal locus of control, and poorer self-perceived health; and not receiving instrumental social support. **(p. 18)**

References

Beekman ATF, Deeg DJH, van Tilberg T, et al: Major and minor depression in later life: a study of prevalence and risk factors. J Affect Disord 36:65–75, 1995

Blazer DG: Psychiatry and the oldest old. Am J Psychiatry 157:1915–1924, 2000

Federal Interagency Forum on Aging Related Statistics: Older Americans 2000: Key Indicators of Well-Being. Washington, DC, Federal Interagency Forum on Aging Related Statistics, 2000

Regier DA, Myers JK, Kramer M, et al: The NIMH Epidemiologic Catchment Area Program: historical context, major objectives and study population characteristics. Arch Gen Psychiatry 41:934–941, 1984

Regier DA, Boyd JH, Burke JD, et al: One-month prevalence of mental disorders in the United States. Arch Gen Psychiatry 45:977–986, 1988

Chapter 2:
Physiological and Clinical Considerations of Geriatric Patient Care

Select the single best response for each question.

1. Falls in the elderly

   A. Are frequently multifactorial.
   B. Involve one-third of all community-dwelling elderly every year.
   C. Predict considerable morbidity.
   D. Promote risk for decline in instrumental activities of daily living.
   E. All of the above.

The correct response is option **E**.

Falls are generally multifactorial and are caused by intrinsic factors, situational factors, extrinsic factors, and medications (Alexander 1999; King and Tinetti 1995). Half of all nursing home residents and one-third of all community-dwelling elderly have a fall every year. These falls produce notable morbidity. Those who fall frequently are at risk for a decline in their instrumental activities of daily living. **(p. 37)**

2. Urinary incontinence in the elderly is

    A. Most frequently stress incontinence in men.
    B. Most frequently overflow incontinence.
    C. Most frequently urge incontinence.
    D. Seen in up to one-half of community-residing elderly.
    E. None of the above.

    The correct response is option **C.**

Half of all nursing home residents and up to one-third of persons older than 65 residing in the community carry the diagnosis of urinary continence (DuBeau 1999; Tannenbaum et al. 2001).

Urge incontinence is the form of incontinence that has the highest prevalence in older patients. Stress incontinence is a frequent form of incontinence among elderly women, ranking second. Overflow incontinence is the second most prevalent type of incontinence in elderly men; often, it is produced by bladder outlet obstruction resulting from urethral strictures, benign prostatic hypertrophy, and prostate cancer. **(p. 38)**

3. The musculoskeletal system is affected in which of the following ways?

    A. Decrease in skeletal muscle mass.
    B. Increase in number of type II fibers.
    C. Age-associated changes in muscle mass and strength may be modified by exercise.
    D. A and B.
    E. A and C.

    The correct response is option **E.**

In the fourth decade, both muscle mass and strength begin to decrease, and exercise may modify these age-associated changes (Loeser and Delbono 2003; Taffet 1999). The number of type II fast-twitch fibers decreases in the elderly. **(pp. 34–35)**

4. Considerations in geriatric prescription should include all of the following *except*

    A. Volume of distribution.
    B. Absorption.
    C. Renal clearance.
    D. Oxidative metabolism in the cytochrome P450 system.
    E. Change in elimination half-life.

    The correct response is option **B.**

Age has no significant effect on absorption, although acid secretion, gastrointestinal perfusion, and membrane transport all may decrease and thereby lower absorption (Schwartz 1999; Semla and Rochon 2002). Gastrointestinal transit time is prolonged and increases absorption, and thus no net change occurs.

The volume of distribution is significantly affected by the changes in body mass and total body water that occur with aging. With age, renal mass and renal blood flow are decreased, resulting in a decline in glomerular filtration rate and creatinine clearance. This decrease in clearance can alter the rate at which drugs are excreted, and dosages must be appropriately adjusted. Oxidative metabolism in the cytochrome P450 system is slower, thereby affecting elimination, but conjugation is not. The elimination half-life—the time required for the drug concentration to decrease by half—of certain drugs increases in the elderly and may be affected by the relation between volume of distribution or clearance; this may require adjustment of the drug dosing interval. **(p. 40)**

5. Which of the following is true of cognition in normal aging?
    A. Crystallized intelligence changes with age.
    B. Fluid intelligence begins to improve in the middle of the sixth decade and thereafter.
    C. Practical intelligence may be stable or even improve with age.
    D. Executive function deteriorates with age.
    E. Long-term memory is affected.

The correct response is option **C**.

Practical intelligence, which tracks procedural skills, may be stable or even improve with age.

Crystallized intelligence, an indication of accumulated knowledge or experience, does not change with age, but fluid intelligence, or novel problem-solving ability, begins to decline in the middle of the sixth decade and accelerates thereafter. Executive function—or the ability to conceive, organize, and carry out a plan or activity—may remain intact in the elderly (Craft et al. 2003; Oskvig 1999). Long-term memory, sensory memory, and procedural memory are generally unchanged. **(p. 30)**

6. Ocular changes include which of the following?
    A. Weakening of the ciliary muscle.
    B. Rigidity of the pupil.
    C. Decline in ability to view objects at rest.
    D. A and B.
    E. A, B, and C.

The correct response is option **E**.

The weakening of the ciliary muscle, combined with the loss of elasticity in the lens, results in presbyopia. The elderly have difficulty adapting to light because of rigidity of the pupil and increased opacity of the lens. In addition, they show a decline in their ability to view objects at rest (static acuity) and in motion (dynamic acuity) (Kalina 1999; Taffet 1999). **(p. 30)**

7. Gastrointestinal system changes of the elderly include

    A. Fewer myenteric ganglion cells.
    B. Diminished acid and pepsin production by the stomach.
    C. Diminished function of liver, gallbladder, and pancreas.
    D. Increased transit of food through the large bowel.
    E. More effective absorption of vitamins and minerals by the small bowel.

The correct response is option **A.**

There are fewer myenteric ganglion cells, which affects the coordination of swallowing and may predispose some elderly patients to aspiration.

The production of acid and pepsin by the stomach is mostly preserved. The liver, gallbladder, and pancreas continue to function well in the elderly patient. Because the stomach and small intestines do not dilate as easily, transit of food through the large bowel may be slower. The small bowel absorbs vitamins and minerals less effectively (Hall and Wiley 2003; Majumdar et al. 1997; Taffet 1999). **(pp. 31–32)**

8. Hormone levels are affected in all of the following ways *except*

    A. Decrease in growth hormone.
    B. Decrease in dehydroepiandrosterone.
    C. Decrease in cortisol.
    D. Increase in parathyroid hormone levels.
    E. Increase in sex-hormone binding globulin levels.

The correct response is option **C.**

Cortisol levels remain the same in the elderly because of a decrease in the cortisol metabolic clearance rate.

Growth hormone (GH) declines because of both a decrease in growth hormone releasing hormone secretion and an increase in somatostatin. Both dehydroepiandrosterone (DHEA) and dehydroepiandrosterone sulfate (DHEA-S) decrease significantly in the elderly. Parathyroid hormone (PTH) levels are higher in the elderly because of increased secretion and decreased renal clearance. An increase in sex-hormone binding globulin levels limits the amount of free testosterone available (Gruenewald and Matsumoto 2003; Oskvig 1999; Perry 1999). **(pp. 32–34)**

References

Alexander NB: Falls and gait disturbances, in Geriatrics Review Syllabus: A Core Curriculum in Geriatric Medicine. Edited by Cobbs E, Duthie EH, Murphy JB. Dubuque, IA, Kendall/Hunt, 1999, pp 145–149

Craft S, Cholerton B, Reger M: Aging and cognition: what is normal? in Principles of Geriatric Medicine and Gerontology, 5th Edition. Edited by Hazzard WR, Blass JP, Halter JB, et al. New York, McGraw-Hill, 2003, pp 1355–1372

DuBeau CW: Urinary incontinence, in Geriatrics Review Syllabus: A Core Curriculum in Geriatric Medicine. Edited by Cobbs E, Duthie EH, Murphy JB. Dubuque, IA, Kendall/Hunt, 1999, pp 115–123

Gruenewald DA, Matsumoto A: Aging of the endocrine system, in Principles of Geriatric Medicine and Gerontology, 5th Edition. Edited by Hazzard WR, Blass JP, Halter JB, et al. New York, McGraw-Hill, 2003, pp 819–836

Hall KE, Wiley JW: Effect of aging on gastrointestinal function, in Principles of Geriatric Medicine and Gerontology, 5th Edition. Edited by Hazzard WR, Blass JP, Halter JB, et al. New York, McGraw-Hill, 2003, pp 593–600

Hanlon JT, Schmader K, Ruby C, et al: Suboptimal prescribing in older inpatients and outpatients. J Am Geriatr Soc 49:200–209, 2001

Kalina R: Aging and visual function, in Principles of Geriatric Medicine and Gerontology, 4th Edition. Edited by Hazzard WR, Blass JP, Ettinger WH, et al. New York, McGraw-Hill, 1999, pp 603–615

King MB, Tinetti ME: Falls in community-dwelling older persons. J Am Geriatr Soc 43:1146–1154, 1995

Loeser RF, Delbono O: Aging of the muscles and joints, in Principles of Geriatric Medicine and Gerontology, 5th Edition. Edited by Hazzard WR, Blass JP, Halter JB, et al. New York, McGraw-Hill, 2003, pp 905–918

Majumdar AP, Jaszewski R, Dubick MA: Effect of aging on gastrointestinal tract and the pancreas. Proc Soc Exp Biol Med 215:134–144, 1997

Oskvig RM: Special problems in the elderly: perioperative cardiopulmonary evaluation and management. Chest 155(suppl):158S–164S, 1999

Schwartz JB: Clinical pharmacology, in Principles of Geriatric Medicine and Gerontology, 4th Edition. Edited by Hazzard WR, Blass JP, Ettinger WH, et al. New York, McGraw-Hill, 1999, pp 303–332

Semla TP, Rochon PA: Pharmacotherapy, in Geriatrics Review Syllabus: A Core Curriculum in Geriatric Medicine. Edited by Cobbs E, Duthie EH, Murphy JB. London, Blackwell Scientific, 2002, pp 37–44

Stewart RB: Drug use in the elderly, in Therapeutics in the Elderly, 3rd Edition. Edited by Delafuente JC, Stewart RB. Cincinnati, OH, Harvey Whitney, 2001, pp 235–256

Taffet GE: Age-related physiologic changes, in Geriatrics Review Syllabus: A Core Curriculum in Geriatric Medicine. Edited by Cobbs E, Duthie EH, Murphy JB. Dubuque, IA, Kendall/Hunt, 1999, pp 10–23

Tannenbaum C, Perrin L, DuBeau CE, et al: Diagnosis and management of urinary incontinence in the older patient. Arch Phys Med Rehabil 82:134–138, 2001

Chapter 3:
The Psychiatric Interview of Older Adults

Select the single best response for each question.

1. Medication history of the older adult

    A. Should involve having the older person bring in all pill bottles.
    B. Should involve a double check between the written schedule and pill containers.
    C. Should assess alcohol intake.
    D. Should assess substance abuse.
    E. All of the above.

    The correct response is option **E.**

    The clinician should ask the older person to bring in all pill bottles as well as a list of medications taken and the dosage schedule. A double check between the written schedule and the pill containers will frequently expose some discrepancy. Older persons are less likely than younger persons to abuse alcohol, but a careful history of alcohol intake is essential to the diagnostic workup. Substance abuse beyond alcohol and prescription drugs is rare in older adults, but not entirely absent. **(p. 52)**

2. Evaluation of the family of the psychiatrically ill older adult would include all of the following parameters of support *except*

    A. Availability of the family member.
    B. Tangible services provided by the family.
    C. Patient's perception of family support.
    D. Tolerance by the family of specific behaviors derived from the psychiatric disorder.
    E. Consideration of only those individuals genetically related to the patient.

    The correct response is option **E.**

    For clinical purposes, the family consists not only of individuals genetically related but also of those who have developed relationships and are living together as if they were related (Miller and Miller 1979).

    At least four parameters of support are important for the clinician to evaluate as the treatment plan evolves. These include 1) availability of family members to the older person over time, 2) the tangible services provided by the family to the disturbed older person, 3) the perception of family support by the older patient (and subsequently the willingness of the patient to cooperate and accept support), and 4) tolerance by the family of specific behaviors that derive from the psychiatric disorder. **(pp. 53–54)**

3. A dementia scale for assessing the probability that dementia is secondary to multiple infarcts was suggested by Hachinski et al. (1975). Among the clinical features noted to be more associated with multi-infarct dementia were all of the following *except*

    A. Stepwise deterioration.
    B. Gradual onset.
    C. Fluctuating course.
    D. Focal neurological symptoms.
    E. Focal neurological signs.

    The correct response is option **B.**

    A dementia scale for assessing the probability that dementia is secondary to multiple infarcts was suggested by Hachinski et al. (1975). In the study, cerebral blood flow in patients with primary degenerative dementia was compared with those who had multi-infarct dementia. Certain clinical features were determined to be more associated with multi-infarct dementia, and each of these features was assigned a score. Those clinical features, along with their scores, are as follows: abrupt onset=2, stepwise deterioration=1, fluctuating course= 2, nocturnal confusion=1, relative preservation of personality=1, depression=1, somatic complaints=1, emotional incontinence = 1, history of hypertension = 1, history of strokes=2, evidence of associated atherosclerosis=1, focal neurological symptoms=2, and focal neurological signs =2. A score of 7 or greater was highly suggestive of multi-infarct dementia. However, given the frequent overlap of multiple small infarcts and primary degenerative dementia, as well as the difficulty of assessing these items effectively, most investigators have ceased to rely on the Hachinski scale for clinical use. **(p. 58)**

4. Barriers to effective communication between the older patient and clinician can include

    A. Physician perceiving the older adult patient incorrectly because of personal fears of aging and death.

    B. The patient's perceptual problems.

    C. Patient taking longer to respond to inquiries, resisting the physician who attempts to hurry through the interview.

    D. Patient perceiving the physician unrealistically.

    E. All of the above.

The correct response is option **E**.

The clinician may perceive the older adult patient incorrectly because of personal fears of aging and death or because of previous negative experiences with his or her own parents. Perceptual problems, such as hearing and visual impairments, may exacerbate disorientation and complicate the communication of problems to the clinician. Elderly persons frequently take longer to respond to inquiries and resist the clinician who attempts to rush through the history-taking interview. The elderly patient may perceive the physician unrealistically, on the basis of previous life experiences (i.e., transference may occur) (Blazer 1978). **(p. 61)**

References

Blazer DG: Techniques for communicating with your elderly patient. Geriatrics 33:79–80, 83–84, 1978

Hachinski VC, Iliff LD, Zilhka E, et al: Cerebral blood flow in dementia. Arch Neurol 32:632–637, 1975

Miller KT, Miller JL: The family as a system. Paper presented at the annual meeting of the American College of Psychiatrists, New York, February 1979

Chapter 4:
Use of the Laboratory in the Diagnostic Workup of Older Adults

Select the single best response for each question.

1. Serum vitamin B_{12} and folate levels

    A. Are rarely important in the evaluation of the elderly patient.

    B. May point to etiologies of a range of neuropsychiatric disturbances.

    C. May produce microcytic anemia when levels are deficient.

    D. Are not related to hyperhomocysteinemia.

    E. Are not related to one-carbon metabolism in brain tissue.

The correct response is option **B**.

Vitamin B_{12} and folate deficiencies may result in neuropsychiatric disturbances, including depression, psychosis, and cognitive deficits (Carmel et al. 1995). Measurement of serum vitamin B_{12} and folate levels is an integral part of the laboratory evaluation as the prevalence of B_{12} deficiency increases with age. B_{12} deficiency may have various clinical signs, including macrocytic anemia and neuropathy. Serum homocysteine levels may serve as a functional indicator of B_{12} and folate status (Selhub et al. 2000), because vitamin B_{12} is needed to convert homocysteine to methionine in one-carbon metabolism in brain tissue. **(p. 68)**

2. Approximately what percentage of persons admitted from the community to a geropsychiatry unit may have a urinary tract infection that may result in a delirium?

   A. 10%.
   B. 20%.
   C. 35%.
   D. 45%.
   E. 55%.

   The correct response is option **B.**

   Identification of a urinary tract infection is critical in the elderly population, particularly in those with dementia. Approximately 20% of people admitted from the community to a geropsychiatry unit may have a urinary tract infection, and in many cases it may result in a delirium; however, the condition improves with appropriate antibiotic treatment (Manepalli et al. 1990). **(p. 69)**

3. Lithium is most likely to demonstrate which of the following ECG changes?

   A. AV block.
   B. Prolonged PR interval.
   C. Sick sinus syndrome.
   D. Bradycardia.
   E. QTc prolongation.

   The correct response is option **C.**

   Lithium appears to most affect the sinus node, and even at therapeutic levels it may result in sick sinus syndrome or sinoatrial block, either of which may occur early or later in treatment. At higher levels, there have been reports of sinus arrest and asystole.

   Individuals with preexisting bundle branch block who take tricyclic antidepressants are at increased risk for AV block. Even therapeutic levels are associated with prolonged PR intervals and QRS complexes; these results may be more pronounced in elderly individuals as the incidence and severity of adverse drug reactions increase with age.

   Antipsychotics also result in ECG changes; about 25% of individuals receiving antipsychotics exhibit ECG abnormalities (Thomas 1994). Although many of these changes have historically been considered benign, there is increased concern that prolongation of the QTc interval may contribute to potentially fatal ventricular arrhythmias, particularly torsades de pointes. Beta-blockers may produce bradycardia. **(pp. 69–70; see Table 4–2)**

4. *APOE* testing has shown that

   A. A homozygous epsilon 4/epsilon 4 genotype is diagnostic for Alzheimer's disease.
   B. It is valuable in modifying the disease course and influencing current supportive treatments for Alzheimer's disease.
   C. It predicts response to cholinesterase inhibitors.

D. It lacks hierarchy of the alleles for prediction or risk for development of Alzheimer's disease.

E. None of the above.

The correct response is option **E**.

Multiple epidemiological studies have documented that the presence of the epsilon 4 allele is a risk factor for Alzheimer's disease (Roses 1997). Additionally, the presence of epsilon 4 alleles increases the specificity of the diagnosis of Alzheimer's disease. Despite these associations, the presence of an epsilon 4 allele, even a homozygous epsilon 4/epsilon 4 genotype, is not diagnostic for Alzheimer's disease. Other causes of dementia would have to be explored as clinically indicated. *APOE* testing is not currently recommended to predict dementia risk in asymptomatic individuals. Current treatments for cognitive dysfunction are limited to cholinesterase inhibitors, but response to these drugs is not dependent on *APOE* status. **(p. 73)**

5. Which of the following statements about genetic testing is *not* true? Genetic testing

A. Results in transient heightened anxiety and depression.

B. Can possibly result in hopelessness.

C. Results in job loss or lack of insurability.

D. Proves to be a valuable tool with untapped potential.

E. Is recommended to predict dementia risk in asymptomatic individuals.

The correct response is option **E**.

Testing can result in transient heightened anxiety and depression; in the long term, a positive test may result in hopelessness (Tibben et al. 1994). The inappropriate release of information could result in job loss or lack of insurability. Genetic testing is a tool with much untapped potential. **(pp. 72–73)**

References

Carmel R, Gott PS, Waters CH, et al: The frequently low cobalamin levels in dementia usually signify treatable metabolic, neurologic and electrophysiologic abnormalities. Eur J Haematol 54:245–253, 1995

Manepalli J, Grossberg GT, Mueller C: Prevalence of delirium and urinary tract infection in a psychogeriatric unit. J Geriatr Psychiatry Neurol 3:198–202, 1990

Pollock BG: Adverse reactions of antidepressants in elderly patients. J Clin Psychiatry 60:4–8, 1999

Roses AD: A model for susceptibility polymorphisms for complex diseases: apolipoprotein E and Alzheimer disease. Neurogenetics 1:3–11, 1997

Selhub J, Bagley LC, Miller J, et al: B vitamins, homocysteine, and neurocognitive function in the elderly. Am J Clin Nutr 71(suppl):614S–620S, 2000

Thomas SHL: Drugs, QT interval abnormalities, and ventricular arrhythmias. Adverse Drug React Toxicol Rev 13:77–102, 1994

Tibben A, Duivenvoorden HJ, Niermeijer MF, et al: Psychological effects of presymptomatic DNA testing for Huntington's disease in the Dutch program. Psychosom Med 56:526–532, 1994

Chapter 5:
Neuropsychological Assessment of Dementia

Select the single best response for each question.

1. The most common cause for cognitive change after age 50 is

   A. Alzheimer's disease.
   B. Frontotemporal dementia.
   C. Normal aging of the nervous system.
   D. Vascular dementia.
   E. None of the above.

   The correct response is option **C**.

   By far the most common cause for cognitive change after age 50 is normal aging of the nervous system (Ebly et al. 1994). Compared to young adults, older individuals show selective losses in functions related to the speed and efficiency of information processing. Particularly vulnerable are memory retrieval abilities, attentional capacity, executive skills, and divergent thinking, such as working memory and multitasking (Cullum et al. 1990; Salthouse et al. 1996). **(pp. 80–81)**

2. The differences underlying memory loss of normal aging and that of Alzheimer's disease include

   A. Consolidation or storage of new information in long-term memory stores.
   B. Efficient accessing of recently stored information.
   C. Difficulty with visuospatial tasks.
   D. A and B.
   E. A, B, and C.

   The correct response is option **D**.

   Different mechanisms underlie the memory loss of aging and that of Alzheimer's disease. In Alzheimer's disease, it is suggested that the problems reside in the consolidation or storage of new information in long-term memory stores. In normal aging, the principal problem appears to be the efficient accessing of recently stored information. Besides memory problems, older adults without dementing disorders also show some decrements compared to younger cohorts on tests of visuoperceptual, visuospatial, and constructional functions (Eslinger et al. 1985; Howieson et al. 1993; Koss et al. 1991). **(pp. 81–84)**

3. The leading cause of dementia in elderly persons is

   A. Vascular disease.
   B. Alzheimer's disease.
   C. Lewy body disease.
   D. Frontotemporal disease.
   E. Corticobasal degeneration.

   The correct response is option **B**.

Alzheimer's disease is the leading cause of dementia in elderly persons. Alone or in combination with other nervous system disorders, Alzheimer's disease accounts for nearly 50%–75% of all cases in Western countries (Ebly et al. 1995; Fratiglioni et al. 1999).

The second most common cause of dementia, accounting for 15%–30% of cases, is vascular dementia, which includes disorders arising from either large- or small-vessel strokes (Lobo et al. 2000). Far less common are the frontal lobe disorders, which include the now well-recognized disorders of frontotemporal dementia, Pick's disease, and forms of progressive aphasia (Geldmacher and Whitehouse 1997). Lewy body dementia and related movement disorders of the basal ganglia—including Parkinson's disease, progressive supranuclear palsy, corticobasal degeneration, Huntington's disease, and multisystem atrophy—together account for 10% of the cases (Hanson et al. 1990; Holman et al. 1995; Savolainen et al. 1999). **(p. 81)**

4. The earliest manifestation of Alzheimer's disease is

    A. Rapid forgetting of new information after very brief delays.
    B. Expressive language difficulty.
    C. Visuospatial difficulty.
    D. Apraxia.
    E. Circumlocution.

The correct response is option **A.**

On formal neuropsychological testing, the memory problem of Alzheimer's disease is manifest as a rapid forgetting of new information after very brief delays (Welsh et al. 1991).

As the disease progresses, other areas of cognition are involved, reflecting the specific spread of neuropathological involvement to the lateral temporal areas, parietal cortex, and frontal neocortical areas (Welsh et al. 1992). Prototypical changes occur in expressive language, visuospatial function, higher executive controls, and semantic knowledge. Visuospatial problems become more prominent in later stages of the illness, resulting in dressing apraxia, difficulty in recognizing objects or people, and problems in performing familiar motor acts (Benke 1993). Word search and circumlocution tendencies are common in conversational speech, whereas speech comprehension itself is better preserved, as are all other fundamental elements of communication (Bayles et al. 1989). **(p. 81)**

5. Patients with vascular dementia could be expected to show all of the following *except*

    A. Memory deficits often patchy in nature.
    B. Impaired recollection of some recent event but surprisingly good memory of some other event occurring during the same time frame.
    C. Flattened learning curve over repeated trials.
    D. Low recall performance as well as rapid forgetting.
    E. Recognition improving dramatically with a recognition format.

The correct response is option **D.**

Recall performance can be quite low—similar to Alzheimer's disease—but is typically without the rapid forgetting shown in Alzheimer's disease (Matsuda et al. 1998).

Memory is involved, but deficits are often patchy in nature. Patients may show impaired recollection of some recent event but show a surprising memory of some other event occurring during the same time frame. On formal neuropsychological testing, the pattern shown in results of memory testing is one of inefficient acquisition of new information, leading to a flattened learning curve over repeating trials (Looi and Sachdev 1999; Padovani et al. 1995). Finally, recognition improves dramatically with a recognition format, suggesting a primary difficulty in retrieval rather than in storage or consolidation of new information (Hayden et al. 2005). **(pp. 84–85)**

6. What percentage of patients with Parkinson's disease are reported to have dementia?

    A. 5%–10%.
    B. 10%–20%.
    C. 20%–40%.
    D. 50%–60%.
    E. 70%–80%.

The correct response is option **C**.

Typically, only 20%–40% of patients with Parkinson's disease are reported to have dementia (Cummings 1988; Pillon et al. 1991), and there is some evidence that younger age at onset is a risk factor for Parkinson's disease dementia (Friedman and Barcikowska 1994; Reid 1992). **(p. 86)**

7. Geriatric depression shows which of the following deficits?

    A. Impairments on tests sensitive to frontal lobe function.
    B. Difficulties on sustained and selective attention.
    C. Set shifting.
    D. Verbal fluency.
    E. All of the above.

The correct response is option **E**.

With treatment, not all the cognitive impairments associated with geriatric depression remit. In older patients, these continuing impairments may be due to the co-occurrence of another disease process, such as Alzheimer's disease or vascular dementia. Although far from conclusive, a number of studies have reported that depression in elderly persons exerts a discernible additional effect on cognition and functional independence and that depression may be a risk factor for later cognitive decline (Steffens et al. 2006)

On formal neuropsychological testing, geriatric depressed patients show impairments on tests sensitive to frontal lobe function. Difficulties can be readily seen on tests of selective and sustained attention, verbal fluency, inhibitory control, and set shifting (Boone et al. 1995; Lockwood et al. 2002). **(pp. 87–88)**

References

Bayles KA, Boone DR, Tomoeda CK, et al: Differentiating Alzheimer's patients from the normal elderly and stroke patients with aphasia. J Speech Hear Disord 54:74–87, 1989

Benke T: Two forms of apraxia in Alzheimer's disease. Cortex 29:715–725, 1993

Boone KB, Lesser I, Miller B, et al: Cognitive functioning in older depressed outpatients: relationship of presence and severity of depression on neuropsychological test scores. Neuropsychology 9:390–398, 1995

Cullum CM, Butters N, Troster AL, et al: Normal aging and forgetting rates on the Wechsler Memory Scale—Revised. Arch Clin Neuropsychol 5:23–30, 1990

Cummings JL: Intellectual impairment in Parkinson's disease: clinical, pathologic, and biochemical correlates. J Geriatr Psychiatry Neurol 1:24–36, 1988

Ebly EM, Parhad IM, Hogan DB, et al: Prevalence and types of dementia in the very old: results from the Canadian Study of Health and Aging. Neurology 44:1593–1600, 1994

Ebly EM, Hogan DB, Parhad IM: Cognitive impairment in the nondemented elderly: results from the Canadian Study of Health and Aging. Arch Neurol 52:612–619, 1995

Eslinger PJ, Damasio AR, Benton AL, et al: Neuropsychologic detection of abnormal mental decline in older persons. JAMA 253:670–674, 1985

Fratiglioni L, De Ronchi D, Aguero-Torres H: Worldwide prevalence and incidence of dementia. Drugs Aging 15:365–375, 1999

Friedman A, Barcikowska M: Dementia in Parkinson's disease. Dementia 5:12–16, 1994

Geldmacher DS, Whitehouse PJ Jr: Differential diagnosis of Alzheimer's disease. Neurology 48 (5, suppl 6):S2–S9, 1997

Hanson L, Salmon D, Galasko D, et al: The Lewy body variant of Alzheimer's disease: a clinical and pathological entity. Neurology 40:1–8, 1990

Hayden KM, Warren LH, Pieper CF, et al: Identification VaD and AD prodromes: The Cache County Study. Alzheimer's & Dementia: The Journal of the Alzheimer's Association 1:19–29, 2005

Holman RC, Khan AS, Kent J, et al: Epidemiology of Creutzfeldt-Jakob disease in the United States 1979–1990: analysis of national mortality data. Neuroepidemiology 14:174–181, 1995

Howieson D, Holm L, Kaye J, et al: Neurologic function in the optimally healthy oldest old: neuropsychological evaluation. Neurology 43:1882–1886, 1993

Koss E, Haxby JV, DeCarli C, et al: Patterns of performance preservation and loss in healthy aging. Dev Neuropsychol 7:99–113, 1991

Lobo A, Launer LJ, Fratiglioni L, et al: Prevalence of dementia and major subtypes in Europe: a collaborative study of population-based cohorts. Neurologic Diseases in the Elderly Research Group. Neurology 54 (11, suppl 5):S4–S9, 2000

Lockwood KA, Alexopoulos GS, Van Gorp WG: Executive dysfunction in geriatric depression. Am J Psychiatry 159:1119–1126, 2002

Looi J, Sachdev PS: Differentiation of vascular dementia from AD on neuropsychological tests. Neurology 53:670–678, 1999

Matsuda O, Saito M, Sugishita M: Cognitive deficits of mild dementia: a comparison between dementia of the Alzheimer's type and vascular dementia. Psychiatry Clin Neurosci 52:87–91, 1998

Padovani A, Di Piero V, Bragoni M, et al: Patterns of neuropsychological impairment in mild dementia: comparison between Alzheimer's disease and multi-infarct dementia. Acta Neurol Scand 92:433–442, 1995

Pillon B, Dubois B, Agid Y: Severity and specificity of cognitive impairment in Alzheimer's, Huntington's, and Parkinson's diseases and progressive supranuclear palsy. Ann N Y Acad Sci 640:224–227, 1991

Reid WG: The evolution of dementia in idiopathic Parkinson's disease: neuropsychological and clinical evidence in support of subtypes. Int Psychogeriatr 4:147–160, 1992

Salthouse TA, Fristoe N, Rhee SH: How localized are age-related effects on neuropsychological measures? Neuropsychology 10:272–285, 1996

Savolainen S, Palijarvi L, Vapalahti M: Prevalence of Alzheimer's disease in patients investigated for presumed normal pressure hydrocephalus: a clinical and neuropathological study. Acta Neurochir (Wien) 141:849–853, 1999

Steffens DC, Otey E, Alexopoulos GS, et al: Perspectives on depression, mild cognitive impairment, and cognitive decline. Arch Gen Psychiatry 63:130–138, 2006

Welsh K, Butters N, Hughes JP, et al: Detection of abnormal memory decline in mild Alzheimer's disease using CERAD neuropsychological measures. Arch Neurol 48:278–281, 1991

Welsh KA, Butters N, Hughes JP, et al: Detection and staging of dementia in Alzheimer's disease: use of the neuropsychological measures developed for the Consortium to Establish a Registry for Alzheimer's Disease (CERAD). Arch Neurol 49:448–452, 1992

Chapter 6:
Cognitive Disorders

Select the single best response for each question.

1. Cognitive deficits of Alzheimer's disease correlate

    A. With density of neurofibrillary tangles.
    B. With hyperphosphorylated tau.
    C. With density of neuritic plaques.
    D. A and B.
    E. A and C.

The correct response is option **D**.

The major constituent of neurofibrillary tangles is a hyperphosphorylated form of the microtubule-associated phosphoprotein tau. The correlation between the density of postmortem neurofibrillary tangles and antemortem cognitive deficits is more robust than that between neuritic plaques and cognitive deficits (Snowdon et al. 1997). **(p. 107)**

2. Serotonin abnormalities of Alzheimer's disease include

    A. Loss of serotonergic neurons in brain stem raphe nuclei.
    B. Decreased concentration of serotonin in brain tissue.
    C. Decreased concentration of serotonin in CSF.
    D. Decreased serotonin receptor concentrations.
    E. All of the above.

The correct response is option **E**.

In patients with Alzheimer's disease, there is a clear deficiency in brain serotonin systems, manifested by loss of serotonergic neurons in the brain stem raphe nuclei (Mann and Yates 1983; Yamamoto and Hirano 1985), decreased concentrations of serotonin and its metabolite in brain tissue (Arai et al. 1984; D'Amato et al. 1987) and CSF (Blennow et al. 1991; Volicer et al. 1985), and decreased serotonin receptor concentrations (Cross et al. 1984). **(pp. 108–109)**

3. Brain presynaptic cholinergic deficit has been demonstrated in which of the following?

    A. Alzheimer's disease.
    B. Vascular dementia.
    C. Lewy body dementia.
    D. All of the above.
    E. None of the above.

The correct response is option **D.**

Whitehouse and colleagues (1982) demonstrated extensive neuronal loss in the cholinergic nucleus basalis of Meynert in patients with Alzheimer's disease. A brain presynaptic cholinergic deficit has also been demonstrated in vascular dementia (Erkinjuntti et al. 2002) and dementia with Lewy bodies (Perry et al. 1994). **(p. 110)**

4. Cholinesterase inhibitors are best conceptualized as drugs
    A. That stabilize cognition, activities of daily living, and behavioral function.
    B. That improve cognitive function greatly.
    C. Only indicated for mild to moderate stages of Alzheimer's disease.
    D. Contraindicated in the treatment of Lewy body dementia.
    E. Predominately associated with the side effect of sedation.

The correct response is option **A.**

Cholinesterase inhibitors are best conceptualized as drugs that stabilize cognition, activities of daily living, and behavioral function and that slow clinical deterioration in Alzheimer's disease. Stabilization of cognition and functioning for approximately 1 year has been demonstrated with both galantamine and donepezil (Raskind et al. 2000; Winblad et al. 2001).

A consensus is emerging that cholinesterase inhibitor therapy should be started as soon as Alzheimer's disease, dementia with Lewy bodies, vascular dementia, or mixed dementia becomes apparent and that treatment should be continued at least into moderately advanced stages of disease, provided the drug is well tolerated. As is the case with all cholinesterase inhibitors, gastrointestinal symptoms—particularly nausea and vomiting (CNS cholinergic effects) and diarrhea—are the most frequent adverse effects. **(p. 110)**

5. Vitamin E and selegiline have *not* been shown to
    A. Have beneficial effects on cognitive function per se.
    B. Delay nursing home placement.
    C. Delay progression to severe dementia.
    D. Be more effective in combination than either agent alone.
    E. Delay loss of basic activities of daily living.

The correct response is option **A.**

Vitamin E and selegiline have no beneficial effects on cognitive function per se.

In a large multicenter trial, the National Institute on Aging–supported Alzheimer's Disease Cooperative Study evaluated two such drugs—vitamin E and selegiline—singly and in combination, in AD outpatients with moderately advanced disease (Sano et al. 1997). The combination of vitamin E and selegiline was no more effective than either agent alone. Neither agent had beneficial effects on cognitive function per se. Both vitamin E and selegiline were more effective than placebo in delaying deterioration to functional end points that included nursing home placement, progression to severe dementia, and substantial loss of basic activities of daily living or death. **(pp. 112–113)**

6. Dementia with a cerebrovascular contribution

    A. Is as common as Alzheimer's disease.
    B. Is most frequently seen as pure vascular dementia.
    C. Lowers the threshold for and increases the magnitude of dementia caused by Alzheimer's disease.
    D. Is associated with an especially high prevalence and severity of dementia with infarcts in the basal ganglia, thalamus, or deep white matter.
    E. C and D.

The correct response is option **E.**

Infarcts lower the threshold for and increase the magnitude of dementia caused by Alzheimer's disease (Snowdon et al. 1997). Infarcts in the basal ganglia, thalamus, or deep white matter are associated with an especially high prevalence and severity of dementia.

Vascular dementia is not as common as Alzheimer's disease. Mixed dementia is more common than previously believed and may make up 10%–30% of late-life dementia (Lim et al. 1999). **(p. 115)**

7. Most forms of frontotemporal dementia involve

    A. Neuronal cell loss.
    B. Gliosis.
    C. Pick bodies.
    D. Abnormal function of tau protein.
    E. Amyloidopathy.

The correct response is option **D.**

It is increasingly clear that abnormal function of the cytoskeletal protein tau ("taupathy") is a central feature of most forms of frontotemporal dementia (Wilhelmsen et al. 1999). Frontotemporal atrophy and microscopic changes are present in Pick's disease; the latter include neuronal cell loss, gliosis, and the presence of massed cytoskeletal elements called Pick bodies. Additional tau mutations were soon described by others (Hutton et al. 1998). Because these tau mutations demonstrated that tau dysfunction is sufficient to cause neurodegenerative dementia even in the absence of brain amyloidopathy, there is increased interest in the role of tau abnormalities in the pathogenesis of the much more common dementia disorder of Alzheimer's disease. **(pp. 116–117)**

8. Hypothyroidism

    A. Can produce a dementia accompanied by irritability, paranoid ideation, and depression.
    B. Can produce a dementia for which aggressive thyroid replacement results in the patient's return to previous level of functioning.
    C. Is similar to vitamin B12 deficiency dementia in that B12 replacement leads to remission of dementia.
    D. A and B.
    E. A, B, and C.

The correct response is option **A.**

Hypothyroidism classically produces a cognitive syndrome of dementia accompanied by irritability, paranoid ideation, and depression. Once the dementia is established, even aggressive thyroid replacement therapy does not result in a return to the patient's previous level of functioning (Larson et al. 1984). Anecdotal reports suggest that B_{12} replacement in dementia that is apparently secondary to B_{12} deficiency may produce some cognitive improvement (Gross et al. 1986; Rajan et al. 2002; Wieland 1986), but dementia persists. **(p. 118)**

9. Delirium in the elderly

   A. Usually persists for months in those hospitalized for medical or surgical reasons.
   B. Rarely results in full resolution of symptoms in a short time.
   C. Is often the initial presentation of an underlying dementia.
   D. Could have an insidious onset.
   E. All of the above.

   The correct response is option **E**.

   Levkoff et al. (1992) demonstrated that incident delirium in elderly persons hospitalized for medical or surgical reasons usually persists for months. Full resolution of symptoms of delirium in a short time was the exception rather than the rule in this study. An episode of delirium often is the initial presentation of an underlying dementia. In the elderly, a delirium secondary to drugs or to illnesses such as renal failure may have an insidious onset. **(p. 119)**

References

Arai H, Kosaka K, Iizuka R: Changes of biogenic amines and their metabolites in postmortem brains from patients with Alzheimer-type dementia. J Neurochem 43:388–393, 1984

Blennow KAH, Wallin A, Gottfries CG, et al: Significance of decreased lumbar CSF levels of HVA and 5-HIAA in Alzheimer's disease. Neurobiol Aging 13:107–113, 1991

Cross AJ, Crow TJ, Ferrier IN, et al: Serotonin receptor changes in dementia of the Alzheimer type. J Neurochem 43:1574–1581, 1984

D'Amato RJ, Zweig RM, Whitehouse PJ, et al: Aminergic systems in Alzheimer's disease and Parkinson's disease. Ann Neurol 22:229–236, 1987

Erkinjuntti T, Kurz A, Gauthier S, et al: Efficacy of galantamine in probable vascular dementia and Alzheimer's disease combined with cerebrovascular disease: a randomised trial. Lancet 359:1283–1290, 2002

Gross JS, Weintraub NT, Neufeld RR, et al: Pernicious anemia in the demented patient without anemia or macrocytosis: a case for early recognition. J Am Geriatr Soc 34:612–614, 1986

Hutton M, Lendon CL, Rizzu P, et al: Association of missense and 5′ splice-site mutations in tau with the inherited dementia FTDP-17. Nature 393:702–705, 1998

Larson EB, Reifler BV, Featherstone HJ, et al: Dementia in elderly outpatients: a prospective study. Ann Intern Med 100:417–423, 1984

Levkoff SE, Evans DA, Liptzin B, et al: Delirium: the occurrence and persistence of symptoms among elderly hospitalized patients. Arch Intern Med 152:334–340, 1992

Lim A, Tsuang D, Kukull W, et al: Clinico-neuropathological correlation of Alzheimer's disease in a community-based case series. J Am Geriatr Soc 47:564–569, 1999

Mann DMA, Yates PO: Serotonin nerve cells in Alzheimer's disease. J Neurol Neurosurg Psychiatry 46:96–98, 1983

Perry EK, Haroutunian V, Davis KL, et al: Neocortical cholinergic activities differentiate Lewy body dementia from classical Alzheimer's disease. Neuroreport 5:747–749, 1994

Raskind MA, Peskind ER, Wessel T, et al: Galantamine in AD: a 6-month randomized, placebo-controlled trial with a 6-month extension. The Galantamine USA-1 Study Group. Neurology 54:2261–2268, 2000

Rajan S, Wallace JI, Beresford SAA, et al: Screening for cobalamin deficiency in geriatric outpatients: prevalence and influence of synthetic cobalamin intake. J Am Geriatr Soc 50:624–630, 2002

Sano M, Ernesto C, Thomas RG, et al: A controlled trial of selegiline, alpha-tocopherol, or both as treatment for Alzheimer's disease. The Alzheimer's Disease Cooperative Study. N Engl J Med 336:1216–1222, 1997

Snowdon DA, Greiner LH, Mortimer JA, et al: Brain infarction and the clinical expression of Alzheimer disease. The Nun Study. JAMA 277:813–817, 1997

Volicer L, Direnfeld LK, Freedman M, et al: Serotonin and 5-hydroxyindoleacetic acid in CSF: differences in Parkinson's disease and dementia of the Alzheimer's type. Arch Neurol 42:127–129, 1985

Whitehouse PJ, Price DL, Struble RG, et al: Alzheimer's disease and senile dementia: loss of neurons in the basal forebrain. Science 215:1237–1239, 1982

Wieland RG: Vitamin B_{12} deficiency in the nonanemic elderly. J Am Geriatr Soc 34:618–619, 1986

Wilhelmsen KC, Clark LN, Miller BL, et al: Tau mutations in frontotemporal dementia. Dement Geriatr Cogn Disord 10:88–92, 1999

Winblad B, Engedal K, Soininen H: A 1-year, randomized, placebo-controlled study of donepezil in patients with mild to moderate AD. Neurology 57:489–495, 2001

Yamamoto T, Hirano A: Nucleus raphe dorsalis in Alzheimer's disease: neurofibrillary tangles and loss of large neurons. Ann Neurol 17:573–577, 1985

Chapter 7:
Movement Disorders

Select the single best response for each question.

1. All of the following are features of Parkinson's disease *except*

   A. Postural instability.
   B. Prevalence increasing with age.
   C. Lewy bodies in the cytoplasm of degenerating neurons.
   D. Resting tremor attenuating at least transiently during voluntary movement, much like that of essential tremor.
   E. Presentation with an akinetic form in which resting tremor is minimal.

   The correct response is option **D.**

   The resting tremor of Parkinson's disease typically attenuates at least transiently during voluntary movement of the affected extremity, such as when the patient picks up an object, and is to be distinguished from the postural, antigravity tremor observed in essential tremor.

   Parkinson's disease is a chronic, progressive, neurodegenerative illness that produces rigidity, slowness of movement (bradykinesia), postural instability, and, often, tremor at rest. The prevalence of Parkinson's disease increases with age, with estimates of 1% at age 60 and up to 2.6% at age 85 or older (Mutch et al. 1986; Sutcliffe et al. 1985). Parkinson's disease is characterized pathologically by abnormal collections of proteins, called Lewy bodies, in the cytoplasm of degenerating neurons (Forno 1996; Golbe 1999). **(pp. 132–133)**

2. Synkinetic movement refers to

   A. Resting tremor.
   B. Cogwheel rigidity.
   C. Involuntary resistance to passive movement of the extremities.
   D. Voluntary movement of contralateral extremity bringing out rigidity in ipsilateral limb.
   E. None of the above.

   The correct response is option **D.**

   Active, voluntary movement of the contralateral extremity (synkinetic movement) can bring out subtle rigidity in an ipsilateral limb.

   In patients with resting tremor, the combination of rigidity and tremor results in cogwheel rigidity—that is, a jerky resistance to passive movement. The stiffness or rigidity of Parkinson's disease is detected clinically by testing for involuntary resistance to passive movement of the extremities. Parkinson's disease can be divided into two clinical forms: 1) tremor-dominant Parkinson's disease, in which tremor at rest is a prominent feature, and 2) postural instability and gait disorder, or akinetic Parkinson's disease, in which resting tremor is minimal, if present at all, and patients exhibit earlier balance difficulty. **(p. 132)**

3. Side effects of dopamine agonists include which of the following?

   A. Hallucinations.
   B. Dyskinesias.
   C. Dystonia.
   D. A and B.
   E. A, B, and C.

   The correct response is option **E.**

   The side effects of dopamine agonists are similar to those of levodopa: hallucinations, dyskinesias (head bobbing and involuntary writhing or twisting movements of the extremities), and dystonia (muscle spasms) are the most common. **(p. 133)**

4. All of the following are features of progressive supranuclear palsy (PSP) *except*

   A. Vertical gaze palsy.
   B. Early postural instability.
   C. Axial rigidity greater than appendicular rigidity.
   D. Good response to levodopa.
   E. Sloppy eating.

   The correct response is option **D.**

   Unlike in Parkinson's disease, there is little or no response to levodopa therapy because of degeneration of secondary neurons downstream from the dopaminergic substantia nigra pars compacta neurons.

   Progressive supranuclear palsy (PSP), or Steele-Richardson-Olszewski syndrome, features parkinsonism without prominent tremor, vertical gaze palsy, axial (midline) more than appendicular (arm and leg) rigidity, early postural instability, and poor response to levodopa (Litvan 2004). PSP is often associated with frequent falling, lack of eye contact, monotonous speech, sloppy eating, and slowed mentation. **(p. 134)**

5. Which of the following is *not* true of essential tremor?
    A. It is the most prevalent movement disorder among the elderly.
    B. Prevalence increases with age.
    C. Frequency may decrease with age.
    D. Early on, tremor is absent at rest.
    E. Usually it is not associated with a family history of tremor.

The correct response is option **E**.

There is usually a clear family history of tremor, and often the tremor attenuates with alcohol use, a phenomenon that can contribute to development of alcoholism in susceptible individuals.

Essential tremor is the most prevalent movement disorder among adults and elderly persons, affecting up to 2% of the general population. The prevalence of essential tremor increases with age, and in individuals older than 70 years, estimates of the prevalence of essential tremor range to more than 10%. A key feature of essential tremor, at least early on, is that the tremor is absent at rest, only occurring during action or when a posture is being held. **(p. 137)**

6. Which of the following attenuates essential tremor?
    A. Propranolol.
    B. Primidone.
    C. Alcohol.
    D. Deep brain stimulation of the ventral intermediate nucleus of the contralateral thalamus.
    E. All of the above.

The correct response is option **E**.

The mainstays of medical treatment for essential tremor are propranolol therapy and primidone therapy. Often the tremor attenuates with alcohol use. Deep brain stimulation targeting the ventral intermediate nucleus of the contralateral thalamus is sometimes helpful in medically refractory cases. **(p. 138)**

References

Forno LS: Neuropathology of Parkinson's disease. J Neuropathol Exp Neurol 55:259–272, 1996
Golbe LI: Alpha-synuclein and Parkinson's disease. Mov Disord 14:6–9, 1999
Litvan I: Update on progressive supranuclear palsy. Curr Neurol Neurosci Rep 4:296–302, 2004
Mutch WJ, Dingwall-Fordyce I, Downie AW, et al: Parkinson's disease in a Scottish city. Br Med J (Clin Res Ed) 292:534–536, 1986
Sutcliffe RL, Prior R, Mawby B, et al: Parkinson's disease in the district of the Northampton Health Authority, United Kingdom: a study of prevalence and disability. Acta Neurol Scand 72:363–379, 1985

Chapter 8:
Mood Disorders

Select the single best response for each question.

1. In contrast to low rates of major depression among older adults in the community, it has been estimated that up to what percentage of hospitalized elders fulfill criteria for a major depressive episode?

    A. 6%.
    B. 11%.
    C. 16%.
    D. 21%.
    E. 31%.

The correct response is option **D.**

In contrast to low rates (1%) of major depression among older adults in the community, it has been estimated that, depending on the diagnostic scheme, up to 21% of hospitalized elders fulfill criteria for a major depressive episode, and an additional 20%–25% have a minor depression (Koenig et al. 1997). **(p. 147)**

2. Mortality among elderly patients is

    A. Increased in older men with physical health problems and depression.
    B. Increased among nursing home patients with depression.
    C. Increased in previously hospitalized depressed women.
    D. A and B.
    E. A, B, and C.

The correct response is option **E.**

Older men with physical health problems and depression are significantly more likely to die than similarly aged, physically ill, nondepressed men. Among depressed women, mortality is twice the expected rate; among the men, it is three times the expected rate. Rovner and colleagues (1991) found greater death rates among elderly nursing home patients with depression. Several subsequent studies involving medically ill patients likewise found greater mortality among those with depression (Arfken et al. 1999; Covinsky et al. 1999; Black and Markides 1999). **(pp. 147–148)**

3. Studies of prognosis of late-life depression show all of the following *except*

    A. Older adults differ from their middle-age counterparts in terms of recovery and remission.
    B. Elders who have recovered appear to experience residual depressive symptoms.
    C. Seventy percent of elderly patients with major depression treated with adequate antidepressant regimens recover from the index episode.
    D. Older patients who have experienced one or more moderate to severe episodes of major depression may need to continue antidepressant therapy permanently to minimize relapse.
    E. Physical illness and cognitive impairment are associated with a worse outcome.

The correct response is option **A.**

In terms of recovery and remission, older adults do not differ from their middle-aged counterparts (Blazer et al. 1992). If they do recover, however, elders appear to experience residual depressive symptoms. Most clinicians and clinical investigators report that more than 70% of elderly patients with major depression who are treated with antidepressant medication (at an adequate dose for a sufficient time) recover from the index episode of depression. Once an older patient has experienced one or more moderate to severe episodes of major depression, he or she may need to continue antidepressant therapy permanently, to minimize the risk of relapse (Greden 1993; Old Age Depression Interest Group 1993). Physical illness, disability, cognitive impairment, and more severe depression are associated with worse outcomes (Baldwin and Jolley 1986; Cole 1983; Koenig et al. 1997; Murphy et al. 1988). **(pp. 148–150)**

4. Bipolar disorder in the elderly may have all of the following characteristics *except*
    A. Tendency toward more rapid recurrences late in the illness.
    B. Stressful events more likely to precede early-onset mania than late-onset mania.
    C. Increased cerebral vulnerability playing a stronger role than life events in precipitating late-onset mania.
    D. Association with low rates of familial affective disorder.
    E. Genetic factors weighing heavily in the etiology.

The correct response is option **E.**

Evidence that genetic factors weigh heavily in the etiology of bipolar disorders in late life is virtually nonexistent, although the biological nature of this disorder would suggest some genetic contribution.

In a review of records of a small number of untreated patients with severe and prolonged bipolar disorder, Cutler and Post (1982) found a tendency toward more rapid recurrences late in the illness, with decreasing periods of normality. Ameblas (1987) emphasized a relationship between life events and onset of mania, noting that stressful events were more likely to precede early-onset mania than late-onset mania. Likewise, Shulman (1989) stressed that increased cerebral vulnerability due to organic insults (stroke, head trauma, other brain insults) played a stronger role than life events in precipitating late-onset mania (a factor that may also play a role in treatment resistance). Young and Klerman (1992) emphasized the low rates of familial affective disorder. **(p. 153)**

5. Reversible dementia due to depression
    A. Predicts poor response to treatment of the depression.
    B. Is associated with patients attempting to conceal disabilities rather than highlighting them on formal mental status exam.
    C. Cannot be differentiated from that of bona fide dementia by way of REM sleep measures.
    D. Often indicates the presence of an early dementing illness.
    E. Should not be treated with a potent anticholinergic antidepressant such as imipramine.

The correct response is option **D.**

The combination of depression and reversible dementia in elderly patients often indicates the presence of an early dementing illness (Alexopoulos et al. 1993). In a study conducted by Reifler et al. (1982), elderly patients with depression and dementia, when treated with an antidepressant, responded with a remission of the depressive symptoms, while cognitive dysfunction persisted. The tendency among depressed patients is to highlight disabilities as opposed to concealing (or attempting to conceal) them. Both depressed and nondepressed Alzheimer's patients were treated with the relatively potent anticholinergic antidepressant imipramine; patients improved whether or not they were in the treatment group, and cognitive function did not decline (Reifler et al. 1989). Dykierek and colleagues (1998) found that nearly all REM sleep measures differentiated significantly in patients with Alzheimer's disease, depressed elderly patients, and healthy controls. REM density, rather than REM sleep latency, was particularly important in separating depressed elders with dementia. **(p. 160)**

6. According to a recent study, what percentage of elders fulfill criteria for definite or questionable alcohol abuse?

   A. Between 2% and 4%.
   B. Between 3% and 6%.
   C. Between 10% and 15%.
   D. Between 20% and 30%.
   E. Between 30% and 40%.

The correct response is option **C**.

Results of a recent study involving more than 10,000 older persons indicate that between 10% and 15% of elders fulfill criteria for definite or questionable alcohol abuse (Thomas and Rockwood 2001). **(p. 161)**

7. ECT

   A. Is less effective in older adults than in younger ones.
   B. Is no more effective than and has more side effects than antidepressants when used in the old-old populace.
   C. Has a relapse rate that may exceed 50% in the year after a course of ECT, without prophylaxis.
   D. Leads to a significant worsening of cognition in the majority of elderly depressed patients with dementia.
   E. Should be avoided in patients with cardiovascular, neurological, endocrine, or metabolic conditions.

The correct response is option **C**.

The relapse rate with no prophylactic intervention may exceed 50% in the year after a course of ECT. This relapse rate can be decreased if antidepressants or lithium carbonate is prescribed after the treatment. Investigators concluded that despite a higher level of physical illness and cognitive impairment, patients age 75 or older who had severe major depression tolerated ECT in a manner similar to the way in which younger patients tolerated the treatment, and the old-old patients demonstrated a similar or even better response (Tew et al. 1999). There is also evidence that ECT may be more effective and have fewer side effects than antidepressants when used to treat depression in old-old patients (Manly et al. 2000). Price and McAllister (1989) examined the efficacy of ECT in elderly depressed patients with dementia and found that only 21% experienced cognition problems; in most cases the problems were transient. Data do support the use of ECT in patients with cardiovascular, neurological, endocrine, or metabolic conditions, as well as a variety of other conditions (Stoudemire et al. 1998). **(pp. 166–167)**

References

Ameblas A: Life events and mania. Br J Psychiatry 150:235–240, 1987

Arfken CL, Lichtenberg PA, Tancer ME: Cognitive impairment and depression predict mortality in medically ill older adults. J Gerontol A Biol Sci Med Sci 54:M152–M156, 1999

Alexopoulos GS, Meyers BS, Young RC, et al: The course of geriatric depression with "reversible dementia": a controlled study. Am J Psychiatry 150:1693–1699, 1993

Baldwin JC, Jolley DJ: The prognosis of depression in old age. Br J Psychiatry 149:574–583, 1986

Black SA, Markides KS: Depressive symptoms and mortality in older Mexican Americans. Ann Epidemiol 9:45–52, 1999

Blazer DG, Hughes DC, George LK: Age and impaired subjective support: predictors of symptoms at one-year follow-up. J Nerv Ment Dis 180:172–178, 1992

Cole MG: Age, age of onset and course of primary depressive illness in the elderly. Can J Psychiatry 28:102–104, 1983

Covinsky KE, Kahana E, Chin MH, et al: Depressive symptoms and 3-year mortality in older hospitalized medical patients. Ann Intern Med 130:563–569, 1999

Cutler NR, Post RM: Life course of illness in untreated manic-depressive patients. Compr Psychiatry 23:101–115, 1982

Dykierek P, Stadtmuller G, Schramm P, et al: The value of REM sleep parameters in differentiating Alzheimer's disease from old-age depression and normal aging. J Psychiatr Res 32:1–9, 1998

Greden JF: Antidepressant maintenance medications: when to discontinue and how to stop. J Clin Psychiatry 54 (suppl 8):39–45, 1993

Koenig HG, George LK, Peterson BL, et al: Depression in medically ill hospitalized older adults: prevalence, characteristics, and course of symptoms based on six diagnostic schemes. Am J Psychiatry 154:1376–1383, 1997

Manly DT, Oakley SP Jr, Bloch RM: Electroconvulsive therapy in old-old patients. Am J Geriatr Psychiatry 8:232–236, 2000

Murphy E, Smith R, Lindsay J, et al: Increased mortality rates in late-life depression. Br J Psychiatry 152:347–353, 1988

Old Age Depression Interest Group: How long should the elderly take antidepressants? A double-blind placebo-controlled study of continuation/prophylaxis therapy with dothiepin. Br J Psychiatry 162:175–182, 1993

Price TR, McAllister TW: Safety and efficacy of ECT in depressed patients with dementia: a review of clinical experience. Convuls Ther 5:61–74, 1989

Reifler BV, Larson E, Henley R: Coexistence of cognitive impairment and depression in geriatric outpatients. Am J Psychiatry 39:623–626, 1982

Reifler BV, Teri L, Raskind M, et al: Double-blind trial of imipramine in Alzheimer's disease patients with and without depression. Am J Psychiatry 146:45–49, 1989

Rovner BW, German PS, Brant LJ, et al: Depression and mortality in nursing homes. JAMA 265:993–996, 1991

Shulman KI: The influence of age and aging on manic disorder. Int J Geriatr Psychiatry 4:63–65, 1989

Stoudemire A, Hill CD, Marquardt M, et al: Recovery and relapse in geriatric depression after treatment with antidepressants and ECT in a medical-psychiatric population. Gen Hosp Psychiatry 20:170–174, 1998

Tew JD Jr, Mulsant BH, Haskett RF, et al: Acute efficacy of ECT in the treatment of major depression in the old-old. Am J Psychiatry 156:1865–1870, 1999

Thomas VS, Rockwood KJ: Alcohol abuse, cognitive impairment, and mortality among older people. J Am Geriatr Soc 49:415–420, 2001

Young RC, Klerman GL: Mania in late life: focus on age at onset. Am J Psychiatry 149:867–876, 1992

Chapter 9:
Schizophrenia and Paranoid Disorders

Select the single best response for each question.

1. Factors distinguishing patients with very late onset schizophrenia from "true" schizophrenia of younger patients include all of the following *except*

    A. Lower genetic load.
    B. Less evidence of early childhood maladjustment.
    C. Relative lack of formal thought disorder and negative symptoms.
    D. Lesser risk of tardive dyskinesia.
    E. Evidence of a neurodegenerative rather than a neurodevelopmental process.

    The correct response is option **D.**

    Factors distinguishing patients with very late onset schizophrenia from "true" schizophrenia patients include a lower genetic load, less evidence of early childhood maladjustment, a relative lack of thought disorder and negative symptoms (including blunted affect), greater risk of tardive dyskinesia, and evidence of a neurodegenerative rather than a neurodevelopmental process (Andreasen 1999; Howard et al. 1997). **(p. 179)**

2. What approximate percentage of Alzheimer's disease patients manifest psychotic symptoms, typically in the middle stages of the disease?

    A. 10%–20%.
    B. 15%–25%.
    C. 25%–30%.
    D. 35%–50%.
    E. 55%–65%.

    The correct response is option **D.**

    Approximately 35%–50% of Alzheimer's disease patients manifest psychotic symptoms, typically in the middle stages of the disease (Ropacki and Jeste 2005). **(p. 181)**

3. Alzheimer's disease patients with and without psychosis differ in all of the following *except*

    A. Alzheimer's disease patients with psychosis show greater impairment in executive functioning.
    B. Alzheimer's disease patients with psychosis have a greater prevalence of extrapyramidal signs.
    C. Alzheimer's disease patients with psychosis have shown increased norepinephrine levels and reduced serotonin levels in subcortical regions.

D. Alzheimer's disease patients with psychosis typically warrant very long term maintenance therapy with antipsychotics.

E. Alzheimer's disease patients with psychosis have more prevalent behavioral disturbances such as agitation than hallucinations and paranoid delusions.

The correct response is option **D**.

Because psychotic symptoms in patients with dementia tend to remit in the late stages of the disease, very long term maintenance therapy with antipsychotics is typically unnecessary.

Alzheimer's disease patients with psychosis and those without psychosis differ in several important ways. Neuropsychologically, Alzheimer's disease patients with psychosis show greater impairment in executive functioning and a more rapid cognitive decline (Jeste et al. 1992; Stern et al. 1994). Psychosis is associated with a greater prevalence of extrapyramidal signs in Alzheimer's disease (Stern et al. 1994). Neuropathologically, dementia patients with psychosis have shown increased neurodegenerative changes in the cortex, increased norepinephrine levels in subcortical regions, and reduced serotonin levels in both cortical and subcortical areas (Zubenko et al. 1991). Devanand and colleagues (1997) found that hallucinations and paranoid delusions were more persistent than depressive symptoms but less prevalent and less persistent than behavioral disturbances, particularly agitation. **(p. 182)**

4. The most important risk factor for tardive dyskinesia is

A. Alcohol abuse.
B. Early extrapyramidal symptoms.
C. Certain ethnicities.
D. Aging.
E. None of the above.

The correct response is option **D**.

Aging appears to be the most important risk factor for tardive dyskinesia (American Psychiatric Association 2000; Yassa and Jeste 1992).

Previous investigators found TD to be associated with early extrapyramidal symptoms (Chouinard et al. 1979; Saltz et al. 1991), diabetes (Caligiuri and Jeste 2004), alcohol abuse or dependence (Dixon et al. 1992; Olivera et al. 1990), and certain ethnicities (Glazer et al. 1994; Jeste et al. 1996; Lawson 1986). **(p. 186)**

References

Andreasen NC: I don't believe in late onset schizophrenia, in Late-Onset Schizophrenia. Edited by Howard R, Rabins PV, Castle DJ. Philadelphia, PA, Wrightson Biomedical, 1999, pp 111–123

Caligiuri MP, Jeste DV: Association of diabetes with dyskinesia in older psychosis patients. Psychopharmacology (Berl) 176:281–286, 2004

Chouinard G, Annable L, Ross-Chouinard A, et al: Factors related to tardive dyskinesia. Am J Psychiatry 136:79–82, 1979

Devanand DP, Jacobs DM, Tang MX, et al: The course of psychopathologic features in mild to moderate Alzheimer disease. Arch Gen Psychiatry 54:257–263, 1997

Dixon L, Weiden PJ, Haas G, et al: Increased tardive dyskinesia in alcohol-abusing schizophrenic patients. Compr Psychiatry 33:121–122, 1992

Glazer WM, Morgenstern H, Doucette J: Race and tardive dyskinesia among outpatients at a CMHC. Hosp Community Psychiatry 45:38–42, 1994

Howard R, Graham C, Sham P, et al: A controlled family study of late-onset non-affective psychosis (late paraphrenia). Br J Psychiatry 170:511–514, 1997

Jeste DV, Wragg RE, Salmon DP, et al: Cognitive deficits of patients with Alzheimer's disease with and without delusions. Am J Psychiatry 149:184–189, 1992

Jeste DV, Lindamer LA, Evans J, et al: Relationship of ethnicity and gender to schizophrenia and pharmacology of neuroleptics. Psychopharmacol Bull 32:243–251, 1996

Lawson WB: Racial and ethnic factors in psychiatric research. Hosp Community Psychiatry 37:50–54, 1986

Olivera AA, Kiefer MW, Manley NK: Tardive dyskinesia in psychiatric patients with substance use disorders. Am J Drug Alcohol Abuse 16:57–66, 1990

Ropacki S, Jeste DV: Epidemiology of and risk factors for psychosis of Alzheimer disease: a review of 55 studies published from 1990 to 2003. Am J Psychiatry 162:2022–2030, 2005

Saltz BL, Woerner MG, Kane JM, et al: Prospective study of tardive dyskinesia incidence in the elderly. JAMA 266:2402–2406, 1991

Stern Y, Albert M, Brandt J, et al: Utility of extrapyramidal signs and psychosis as predictors of cognitive and functional decline, nursing home admission, and death in Alzheimer's disease: prospective analyses from the Predictors Study. Neurology 44:2300–2307, 1994

Zubenko GS, Moossy J, Martinez AJ, et al: Neuropathologic and neurochemical correlates of psychosis in primary dementia. Arch Neurol 48:619–624, 1991

Chapter 10:
Anxiety and Panic Disorders

Select the single best response for each question.

1. According to the Epidemiologic Catchment Area (ECA) study of the 1980s, the combined prevalence of phobia, panic disorder, and obsessive-compulsive disorder in people over age 65 is approximately what percentage?

   A. 2.5%.
   B. 3.5%.
   C. 5.5%.
   D. 6.5%.
   E. 7%.

The correct response is option **C**.

The combined prevalence of phobia, panic disorder, and obsessive-compulsive disorder in people older than age 65 years was 5.5% according to the ECA study of the 1980s (Regier et al. 1990). **(p. 193)**

2. Panic disorder in those older than 65

   A. Has a point prevalence of 0.4%.
   B. Is not uncommonly ascribed to other causes by the elderly.
   C. May present with fewer symptoms.
   D. Is a relatively uncommon development in late life.
   E. All of the above.

The correct response is option **E**.

In the ECA study, the point prevalence among middle-age subjects was 1.1%, whereas among those age 65 or older, the point prevalence was 0.4% (Regier et al. 1988). Development of panic disorder in late life is relatively uncommon, but it does occur (Luchins and Rose 1989; Sheikh and Cassidy 2000). It is not uncommon for elderly adults to ascribe the symptoms to other causes, and the frequent waxing and waning of symptoms may make correct diagnosis difficult. Elderly individuals with late-onset panic attacks may have fewer symptoms and may do less to avoid the attacks (Sheikh et al. 1991). **(p. 194)**

3. In at least one study, what percentage of elderly Holocaust survivors met criteria for posttraumatic stress disorder more than 40 years after the war?

    A. 10%.
    B. 20%.
    C. 30%.
    D. 40%.
    E. 50%.

The correct response is option **E.**

Nearly half of the elderly Holocaust survivors studied met criteria for posttraumatic stress disorder more than 40 years after the war (Kuch and Cox 1992). **(p. 196)**

4. The most common anxiety disorder of the elderly population is

    A. Generalized anxiety disorder.
    B. Posttraumatic stress disorder.
    C. Social phobia.
    D. Specific phobia.
    E. Obsessive-compulsive disorder.

The correct response is option **D.**

Generalized anxiety disorder is the second most common anxiety disorder in the elderly population (phobias are the most common) (Blazer et al. 1991). **(p. 196)**

5. Which of the following factors could pertain to medical illnesses and anxiety among the elderly?

    A. The older adult may worry about the effect and meaning of physical illness.
    B. Anxiety may contribute to medical problems and complications.
    C. Many anxiety symptoms may masquerade as medical illness.
    D. Anxiety symptoms may be caused by medications given to elderly persons.
    E. All of the above.

The correct response is option **E.**

There is a complex interaction among anxiety, medical illness, and the medications used to treat these conditions (Flint 1999). First, medical illness may masquerade as anxiety symptoms, and many anxiety symptoms may masquerade as medical illness. Seccond, the presence of anxiety may contribute to medical problems and complications. Third, older adults may have the realistic worry about the effect and meaning of physical illness. Finally, anxiety symptoms may be caused by the medications given to elderly persons to treat either physical or mental diseases. **(pp. 197–198)**

6. Which of the following pharmacological agents has become the mainstay treatment of anxiety disorder in the elderly?

    A. Tricyclic antidepressants (TCAs).
    B. Monoamine oxidase inhibitors (MAOIs).
    C. Selective serotonin reuptake inhibitors (SSRIs).
    D. Benzodiazepines.
    E. Buspirone.

    The correct response is option **C**.

    SSRIs have become the mainstay of anxiety disorder treatment, for several reasons. First, various SSRIs have obtained U.S. Food and Drug Administration–approved indications for use in the treatment of panic disorder, GAD, social phobia, and OCD in the general population. Second, anxiety disorders and depressive disorders are frequently comorbid, and use of a single agent to treat both conditions decreases the rate of polypharmacy, a situation often occurring with the elderly. Finally, the side-effect profiles of SSRIs are much more acceptable than those of many older medications. **(pp. 198–199)**

References

Blazer DG, Hughes D, George LK, et al: Generalized anxiety disorder, in Psychiatric Disorders in America: The Epidemiologic Catchment Area Study. Edited by Robins LN, Regier DA. New York, Free Press, 1991b, pp 180–203

Flint AJ: Anxiety disorders in late life. Can Fam Physician 45:2672–2679, 1999

Kuch K, Cox BJ: Symptoms of PTSD in 124 survivors of the Holocaust. Am J Psychiatry 149:337–340, 1992

Luchins DJ, Rose RP: Late-life onset of panic disorder with agoraphobia in three patients. Am J Psychiatry 146:920–921, 1989

Regier DA, Boyd JH, Burke JD Jr, et al: One-month prevalence of mental disorders in the United States. Based on five Epidemiologic Catchment Area sites. Arch Gen Psychiatry 45:977–986, 1988

Regier DA, Narrow WE, Rae DS: The epidemiology of anxiety disorders: the Epidemiologic Catchment Area (ECA) experience. J Psychiatr Res 24 (suppl 2):3–14, 1990

Sheikh JI, Cassidy EL: Treatment of anxiety disorders in the elderly: issues and strategies. J Anxiety Disord 14:173–190, 2000

Sheikh JI, King RJ, Taylor CB: Comparative phenomenology of early onset versus late-onset panic attacks: a pilot study. Am J Psychiatry 148:1231–1233, 1991

Chapter 11:
Somatoform Disorders

Select the single best response for each question.

1. Somatization disorder is a psychiatric illness characterized by numerous physical complaints that are in excess of examination findings. This may be an especially challenging problem in the older patient with other chronic medical conditions. Which of the following is also true regarding somatization disorder?

    A. Patients with somatization disorder have pain localized to one site.
    B. Somatization disorder is seen almost exclusively in women.

C. As somatization disorder patients age, their reported symptoms tend to change.

D. The prevalence rate has been estimated to be 8%–10%.

E. Another term for somatization disorder is Munchausen syndrome.

The correct response is option **B.**

Somatization disorder is seen almost exclusively in women and may have a prevalence rate ranging from 1% to 3% (Faravelli et al. 1997; Martin and Yutzy 1994). The majority of individuals with somatization disorder demonstrate consistent symptom patterns as they age (Cloninger et al. 1986; Pribor et al. 1994). Somatization disorder is characterized by multiple physical complaints that include pain at four or more sites, two gastrointestinal symptoms, one sexual symptom, and one pseudoneurological symptom (other than pain). Another term used to describe somatization disorder is *Briquet's syndrome* (Liskow et al. 1986; Orenstein 1989). **(p. 208)**

2. Undifferentiated somatoform disorder and hypochondriasis may present in the geriatric psychiatric patient. Distinguishing between these two conditions may be difficult in the clinical setting. Which of the following statements is true?

    A. Undifferentiated somatoform disorder requires the presence of persistent physical complaints for at least 12 months.

    B. Patients with chronic pain rarely also qualify for a diagnosis of undifferentiated somatoform disorder.

    C. The psychological preoccupation in hypochondriasis relates to the symptoms experienced, rather than the possible disease "represented" by the symptoms.

    D. It has been clearly established that high educational level and high socioeconomic status lead to a predisposition to hypochondriasis, because individuals with these factors may be more aware of medical conditions and have greater access to information.

    E. Comorbid depressive and anxiety disorders are common in hypochondriasis.

The correct response is option **E.**

Comorbid psychiatric disorders, especially major depression, panic disorder, and obsessive-compulsive disorder, are common in hypochondriasis (Barsky et al. 1992).

Undifferentiated somatoform disorder requires the presence of persistent physical pain for at least 6 months. Patients with chronic pain have been found to have quite high rates of undifferentiated somatoform disorder (Aigner and Bach 1999). Hypochondriasis is characterized by a preoccupation with fears of having a serious illness. There is some debate regarding whether factors such as low education level, low socioeconomic status, and old age increase the risk of hypochondriasis (Barsky et al. 1991; Brink et al. 1981; Kellner 1986; Rief et al. 2001). **(pp. 208–209)**

3. Conversion disorder is characterized by motor and/or sensory deficits that suggest neurological illness(es) but that cannot be elucidated by the appropriate neurological and neuroimaging evaluations. Which of the following is true regarding this syndrome?

    A. Conversion disorder is more common in elderly than in young patients.

    B. Conversion disorder is seen almost exclusively in women.

    C. A risk factor for conversion disorder is sexual abuse.

D. Although nonepileptic seizures (often referred to as pseudoseizures) are a subtype of conversion disorder, they are rarely seen in patients with a bona fide seizure disorder.

E. Conversion disorder in late life is rarely associated with a comorbid neurological disorder.

The correct response is option **C**.

Sexual abuse (Martin 1994), personality disorders, and other neurological disorders (Ford and Folks 1985; Slater and Glithero 1965) are risk factors for conversion disorder.

Conversion disorder is more common in young women, although it has also been reported in the elderly population (Weddington 1979). Nonepileptic seizures are seen in 5%–20% of outpatients with epilepsy (Chabolla et al. 1996). Conversion disorder in late life is likely associated with an actual comorbid neurological disorder. **(p. 209)**

4. The etiology of somatoform disorders has been subject to much theoretical speculation. Which of the following is true?

    A. The prevalence of all definitively diagnosed somatoform disorders increases with age.

    B. When somatoform disorders present in the older patient, comorbid neurological illness may be associated with them, but neuropsychological (cognitive) impairment is not.

    C. Somatoform disorders are associated with a history of serious illness of a parent, but not in the patient, early in life.

    D. Comorbid panic disorder is common in somatoform disorders, but other anxiety disorders are not.

    E. The personality trait of neuroticism, wherein the subject experiences more negative emotions, is associated with the development of somatoform disorders.

The correct response is option **E**.

The personality trait of neuroticism is associated with the development of somatoform disorders (Affleck et al. 1992; Chaturvedi 1986; Costa and McCrae 1980; Phillips and McElroy 2000).

The prevalence of somatoform disorders does not increase with age, with the exception of hypochondriasis. When present in late life, somatoform disorders may be associated with neuropsychological impairment and/or comorbid neurological illness (Sheehan and Banerjee 1999). Somatoform disorders have been associated with the experience of serious illness early in life (Stuart and Noyes 1999), childhood abuse (Martin 1994; Walker et al. 1992), and significant psychological stress (Hollifield et al. 1999; Ritsner et al. 2000). Comorbid depression, anxiety and panic disorders, substance abuse, and personality disorders are common in somatoform disorders (Noyes et al. 2001). **(pp. 211–212)**

5. Treatment of somatoform disorders calls for an integrative biopsychosocial approach by the physician. Which of the following approaches is recommended?

    A. The physician should arrange appointments on an as-needed basis.

    B. A focus on obtaining insight into the psychological context of somatoform symptoms should be the first priority for intervention.

C. The physician should not offer to review all prior medical records, as this merely reinforces maladaptive somatization behavior.

D. Hypochondriasis has been shown to respond to antidepressants and anxiolytics.

E. The clinician should avoid forming a therapeutic alliance, since doing so would reinforce preexisting systems.

The correct response is option **D**.

Hypochondriacal symptoms have responded to antidepressant medications, especially to selective serotonin reuptake inhibitors (SSRIs) and anxiolytics (Barsky 2001; Fallon et al. 1996; Oosterbaan et al. 2001).

The physician should arrange periodic but regularly scheduled appointments (Smith et al. 1986) and should focus on symptom reduction and rehabilitation (Kellner 1987). The clinician must form a therapeutic alliance through empathetic listening and acknowledgment of physical discomfort. Offering to review all available medical records can be a tangible way for the physician to convey the seriousness given to the patient's symptoms. In conversion disorders, hypnosis is sometimes used as both a diagnostic and a therapeutic tool. **(pp. 212–213)**

References

Affleck G, Tennen H, Urrows S, et al: Neuroticism and the pain-mood relation in rheumatoid arthritis: insights from a prospective daily study. J Consult Clin Psychol 60:119–126, 1992

Aigner M, Bach M: Clinical utility of DSM-IV pain disorder. Compr Psychiatry 40:353–357, 1999

Barsky AJ: The patient with hypochondriasis. N Engl J Med 345:1395–1399, 2001

Barsky AJ, Frank C, Cleary P, et al: The relation between hypochondriasis and age. Am J Psychiatry 148:923–928, 1991

Barsky AJ, Wyshak G, Klerman G: Psychiatric comorbidity in DSM-III-R hypochondriasis. Arch Gen Psychiatry 49:101–108, 1992

Brink T, Janakes C, Martinez N: Geriatric hypochondriasis: situational factors. J Am Geriatr Soc 29:37–39, 1981

Chaturvedi SK: Chronic idiopathic pain disorder. J Psychosom Res 30:199–203, 1986

Chabolla DR, Krahn LE, So EL, et al: Psychogenic nonepileptic seizures. Mayo Clin Proc 71:493–500, 1996

Cloninger CR, Martin RL, Guze SB, et al: A prospective follow-up and family study of somatization in men and women. Am J Psychiatry 143:873–878, 1986

Costa PT Jr, McCrae RR: Somatic complaints in males as a function of age and neuroticism: a longitudinal analysis. J Behav Med 3:245–257, 1980

Fallon BA, Schneier FR, Marshall R, et al: The pharmacotherapy of hypochondriasis. Psychopharmacol Bull 32:607–611, 1996

Faravelli C, Salvatori S, Galassi F, et al: Epidemiology of somatoform disorders: a community survey in Florence. Soc Psychiatry Psychiatr Epidemiol 32:24–29, 1997

Ford CV, Folks DG: Conversion disorders: an overview. Psychosomatics 26:371–383, 1985

Hollifield M, Tuttle L, Paine S, et al: Hypochondriasis and somatization related to personality and attitudes towards self. Psychosomatics 40:387–395, 1999

Kellner R: Somatization and Hypochondriasis. New York, Praeger, 1986

Kellner R: Hypochondriasis and somatization. JAMA 258:2718–2722, 1987

Liskow B, Othmer E, Penick EC, et al: Is Briquet's syndrome a heterogeneous disorder? Am J Psychiatry 143:626–629, 1986

Martin RL: Conversion disorder, proposed autonomic arousal disorder, and pseudocyesis, in DSM-IV Sourcebook, Vol 2. Edited by Widiger TA, Frances AJ, Pincus HA, et al. Washington, DC, American Psychiatric Association, 1994, pp 893–914

Martin RL, Yutzy SH: Somatoform disorders, in The American Psychiatric Press Textbook of Psychiatry, 2nd Edition. Edited by Hales RE, Yudofsky SC, Talbott JA. Washington, DC, American Psychiatric Press, 1994, pp 591–622

Noyes R Jr, Langbehn DR, Happel RL, et al: Personality dysfunction among somatizing patients. Psychosomatics 42:320–329, 2001

Orenstein H: Briquet's syndrome in association with depression and panic: a reconceptualization of Briquet's syndrome. Am J Psychiatry 146:334–338, 1989

Oosterbaan DB, van Balkom AJ, van Boeijen CA, et al: An open study of paroxetine in hypochondriasis. Prog Neuropsychopharmacol Biol Psychiatry 25:1023–1033, 2001

Phillips KA, McElroy SL: Personality disorders and traits in patients with body dysmorphic disorder. Compr Psychiatry 41:229–236, 2000

Pribor EF, Smith DS, Yutzy SH: Somatization disorder in elderly patients. J Geriatr Psychiatry 2:109–117, 1994

Rief W, Hessel A, Braehler E: Somatization symptoms and hypochondriacal features in the general population. Psychosom Med 63:595–602, 2001

Ritsner M, Ponizovsky A, Kurs R, et al: Somatization in an immigrant population in Israel: a community survey of prevalence, risk factors, and help-seeking behavior. Am J Psychiatry 157:385–392, 2000

Sheehan B, Banerjee S: Review: somatization in the elderly. Int J Geriatr Psychiatry 14:1044–1049, 1999

Slater ETO, Glithero E: A follow-up of patients diagnosed as suffering from "hysteria." J Psychosom Res 9:9–13, 1965

Smith GR Jr, Monson RA, Ray DC: Psychiatric consultation in somatization disorder: a randomized controlled study. N Engl J Med 314:1407–1413, 1986

Stuart S, Noyes R Jr: Attachment and interpersonal communication in somatization. Psychosomatics 40:34–43, 1999

Walker EA, Katon WJ, Hansom J, et al: Medical and psychiatric symptoms in women with childhood sexual abuse. Psychosom Med 54:658–664, 1992

Weddington WW: Conversion reaction in an 82 year old man. J Nerv Ment Dis 167:368–369, 1979

Chapter 12:
Bereavement and Adjustment Disorders

Select the single best response for each question.

1. Bereavement is a common focus of clinical inquiry in geropsychiatry. The epidemiology of partner loss as a locus for bereavement has led to some conclusions that are of interest to the practicing clinician. Which of the following is true regarding widowhood and widowerhood in the United States?

   A. The mean age of spousal loss is 69 years for women and 66 years for men.
   B. The mean duration of widowhood is longer than the mean duration of widowerhood.
   C. The rates of widowhood among persons older than 65 are much higher for Hispanic and Asian Americans than for Caucasians.
   D. Among those older than 65, about 15% of women have lost a spouse.
   E. None of the above.

   The correct response is option **B**.

The mean duration of widowhood is longer than the mean duration of widowerhood.

The mean age at spousal loss is 69 years for men and 66 years for women (Centers for Disease Control and Prevention 2002). Among people age 65 or older, about 45% of women and 15% of men have lost a spouse (Federal Interagency Forum on Aging Related Statistics 2000). The rates of widowhood among people age 65 or older are similar for whites, Hispanics, and Asian Americans and are slightly higher for African Americans (U.S. Census Bureau 1998). After the loss of a spouse, older men are at higher risk for mortality than are women. **(pp. 219–220)**

2. Stroebe and Schut are notable for their recent work on a dual-process model of bereavement. According to this model, which of the following is considered to be a restoration-oriented rather than a loss-oriented stressor?

    A. Emotional symptoms.
    B. Behavioral symptoms.
    C. New identity development.
    D. Physiological symptoms.
    E. Cognitive symptoms.

    The correct response is option **C**.

    Restoration-oriented stressors include developing new identities and learning new skills to perform tasks previously done by the deceased. Loss-oriented stressors are manifested as emotional, behavioral, physiological, and cognitive symptoms (Stroebe and Schut 1999, 2001). **(pp. 223–224)**

3. In clinical classification of cases that present with depressive symptoms in the context of interpersonal loss or grief, the physician often faces the task of deciding when symptoms cross the threshold of becoming complicated bereavement. This distinction is not always simple. To address this, DSM-IV-TR includes several specific symptoms that are not considered to be characteristic of a "normal" grief reaction. Which of the following symptoms would *not* be considered evidence of complicated bereavement?

    A. Guilt about actions not taken at the time of death.
    B. Preoccupation with personal worthlessness.
    C. Marked psychomotor retardation.
    D. Prolonged and marked functional impairment.
    E. Hallucinations not containing imagery of the dead person.

    The correct response is option **A**.

    Guilt about actions not taken by the survivor at the time of death would not be considered evidence of complicated bereavement.

    Several specific symptoms that are not considered to be characteristic of a normal grief reaction are also listed in DSM-IV-TR. These include "1) guilt about things other than actions taken or not taken by the survivor at the time of the death; 2) thoughts of death other than the survivor feeling that he or she would be better off dead or should have died with the deceased person; 3) morbid preoccupation with worthlessness; 4) marked psychomotor retardation; 5) prolonged and marked functional impairment;

and 6) hallucinatory experiences other than thinking that he or she hears the voice of, or transiently sees the image of, the deceased person" (American Psychiatric Association 2000a, p. 741). **(p. 221)**

4. Several longitudinal studies of late-life bereavement have revealed some specific findings. Which of the following is true?

    A. Symptoms of anxiety and depression among bereaved subjects differ from controls only in the first 2 months following the loss.
    B. All studies have shown a higher psychological symptom burden among bereaved men than among bereaved women.
    C. When separated operationally from other symptoms such as anxiety and depression, grief has been found to remain for longer time periods.
    D. Women have been found to have higher rates of persistent grief than men.
    E. Older women who have lost their spouses have a higher risk of death than older bereaved men.

    The correct response is option **C.**

    The level of grief remains high for at least 30 months after a spouse's death, and the experience of grief is distinct from the experience of depressed mood and related symptoms, which lessen significantly over that same interval (Thompson et al. 1991).

    Symptoms of anxiety and depression among bereaved subjects and nonbereaved controls differ significantly in the first 2–6 months after a spouse's death (Harlow et al. 1991; Lund et al. 1989; Thompson et al. 1991). Although, typically, bereaved women report more psychological distress than bereaved men, no gender differences have been found in the level of grief reported by individuals. Older bereaved men who have lost their spouses are at higher risk for death than bereaved women (Bowling 1988–1989; Stroebe and Stroebe 1993; Thompson et al. 1984). **(pp. 225–226)**

5. Which of the following is true regarding clinical interventions for complicated bereavement in older patients?

    A. If depression is present, it should not be treated first. The grieving process must first be addressed.
    B. Even if major depression is present, it should not be treated for at least 6 months.
    C. Since most deaths of elderly patients are due to chronic illness, posttraumatic stress disorder in survivors is rare.
    D. Combined pharmacological and psychotherapeutic treatment has been shown to be more effective than either intervention alone.
    E. Bereavement-related anxiety disorders are rare.

    The correct response is option **D.**

    Pharmacological treatments combined with psychotherapy appear to be more effective than either intervention alone in reducing depressive symptoms in the context of bereavement (Miller et al. 1997; Reynolds et al. 1999), although this conclusion is based on a small number of studies at present. If a clinical level of depression is present, it should be treated first, as early as 2 months after the loss (American Psychiatric Association 2000). Posttraumatic stress disorder, bereavement-related anxiety disorders, and subsyndromal depression are common complications that require treatment (Reynolds et al. 1999; Rosenzweig et al. 1997; Schut et al. 1997). The presence of clinically significant symptoms of depression within the first 2 months after a spouse's death is a significant risk factor for continued depression (Stroebe et al. 2001). **(pp. 227–228)**

References

American Psychiatric Association: Practice Guideline for the Treatment of Patients With Major Depressive Disorder, 2nd Edition. Washington, DC, American Psychiatric Association, 2000

Bowling A: Who dies after widow(er)hood? a discriminant analysis. Omega (Westport) 19:135–153, 1988–1989

Centers for Disease Control and Prevention: U.S. life tables, 2002. Hyattsville, MD, National Center for Health Statistics, 2002. Available at http://www.cdc.gov/nchs/data/dvs/life2002.pdf. Accessed March 1, 2006.

Federal Interagency Forum on Aging Related Statistics: Older Americans 2000: Key Indicators of Well-Being. Washington, DC, Federal Interagency Forum on Aging Related Statistics, 2000

Field NP, Nichols C, Holen A, et al: The relation of continuing attachment to adjustment in conjugal bereavement. J Consult Clin Psychol 67:212–218, 1999

Harlow SD, Goldberg EL, Comstock GW: A longitudinal study of the prevalence of depressive symptomatology in elderly widowed and married women. Arch Gen Psychiatry 48:1065–1068, 1991

Lund DA, Caserta M, Dimond M: Impact of spousal bereavement on the subjective well-being of older adults, in Older Bereaved Spouses. Edited by Lund DA. New York, Hemisphere, 1989, pp 3–15

Miller MD, Wolfson L, Frank E, et al: Using interpersonal psychotherapy (IPT) in a combined psychotherapy/medication research protocol with depressed elders. A descriptive report with case vignettes. J Psychother Pract Res 7:47–55, 1997

Reynolds CF 3rd, Miller MD, Pasternak RE, et al: Treatment of bereavement-related major depressive episodes in later life: a controlled study of acute and continuation treatment with nortriptyline and interpersonal psychotherapy. Am J Psychiatry 156:202–208, 1999

Rosenzweig A, Prigerson H, Miller MD, et al: Bereavement and late-life depression: grief and its complications in the elderly. Annu Rev Med 48:421–428, 1997

Schut HA, Stroebe MS, van den Bout J: Intervention for the bereaved: gender differences in the efficacy of two counselling programmes. Br J Clin Psychol 36:63–72, 1997

Stroebe M, Schut H: The dual process model of coping with bereavement: rationale and description. Death Stud 23:197–224, 1999

Stroebe MS, Schut H: Models of coping with bereavement: a review, in Handbook of Bereavement Research: Consequences, Coping, and Care. Edited by Stroebe MS, Hansson RO, Stroebe W, et al. Washington, DC, American Psychological Association, 2001, pp 375–403

Stroebe MS, Stroebe W: The mortality of bereavement: a review, in Handbook of Bereavement. Edited by Stroebe MS, Stroebe W, Hansson R. Cambridge, UK, Cambridge University Press, 1993, pp 175–195

Thompson LW, Breckenridge JN, Gallagher D, et al: Effects of bereavement on self-perceptions of physical health in elderly widows and widowers. J Gerontol 39:309–314, 1984

Thompson LW, Gallagher-Thompson D, Futterman A, et al: The effects of late-life spousal bereavement over a 30-month interval. Psychol Aging 6:434–441, 1991

U.S. Census Bureau: Current Population Survey Report. Marital and Living Arrangements: March 1998 (Update) (P20-514). Available at http://www.census.gov/prod/99pubs/p20-514u.pdf. Accessed November 3, 2003.

Chapter 13:
Sleep and Circadian Rhythm Disorders

Select the single best response for each question.

1. Sleep disorders are an important and often obscure cause of clinical distress in elderly patients. As such, their full evaluation and thoughtful management may enhance patients' quality of life substantially. Which of the following is true?

    A. One-quarter of noninstitutionalized persons older than 65 report chronic sleep problems.
    B. Despite clinical distress due to sleep disorders, they are an infrequent reason for long-term care placement.
    C. Most age-related sleep disturbances are caused by primary, as opposed to secondary, sleep-related symptoms.
    D. Sleep and circadian rhythm changes in elderly patients are absent unless there is a sleep disorder.
    E. With increasing age, an increased number of arousals is causative in the increased amount of nocturnal wake time.

    The correct response is option **E**.

    With increasing age, nocturnal sleep time steadily decreases and nocturnal wake time increases because of an increase in arousals.

    More than half of noninstitutionalized individuals age 65 or older report chronic sleep difficulties (Foley et al. 1995; "National Institutes of Health Consensus Development Conference Statement" 1991; Prinz et al. 1990). Sleep disturbances are among the leading reasons for long-term care placement (Pollack and Perlick 1991; Pollack et al. 1990; Sanford 1975). Most age-related sleep changes stem from an increased incidence of sleep disturbances that lead to secondary sleep-related symptoms (Bliwise 1993; Foley et al. 1995; Gislason and Almqvist 1987; Prinz 1995; Prinz et al. 1990). Changes in sleep and circadian rhythms also occur in healthy elderly individuals (Bliwise 2000; Czeisler et al. 1999). **(pp. 241–242)**

2. Sleep apnea (SA), periodic limb movement disorder (PLMD), and restless legs syndrome (RLS) are relatively commonly encountered in older patients. Which of the following is true?

    A. The more common form of SA in elderly patients is central rather than obstructive.
    B. SA, even in mild cases, is not associated with insomnia.
    C. Referral to a sleep disorder specialist is not required to diagnose SA.
    D. Clinically significant PLMD is five to six times more common in elderly patients, when compared to younger adults.
    E. Polysomnography is required for the diagnosis of both PLMD and RLS.

    The correct response is option **D**.

    Clinically significant PLMD is seen in 30%–45% of adults age 60 years or older, compared with 5%–6% of all adults (Ancoli-Israel et al. 1991).

The predominant type of sleep apnea seen in elderly persons is obstructive (oropharynx collapses during attempts to breathe) (Ancoli-Israel et al. 1987). Apnea generally causes excessive sleepiness, although mild to moderate apnea can be associated with insomnia. Referral to a sleep disorder specialist is required for diagnosis and treatment. Polysomnography is not needed for an RLS diagnosis, which is made through history taking. **(pp. 243–244)**

3. Alzheimer's disease and Parkinson's disease are associated with many neuropsychiatric complications. Among these is disturbed sleep; when sleep disturbance is associated with behavioral agitation, the term "sundowning" is used. Which of the following is true regarding sleep disorders and their management in these neurodegenerative conditions?

    A. Alzheimer's disease patients have increased arousals and awakenings, and increased amounts of REM and slow-wave sleep.
    B. Benzodiazepines are the treatment of choice for the sundowning in Alzheimer's disease.
    C. Antipsychotics may be helpful for the treatment of Alzheimer's disease patients with sundowning, and the atypical agents are generally well tolerated.
    D. Sleep complaints are notable in less than one-half of Parkinson's disease patients.
    E. Although carbidopa/levodopa combinations may cause initial insomnia, they do not increase risk of nightmares.

    The correct response is option **C.**

    Of all medications prescribed for sundowning, antipsychotics have the most evidence of efficacy (Bliwise 2000).

    Individuals with Alzheimer's disease have increased arousals and awakenings and a diminished amount of REM and slow-wave sleep (Prinz et al. 1982). Benzodiazepines are ineffective in the treatment of sundowning in Alzheimer's disease (Bliwise 2000). Sleep complaints are noted in 60%–90% of individuals with Parkinson's disease (Trenkwalder 1998). Carbidopa/levodopa may cause initial insomnia and cause nightmares (Trenkwalder 1998). **(pp. 245–246)**

4. Comorbid medical conditions are common in older patients with sleep complaints, and the management of the chronic illness may be of great utility in assisting these patients. Which of the following is true for those patients with chronic obstructive pulmonary disease (COPD)?

    A. In COPD, the degree of sleep disruption is correlated with the degree of hypoxemia.
    B. Daytime sleepiness is typical in COPD.
    C. Polysomnography is routinely necessary to evaluate sleep complaints in COPD because sleep apnea is much more common in these patients.
    D. Oral theophyllines are adenosine receptor antagonists and may themselves disrupt sleep in COPD.
    E. Benzodiazepines are the treatment of choice for COPD patients with sleep complaints.

    The correct response is option **D.**

    Oral theophyllines may have a sleep-disruptive effect in COPD treatment (Douglas 2000).

In COPD, the degree of sleep disruption is unrelated to hypoxemia (Douglas 2000). Daytime sleepiness does not appear in COPD. Polysomnography is not routinely indicated for individuals with COPD with sleep difficulties (Connaughton et al. 1988). Sleep apnea is not more common in persons with COPD than in the general population. Benzodiazepines should be used with great caution because they may worsen nocturnal hypoxemia in COPD patients (Douglas 2000). **(p. 246)**

References

Ancoli-Israel S, Kripke DF, Mason W: Characteristics of obstructive and central sleep apnea in the elderly: an interim report. Biol Psychiatry 22:741–750, 1987

Ancoli-Israel S, Kripke D, Klauber M, et al: Periodic limb movements in sleep in the community-dwelling elderly. Sleep 14:496–500, 1991

Bliwise DL: Sleep in normal aging and dementia. Sleep 16:40–81, 1993

Bliwise DL: Normal aging, in Principles and Practice of Sleep Medicine, 3rd Edition. Edited by Kryger MH, Roth T, Dement WC. Philadelphia, PA, WB Saunders, 2000, pp 26–42

Connaughton JJ, Catterall JR, Elton RA, et al: Do sleep studies contribute to the management of patients with severe chronic obstructive pulmonary disease? Am Rev Respir Dis 138:341–344, 1988

Czeisler CA, Duffy JF, Shanahan TL, et al: Stability, precision, and near-24-hour period of the human circadian pacemaker. Science 284:2177–2181, 1999

Foley DJ, Monjan AA, Brown SL, et al: Sleep complaints among elderly persons: an epidemiologic study of three communities. Sleep 18:425–432, 1995

Gislason T, Almqvist M: Somatic diseases and sleep complaints. An epidemiological study of 3,201 Swedish men. Acta Med Scand 221:475–481, 1987

National Institutes of Health Consensus Development Conference Statement: Treatment of sleep disorders in older people March 26–28, 1990. Sleep 14:169–177, 1991

Pollack CP, Perlick D: Sleep problems and institutionalization of the elderly. J Geriatr Psychiatry Neurol 4:204–210, 1991

Pollack CP, Perlick D, Lisner JP, et al: Sleep problems in the community elderly as predictors of death and nursing home placement. J Community Health 15:123–135, 1990

Prinz PN: Sleep and sleep disorders in older adults. J Clin Neurophysiol 12:139–146, 1995

Prinz PN, Peskind ER, Vitaliano PP, et al: Changes in the sleep and waking EEGs of nondemented and demented elderly subjects. J Am Geriatr Soc 30:86–93, 1982

Prinz PN, Vitiello MV, Raskind MA, et al: Geriatrics: sleep disorders and aging. N Engl J Med 323:520–526, 1990

Sanford JRA: Tolerance of debility in elderly dependants by supporters at home: its significance for hospital practice. Br Med J 3:471–473, 1975

Trenkwalder C: Sleep dysfunction in Parkinson's disease. Clin Neurosci 5:107–114, 1998

Chapter 14: Alcohol and Drug Problems

Select the single best response for each question.

1. Substance abuse and dependence problems may cause significant distress for the older patient and need to be evaluated fully by the geropsychiatrist. Which of the following is true regarding substance use disorders in this population?

    A. The prevalence of substance use disorders in patients over 65 ranges from 0.1% to 0.7% for men.

    B. Risk factors for elder substance abuse are similar to those for younger adults (e.g., male gender, lower educational attainment, and comorbid mood disorder).

C. The comorbidity of alcohol problems and psychiatric illness in late life is 5%–7%.
D. In the United States, the lifetime prevalence of alcohol problems in older adults is higher than in younger persons.
E. Some studies suggest that the prevalence of alcohol abuse among older persons is higher in African Americans than in whites.

The correct response is option **B**.

The risk factors for alcohol abuse (e.g., male gender, poor education, low income, and a history of other psychiatric disorders, especially depression) in the elderly are similar to those for the general population.

The prevalence of substance use disorder in patients over 65 ranges from 1.9% to 4.6% for men and from 0.1% to 0.7% for women (Myers et al. 1984). The comorbidity of alcohol problems and psychiatric illness in late life has been estimated to be between 10% and 15% (Finlaysen et al. 1988). In the United States, the lifetime prevalence of alcohol problems is lower in older adults than in younger persons. Some studies suggest that alcohol abuse in later life is higher among whites than among African Americans (Ruchlin 1997). **(pp. 257–259)**

2. The physician may be consulted to manage some of the chronic effects of alcohol on neurophysiology and cognitive function in the elderly patient. Which of the following is true regarding alcohol's chronic effects?

   A. Peripheral neuropathy in persons with alcoholism, which often follows deficiency states of thiamine and other B-complex vitamins, is seen in 25% of individuals with chronic alcoholism.
   B. The cognitive effects of alcohol typically result in a decreased overall level of intelligence as reflected in the IQ on formal testing.
   C. Focal cognitive deficits with chronic alcoholism include deficits in visuospatial analysis and nonverbal abstraction.
   D. The use of alcohol for sleep may produce prolonged sleep (8–10 hours) in the elderly.
   E. Alcoholic dementia deficits are permanent; abstinence does not reverse deficits in short-term memory.

The correct response is option **C**.

The most common deficits in persons with alcoholism include visuospatial analysis, tactual spatial analysis, nonverbal abstraction, and set flexibility.

Peripheral neuropathy may occur in as many as 45% of chronic alcoholic patients. Although specific clusters of cognitive functions are affected in the older alcoholic patient, intelligence remains relatively unaffected. End-stage alcoholic dementia features severe anterograde and retrograde amnesia. Patients with alcoholic dementia who abstain may exhibit stable or improved short-term memory. The relatively rapid metabolism of alcohol, in contrast to most sedative-hypnotics, may produce a rebound awakening at a point 3–4 hours into sleep. Even though the older adult using alcohol may fall asleep without difficulty, his or her sleep is disrupted during the night. **(pp. 259–261)**

3. The useful mnemonic **FRAMES** (Miller and Sanchez) can be used to organize clinical interventions for substance abuse in the elderly patient. Which of the following statements is *not* part of the **FRAMES** schema?

   A. Feedback about substance use.
   B. Responsibility to address the problem of substance use.
   C. Abstinence as an early requirement.
   D. Menu of patient options.
   E. Empathy for the patient's ambivalence and challenge.

   The correct response is option **C**.

   "Advice with regard to what the patient might reasonably do" is the correct statement for letter A in the **FRAMES** mnemonic (Miller and Sanchez 1994). (The letter **S** in the mnemonic corresponds to the following statement: "Self-efficacy of the patient to do something about the problem.") **(p. 264)**

References

Finlaysen RE, Hunt RD, Davis LJ, et al: Alcoholism in elderly persons: a study of the psychiatric and psychosocial features of 216 inpatients. Mayo Clin Proc 63:761–768, 1988

Miller WR, Sanchez VC: Motivating young adults for treatment and lifestyle change, in Alcohol Use and Misuse by Young Adults. Edited by Howard GS, Nathan PE. South Bend, IN, University of Notre Dame Press, 1994

Myers JK, Weissman MM, Tischler GL, et al: Six-month prevalence of psychiatric disorders in three communities: 1980 to 1982. Arch Gen Psychiatry 41:959–967, 1984

Ruchlin HS: Prevalence and correlates of alcohol use among older adults. Prev Med 26 (5 pt 1): 651–657, 1997

Chapter 15:
Agitation and Suspiciousness

Select the single best response for each question.

1. Which of the following is true regarding the psychotic disorder of late life referred to as late-life paraphrenia?

   A. It is the late-life recurrence of an earlier onset of schizophrenia in a patient who had been symptom-free for many years.
   B. According to Kraepelin's original description, most patients were male.
   C. Psychotic symptoms of the late-life episode typically include delusions, but hallucinations are not experienced.
   D. Patients have been reported to have simultaneous sensory deficits.
   E. Antipsychotics have been shown to be effective for late-life delusional disorder.

   The correct response is option **D**.

   Patients with late-life paraphrenia may have comorbid sensory deficits, especially visual or hearing loss.

   Late-life paraphrenia identifies psychosis that has a late age at onset. According to Kraepelin, most patients were women, usually living alone. Paranoid ideation is sometimes accompanied by hallucinations. Neuroleptics are usually the first-line treatment. **(p. 279)**

2. The clinical evaluation of the suspicious and/or paranoid older patient requires consideration of specific concerns about psychotic disorders in older patients. Which of the following is true?

   A. Because of tendency of patients with schizophrenia to isolate and have a shorter life expectancy, chronic paranoid schizophrenia is an infrequent cause of suspiciousness in elderly patients.
   B. Elderly patients with schizophrenia are best managed with medication alone, rather than comprehensive treatment models.
   C. Agitation in elderly patients with chronic paranoid schizophrenia is rare.
   D. Agitation may follow family members' challenging of the patient's delusions.
   E. None of the above.

   The correct response is option **D.**

   Agitation may become an issue in the elderly when they are confronted by family or clinicians about their delusions. Chronic paranoid schizophrenia is a major cause of suspiciousness and agitation in elderly patients. Multimodal treatment—including neuroleptic medication, case management, and family education and involvement—is essential for ensuring adequate care. Chronic paranoid schizophrenia persisting into late life is a major cause of suspiciousness and agitation in elderly persons. The occurrence of agitation in patients with chronic paranoid schizophrenia is common and may indicate a need for an adjustment in neuroleptic dosing. **(p. 280)**

3. When the physician evaluates the older patient with suspicious and/or paranoid complaints, which of the following is *not* recommended?

   A. Determine whether suspicious behavior is warranted; for example, consider the possibility of neglect or abuse.
   B. Challenge the delusion to verify that it is indeed fixed in the patient's mind.
   C. Obtain routine laboratory studies, including chemistry and complete blood count.
   D. Consider use of neuroimaging (e.g., CT or MRI of the head).
   E. Consider specialty referrals for vision and hearing examination and correction.

   The correct response is option **B.**

   Challenging the delusional patient is usually not recommended.
   Routine laboratories needed in new cases of paranoia include blood chemistry, a complete blood count, and a thyroid profile. Use of neuroimaging and examinations of vision and hearing may be indicated to identify potential areas for intervention. **(p. 280)**

4. Agitation in dementia is a common clinical problem, for both the patient and the family. Which of the following is true regarding behavioral approaches to agitation in dementia?

   A. Pharmacological approaches should precede nonpharmacological ones.
   B. Patients with dementia are more likely to act out frustration with strangers than with family members because strangers are unfamiliar.
   C. Agitation often correlates with other areas of impulsive behavior.

D. Because of their cognitive impairments, patients with dementia are usually non-responsive to nonverbal behavior of caregivers.

E. Excessively calm, familiar surroundings and predictable routines unnecessarily understimulate the patient with dementia and thus should be avoided.

The correct response is option **C**.

Agitation is often accompanied by a loss of impulse control.

Nonpharmacological strategies are recommended as a first-line approach. Persons with dementia are more likely to take out their frustration on those closest to them while behaving appropriately with strangers. Although people with dementia may seem insensitive to others' feelings, they are extremely sensitive to and will respond negatively to patronizing, angry, tense, rushed, or demanding nonverbal communication from family members. Agitated patients with dementia usually respond well to calm, familiar settings with predictable routines. **(pp. 281–283)**

5. Communication strategies in dementia may facilitate the patient's maintenance of behavioral control and avoidance of escalation into agitation. All of the following communication strategies are helpful *except*

A. Ensuring adequate vision and hearing correction.

B. Maintaining good eye contact and approaching the patient slowly.

C. Decreasing "clutter" in the sensory milieu (e.g., turning off noisy electronic equipment).

D. In assisting understanding, paraphrasing, rather than simply repeating, ideas that are not apparently understood.

E. Using specific names and references and avoiding pronouns and other nonspecific language devices.

The correct response is option **D**.

To assist understanding between patient and clinician, the clinician should speak slowly and give the patient time to respond. Words should be repeated exactly and not paraphrased. Ask questions if the patient's meaning is unclear; be patient and reassuring. **(p. 283)**

Chapter 16:
Psychopharmacology

Select the single best response for each question.

1. Psychopharmacological treatment of late-life psychiatric illness has significantly improved clinical function and quality of life for patients. However, systemic side effects from psychotropic medications are a vexing problem in this population. Many side effects are due to anticholinergic, antihistaminic, and antiadrenergic effects. All of the following clinical problems are referable to anticholinergic effects *except*

A. Constipation.

B. Urinary retention.

C. Sedation.

D. Delirium.
E. Cognitive dysfunction.

The correct response is option **C**.

Sedation is an antihistaminergic effect. **(p. 293)**

2. The selective serotonin reuptake inhibitors (SSRIs) have become the first-line agents in the treatment of mood disorders in older adults. Which of the following is true regarding the use of SSRIs in older patients?

A. Due to their pharmacokinetic profiles and low risk for drug-drug interactions, sertraline and fluoxetine are the preferred SSRIs.
B. Several controlled trials have demonstrated the effectiveness of SSRIs in anxiety disorders in elderly patients.
C. Despite not being technically "antipsychotic," SSRIs have been shown to be efficacious in treating delusions and hallucinations in dementia.
D. SSRIs may cause the syndrome of inappropriate secretion of antidiuretic hormone (SIADH) with hypernatremia, which may lead to delirium.
E. SSRIs are poorly tolerated in Parkinson's disease.

The correct response is option **C**.

SSRIs are effective in the treatment of behavioral disturbances with dementia, including not only agitation and disinhibition but also delusions and hallucinations (Nyth and Gottfries 1990; Nyth et al. 1992; Pollock et al. 1997, 2002).

Escitalopram, citalopram, and sertraline are the preferred SSRIs in the treatment of depression (Alexopoulos et al. 2001; Mulsant et al. 2001); however, their efficacy in older patients with anxiety disorders has not been proven. A rare but dangerous adverse effect in the elderly is SIADH with significant hyponatremia (Fabian et al. 2004). SSRIs are well tolerated by most patients with Parkinson's disease (Richard and Kurlan 1997). **(pp. 293–296)**

3. Other contemporary antidepressants may be clinically indicated in the older patient for various psychiatric symptoms. Which of the following is true?

A. Bupropion is contraindicated in seizure disorder patients, but it is recommended for poststroke depression.
B. Because it may energize a fatigued depressed patient, bupropion is the antidepressant of choice in psychotic depression.
C. Venlafaxine has different pharmacokinetic properties depending on the patient's age; thus, lower doses are typically effective for older patients.
D. Venlafaxine significantly reduces the risk for a withdrawal syndrome when treatment is interrupted or discontinued.
E. Mirtazapine inhibits 5-HT$_2$ and 5-HT$_3$ receptors, making it an attractive choice for elderly depressed patients with severe nausea.

The correct response is option **E**.

Mirtazapine is the chosen SSRI for patients with severe nausea (Pedersen and Klysner 1997), tremor (Pact and Giduz 1999), or sexual dysfunction (Gelenberg et al. 2000; Montejo et al. 2001).

Bupropion is contraindicated in patients with seizure disorders and in poststroke patients and should be avoided in psychotic patients because of its dopaminergic action. Higher doses of venlafaxine are required in geriatric patients. The use of extended-release venlafaxine does not seem to reduce the incidence or severity of withdrawal symptoms (Fava et al. 1997). **(pp. 296–303)**

4. Newer agents have largely supplanted the tricyclic antidepressants (TCAs). However, some TCAs may be useful for certain patients. The secondary, rather than tertiary, amine structures are associated with less side-effect burden. Which of the following TCAs is a secondary amine and thus likely to be more tolerable by older patients?

   A. Amitriptyline.
   B. Desipramine.
   C. Imipramine.
   D. Doxepin.
   E. Clomipramine.

   The correct response is option **B.**

   Desipramine, as well as nortriptyline, is a secondary amine. **(p. 303)**

5. The atypical antipsychotic agents have been quickly integrated into geriatric psychiatric practice, as they are in general more tolerable than the older typical agents. Which of the following is true regarding this group of antipsychotic agents?

   A. When used for drug-induced psychosis in Parkinson's disease, clozapine should be used at dosages between 100 and 200 mg/day.
   B. Olanzapine has been associated with elevated glucose and lipids, but only when there is simultaneous weight gain.
   C. Because of risk of extrapyramidal symptoms in elderly patients, the dosage of risperidone should be limited to less than 1 mg/day.
   D. Quetiapine does not show affinity for muscarinic receptors and is a viable alternative to clozapine for drug-induced psychosis in Parkinson's disease.
   E. Ziprasidone's use in elderly patients is limited by its high degree of muscarinic receptor affinity and resultant risk of cognitive impairment.

   The correct response is option **D.**

In patients with Parkinson's disease and drug-induced psychosis, quetiapine is a useful alternative to clozapine (Fernandez et al. 1999, 2002; Menza et al. 1999; Targum and Abbott 2000).

Clozapine should be used at low dosages (between 12.5 and 50 mg/day) for drug-induced psychosis in Parkinson's disease (Parkinson Study Group 1999). Elevated glucose and lipids with the use of olanzapine occur even in the absence of weight gain but appear to be reversible on discontinuation of the drug (Lindenmayer et al. 2001). Risperidone is efficacious and safe at low dosages (0.5–1.5 mg/day). Ziprasidone has low potential to cause cognitive impairment and minimal impact on glucose and lipid concentrations and on weight (American Diabetes Association et al. 2004); however, its use in older patients has been limited due to the almost total lack of geriatric data and lingering concerns regarding its potential effects on cardiac conduction (Alexopoulos et al. 2004). **(pp. 304–310)**

6. Mood stabilizers may be useful in elderly patients, both for patients with long-established bipolar disorders and for behavioral acting-out in dementing illness. Which of the following is true?

   A. Because of their greater safety profile in older patients, anticonvulsants are now prescribed much more commonly than lithium for elderly bipolar patients.
   B. Older patients are subject to lithium toxicity at lower serum lithium levels than younger adults, with cognitive impairment reported at levels even lower than 1 mEq/L.
   C. Thrombocytopenia is a rare complication of valproate use in elderly patients.
   D. Aging alone typically increases the half-life of valproate metabolism by a factor of 2 to 3.
   E. Carbamazepine is a cytochrome P450 inhibitor and thus can inhibit its own metabolism, increasing serum levels.

The correct response is option **B**.

Lithium neurotoxicity in the elderly has manifested with cognitive impairment with levels well below 1 mEq/L (Sproule et al. 2000).

Despite its age-associated risks, lithium is still used more commonly than anticonvulsant medication in elders with bipolar disorder (Umapathy et al. 2000). Aging alone does not increase the half-life of valproate. Thrombocytopenia is possible in more than half of elderly patients treated with valproate and may ensue at lower total drug levels than in younger patients (Conley et al. 2001). Carbamazepine concentrations are increased to potential toxicity by cytochrome P450 inhibitors but decreased by cytochrome P450 inducers (Spina et al. 1996). **(pp. 310–312)**

7. Which of these cholinesterase inhibitors is notably affected by renal function and carries an FDA warning about dose titration?

   A. Tacrine.
   B. Donepezil.
   C. Rivastigmine.
   D. Galantamine.
   E. Physostigmine.

The correct response is option **C**.

Rivastigmine must be titrated to prevent severe vomiting (Chew et al. 2005; Mulsant et al. 2003). **(p. 314)**

References

Alexopoulos GS, Katz IR , Reynolds CF 3rd, et al: Pharmacotherapy of depression in older patients: a summary of the expert consensus guidelines. J Psychiatr Pract 7:361–376, 2001

Alexopoulos GS, Streim J, Carpenter D, Docherty JP, Expert Consensus Panel for Using Antipsychotic Drugs in Older Patients: Using antipsychotic agents in older patients. J Clin Psychiatry 65 (suppl 2):5–104, 2004

American Diabetes Association, American Psychiatric Association, American Association of Clinical Endocrinologists, et al: Consensus development conference on antipsychotic drugs and obesity and diabetes. Diabetes Care 27(2):596–601, 2004

Chew ML, Mulsant BH, Rosen J, et al: Serum anticholinergic activity and cognition in patients with moderate to severe dementia. Am J Geriatr Psychiatry 13:535–538, 2005

Conley EL, Coley KC, Pollock BG, et al: Prevalence and risk of thrombocytopenia with valproic acid: experience at a psychiatric teaching hospital. Pharmacotherapy 21:1325–1330, 2001

Fabian TJ, Amico JA, Kroboth PD, et al: Paroxetine-induced hyponatremia in older adults: a 12-week prospective study. Arch Intern Med 164(3):327–332, 2004

Fava M, Mulroy R, Alpert J, et al: Emergence of adverse events following discontinuation of treatment with extended-release venlafaxine. Am J Psychiatry 154:1760–1762, 1997

Fernandez HH, Friedman JH, Jacques C, et al: Quetiapine for the treatment of drug-induced psychosis in Parkinson's disease. Mov Disord 14:484–487, 1999

Fernandez HH, Trieschmann ME, Burke MA, et al: Quetiapine for psychosis in Parkinson's disease versus dementia with Lewy bodies. J Clin Psychiatry 63(6):513–515, 2002

Gelenberg AJ, Laukes C, McGahuey C, et al: Mirtazapine substitution in SSRI-induced sexual dysfunction. J Clin Psychiatry 61:356–360, 2000

Lindenmayer JP, Nathan AM, Smith RC: Hyperglycemia associated with the use of atypical antipsychotics. J Clin Psychiatry 62 (suppl 23):30–38, 2001

Melkersson KI, Hulting AL: Insulin and leptin levels in patients with schizophrenia or related psychoses—a comparison between different antipsychotic agents. Psychopharmacology 154:205–212, 2001

Menza MM, Palermo B, Mark M: Quetiapine as an alternative to clozapine in the treatment of dopamimetic psychosis in patients with Parkinson's disease. Ann Clin Psychiatry 11:141–144, 1999

Montejo AL, Llorca G, Izquierdo JA, et al: Incidence of sexual dysfunction associated with antidepressant agents: a prospective multicenter study of 1022 outpatients. Spanish Working Group for the Study of Psychotropic-Related Sexual Dysfunction. J Clin Psychiatry 62 (suppl 3):10–21, 2001

Mulsant BH, Alexopoulos GS, Reynolds CF 3rd, et al: The PROSPECT Study Group. Pharmacological treatment of depression in older primary care patients: the PROSPECT algorithm. Int J Geriatr Psychiatry 16:585–592, 2001

Mulsant BH, Pollock BG, Kirshner M, et al: Serum anticholinergic activity in a community-based sample of older adults: relationship with cognitive performance. Arch Gen Psychiatry 60:198–203, 2003

Nyth AL, Gottfries CG: The clinical efficacy of citalopram in treatment of emotional disturbances in dementia disorders. A Nordic multicentre study. Br J Psychiatry 157:894–901, 1990

Nyth AL, Gottfries CG, Lyby K, et al: A controlled multicenter clinical study of citalopram and placebo in elderly depressed patients with and without concomitant dementia. Acta Psychiatr Scand 86:138–145, 1992

Pact V, Giduz T: Mirtazapine treats resting tremor, essential tremor, and levodopa-induced dyskinesias. Neurology 53:1154, 1999

Parkinson Study Group: Low-dose clozapine for the treatment of drug-induced psychosis in Parkinson's disease. N Engl J Med 340:757–763, 1999

Pedersen L, Klysner R: Antagonism of selective serotonin reuptake inhibitor-induced nausea by mirtazapine. Int Clin Psychopharmacol 12:59–60, 1997

Pollock BG, Mulsant BH, Sweet R, et al: An open pilot study of citalopram for behavioral disturbances of dementia. Am J Geriatr Psychiatry 5:70–78, 1997

Pollock BG, Mulsant BH, Rosen J, et al: Comparison of citalopram, perphenazine, and placebo for the acute treatment of psychosis and behavioral disturbances in hospitalized, demented patients. Am J Psychiatry 159:460–465, 2002

Richard IH, Kurlan R: A survey of antidepressant drug use in Parkinson's disease. Parkinson Study Group. Neurology 49:1168–1170, 1997

Spina E, Pisani F, Perucca E: Clinically significant pharmacokinetic drug interactions with carbamazepine. An update. Clin Pharmacokinet 31:198–214, 1996

Sproule BA, Hardy BG, Shulman KI: Differential pharmacokinetics of lithium in elderly patients. Drugs Aging 16:165–177, 2000

Targum SD, Abbott JL: Efficacy of quetiapine in Parkinson's patients with psychosis. J Clin Psychopharmacol 20:54–60, 2000

Chapter 17:
Individual and Group Psychotherapy

Select the single best response for each question.

1. Psychotherapy may be a preferred model for certain geropsychiatric conditions. Which of the following is true regarding the general issue of psychotherapy for older patients?

   A. Because of the availability of Medicare, over 50% of older patients with psychiatric illnesses receive professional mental health care, unlike younger patients for whom insurance coverage is often problematic.

   B. Descriptive research regularly shows that older patients prefer psychopharmacological treatment to psychotherapy.

   C. Part of older patients' preference for psychopharmacological therapy is because few elders are concerned about "addiction" to antidepressants.

   D. Objective research confirms that "relationship factors" account for 80% of the variance in treatment outcomes with psychotherapy.

   E. None of the above.

   The correct response is option **E**.

   It has been estimated that only 10% of older adults in need of psychiatric services actually receive professional care (Abrahams and Patterson 1978; Friedhoff 1994; Weissman et al. 1981), and there has been minimal utilization of mental health services in this age group. Although research on attitudes toward treatment in elderly samples is not conclusive, contrary to clinical lore, growing descriptive research suggests that older adults may prefer counseling over medication treatment (Vitt et al. 1999). Interestingly, 56% of the same sample reported that they believed antidepressant medications to be addictive, and only 4% disagreed. Therapy also typically occurs within the context of some type of interpersonal relationship. Some have argued that relationship factors account for as much as 80% of the variance in treatment outcomes (Andrews 1998); however, research has not confirmed this assertion. **(p. 337)**

2. In conducting psychotherapy with older patients, several factors specific to this age group should be taken into close account. All of the following are true *except*

   A. Older adults rarely respond to therapeutic interventions used with younger patients.

   B. Medical illnesses or medications may exacerbate psychiatric symptoms.

   C. The clinician must work against stereotypes about elderly patients.

   D. Older adults may not easily remember troubling earlier life events.

   E. Cognitive deficits may affect the progress of psychotherapy.

The correct response is option **A**.

In general, older adults will respond to many of the therapeutic interventions used with younger populations.

Medical illness or problematic medicines can exacerbate symptoms of a mental disorder. The clinician should actively work against stereotypes of elderly persons as being withdrawn, rigid, lonely, dependent, or unable to learn. Older adults may have difficulty remembering troublesome events. The clinician should consider consulting family members or longtime friends. Cognitive deficits can impede learning speed and memory. **(p. 338)**

3. Cognitive-behavioral psychotherapy models may be considered for older patients. Which of the following is true?

   A. The Thompson et al. study (1987) showed cognitive and behavioral therapy to be superior to brief psychodynamic therapy in reducing depression symptoms.
   B. The studies by Thompson et al. (2001) and Reynolds et al. (1999) both concluded that combined medication and psychotherapy were optimal in the treatment of depression in older adults.
   C. A logistical limitation of social problem-solving therapy is that it is not adaptable to the primary care clinic.
   D. All of the above.
   E. None of the above.

The correct response is option **B**.

The 2001 study by Thompson et al. supports conclusions by Reynolds et al. (1999) that a combined medication plus psychotherapy approach may be optimal for the treatment of depression in older adults.

There were no significant differences between treatment groups, suggesting that exercise training might be comparable to the use of medication in older adults. In a study comparing cognitive, behavioral, and brief psychodynamic therapy to waiting-list control subjects, Thompson and colleagues (1987) found that all of the treatment modalities led to comparable and clinically significant reductions of depression. Problem-solving therapy can be delivered in a limited space of time; thus it can be adapted to use in primary care facilities. **(pp. 339–340)**

4. Another useful model of psychotherapy for depressed older adults is interpersonal psychotherapy (IPT). This model is based on four components of interpersonal relationships that lead to and maintain depressive states. These four components include all of the following *except*

   A. Grief.
   B. Interpersonal disputes.
   C. Role transitions.
   D. Interpersonal deficits.
   E. Intrapsychic or psychodynamic conflict.

The correct response is option **E**.

Interpersonal psychotherapy (IPT) is a manualized treatment that focuses on four components that are hypothesized to lead to or maintain depression. Whatever its etiology, depression is seen to persist in a social context. Components of treatment are 1) grief (e.g., death of spouse), 2) interpersonal disputes (e.g., conflict with adult children), 3) role transitions (e.g., retirement), and 4) interpersonal deficits (e.g., lack of assertiveness skills). **(p. 341)**

5. Various psychotherapy models can be utilized for the management of anxiety disorders in older patients. Which of the following is true?

    A. The most frequently used and well-substantiated psychotherapy model for geriatric anxiety symptoms is cognitive-behavioral therapy (CBT).
    B. Behavioral therapy such as progressive muscle relaxation training is contraindicated for patients with cognitive impairment.
    C. CBT appears to be the best-equipped psychotherapy model for generalized anxiety disorder (GAD) in older patients.
    D. A major limitation of CBT for geriatric anxiety states is that it cannot be conducted in the primary care clinic.
    E. Elderly patients with GAD infrequently exhibit simultaneous depressive symptoms.

The correct response is option **C**.

CBT appears to be the best-equipped form of psychotherapy to manage the diagnostic and treatment issues that exist in older populations with GAD. Treatment research on GAD in late life is limited. Not surprisingly, though, the bulk of this literature focuses on the efficacy of CBT in this population (Mohlman and Gorman 2005; Stanley and Novy 2000; Stanley et al. 1996, 2004; Wetherell et al. 2003).

The most frequently used and the most well-substantiated treatments for anxiety in older adults are based on behavioral therapies. Specifically, a variety of relaxation training techniques have been pilot-tested as a treatment strategy for older adults. Patients with cognitive deficits, who may have difficulty with more cognitive strategies, may benefit from purely behavioral strategies. A pilot study by Stanley and associates (2004) presents a shortened CBT protocol for use in a primary care setting. In a sample of older adults, 60% of those who met criteria for GAD also endorsed comorbid depressive episodes. **(pp. 343–345)**

References

Abrahams RB, Patterson RD: Psychological distress among the community elderly: prevalence, characteristics and implications for service. Int J Aging Hum Dev 9:1–18, 1978

Blumenthal JA, Babyak MA, Moore KA, et al: Effects of exercise training on older patients with major depression. Arch Intern Med 159:2349–2356, 1999

Friedhoff AJ: Consensus Development Conference statement: diagnosis and treatment of depression in late life, in Diagnosis and Treatment of Depression in Late Life: Results of the NIH Consensus Development Conference. Edited by Schneider LSM, Reynolds CF III, Lebowitz BD, et al. Washington, DC, American Psychiatric Press, 1994, pp 491–511

Luborsky L, Rosenthal R, Diguer L, et al: The dodo bird verdict is alive and well—mostly. Clinical Psychology Science and Practice 9:2–12, 2002

Mohlman J, Gorman JM: The role of executive functioning in CBT: a pilot study with anxious older adults. Behav Res Ther 43:447–465, 2005

Reynolds CF 3rd, Frank E, Perel JM, et al: Nortriptyline and interpersonal psychotherapy as maintenance therapies for recurrent major depression: a randomized controlled trial in patients older than 59 years. JAMA 281:39–45, 1999

Stanley MA, Novy DM: Cognitive-behavior therapy for generalized anxiety in late life: an evaluative overview. J Anxiety Disord 14:191–207, 2000

Stanley MA, Beck JG, Glassco JD: Treatment of generalized anxiety in older adults: a preliminary comparison of cognitive-behavioral and supportive approaches. Behav Ther 27:565–581, 1996

Stanley MA, Diefenbach GJ, Hopko DR: Cognitive behavioral treatment for older adults with generalized anxiety disorder: a therapist manual for primary care settings. Behav Modif 28:73–117, 2004

Thompson LW, Gallagher D, Breckenridge JS: Comparative effectiveness of psychotherapies for depressed elders. J Consult Clin Psychol 55:385–390, 1987

Thompson LW, Coon DW, Gallagher-Thompson D, et al: Comparison of desipramine and cognitive/behavioral therapy in the treatment of elderly outpatients with mild-to-moderate depression. Am J Geriatr Psychiatry 9:225–240, 2001

Vitt CM, Idler EL, Leventhal H, et al: Attitudes toward treatment and help-seeking preferences in an elderly sample. Poster presented at the 52nd Annual Meeting of the Gerontological Society of America, San Francisco, CA, November 19–23, 1999

Weissman MM, Myers JK, Thompson WD: Depression and its treatment in a U.S. urban community—1975–1976. Arch Gen Psychiatry 38:417–421, 1981

Wetherell JL, Gatz M, Craske MG: Treatment of generalized anxiety disorder in older adults. J Consult Clin Psychol 71:31–40, 2003

Chapter 18:
Working With the Family of the Older Adult

Select the single best response for each question.

1. Which of the following is true regarding care of elderly patients with dementia in the community?

   A. Fifty percent of older patients with moderate or severe dementia live alone with some level of supervision.

   B. Spousal caregiver strain from care for patients with dementia is associated with increased risk of premature death.

   C. Anxiety symptoms are the most commonly reported psychiatric symptoms in caregivers of patients with dementia.

   D. Dependent elders are much more likely to engage in manipulative behavior than to have legitimate unmet dependency needs.

   E. Defensive denial of inevitable bad outcomes in dementia must be discouraged and avoided for caregivers to give appropriate dementia care.

The correct response is option **B**.

Research documents that premature death is associated with spousal caregiver strain in the care of persons with Alzheimer's disease, suggesting an urgent public health preventive or protective focus for work with spouses of older adults with dementia (Schulz and Beach 1999).

Despite the high rates of shared residence, there is increasing evidence that 20% of older adults with moderate to severe dementia live alone, often with extensive supervision and assistance from local and long-distance family caregivers. Although depression is the most frequently reported psychiatric symptom among caregivers of Alzheimer's disease patients, some families express pride in their care as a legacy of commitment to family values. There is much less manipulation by dependent elders than there are real unmet dependency needs. There is more underreporting of burden and underutilization of services than the reverse. Denial is a common defense of family caregivers. Some people need to deny the inevitable outcome (loss of a beloved spouse or eventual placement of a parent in a nursing home) to provide hopeful consistent daily care. **(pp. 358–359)**

2. In working with dementia patients and their families, psychiatrists are advised to attend to many parallel issues in both patients and family members. All of the following are true *except*

    A. Psychiatrists should monitor the mental health, capacity, and vulnerability of caregivers as well as patients.
    B. Caregivers' self-neglect and patient neglect by caregivers are both important areas for surveillance.
    C. A common goal in working with families of older adults with dementia is to address safety and security issues.
    D. Affective, anxiety, and substance abuse disorders of primary caregivers do not predict breakdown of family care.
    E. Major precipitants of patient placement include both patient and caregiver factors.

    The correct response is option **D.**

    Predictors of family care breakdown are affective, substance abuse, or anxiety disorders of the primary caregiver and unresolved family conflict (Yaffe et al. 2002), all of which are amenable to psychiatric treatment of families of older adults.

    A common goal in working with families of older adults with dementia is to address safety and security issues. Psychiatrists working with family caregivers over time will monitor the quality of family care; the mental health, capacity, and vulnerability of caregivers; and the impact of the demands of care on family relationships (Yates et al. 1999). Psychiatrists should be especially alert to escalating anxiety, self-neglect, suicidal ideation, depression, or anger in caregivers and abuse or neglect of the patient. Major precipitants of placement include both patient and caregiver factors. Changes in behavior and personality are also major causes of caregiver burden and depression (Yaffe et al. 2002). **(pp. 359–360)**

3. The conduct of office visits with dementia patients and family caregivers calls for the psychiatrist to make certain commonsense changes to clinical routine. Which of the following is true?

    A. The psychiatrist should rigorously preserve patient confidentiality and not speak to family members unless the patient is present.
    B. The patient should not be accompanied to the physician's office by more than one family member as this confuses the patient and leads to excessive boundary management challenges.
    C. Older couples with long relationships often prefer to face medical challenges together rather than singly.
    D. Psychiatrists should not encourage family members to remove weapons from the home of patients with dementia, as this is an invasion of privacy.
    E. The psychiatrist should not encourage physical activity for the patient with dementia as the patient needs to preserve energy for cognitive tasks.

The correct response is option **C**.

Older couples in first marriages are generally more comfortable facing threatening health information together.

Although the older adult is entitled to initial time alone with the psychiatrist, later time alone with family informants will be invaluable in assessing the impact of functional loss and other family stressors. It may be helpful to have two family members accompany the patient for an evaluation. One family member can distract or sit with the older adult while another family member has a private conversation with the psychiatrist. A family concerned about the increasingly combative behavior of an older adult male may be helped by a psychiatrist who responds, "First, let's get the guns out of the house" (Spangenberg et al. 1999). Increasing evidence shows that encouraging physical activity (King and Brassington 1997) and actively assessing and treating sleep disorders in older adults and their family caregivers are associated with positive care and family outcomes (McCurry et al. 2005). **(pp. 362–363)**

4. The psychiatrist caring for patients with dementia also needs to assess the family members of the patient. Which of the following is *not* true?

   A. Older husbands who are caregivers are at increased risk of alcohol abuse.
   B. Caregivers should be encouraged to pursue regular exercise.
   C. The caregiver has a need for social stimulation while caring for a dependent elder.
   D. Secondary family support should be assessed.
   E. The psychiatrist should not directly address the caregiver's own health, as this is a matter for that person's own physician.

   The correct response is option **E**.

   The psychiatrist should ask specifically about the primary caregiver's health.

   Older husband caregivers are particularly at risk of increased alcohol use in response to care demands. The psychiatrist should be alert for positive activities such as regular exercise, social stimulation, and secondary family support. **(pp. 363–365)**

5. Driving is often a contentious issue in dementia. Which of the following is *not* true regarding driving by cognitively impaired patients?

   A. Dementia leads to decreased judgment.
   B. Increased reaction time is common in dementia.
   C. Patients with dementia will respect the loss of their driver's license and cease to try to drive.
   D. Mechanically disabling the car reduces the need to confront the patient with his or her lost skills.
   E. Families should proactively arrange for alternative transportation to decrease the incentive for the patient to try to drive.

   The correct response is option **C**.

   Anonymous reports to the department of motor vehicles may lead to required testing or removal of the patient's license, but the absence of a license rarely stops a determined older adult with dementia.

Families can be encouraged to assess driving capacity based on observations of current driving, with reminders that dementia affects judgment, reaction time, and problem solving. Shaving the patient's keys, substituting another key, removing a distributor cap, or otherwise disabling a car can sometimes reduce the need to confront the patient with lost skills. The family can also work on solutions that limit the need for driving—delivery services, senior vans, or offers of regular rides to church or for visits. **(p. 368)**

References

McCurry SM, Gibbons LE, Logsdon RG, et al: Nighttime insomnia treatment and education for Alzheimer's disease: a randomized controlled trial. J Am Geriatr Soc 53(5):793–802, 2005

Schulz R, Beach SR: Caregiving as a risk factor for mortality: the Caregiver Health Effects Study. JAMA 282:2215–2219, 1999

Spangenberg KB, Wagner MT, Hendrix S, et al: Firearm presence in households of patients with Alzheimer's disease and other dementias. J Am Geriatr Soc 47:1183–1186, 1999

Yaffe K, Fox P, Newcomer R, et al: Patient and caregiver characteristics and nursing home placement in patients with dementia. JAMA 287:2090–2097, 2002

Yates ME, Tennstedt S, Chang BH: Contributors to and mediators of psychological well-being for informal caregivers. J Gerontol B Psychol Sci Soc Sci 54:P12–P22, 1999

Chapter 19:
Clinical Psychiatry in the Nursing Home

Select the single best response for each question.

1. The prevalence of psychiatric disorders in nursing home residents has been the subject of several studies. Which of the following is *not* true?

    A. Interview-based studies have found prevalence rates of psychiatric illness in nursing home residents as high as 94%.
    B. The Rovner et al. study (1990) found that two-thirds of nursing home residents had dementia.
    C. The Medical Expenditures Panel Survey (MEPS) found a rate of depressive disorders in nursing home residents of 20%.
    D. The MEPS study was based on clinical interviews.
    E. Rovner et al. (1990) found a prevalence of psychiatric illness of 80% in new nursing home admissions.

    The correct response is option **D**.

    The Medical Expenditures Panel Survey (Krauss and Altman 1998) was not derived from clinical interviews.

    On the basis of psychiatric interviews of subjects in randomly selected samples, investigators found prevalence rates of psychiatric disorder to be as high as 94% (Chandler and Chandler 1988; Rovner et al. 1986; Tariot et al. 1993). The study by Rovner and colleagues (1990) found that 67.4% of residents had dementia. The MEPS study revealed that 70%–80% of residents had cognitive impairment and 20% had a diagnosis of depressive disorder (Krauss and Altman 1998). Rovner et al. (1990) reported that the prevalence of psychiatric disorder among persons newly admitted to a nursing home was 80.2%. **(pp. 375–376)**

2. Among psychiatric illnesses in nursing home residents, disorders of cognitive impairment are of great importance. Which of the following is true?

   A. Among dementia subtypes, Alzheimer's disease accounts for 75% of cases, with Lewy body dementia the second most common dementia.
   B. Delirium has been found in 20% of nursing home residents, primarily due to underlying dementia.
   C. Psychotic symptoms are seen in 25%–50% of dementia patients in nursing homes.
   D. Most psychiatric consultations in nursing homes are for psychotic episodes.
   E. Behavioral disturbance in dementia is solely due to cognitive impairment.

   The correct response is option **C**.

   Psychotic symptoms have been reported in approximately 25%–50% of residents with a primary dementing illness (Berrios and Brook 1985; Chandler and Chandler 1988; Rovner et al. 1986, 1990; Teeter et al. 1976).

   Among dementia subtypes, Alzheimer's disease accounts for about 50%–60% of cases and vascular dementia accounts for about 25%–30% (Barnes and Raskind 1980; Rovner et al. 1986, 1990), while Lewy body dementia has not been ascertained in nursing home populations. Delirium is common in nursing homes and occurs primarily in patients made more vulnerable by a dementing illness. Available studies indicated that approximately 6%–7% of residents were delirious at the time of evaluation (Barnes and Raskind 1980; Rovner et al. 1986, 1990). The majority of psychiatric consultations in long-term-care settings are for evaluation and treatment of behavioral disturbances such as pacing and wandering, verbal abusiveness, disruptive shouting, physical aggression, and resistance to necessary care (Loebel et al. 1991). **(pp. 376–377)**

3. In addition to cognitive disorders, mood disorders are common psychiatric illnesses in nursing home residents. Which of the following is true?

   A. Depressive disorders are the second most common psychiatric illness in nursing home residents.
   B. The rate of mood disorders in nursing home residents in the United States is substantially higher than in other industrialized nations.
   C. Depression in nursing home residents increases morbidity, but not mortality, rates.
   D. Because of concurrent chronic medical illnesses, the DSM-IV-TR diagnostic criteria for mood disorders are not clinically valid in nursing home residents.
   E. There is a subtype of depression in nursing home residents featuring low serum albumin, high levels of psychosocial disability, and prompt response to treatment with nortriptyline.

   The correct response is option **A**.

   Depressive disorder represents the second most common psychiatric diagnosis in nursing home residents (Tariot et al. 1993). Most studies in U.S. nursing homes show depression prevalence rates of 15%–50%. Studies from other countries (Ames 1991) have shown similar rates.

In addition to its association with morbidity, depression has been found to be associated with an increase in mortality rates (Ashby et al. 1991; Katz et al. 1989; Parmelee et al. 1992; Rovner et al. 1991). DSM-IV-TR diagnostic criteria remain valid as predictors of treatment response, since the symptoms of major depression in frail elderly patients characterize a disease similar to that which occurs among younger psychiatric patients (Katz et al. 1990), even though most nursing home patients have concurrent medical illnesses and disabilities that complicate diagnosis and treatment. There is evidence for a clinically relevant subtype of depression in nursing home residents that is characterized by low levels of serum albumin and high levels of self-care deficits—it is not responsive to treatment with nortriptyline (Katz et al. 1990). **(pp. 377–378)**

4. Intervention for psychiatric illnesses in nursing home residents is a major clinical focus of the geropsychiatrist. Which of the following is true?

    A. A program of daytime physical activity and nursing interventions to promote nighttime sleep may decrease depression, but not agitation.
    B. Outcome studies on psychotherapy models in nursing home residents are derived from illness-specific interventions.
    C. Risperidone has been shown to have a beneficial effect on psychotic symptoms but not independent effects on agitation or aggression.
    D. Risperidone has been repeatedly demonstrated to have beneficial long-term effects on psychosis in nursing home residents.
    E. The majority of nursing home residents who are withdrawn from antipsychotic agents do not experience a reemergence of psychosis.

The correct response is option **E**.

Two double-blind, placebo-controlled studies of antipsychotic drug discontinuation demonstrated that the majority of patients who had been receiving longer-term treatment with antipsychotic agents could be withdrawn from these agents without reemergence of psychosis or agitated behaviors (Bridges-Parlet et al. 1997; Cohen-Mansfield et al. 1999).

Reductions in agitation were observed in a study of a daytime physical activity intervention combined with a nighttime program to decrease noise and sleep-disruptive nursing care practices (Alessi 1999). Patients in most outcome studies on psychotherapeutic interventions were not selected on the basis of specific psychiatric symptoms or syndromes, but rather on the basis of age, cognitive status, or mobility. Risperidone has been shown to have antipsychotic effects and also independent effects on agitation or aggression (Brodaty et al. 2003; DeDeyn et al. 1999; Katz et al. 1999). **(pp. 379–381)**

5. Several concerns noted in the 1970s and 1980s in the United States led to various legal and regulatory initiatives to improve the psychiatric care in nursing homes. Which of the following is true?

    A. A 1977 survey in the United States revealed that 10% of nursing home residents were physically restrained.
    B. Mechanical restraints independently decrease physical agitation.
    C. Nursing home patients with nonpsychotic causes of agitation nonetheless require antipsychotic medications.

D. The 1986 Institute of Medicine report found that antipsychotic drugs were being overused in nursing homes.

E. The 1986 Institute of Medicine report found that antidepressant drugs were being overused in nursing homes.

The correct response is option **D**.

The 1986 Institute of Medicine report highlighted problems in the overuse of antipsychotic drugs and the underuse of antidepressants for the treatment of affective disorders.

A 1977 U.S. survey of nursing home residents showed that 25% were restrained by geriatric chairs, cuffs, belts, or similar devices, primarily to control behavioral symptoms (National Center for Health Statistics 1979). Mechanical restraints have often been used in attempts to control agitation, but they do not, in fact, decrease behavioral disturbances (Werner et al. 1989). Patients with nonpsychotic behavioral problems may be appropriately managed with medications other than antipsychotics, behavioral treatments, interpersonal approaches, or environmental interventions. **(p. 383)**

6. Concern had been raised about the use of "unnecessary drugs" in psychiatrically ill nursing home patients. All of the following constitute an "unnecessary drug" use *except*

A. Drug used at an excessive dose.

B. Drug used for excessive duration.

C. Drug used with inadequate monitoring.

D. Drug used despite adverse consequences.

E. Drug used for other than FDA-approved indications ("off-label").

The correct response is option **E**.

"Unnecessary drugs" are described as any drug used in excessive dose, for excessive duration, without adequate monitoring, or in the presence of adverse consequences (Health Care Financing Administration 1991). Physicians may prescribe off-label medication if the clinical rationale is clearly documented in the medical record. **(p. 385)**

References

Alessi CA: A randomized trial of a combined physical activity and environmental intervention in nursing home residents: do sleep and agitation improve? J Am Geriatr Soc 47:784–791, 1999

Ames D: Epidemiological studies of depression among the elderly in residential and nursing homes. Int J Geriatr Psychiatry 6:347–354, 1991

Ashby D, Ames D, West CR, et al: Psychiatric morbidity as prediction of mortality for residents of local authority homes for the elderly. Int J Geriatr Psychiatry 6:567–575, 1991

Barnes RD, Raskind MA: DSM-III criteria and the clinical diagnosis of dementia: a nursing home study. J Gerontol 36:20–27, 1980

Berrios GE, Brook P: Delusions and psychopathology of the elderly with dementia. Acta Psychiatr Scand 75:296–301, 1985

Bridges-Parlet S, Knopman D, Steffes S: Withdrawal of neuroleptic medications from institutionalized dementia patients: results of a double-blind, baseline-treatment-controlled pilot study. J Geriatr Psychiatry Neurol 10:119–126, 1997

Brodaty H, Ames D, Snowdon J, et al: A randomized placebo-controlled trial of risperidone for the treatment of aggression, agitation, and psychosis of dementia. J Clin Psychiatry 64:134–143, 2003

Chandler JD, Chandler JE: The prevalence of neuropsychiatric disorders in a nursing home population. J Geriatr Psychiatry Neurol 1:71–76, 1988

Cohen-Mansfield J, Lipson S, Werner P, et al: Withdrawal of haloperidol, thioridazine, and lorazepam in the nursing home: a controlled, double-blind study. Arch Intern Med 159:1733–1740, 1999

DeDeyn PP, Rabheru K, Rasmussen A, et al: A randomized trial of risperidone, placebo, and haloperidol for behavioral symptoms of dementia. Neurology 53:946–955, 1999

Health Care Financing Administration: Medicare and Medicaid: Requirements for Long Term Care Facilities, Final Regulations. Fed Regist 56:48865–48921, 1991

Institute of Medicine, Committee on Nursing Home Regulation: Improving the Quality of Care in Nursing Homes. Washington, DC, National Academy Press, 1986

Katz IR, Lesher E, Kleban M, et al: Clinical features of depression in the nursing home. Int Psychogeriatr 1:5–15, 1989

Katz IR, Simpson GM, Curlik SM, et al: Pharmacological treatment of major depression for elderly patients in residential care settings. J Clin Psychiatry 51(suppl):41–48, 1990

Katz IR, Jeste DV, Mintzer JE, et al: Comparison of risperidone and placebo for psychosis and behavioral disturbances associated with dementia: a randomized, double-blind trial. J Clin Psychiatry 60:107–115, 1999

Krauss NA, Altman BM: Characteristics of Nursing Home Residents—1996. MEPS Research Findings No 5 (AHCPR Publ No 99-0006). Rockville, MD, Agency for Health Care Policy and Research, 1998

Loebel JP, Borson S, Hyde T, et al: Relationships between requests for psychiatric consultations and psychiatric diagnoses in long-term care facilities. Am J Psychiatry 148:898–903, 1991

National Center for Health Statistics: The National Nursing Home Survey (DHEW Publ No PHS-79-1794). Hyattsville, MD, National Center for Health Statistics, 1979

Parmelee PA, Katz IR, Lawton MP: Incidence of depression in long-term care settings. J Gerontol 47:M189–M196, 1992b

Rovner BW, Kafonek S, Filipp L, et al: Prevalence of mental illness in a community nursing home. Am J Psychiatry 143:1446–1449, 1986

Rovner BW, German PS, Broadhead J, et al: The prevalence and management of dementia and other psychiatric disorders in nursing homes. Int Psychogeriatr 2:13–24, 1990

Rovner BW, German PS, Brant LJ, et al: Depression and mortality in nursing homes. JAMA 265:993–996, 1991

Tariot PN, Podgorski CA, Blazina L, et al: Mental disorders in the nursing home: another perspective. Am J Psychiatry 150:1063–1069, 1993

Werner P, Cohen-Mansfield J, Braun J, et al: Physical restraint and agitation in nursing home residents. J Am Geriatr Soc 37:1122–1126, 1989

Index

Page numbers printed in **boldface** type refer to tables or figures.